Jenn Wal

The Neurological Boundaries
of Reality

# The Neurological Boundaries of Reality

*Edited by*

E.M.R. Critchley

JASON ARONSON INC.
*Northvale, New Jersey*
*London*

US EDITION 1995

Copyright © 1994 by Farrand Press

All rights reserved. Printed in the United States of America. No part of this book may be used or reproduced in any manner whatsoever without written permission from Jason Aronson Inc. except in the case of brief quotations in reviews for inclusion in a magazine, newspaper, or broadcast.

Library of Congress Cataloging-in-Publication Data

    The neurological boundaries of reality / edited by E. M. R. Critchley.
       p.   cm.
    Originally published : London : Farrand Press, 1994.
    Includes bibliographical references and index.
    ISBN 1-56821-739-0 (alk. paper)
    1. Cognitive neuroscience.  2. Reality.  I. Critchley, E. M. R. (Edmund Michael R.)
    [DNLM: 1. Mental Processes.   BF 455 N494  1994a]
QP360.5.N48    1995
616.89--dc20
DNLM/DLC
for Library of Congress                                      95-36649

Manufactured in the United States of America. Jason Aronson Inc. offers books and cassettes. For information and catalog write to Jason Aronson Inc., 230 Livingston Street, Northvale, New Jersey 07647.

# Preface

> What can we reason, but from what we know?
> Of Man what see we?
> *Alexander Pope (1688-1744)*
> *An Essay on Man*

Anyone intrigued by the question implicit in the title of this book, The Neurological Boundaries of Reality, can be presumed to possess the curiosity and intellectual vigour to read further. The more familiar lines from Pope's "Essay on Man", beginning "Know then thyself, presume not God to scan, the proper study of Mankind is Man", would normally be addressed in today's world at the Natural Sciences. Although physicists have been concerned to define the essence of the material world, and philosophers – some with remarkable penetration – have attempted to determine the meaning of reality, there has been no comparable undertaking by those whose daily concern is with patients experiencing difficulties involving the borderlands of reality.

The purpose of this book is to redress this serious omission in the writings of neuroscientists by examining in detail various aspects of human awareness. The text is intended to be read at many levels. The emphasis has been on simplicity of expression and clarity of thought. A critical examination of the boundaries of reality has meant that many cherished myths have been discarded, newer concepts have been introduced, and the work should prove invigorating for those seeking a deeper understanding of their speciality. The choice of the syntactic phrase "neurological boundaries" is to emphasize that many apparent distortions encroaching on the borderland of reality are not necessarily aberrations and are best explained in neurological rather than psychological or psychiatric terms.

Every one of the galaxy of authors – representing psychiatrists, psychologists, philosophers and neurologists – has risen to the challenge, examining how we recognize what is real or unreal, correlating scientific knowledge, unusual experiences, examples from literature and elsewhere, and the many hypotheses advanced to provide an exciting, stimulating and thought-provoking text. "True Science then, with modesty thy guide, deduct what is". It is left to the reader to discern any central theme, and in this respect, the book can be treated as a comprehensive series of individual essays on which to browse, rather than as a sequence to be followed dogmatically.

# PREFACE

I wish to thank all those who have helped to stimulate the ideas upon which the book is based, the many secretaries who have been concerned with its production, and in particular our publisher, Farrand Press, for the stability of support necessary for a work of unusual character. Finally I would like to dedicate it to my uncle, Dr Macdonald Critchley, Ex-President of the World Federation of Neurology, who has inspired many with an interest in higher cerebral functions.

*Edmund M.R. Critchley*
*January 1994*

# Contributors

**Dr Michael Ayers,** Philosopher, Wadham College, Oxford, OX1 3PN, England.

**Dr David Bates,** Consultant and Senior Lecturer, Royal Victoria Infirmary, Queen Victoria Road, Newcastle-upon-Tyne, NE1 4LP, England.

**Dr G.E. Berrios,** Consultant Psychiatrist, University Lecturer in Psychiatry, Addenbrookes Hospital, Cambridge, CB2 2QQ, England.

**Dr N.E.F. Cartlidge,** Consultant and Senior Lecturer, Royal Victoria Infirmary, Queen Victoria Road, Newcastle-upon-Tyne, NE1 4LP, England.

**Dr E.M.R. Critchley,** Consultant Neurologist, Royal Preston Hospital, Sharoe Green Lane, Preston, Lancashire, PR2 4HT and Hon. Professor, University of Central Lancashire, England.

**Dr W.J.K. Cumming,** Consultant Neurologist, Neuroscience Unit, Alexandra Hospital, Mill Lane, Cheadle, Cheshire, SK8 2PX, England.

**Dr W. Falkowski,** Consultant Psychiatrist, St George's Hospital Medical School, Level 01, Jenner Wing G2, Cranmer Terrace, Tooting, London SW17 ORE, England.

**Dr Peter B.C. Fenwick,** Consultant Neuropsychiatrist, The Maudsley Hospital, Denmark Hill, London SE5 8AZ, England.

**Dr John Harrison,** Academic Unit of Neuroscience, Charing Cross and Westminster Medical School, 10 East, Charing Cross Hospital, Fulham Palace Road, London W6 8RF, England.

**Dr C.H. Hawkes,** Consultant Neurologist, Ipswich Hospital, Heath Road, Ipswich, Sulfolk IP4 5PD, England.

**Dr Maggie Hilton,** Clare House, St George's Hospital Medical School, London SW17 ORE, England.

**Dr J.M. Kellett,** Consultant Psychiatrist, St George's Hospital Medical School, Level 01, Jenner Wing G2, Cranmer Terrace, Tooting, London SW17 ORE, England.

**Dr Christopher Kennard,** Academic Unit of Neuroscience, Charing Cross and Westminster Medical School, 10 East, Charing Cross Hospital, Fulham Palace Road, London W6 8RF, England.

**Ms Alison M. Macdonald,** Research Worker, Genetics Section, Institute of Psychiatry, De Crespigny Park, Denmark Hill, London SE5 8AF, England.

**Dr Christopher J. Mace,** Hon. Lecturer in Neuropsychiatry, Institute of Neurology, The National Hospital, Queen Square, London WC1N 3BG and Consultant Psychotherapist and Senior Lecturer in Psychotherapy, The University of Warwick, Coventry CV4 7AL, England.

**Professor Andrew R. Mayes,** Department of Psychology, Eleanor Rathbone Building, P.O. Box 147, University of Liverpool, Liverpool L69 3BX, England.

**Dr J.D. Mitchell,** Consultant Neurologist, Royal Preston Hospital, Sharoe Green Lane, Preston, Lancashire, PR2 4HT and Hon. Professor, University of Central Lancashire, England.

**Dr B. Monteiro,** Consultant Psychiatrist for the Deaf, Prestwich Hospital, Bury New Road, Prestwich, Manchester M25 7BL, England.

**Dr A.P. Moore,** Senior Registrar in Neurology, Walton Hospital, Rice Lane, Liverpool L9 1AE, England.

**Dr Alice M. Parshall,** Senior Registrar in Psychiatry, Maudsley Hospital, Denmark Hill, London SE5 8AZ. England.

**Dr T.M. Reilly,** Consultant Psychiatrist, The Retreat, York YO1 5BN, England.

**Dr Elise Rivlin,** Head of Childrens/Adolescent Clinical Psychology Specialty, Central Manchester Healthcare Trust, St Mary's Hospital; and The Winnicott Centre, 195-197 Hathersage Road, Manchester, M13 OJE; and University of Manchester Teacher to the Depts Child Health and Psychiatry, England.

**Professor J.R. Smythies,** Department of Neurosciences, UCSD, La Jolla, California 92030-0201, USA.

**Dr G.J. Turnbull,** former Wing Commander, Royal Air Force, Consultant Psychiatrist, Ridgeway Hospital, Moorhead Road, Wroughton, Swindon, Wiltshire SN4 9DD, England.

**Dr Andrew W. Young,** MRC Applied Psychology Unit, 15 Chaucer Road, Cambridge CB2 2EF. England.

**Dr Dahlia W. Zaidel,** Department of Psychology, University of California at Los Angeles, Los Angeles, California 90024, USA.

# Contents

| | | |
|---|---|---|
| Preface | | v |
| Contributors | | vii |
| Introduction | | xiii |
| 1. | Touch<br>E.M.R. Critchley | 1 |
| 2. | Balance and tilt<br>A.P. Moore | 17 |
| 3. | Olfaction<br>C.H. Hawkes | 43 |
| 4. | Deafness and communication<br>Brendan Monteiro and E.M.R. Critchley | 55 |
| 5. | Sensory deprivation and hostage situations<br>Gordon Turnbull | 67 |
| 6. | Recognition and reality<br>Andrew W. Young | 83 |
| 7. | The neurological boundaries of visual reality<br>John Harrison and Christopher Kennard | 101 |
| 8. | Synaesthesia<br>E.M.R. Critchley | 111 |
| 9. | Alterations in conscious awareness<br>Peter Fenwick | 121 |

# CONTENTS

10. On the nature of consciousness and the unconscious from the point of view of neuroscience and neurophilosophy  143
    *J.R. Smythies*

11. A view of the world from a split-brain perspective  161
    *Dahlia W. Zaidel*

12. Art and reality  175
    *E.M.R. Critchley*

13. The nature of music and musical hallucinations  191
    *J.D. Mitchell*

14. Philosophy, knowledge and reality  207
    *Michael Ayers*

15. Hallucinations: selected historical and clinical aspects  229
    *G.E. Berrios*

16. Delusions: selected historical and clinical aspects  251
    *G.E. Berrios*

17. Delusions, schizophrenia (as illustrating a breakdown in the boundaries of reality), psychosis and neurosis  269
    *Alice M. Parshall*

18. Hysteria and conversion  287
    *Christopher J. Mace*

19. The psychology and inter-relationship of twins  299
    *Alison M. Macdonald*

20. Perception of sexuality  323
    *John M. Kellett, Maggie Hilton and W. Falkowski*

21. Awareness of body image, parietal lobe disturbances, neglect and agnosias  341
    *W.J.K. Cumming*

22. Childhood development of awareness of self  349
    *E. Rivlin*

| | |
|---|---|
| 23. Psychological correlates of disordered body image<br>    *T.M. Reilly* | 369 |
| 24. Disorders of consciousness<br>    *David Bates and Niall Cartlidge* | 383 |
| 25. Memory, disturbances of memory and human knowledge of reality and ourselves<br>    *Andrew R. Mayes* | 401 |
| 26. The constraints of language<br>    *E.M.R. Critchley* | 419 |
| Index | 431 |

# Introduction

The success of Stephen Hawking's "A Brief History of Time" is confirmation that people are prepared to read scientific material that places accuracy of detail and argument above concessions to journalistic ease, provided that the purpose is to address important questions of today. There can be few astronomers who have not read his book; though not all of them have agreed with his thesis and many have used his explanations to sharpen their arguments in contradiction. At the same time a vast reading public has been made aware of the issues surrounding the destiny of our cosmic system. There is no one of the stature of Hawking to address the issue of our own reality but, by collating the work of experts in the Neurosciences and balancing their contributions against that of an eminent philosopher, there is hope for greater understanding. Do we take the limits of our own field of vision for the limits of the world: or do we, along with Samuel Johnson, believe that curiosity is one of the permanent and certain characteristics of a vigorous mind?

The various approaches in this book to an understanding of reality differ widely in the ease with which they may be grasped. The excellent essay by Macdonald on twins will appeal even to those who do not appreciate the value of twin-studies when comparing the effects of nature and nurture. The essence, though not the detail, of the chapters on the special senses will be readily understood. Wing Commander Turnbull has written on sensory deprivation, not surprisingly influenced by his recent work with released hostages. Indeed his chapter will gain meaning if it can be read in conjunction with Waite (1993). The chapters on Art and Music will have their special appeal. But even for those specialists who are directly involved in aspects of the subject matter – neurologists, psychologists and psychiatrists – there will be large areas of comparative ignorance. What can be more specialized than a view of the world from a split-brain perspective – from patients whose connecting neurons between their cerebral hemispheres have been divided in order to control otherwise intractable epilepsy?

Much progress has been made into recognition and disorders of recognition and memory, and disorders of memory. Both require an intricate system of modulation and integration of information. Clues dependent upon the familiar differ from those used with the unfamiliar, and the mistakes made differ in consequence. Memory is not only viewed in the context of the moment but takes into account the environment, what has happened, what may happen, and even preconceived notions, myths and predictions. To the question, what is truth? Wilson (1992) answers: "Supposing there were such a thing as dispassionate memory, colourless memory, memory which made no interpretation of the facts: If there were such a transparent camera-brain in a human head, it was not in the head that conceived the Fourth Gospel".

Many of the chapters written by psychiatrists debate issues which have been in hot dispute for years: the definition of psychoses, what are delusions, can pseudo-hallucinations be separated from true hallucinations, can illusions, delusions and hallucinations be separated from each other? One of the fascinations of the work is that Drs Berrios and Parshall discuss delusions from totally different perspectives. There is a third aspect. Delusions become delusions when they are not culturally accepted. We allow that the man who dare not micturate lest he flood the whole world or the lady who believes that she is Mary, Queen of Scots is the subject of alien notions that have captured that person's mind. But why do some people have a St Christopher with them when they travel? If a non-conformist minister born before the end of the 19th century declared from the pulpit that he always felt he had an angel on his shoulder he would have evoked no more comment that a few Amens from the High Seat. It would not be so with a present-day clergyman but it was acceptable for a man who travelled the oceans on a raft to entitle a book published in 1966 "An Angel on Each Shoulder".

Explanations of voices in dreams, for example, can become more and more complex according to culture, as with born again Christians. The Gospel story of the Nativity (Matthew 1:18) can be interpreted in many ways:

> Now the birth of Jesus Christ was on this wise. When as his mother Mary was espoused to Joseph before they came together she was found with child of the Holy Ghost. Then Joseph her husband being a just man and not willing to make her a public example was minded to put her away privily. But while he thought on these things, behold, the angel of the Lord appeared unto him in a dream saying Joseph thou son of David fear not to take unto thee Mary thy wife for that which is conceived in her is of the Holy Ghost. And shall bring forth a son and thou shalt call his name Jesus for he shall save his people from their sins.

How we interpret this story depends on our own culture. A few years ago it was required that every Christian accept the story absolutely. Did Joseph dream, or was his account of the angel speaking to him a socially necessary explanation at that time of his change in attitude? Gould (1949) and Green and Preston (1981) would argue on scientific evidence that the angelic voice was almost certainly accompanied by an activation of the hearer's muscles of phonation and perhaps even by actual subvocal speech.

Differences in the degree of insight or substantiality, the presentations in external objective space or internal subjective space, the consciousness of the real environment, and the ego content of the event have all been invoked to separate pseudo-hallucinations from hallucinations proper. Thus, it is claimed that as pseudo-hallucination is usually ego-centric and arises as a result of cogitation, e.g. wishing a dream to continue: true hallucinations are perceptions of a memory abnormally released or excited by an unusual stimulus, possibly due to instability of brain cells. Three examples will suffice to explain just how difficult it is to quantify the degree of insight:

1   A worker on a production line started to hear voices. He knew they were nonsensical because they kept telling him to work overtime.

2   A deaf patient saw a figure he called Molly, who signed to him. The doctors were trying to persuade him to stay in the unit; he wanted to leave to go to London. In desperation they asked him what Molly said. He signed to her and she signed back, "Stay here".

3   The assessment of degree of insight may rest heavily upon the examiner. One patient described two hallucinations. She saw St Theresa who said that she would go to Heaven and she felt elated. She also saw the devil who said she would go to Hell and she then became depressed. The social worker, a nun, was asked what supportive treatment should be given. She answered, send for the priest. "What for?" "To exorcise the devil". "What about St Theresa?" "Oh, that's just lovely."

There are many diseases, both psychiatric and medical, on the borderland of reality, with impairment or loss of ability to test reality. Antipsychiatrists would suggest that a delusion was an adaptive response to intolerable psycho-social stress. In the psychoses, patients may opt out of an unexceptable reality. In the neuroses, they may seek solace in fantasy. In hysteria, there may be a conversion or somatatizisation of an unacceptable reality. In all these there may be a failure of communication between the individual and society (society often being personified in the doctor). Competitive athletes or ballet dancers are prepared to accept pain and fatigue in their performance but there is a balance in what they perceive and can accept in relation to the rewards they get. One explanation for some of those who suffer from the chronic fatigue syndrome (which is essentially a heterogenous condition) is that there has been an "information overload" breakdown in this perceived balance (Edwards, 1993)

There is also an awareness of how we view ourselves – our body image. This may achieve importance in neurological disease as with disorders of the parietal lobe or the presence of a phantom limb after amputation. There may be denial of illness or infirmity. Diseases such as anorexia or bulimia arise from one's self-perception. Dr Rivlin, who writes on childhood awareness of self, is an expert on the psychology of abused and burnt children. We all have a horror of the abnormal and have difficulty accepting disability in ourselves and others. Although improved communications in the modern world have helped remove prejudices, video games have been challenged as placing children in a situation of virtual reality attacking and destroying anything in their sights which is in anyway abnormal. Society has need to examine our perception of sexuality and sexual aberrations. In terms of reality, what is the importance of "fantasy" to sex? Can this be turned around and become part of "imagination" in all aspects of life or is it merely a prolongation of a prepubescent capacity to dream?

The child explores its enlarging environment, often acting out through fantasy and play. He/she may step into his/her own drawing and act out the situation. Dreams may be rehearsals or replays of psychologically important material.

Increasingly there is a search for stability and the importance of identity. The adult may seek stability within the pack, acknowledging a pecking order. Failure to retain status may lead to stress disorders. The capacity to play diminishes. Heart attacks have been known to punctuate management games.

The neurological basis of consciousness is examined by Drs Bates and Cartlidge. Consciousness is the state of arousal or vigilance. It is also awareness of self and environment, the capacity for higher cognitive functions, for motivated and intellectualized behaviour, delayed response solutions and intentionality. Absence of consciousness and even the definition of death merit critical attention. With drugs and sleep the constraints are loosened. A child when sleeping displays more unstable electrophysiological patterns than an adult and is more prone to abnormalities of sleep – night terrors, somnambulism, and nightmares. Dr Fenwick is also concerned with sleep walking, epileptic phenomena, ecstatic and near death experiences. Professor Smythies discusses the nature of consciousness and unconsciousness from a neuro-psychiatric viewpoint advancing beyond most people's concept of ego, id and superego. Many of his hypotheses of reverberating neuronal circuits and a return to the concepts of Hughlings-Jackson are accepted as interesting rather than established but recur to a surprising extent in other sections of the book. His chapter provides an excellent introduction to that of Ayers on philosophy, knowledge and reality. To many scientists, metaphysical concepts are difficult to understand but Dr Ayers has succeeded magnificently in integrating natural philosophy with natural science.

## References

Edwards, R.H.T. (1993). Muscle histopathology and physiology in chronic fatigue syndrome. *In* "Chronic Fatigue Syndrome". (Eds G.R. Bock and J. Whelan). pp. 102-103. Ciba Foundation Symposium 173, Wiley, Chichester.

Gould, L.N. (1949). Auditory hallucinations in schizophrenia. *Journal of Neurology, Neurosurgery, and Psychiatry*, **109**, 418-427.

Green, P. and Preston, P. (1981). Electromyography in the study of auditory hallucinations. *British Journal of Psychiatry*, **139**, 204-208.

Johnson, S. (1751). "The Rambler".

Waite, T. (1993). "Taken on Trust". Hodder & Stoughton, London.

Wilson, A.N. (1992)." Jesus". Sinclair-Stevenson, London.

# 1. Touch

E.M.R. Critchley

---

In this chapter "touch" is used in a generic, Aristotelean, connotation as the fifth human sense. It differs from the other special senses in that it is diffusely represented over the surface of the body whereas vision, hearing, taste and smell require the mediation of specifically developed and circumscribed sensory receptor organs. The skin is also a diffuse, multipurpose organ providing thermal stability, support and protection to other deeper structures; in effect serving as a functional unit of the body comparable to the brain, liver, skeleton or heart. It is not the only organ of "touch" sensation: other membranes such as those of the cornea, lips and tongue can respond to touch. Physiologists prefer the generic term "somaesthesia" for cutaneous and sensory information arising from the skin, viscera, joints, semicircular canals and static postural organs.

The examination of "touch" and "somaesthesia" provides a clear indication of how the body is able to identify objects within its vicinity by means of a limited number of modalities of sensation. The appearance of the object to some extent reflects the modalities available with which it may be studied. The resulting impulses travel up the peripheral nerves, pass through various synapses in the spinal cord and are relayed to the thalamus and brain, and whilst in transit they undergo repeated examination and modification. In effect the reality of the object is "sensed" by limited sensory modalities, competes and mingles with other sensory data from the outside and from within the body, and if the impulses are strong enough will eventually reach consciousness. Many factors can adjust and confuse "reality". Perhaps more is known about the way touch is assessed than about any other form of sensation, partly because the pathways for transmission are spread out rather than being tightly compact. There is every reason to assume that other human senses are treated and interpreted in a similar fashion.

The dictionary definition of "touch" is "a sense by which the texture and other qualities of objects can be experienced when they come in contact with a part of the body surface". Thus touch given its narrowest meaning is a contact signal, received at the periphery, from which deductions are drawn. The contact may be ignored. It may need reinforcement before recognition occurs. The initial response at the periphery may be negative, i.e. passive; though this may not reflect the interpretation placed upon the sensation by the brain. Alternatively, the peripheral response may be positive but contained within the skin. It may lead to an involuntary reflex avoiding-action, produce a pleasureable reaction increasing the degree of contact, or activate muscles in close contact with the touch stimulus as with orgasm or the sucking response of the infant to the teat.

Touch as a contact signal is given a quantitative dimension by means of temporal and spatial summation; but qualitative information is also provided to the body as a result of contact with an object. Von Helmholtz states that there are four major dissociable sensory categories: touch, warmth, cold and pain; and Blix (1984) postulated the existence in normal skin of a sensory mosaic of tiny "spots" each of which reacts preferentially to these four "modalities" of sensation. The spots for warmth and cold are clear cut and easily separable, those for touch more numerous, and pain spots so closely set together that Blix later doubted their individuality. Between 1894 and 1896 von Frey examined the peripheral terminations of nerves under the skin at each sensory spot, concluding that there are specialized end-organs that respond preferentially to particular types of stimuli. Pain is mediated by free nerve endings, cold by Krause's end bulbs, warmth by Ruffini corpuscles and touch by basket formations forming free nerve endings around hair follicles and Messner's corpuscles in glabrous skin.

Different cutaneous areas vary in their sensitivity. A mother testing the temperature of the bath water for her babe will use her elbow rather than her hand as being more sensitive and closer in feel to the baby's skin. If touch is tested for by 2 point discrimination it will be found that the finger tips and lips are two of the most sensitive areas; thus a person feeling in his pockets with his finger tips can identify by stereognosis the shape of different coins. Areas of skin will thicken with use as in manual work but the basic mechanism is similar. Although by training a blind person may learn to read Braille, the arrangement and sensitivity of nerve endings in the skin is no different from that of other people. What change has occurred has been in the ability to interpret what is felt at cortical level.

From the recognition of different nerve endings in the skin has arisen the stimulus specificity hypothesis. Each end-organ preferentially responds to a specific sensory energy or modality which is recognized and transmitted centrally. However, the stimulus specificity hypothesis does not explain how glabrous and hairy skin are equally sensitive or how the cornea, with only free nerve endings, can also transmit the full range of sensory modalities. The alternative, and not mutually incompatible pattern theory, is that the pattern of discharge from any given nerve fibre could at one time contribute towards the sensation of touch, and at another towards the experience of pain, cold or warmth. Rather than being restricted to a limited number of sensory modalities, the concept of preferential receptivity based on the pattern theory can account for other sensory experiences such as roughness, stickiness, hardness, greasiness and clamminess. This wider interpretation of any stimulus is dependent upon modulation of the information at many sites between the periphery and the brain and upon the concept of the plasticity of central pathways subserving sensation with preferential though not exclusive functions.

Modulation is the key-word in considering any form of cutaneous sensation. As

Sir Charles Sherrington observed, any single spot on the trunk is innervated by nerve fibres running into several neighbouring posterior roots, providing a vertical spread of stimuli, as they enter the spinal cord. Some of these afferent fibres will be fast transmitters and others slow. Thus the impulses reaching the spinal cord will be spread spatially and temporally, merging at that site with the background activity received by and generated within the substantia gelatinosa and other cellular grey matter within the spinal cord. The interaction of fibre sizes, speeds of transmission and possibly other factors will "gate" or edit the information received from the periphery. Other processes of selection, modification and alteration of the stimulus will be re-enacted at many sites of stimulus-convergence between the spinal cord and brain.

The outcome is that no stimulus reaches the brain in an unaltered form. In the course of transmission certain stimuli such as those subserving itch or tickle may excite local reflexes whereas others, such as pain or pleasure, probably depend more upon the interpretation placed upon the stimulus by the brain itself rather than upon the basic nature of the primary stimulus. Pain is essentially an imprecise symptom that achieves recognition as a percept within the mind. It was thought that excessive stimulation of any specific nerve ending could cause pain, but more recent studies have shown that individual primary afferent nerves and their peripheral endings are so sharply tuned that they respond well to certain stimuli only and poorly to others, irrespective of the size of their fibres (Hoffert, 1989).

## Pain

Pain is a percept of the central nervous system derived from a nociceptive stimulus at the periphery. It is, as Aristotle called it, "A Passion of the Soul", or a defence of the body against harm or potential danger. Leriche put its dubious characteristics succinctly in the phrase: "a sinister gift which diminishes man, which makes him sicker than he would be without it". Pain is primarily associated with physical damage and often described in terms relating to injury (Merskey and Spear, 1967). The damage may be assumed or real. Thus, there is a psychological component as interpretation takes place only in the mind and the information recorded there is entirely personal – a private matter that cannot be shared by any one or described in terms that mean the same thing to another person (Mehta, 1973). The significance of pain to an individual may take many forms: as a signal of damage or danger to a bodily structure, a means of expressing a need for help, evidence of unfair treatment, a means of manipulation, or a threat to the individual arousing guilt feelings as a punishment for real or imagined misdemeanours. Such interpretations may be far removed from the recognition of noxious stimuli, and a particular individual may benefit as much from psychological support as from analgesia.

There is evidence of a maturation, and development, of the experience of pain. Infants and the newborn have high thresholds for noxious stimulation and young animals reared in an environment of restricted sensory stimulation have considerably increased thresholds for pain. After the early years, however, the pattern of behaviour exhibited by a child in pain reflects both familial and cultural influences, disturbed homes and socio-economic factors. The truth of this statement may be observed when a child is taken to the dentist; and many of us retain throughout life differing responses to pains at various sites depending upon our early experiences of such pains. In later life there is a gradual lessening of pain experienced in most situations and this may be but one aspect of a general decline in sensitivity to sensory stimuli associated with increasing age.

For most of us the appreciation of pain is dependent upon the whole complex of events forming the subjective experience: both the primary painful sensation and the reaction to that sensation. We may attempt to list the relevant factors: the integrity of the nervous system, the total pain load, previous experience of its origin and significance, our state of consciousness, training, fatigue, anxiety, tension, fear, knowledge and understanding, attention and distraction, suggestibility and whether the pain is associated with pleasurable, emotional, religious or hysterical mental states.

When examining the impact of noxious, painful stimuli felt at the periphery we do well to consider acute pain separately from chronic or continuous pains. At the periphery the information obtained is dependent on the groups and sizes of the afferent fibres stimulated, the arrangement of the fibres in the tissues, and the layers and structures stimulated. The stimulus is irritative or later destructive. Thus the stimulus becomes noxious because additional bursts of activity are triggered by tissue damage and the release of nociceptive chemical substances. Local tenderness (primary hyperaesthesia) will result from the sensitization of previously high threshold endings to the products of tissue breakdown. The resulting stimulus is thus more intense and more prolonged. Most of the fibres conducting the information will be small, unmyelinated nerves but some will be fast conducting myelinated fibres and, according to the gate-control theory of Melzack and Wall (1965), the imbalance of inhibitory small fibres and excitatory large fibres on the substantia gelatinosa in the spinal cord will bias the onward relay by T (or transmission) cells centrally to the reticular formation and cortex. A reduction in the number of peripheral nerve fibres can cause a change in the character of a sensation, apart from a diminution in its intensity. The smaller myelinated (delta) and unmyelinated (C) fibres are not an homogeneous group, and the presence or absence of pain in any particular disorder of peripheral nerves (neuropathy) cannot be forecast from the preferential loss of large or small fibres or from the acuteness or severity of the degenerative change. For example, the loss of large fibres in alcoholic neuropathy or myelomatosis and of small fibres in Fabry's disease causes pain; but a similar loss of large fibres in Friedreich's ataxia or in the polyneuropathy of renal failure, or of small fibres in familial amyloidosis or Tangier disease, does not.

The gate-control theory, though subject to much debate, is one of the major concepts of the function of the nervous system to emerge in this century. The principal features of the theory are that: information about the presence of injury is transmitted to the central nervous system by peripheral nerves; certain small diameter fibres respond only to injury while others with lower thresholds increase their discharge frequency if the stimulus reaches noxious levels; cells in the spinal cord or fifth cranial nerve nucleus which are excited by these injury signals are also facilitated or inhibited by other peripheral nerve fibres which carry information about innocuous events; descending control systems originating in the brain modulate the excitability of the cells which transmit information about injury.

In summary, the brain receives messages about injury by way of a gate-controlled system which is influenced by injury signals, other types of afferent impulses, and descending control.

Afferent nerves enter the spinal cord via the dorsal roots. The primary "gating" occurs within the spinal cord at the level of entry. The bias of the gate is influenced not only by fibre size but by the state of degeneration of the fibres as a result of injury. Reflexes controlling the tone of muscles arise from efferent nerves within the spinal cord and their stimulation will, in turn, affect the inward flow of sensations from peripheral nerves of the same segment. There is also evidence that electrical activity, originating in the spinal cord, passes along the posterior roots antidromically to the peripheral nerves, presumably to exert some form of descending control.

The nerve cell bodies of the afferent peripheral nerves lie outside the spinal cord in the dorsal root ganglia. Within the spinal cord, the peripheral nerves make contact with other cell bodies by means of synapses. The central grey matter of the cord is composed of closely packed cell bodies in synaptic contact with each other, providing the means for mutual inhibition or facilitation, and eventually projecting onto relay fibres which transmit impulses to higher levels of the central nervous system. Each cell has its own electrical energy, secretes its own neurotransmitters, and may be modulated by the presence of other chemicals such as substance P and endogenous opioids in its vicinity. The role of many of these substances has yet to be defined. In addition, incoming impulses may undergo presynaptic facilitation or inhibition before reaching the relay cells, or post-synaptic facilitation or inhibition after doing so. The architectonics of this area, and particularly the major part of substantia gelatinosa, have been examined cytologically, by microelectrodes and the humoral microenvironment examined by immunohistochemical studies.

The upward, afferent projects from the spinal cord, carrying sensory information, ascend towards the cortex as two main systems. The lemniscal system deals with tactile and kinaesthetic impulses, which are conducted by large myelinated fibres via the posterior columns to the cuneate and gracile nuclei of the medulla. Here second order afferents arise and pass after crossing over to the opposite side (decussation) to the ventrobasal complex of the thamalus, whence nerve cells project to the primary somatic sensory area in the post-central cortex. Thus tactile and kinaesthetic stimuli represent the contralateral aspect of the body in the ventrobasal complex of the thalamus. The image of the body is distorted, the volume representation of a part being related to the density of innervation. Each thalamic cell is related to a specific receptive field in the opposite side of the body and as far as possible modality specificity is retained.

The spinothalamic or anterolateral system conducts impulses associated with the evocation of pain, heat, cold and sexual sensations. Fibres run through and relay in the central reticular core of the brainstem. Unlike lemniscal fibres they show very little spatial organization and are finally distributed to both cerebral hemispheres by the so-called diffuse thalamocortical projection. They converge on and relay in certain of the intralaminar nuclei of the thalamus, and possibly also in other regions of the diencephalon. By cutting the anterolateral tracts of the cervical spinal cord, either by an open operation or using a needle under X-ray control, some relief of pain down the same side of the body can be obtained. A unilateral cordotomy will relieve pain in 70-75% of patients, raising the threshold to pain by 40%-50%. If bilateral cordotomy is required the second operation should be performed at a different spinal level in order to avoid respiratory distress. The fact that pain perception can return despite the irreversible nature of the neurosurgical operation is of great theoretical importance, and would indicate that the relationship of pain perception to its preferred spinal cord projection system is plastic.

The effect of descending neural activity upon the spinal cord is well demonstrated by experiments in which morphine is administered intracerebrally into the periaqueductal grey matter of the midbrain or from electrophysiological studies in the same area. The result is a profound analgesia in animals and man.

The dorsal root entry zone, Lissauer's tract, substantia gelatinosa, and large cells of the posterior grey matter, are areas of convergence and pooling of sensory information arising not only from the skin but from the muscles and deeper tissues, the autonomic nervous system controlling the smaller blood vessels of the body, and from the viscera – heart, lungs, liver, and other organs.

This convergence or pooling results in the phenomenon of *referred pain,* where pain derived from one part of the body is experienced in a comparatively remote area. The localization of visceral pain which enters this sensory pool from sympathetic afferents of the autonomic nervous system is diffuse and reference is often made to a presumed body-schema based on the embryonic division of the body into dermatomes. The threshold for pain may be altered over the area of reference and infiltration of this trigger area with local anaesthetic agents can bring partial relief of symptoms. Pain from an abscess under the diaphragm may be felt in the shoulder, anginal pain from the heart transmitted to the jaw and down the left arm, and pain at the wrist from compression of the median nerve may be felt higher up the arm (Tinel's sign).

Other forms of mixing of pain stimuli occur in addition to so-called referred pain. Jones (1907) applied the term *synaesthesia* to the sensation of a double stimulation when only one is applied; thus a sensation of pain may be felt at the site of stimulation and also remotely at another place well away from it, most commonly on the opposite side of the body. Such diverse pains are most likely to arise following spinal injury or amputation of limbs. Abnormal spread of sensation can occur, and a complex terminology has been developed to cover all eventualities. Synchiria is applied when a stimulus, such as a pin prick applied to the unaffected side of the body, produces an unpleasant feeling bilaterally; allaesthesia or allochiria when the stimulus is felt only over the opposite affected side and synaesthesialgia to causalgia when a unilateral stimulus to the affect side causes pain in the unaffected side.

Stimuli from the periphery reaching the cord may be divided into three sensory systems. Such division is essentially artificial but Head and others have claimed that there is an evolutionary or phylogenetic separation of afferent fibres. Those from deep structures represent pressure and movement on joints, tendons and muscles. There is then a protopathic or relatively crude cutaneous sensation of pain and extremes of heat and cold which is poorly localized to its origin. And finally an epicritic, accurately localized, discriminative sensation, especially for touch. Whatever their origin these sensations in combination convey an image of the body schema and alert the body as a whole. Frederiks believes that the normal body schema is the peripheral, schematically conscious, structured, plastically bordered spatial perception of one's own body, constructed from previous and current (especially somaesthetic) sensory information. Others have argued that visual sensations, along with tactile and postural sensations, also play a role (though no one sensation is essential).

*Vigilance* is dependent upon the central flow of impulses from all the sense organs. These sensations have an arousing effect, altering the degree of alertness and often reaching consciousness. Impairment of transmission as when the nerve is compressed by crossing the legs may give a sensation of numbness which obscures the schema of the limb and is often described as the limb going to sleep. Particular stimuli may alert other reactions: a sensation of cold may cause shivering and noxious stimuli reaching the spinal cord may initiate a reflex avoidance response at spinal level and at the same time be transmitted rostrally as impulses alerting the sensorium producing pain and even suffering. Loss of affective reactions to pain can follow operations on the frontal lobe (e.g. prefrontal lobotomy). Thus the integrity of the cerebral cortex is necessary for the full appreciation of pain; but it is still possible for violent motor reactions to painful stimuli to occur in the absence of any conscious sensation of pain.

The recognition of pain requires awareness: diffusely at brainstem level, and becoming more specifically appreciated at higher levels. Counter-irritants such as Tiger balm at other sites may drown the appreciation of a particular pain. Immobilizing an injured limb may result in a reduction of pain by lessening the tension of muscles in the neighbourhood of the wound thereby diminishing input of neural signals from the affected part. Impairment of the nervous system may render the transmission of the pain ineffective. Many peripheral neuropathies result from compression or destruction of nerves or from alteration of their nutrition, either from vascular impairment of the feeding blood vessels, or from lack of nutrients which normally pass along the axons in either direction. In syringomyelia cavitation of the spinal cord presses upon and damages nerve pathways. The centre of the cord is most vulnerable so that nerves transmitting pain and temperature may be affected and those for touch remain unimpaired. Patients with syringomyelia often: (a) give anecdotal stories of indulgence in parlour games in which their ability to withstand pain is clearly better than that of their friends, or (b) present with burns which they have failed to recognize at the time.

As already stated, the appreciation of pain occurs within the brain. Melzack (1989) has postulated the presence of a central neuromatrix or central generating mechanism for pain. This hypothesis remains controversial but the experience of noxious stimuli can be blunted by drugs, psychoses or training the psyche through yoga or meditation. Acupuncture can be regarded as a form of priming of the nervous system, altering the gate mechanisms of pain appreciation. But there are many instances when pain passes unrecognized because vigilance is directed elsewhere: a rugby player may not realize his injury until after the match, the person hit by a stray bullet may be aware of blood on his clothes before complaining of pain, e.g. the Marquis of Anglesea, Henry William Paget, at Waterloo who had his horse shot from under him and afterwards realized that he had also lost a leg.

These examples of failure to appreciate pain immediately may be matched by examples of pains arising spontaneously within the body. A wound which has not previously been painful may become infected and the consequent irritation gives rise to pain. Treatment of painful conditions by sectioning the nerve from that area is frequently unsuccessful. The result may not be loss of pain sensation but rather a spontaneous dysaesthesia arising from the damaged axons. Shingles (Herpes zoster) has a predilection for damaged areas of the body, for example the site of previous disc disease, or may be dormant but alighted by other disease such as myelitis affecting the same area. Chronic pain circuits which have been quiescent for years may erupt following trivial injury.

## Chronic Pain

Chronic pain conditions can arise when damaged end-organs, as in the stump of an amputated limb, continue to discharge; where the tissues remain particularly sensitive as in sympathetic dystrophies, through any permanent bias of the "gate", or through reverberating cycles of multi-synaptic afferent nerve circuits within the spinal cord (see Chapter 10, "neuronal cell assemblies"). Spontaneous or thalamic pain can arise from damage to pain pathways in the deeper structures of cerebral hemispheres. Conversely, other people may lack sensitivity to pain. Damage to nerves as in leprosy or syringomyelia may render a part of the body insensitive to pain. A patient with paraplegia due to transection of the cord as may happen in a road traffic accident – will be unable to appreciate sensation of any kind, including pain, below the level of the spinal injury. Several forms of congenital insensitivity to pain are recognized. Some result from disturbances of the autonomic nervous system which normally subserves temperature and sweating control within the muscles and skin. Others are caused by an over-activity of the endogenous opioid system. A third variety of congenital or acquired imperception of pain involves lesions or damage to the dominant parietal lobe of the brain.

The best known form of *spontaneous pain* is that described by Dejerine and Roussy. The pain is presumed to arise within the thalamus as a result of damage to its lateral nucleus. This is a severe form of pain or hyperpathia referred to the opposite half of the body. Usually such pain fails to respond to analgesic drugs including morphine. Intolerable burning pains occur spontaneously yet the threshold for peripheral pain sensation over the affected area is raised. If the skin is pricked by a needle it may not be felt at first but repeated pricking after a while gives rise to a more intense sensation which is not confined to the spot pricked but spread over a wider area. This thalamic syndrome is often referred to as an over-reaction. Occasionally the spontaneous sensation may not be one of pain but of pleasure and a different emotional response my be triggered by pleasurable stimuli such as a warm object applied to the skin on the opposite half of the body.

Certain forms of spontaneous pain, such as thalamic pain, such as the *neuralgias*, have nothing to do with reality with-out the body nor with the state of non-neural tissues with-in the body but arise as a defect or aberration of the nervous system which transmits sensation. It is uncertain whether migraine originates within the brain or within blood vessels (the latest theory is that chemicals are released from the trigeminal nerve) but pain is produced by distension of blood vessels in the lining membranes of the brain thereby triggering off nerve endings which are particularly sensitive to stretch. With epilepsy the irritation spreads among and is confined to nerve cells. The most common sensations produced are of fear or pain, but occasionally, as in the fits described by Dostoevsky in "The Idiot" (he himself suffered from epilepsy), the predominant feeling may be one of pleasure.

Neuralgias arising solely within the nervous system respond poorly to the usual forms of analgesia and best to drugs which diminish the brain's recognition of the stimulus. Unpleasant explosive pains can occur in relation to many medical conditions such as tabes dorsalis (a form of syphilis of the nervous system), shingles or post-herpetic neuralgia, and trigeminal neuralgia. Some pains can be continuous but others are paroxysmal. Over the affected area the threshold for all forms of cutaneous sensibility is raised with a painful over-reaction to such stimuli as are able to cross the threshold. A dying or degenerating nerve is abnormally irritable: a nerve which is completely destroyed has no such reaction. Many of the drugs used to treat these conditions are also used in the treatment of epilepsy.

The term *causalgia* was coined by Dr Weir Mitchell during the American Civil War to denote a burning quality of pain occurring as a result of traumatic injury. Though the severity of the pain may be variable, its description always includes a burning, scalding, searing or hot quality. In peace-time similar disturbances are seen among industrial injuries, road traffic accidents or even as the result of relatively minor trauma. The essential lesion in causalgia is thought to be damage to the sympathetic fibres along a peripheral nerve or nerve plexus; possibly with the development of abnormal synapses between afferent sympathetic and afferent somatic fibres at the site of injury. Gerrard (1951) has shown how damage to nerves at any level of the nervous system, especially if they are in synaptic connection with each other, can disrupt their firing sequences. Synchronously firing neurone pools could recruit additional units, move along the grey matter, be further sustained by impulses different from and feebler than those needed to initiate them, and could discharge excessive, and abnormally patterned, volleys to the higher centres.

Intense pain begins almost immediately after the accident, but occasionally may be delayed for weeks or months. The pain may be spontaneous but may be aggravated or precipitated by touch, movement or psychological factors. New pains and trigger zones may spread unpredictably to other parts of the body where no pathology exists. It is presumed that constant stimulation either alters the gating of sensation at spinal level or leads to abnormal pain circuits developing at sites of convergence of sensory stimulation within the spinal cord. Involuntary jerkings may occur. The limb may show typical skin changes with tightness, redness and sweating. If the pain is severe enough to prevent the full use of the limb, wasting, contractures and other trophic changes appear in the skin and nails, and the bones become osteoporotic. Overall the most successful operations to relieve the pains are sympathectomy or sympathetic blockade but the results can be disappointing. Patients often become demoralized by the persistence and severity of symptoms and the failure of treatment to relieve suffering.

"Phantom limb" was yet another term coined by Weir Mitchell in order to describe the persistent sensation of the missing limb as an almost invariable consequence of amputation. His study of 90 American Civil War amputees was published in 1872. Further experience over the years has confirmed his original observations that phantoms are almost invariable in adults following trauma but are rare in those with mutilating diseases such as leprosy or gangrene or in children before reaching four years of age. Thus, children born with phocomelia (absent limbs) do not get phantom sensations. A phantom may last for years, and even when lost may return under stress. A phantom is an illusory awareness of the missing part. With time the phantom tends to weaken in intensity and the limb appears to telescope in towards the stump until the fingers or toes of the phantom merge into its substance.

Phantom limb sensations after amputation constitute the best known evidence of body image and as such will be discussed in Chapter 21. A missing phantom limb may share other bodily sensations. Disease of the peripheral nerves (polyneuritis) may produce a similar numbness, tingling, and pins and needles sensations in the phantom limb as elsewhere. Even sensations of heat, or of coldness, environmentally determined, will be referred to the missing limb. A phantom limb will appear to move. Other parts of the body, deprived of sensation, may generate phantom limb sensations. This may happen in a limb made numb by local anaesthesia, with avulsion of the brachial plexus when the nerve roots from a limb are severed traumatically though the limb is still attached to the body, and with gross sensory loss to parts of the body as with sensory peripheral neuropathy or the Guillain Barré syndrome. A doctor affected by the Guillain Barré syndrome of post-infective neuritis described how he appeared to be suspended above the bed when sitting on a bedpan and how his legs would feel as though they were at right angles to his body. Such phenomena would appear to indicate that the phantom can be generated centrally in the absence of neural impulses from affected dermatomes. However, this does not mean that the periphery is irrelevant to all phantoms, as electrical stimulation of the stump invariably exaggerates the phantom.

Phantom phenomena affecting other organs have also been described, e.g. following castration, enucleation, tooth extraction, facial mutilation or mastectomy. A phantom anus may occur after a lesion of the lowest part of the spinal cord (conus medullaris). In contrast to the 100% occurrence following limb amputation, phantom pain and non-painful phantom sensations rarely affect more than 20-30% at other sites. However the incidence of phantoms varies, such feelings are rare after removal of a breast or ear, but common after enucleation of an eye, excision of the rectum, or removal of the larynx. The phenomenon in paraplegics after transection of the spinal cord lacks the vividness obvious from discussion with any amputee. They may feel that the lower half of their body is missing but may require considerable concentration to describe exactly what they feel, often talking of a bizarre continuity or a vague awareness. Telescoping does not occur and painful phenomena are absent.

The one aspect common to all phantom phenomena is that there has been some trauma or mutilation. There are in effect three phenomena: phantom sensations affecting the body schema, phantom limb pains and pains in the stump – the latter being a form of causalgia. Phantom limb pains are more likely to develop in patients who have suffered pain in the limb for some time prior to the amputation. The subsequent pain may resemble closely that which was present before the amputation in both quality and localization and a painful phantom is less likely to shrink in size with the passage of time. Approximately 5 to 10% of patients continue to suffer disagreeable sensations which cripple and oppress. Such sensations may be variously described as cramp, shooting, burning and crushing. The phantom may appear to be frozen in distorted attitudes reflecting the posture of the limb at the time of the accident, e.g. tightly clenched fingers digging into the palm of the hand or the arm locked in a half-Nelson behind the back. Relief of pain by local nerve blocks may be accompanied by release and movement of the phantom finger or arm. Conversely drug-induced movement disorders – dyskinesias or dystonias – may affect a phantom limb. Pain from a phantom limb emanates from pressure on specially sensitive areas, trigger zones which are situated initially in the injured part but gradually spreads to other areas of the body which are healthy and unrelated to the injury; so much so that micturition, straining at stool and ejaculation may be accompanied by a burning sensation in both the phantom and the stump end.

Controversy still remains as to the site of recognition of phantom phenomena. There is clearly a peripheral component in the more obvious instances; but phantoms can occur with migraine, schizophrenia, epilepsy, tumours of the brain or spinal cord, with strokes and lesions of the parietal lobes. They can be modified or abolished by electro-cortical therapy (ECT) or cordotomy, by tapping on the stump with a blunt hammer or by transcutaneous electrical stimulation. Although almost all amputees experience phantom limb sensations, they differ widely in their reaction to these experiences, so much so that experienced observers who have dealt with many patients following amputation believe that much of the response is generated by factors such as their underlying personality, the degree of attention paid to bodily sensation, previous occupations, and the general threshold of the individual to pain, injury or other menacing situations.

**Treatment of Pain**

The psychological adjustment of people with neuralgic pains is all important. This includes the surroundings in which they are treated, attention paid to cleansing any wounds, counselling, and using drugs in the acute stages for pain relief, lifting depression and altering the threshold of awareness of pain. Physiotherapy with reduction of spasticity and gradual mobilization is vital to the relief of symptoms and the development of a positive attitude. Treatments have varied from ECT, leucotomies, stereotactic surgery and cordotomy to section of nerve roots, sympathectomies and peripheral nerve blocks. As stated, pain may return after cordotomy. Section of the dorsal roots may not relieve pain. It is nowadays realized that man does not follow the Bell Magendie law which stated that all sensation enters by the dorsal roots and all motor activities emerge by the ventral roots. One third of the ventral root fibres are probably sensory so that the ventral roots contain a mixture of motor and sensory fibres.

Much attention has been given to the treatment of pain by low frequency transcutaneous electrical stimulation. Such stimulation is believed to modify the bias of the "gate" and also has a chemical effect activating the endorphin system within the spinal cord. Most Western observers believe that acupuncture works in a similar way. There are, however, four theories in vogue among Chinese physicians. The neurological theory implies that acupuncture impulses travel via neural pathways. This theory has been confirmed in rats observing the response of the electroencephalogram to pain and to pain treated with acupuncture. However, pain was also relieved in a second rat with a cross-circulation link suggesting the presence of a humoral component of acupuncture treatment. The Chinese also presume that there may be a competitive block very similar in practice to the gate-control theory of Melzack and Wall. This theory supposes that acupuncture stimuli act upon and may close a hypothetical gate in the spinal cord thereby preventing pain impulses from travelling up the spinal cord to reach the pain centre in the brain. Finally, traditionalists subscribe to a meridian theory based on the Taoist concept of the flow of life force, or Ch'i, within the body. The health of the body depends on the balance of Yang and Yin in life force. The Ch'i is presumed to flow over a network of Ching-lo or meridians. Needling the correct points restores any imbalance of Yang and Yin forces in ill-health. There are 12 meridians and over 800 acupuncture points. Amazingly the charts of the acupuncture points of the traditionalists have been found to be both useful and accurate.

**Pressure, Vibration and Itch**

Other forms of sensation besides touch are registered as impact or contact signals. Whereas touch results from stimulation of tactile receptors in the skin and the tissues immediately deep to the skin, pressure results from impingement and deformity of deeper tissues and their receptors. In all, six different receptors have been identified which respond to various forms of contact signal: free nerve endings, Meissner's corpuscles, Iggo's dome receptors, hair and organs, Merkel's discs and pacinian corpuscles. Not all are present in every area of skin. Vibration is best felt over the skin surfaces. By means of vibration a deaf person can follow the rhythm of music from the resonance of the dance floor. Pacinian corpuscles respond extremely rapidly to minute, rapid deformation of tissues from 60 to 500 Hz and Messner's corpuscles to less rapid changes up to 80 Hz. Tickle and itch arise from very mild stimulation on rapidly adapting free nerve endings in the superficial layers of the epidermis, resulting in the release of kinins and histamine into the skin. Itching powders such as cowhage contain proteolytic enzymes liberating itch-producing peptides.

A sensation of pleasure can be obtained by stimulating parts of the hypothalamus and the limbic system and certain kinds of stimulus, such as demonstrable in cats by stroking, elicit pleasure over the body surface. In this respect it is possible to identify certain sites – erogenous zones – which are more susceptible than elsewhere. These zones often contain specially adapted sweat glands for the release of sexually attracting odours in animals, though an excess of such odours in man is no longer regarded as socially acceptable. There are no apparently different features of the sensory receptors, except perhaps that they are connected to reflex circuits which are particularly liable to signify pleasure rather than pain or other modalities of sensation.

**Magnetic and Electrical Phenomena**

That electrical phenomena can affect the organization of crystals and the growth of cells is well known. Inhibition of rapidly growing cell populations may be produced by high gradient fields, and the alteration of normal cyclic behaviour caused by low field strengths indicates the possibility of organisms being regulated in part by the natural biomagnetic field. The effects of implanted electrodes or pulsed electrical currents on orthopaedic practice have been examined in detail. An article in the *United States Medical Times and Gazette* in 1853 suggested the successful use of electrical treatment in healing an ununited fracture. A controlled study by Becker in 1984 was less successful. The streaming potential of the electromagnetic responses of physiologically moist bone have been studied experimentally suggesting 50% faster healing, increased bone growth and 30% less time to stability. Electrical changes have also been invoked in the strengthening of bone. Bone itself develops electrical charges under load conditions. The attempt to bend a long bone will cause a build up of positive charge on the convex or tensile surface and a transient negative charge on the compressed or concave side. Wolff's law states that bone subjected to compression becomes stronger, and it has been widely suggested that electrical phenomena underlie the physiology of adaptive remodelling, though the direct evidence for this is scant.

Geomagnetic and electrical phenomena have an influence upon human skin along with X-rays and ultraviolet light. They are properties of our environment which affect us even though we lack sense receptors able to detect their presence. In 1984 I answered a question in the *British Medical Journal*: why were certain people unable to wear watches. This article attracted world wide media attention and I received nearly 150 anecdotal letters. I will try to present the information as scientifically as possible.

Some people were unable to wear jewellery either because of an allergy, often leading to eczema, or because the jewellery will tarnish if they wear it. Several factors were thought to cause watches to go wrong. These included ill-health, vibration, temperature and magnetism. Spring watches may be affected by changes in magnetic fields, temperature, atmospheric pressure, alterations in position, lubrication and wear on moving parts. Vibration effects, as with thyrotoxicosis, may cause inaccurate escapement. Sometimes the onset of an illness such as thyrotoxicosis can be dated from failure of a watch to keep accurate time. Rises in temperature are more likely to cause slowing due to expansion of the hairspring and watches commonly go slightly faster in winter than in summer. Quartz watches, with no moving parts, may be influenced by aging of the crystal, thermal drift and cleanliness. Self-wind watches are affected by the immobility of the wearer, as with akinesia or serious disability.

These recognizable causes do not explain each individual circumstance: anecdotal accounts of altered behaviour of watches in pathological circumstances (during periods of sleep deprivation, hypokinesia, fatigue following arduous exertion or prolonged emotional stress), temporary changes in the geophysical environment – solar activity, magnetic fields – or even with unusual work/rest patterns appear to share a common factor in alterations in the person's geomagnetic field. Changes in a person's biomagnetic field can be measured in picoteslas either by an ultrasensitive vibrating probe which can only function in a liquid environment or by SQUID – a superconductivity quantum interference device – which requires the presence of liquid helium. Using such apparatus it is possible to show:
1   increased heterogeneity of skin potentials, with areas of high electrical conductivity;
2   desychronized or weakened amplitude of circadian fluctuations; and

3 short period oscillations in sympathetic/parasympathetic tone.

Neurologists might be interested to determine whether people complaining of subjective pins and needles also have similar changes. This much is factual. It would be interesting to know how far changes in biomagnetic fields account for the more varied phenomena described.

From the correspondence it was clear that the majority of people unable to wear watches without influencing the working of their watch was perfectly healthy. Occasionally several members of the same family were similarly affected. Twenty-five healthy children and 77 healthy adults were unable to wear watches and 5 others reported aberration in time keeping during pregnancy or immediately after childbirth, 2 were able to tell the time of ovulation by the behaviour of their watch but this experience was not shared by their friends. Depression, anxiety, having an affair and nightmares accounted for 13 reports and 30 were associated with various forms of physical illness including raised blood pressure (2), changes in cardiac rhythm (4), cancer (5), abdominal surgery (3) and neurological illness (6) – 3 with fits, 1 with multiple sclerosis and 1 with Parkinsonism.

Particular attention was paid to the wearing of quartz watches. These were trouble free in 10 instances, but no better than other watches in 31. Travel clocks (3) and electrical appliances (5) could also be affected when the susceptible individual was in their vicinity but others found that they could carry a watch provided it was on a chain and children could wear a wrist watch provided they wore some rubber between the watch and their wrist. A different form of interaction was experienced by some individuals reacting adversely to electrical activity around them. Two had blurred vision when near electrical appliances, 7 could not wear nylon clothing because of electric shocks from static electricity and 8 others experienced electric shocks from other sources. Two individuals could not wear electronic watches without experiencing tenseness. One stated that he had shoulder pain on which ever side he wore the watch. Biomagnetic environments are a form of reality the body cannot sense, a borderland of reality largely unexplored and unexplained but which carries potential advantage in relation to wound healing, the treatment of burns and regeneration of tissues.

## References

Barker, A.T., Dixon, R.A., Sharrard, W.J.W. and Sutcliffe, M.L. (1984). Pulsed magnetic field therapy for tibial non-union. *Lancet*, i, 994-996.

Becker, R.O. (1982). Electrical control system and regenerative growth. *Journal of Bioelectricity*, 1, 239-264.

Critchley, E.M.R. (1984). Stop watch phenomenon. *British Medical Journal*, 289, 810.

Critchley, E.M.R. and Isaac, M.T. (1992). Spinal modulation of noxious stimuli. *In* "Diseases of the Spinal Cord". Chapter 3, (Eds E.M.R. Critchley and A.A. Eisen), pp. 15-30. Springer Verlag, London.

Frederiks, J.A.M. (1980). Phantom limb and phantom limb pain. *In* "Handbook of Clinical Neurology 45". (Eds P.J. Vinken, G.W. Bruyn and H.L. Klawans). pp. 395-404. Elsevier,

Amsterdam.
Gerrard, R.W. (1951). A new theory of causalgic pain. *Anesthesiology*, **12**, 1-16.
Hoffert, M.J. (1989). The neurophysiology of pain. *Neurology Clinics*, **7**, 183-204.
Jones, E. (1907). Spinal synaesthesia. *Brain*, **30**, 490-532.
Lele, P.P. and Weddell, G. (1956). The relationship between neurohistology and corneal sensitivity. *Brain*, **79**, 119-154.
Mehta, M. (1973). "Intractable Pain". Saunders, London.
Melzack, R. (1989). Phantom limbs, the self and the brain. *Canadian Journal of Psychology*, **30**, 1-16.
Melzack, R. and Wall, P.D. (1965). Pain mechanisms: a new theory. *Science*, **150**, 971-979.
Merskey, H. and Spear, F.G. (1967). "Pain: Psychological and Psychiatric Aspects". Bailliere Tindall, Cassell, London.
Mitchell, S.W., Morehouse, G.R. and Keen, W.W. (1864). "Gunshot Wounds and Other Injuries of Nerves". Lippincott, Philadelphia.
Nixon, J. (1985). Electromagnetic induction of bone. (Leader). *British Medical Journal*, **290**, 490-1.
Ryzhikov, G.V., Kuz'menko, V.A. and Buluev, A.B. (1982). Effect of disturbances of the geomagnetic field on the circadian rhythms of physiological functions. *Human Physiology*, **8**, 87-93.
Ryzhikov, G.V., Raevskaya, O.S., Gumenyuk, V.H. and Kaptsov, A.N. (1983). Effect of the geomagnetic field and nervous and mental state on electric resistance on biologically active skin points. *Human Physiology*, **8**, 452-455.
Sinclair, D. (1981). "Mechanisms of Cutaneous Sensation". Oxford University Press, Oxford.
Wall, P.D. (1978). The gate control theory of pain mechanisms – a re-examination and a re-statement. *Brain*, **101**, 1-18.

# 2. Balance and tilt

A.P. Moore

**Introduction**

The rebellious sheep in George Orwell's "Animal Farm" were taught to bleat "Two legs bad, four legs good". Their masters, the pigs, used the phrase as propaganda until they realized that standing upright was a key ingredient in Man's success. The final chilling slogan which the sheep chanted was "Four legs good, two legs better" (Orwell, 1972).

Our ability to balance is remarkable: and the sense of balance is one of our most primitive faculties. Any loss of balance is alarming. When severe it is terrifying and disabling. Balance is a complicated feat. Analysis of the fascinating machinery which makes it possible and the ways in which it goes wrong has explained many common symptoms and illusions.

Balance keeps us upright and allows us to move around or cope with movement of our surroundings without injury. The vestibular system also adjusts our eyes so that we can maintain our gaze despite movements of the head, especially during walking. This prevents the illusion that the world is moving rather than us. The system which does all this has been compared to an all-seeing, all-feeling, quick-acting computer trying to balance on a pair of stilts (Wright, 1991).

Balance is a dynamic art which we learn by trial and error in childhood. It can be thought of as a reflex in which the senses tell a central processing unit how the body's posture, orientation and movement and the visual scene are changing with relation to the environment. Motor output from the central unit then acts to maintain balance and the direction of gaze. If we get false information or put it together incorrectly we fall over – a powerful incentive to get it right. Understanding how it is done requires knowledge of the ways we gather and interpret the information and how we integrate it with movement.

## Sensory systems contributing to balance

We can take intelligent conscious decisions on only a limited number of factors at any one moment. In computer terms our sensory systems are "hard-wired" and able to filter and process enormous amounts of information automatically. They code it, concentrating or compressing it before it reaches consciousness. Many of the illusions and symptoms discussed below are part and parcel of this process whose job is to present ready digested or interpreted information about the outside world and on the state of our own bodies. The software controlling all this is impressively flexible, but has to work within the limits imposed by the anatomy and physiology of each system.

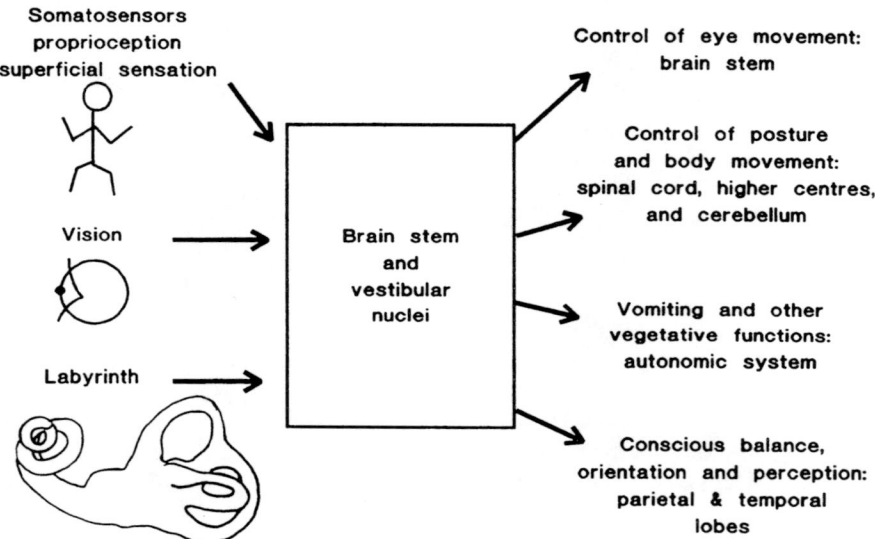

FIG. 1. The vestibular system showing the main senses involved in balance, and central connections.

*Somatosensory system*

Touch and pressure sensors lie in the skin and soft tissues. Joint position sense (proprioception) comes mainly from specialized cells called muscle spindles embedded in the muscles stretched across the joint. They measure the length, force and rate of contraction of the muscle. The brain interprets the information in terms of the joint's position and movement and thus knows where parts of the body are relative to each other.

*Vision*

The eyes tell us about the movement and orientation of the environment. Many visual clues help orientation. Floors and the horizon are horizontal, walls are vertical, shadows are usually cast downward. We learn to judge the direction and orientation of external objects relative to each other and to ourselves. Sometimes vision provides the only reliable cues, such as when divers in poor visibility rely on the fact that bubbles ascend.

## Labyrinthine or vestibular function
Is probably the most important of the senses for balance and tells the brain about linear and angular acceleration (change in velocity or in rate of rotation) of the head in any direction. Gravity is a special form of linear acceleration which applies even when the head is stationary, and the brain detects any deviation from the upright position as tilt.

*The central processor, vertigo and the mismatch concept* (Fig. 2 (Brandt, (1990a)), and see also Fig. 16)

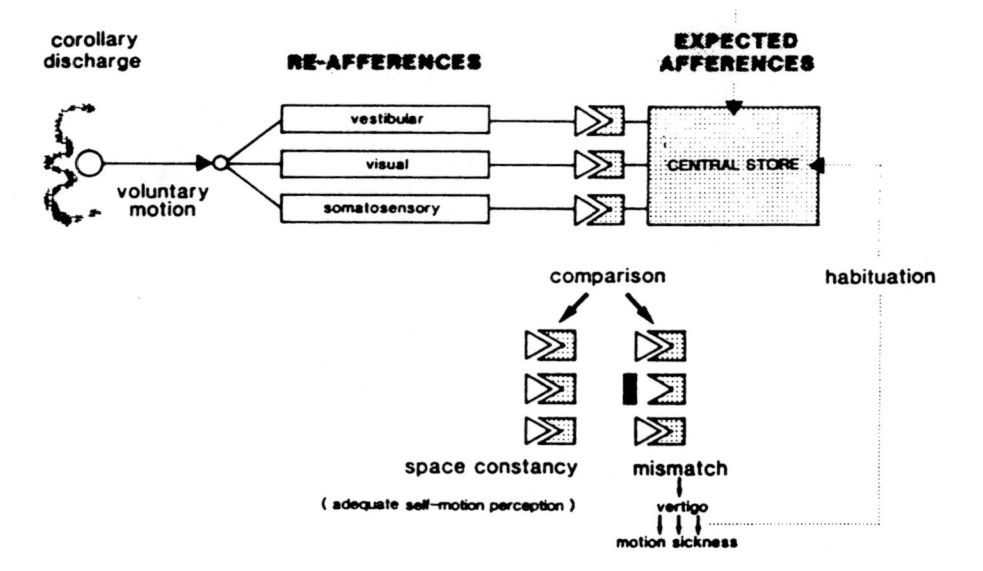

FIG. 2. The central processor and the concept of matching. When the brain commands an active movement it keeps a record, or corollary discharge. The brain uses this together with its own experience to predict the sensations which the movement should evoke, the expected afferences (shown as shaded). When the movement has occurred the sensations it actually evokes, or re-afferent sensations, are compared with the stored expected afferences. If they match then the movement has been performed according to plan, with no unexpected external interference, and the brain perceives the body's movement correctly. If they fail to match there may be a feeling of disorientation, vertigo and eventually motion sickness.

The various senses produce incoming (or afferent) signals which converge on a central processor in the brain. The brain has no problem when they all match, but when they disagree it has to choose between them.

A further refinement applies during active movement. The central processor contains a store of accumulated experience. It knows what sensations should accompany any movement or lack of movement. The brain records the efference copy or corollary discharge, of any motor commands and anticipates which sensations should occur as the movement is performed. The actual sensations experienced (re-afference) are compared with the expected pattern. Normally all these signals match and there is "space constancy" and adequate perception of self-motion. Passive movements are detected because the afferent sensations have no matching efference copy.

Sometimes the sensory signals do not match, such as when reading in a car. The car's motion is detected by the vestibular and somatosensory systems but vision is concentrated on the apparently stationary book. Persistent mismatch produces vertigo and motion sickness.

Vertigo is an unpleasant distortion of apparent gravity or an erroneous feeling of movement of oneself or one's surroundings. It occurs much more readily when there is a *mismatch* of sensory information than when any one of the senses is simply missing. Repeated stimulation eventually causes the system to adapt by rearranging the pattern of information stored in the central processor, a process called habituation.

### Where is the central processor?

The short answer is that no-one knows. It may not be in one place at all, and perhaps there are many centres in the brain and spinal cord able to compare efference copy with sensory signals. These may lie in multiple levels called hierarchies. Higher tiers of control undertake more general, conscious and voluntary decisions, and direct the activity of lower tiers. Lower tiers process more specific details. Each level receives information about evolving motor commands, the state of other levels, and ascending sensory signals.

### Why is matching important?

The strength of the simple principle of matching and progressively modifying motor and sensory signals is its great flexibility. The emphasis given to each level could be modified, or levels by-passed by motor commands. Tiers which are unreliable may be detected and corrected or ignored. However, if errors are not detected they may result in faulty movement or perception (Moore, 1987).

Learning is achieved by trial and error, with refinement of crude and often purely reflex movements and automatic perceptions in infancy. New skills and adaptation are honed by constant checking and modification of the activity of different tiers, with most reliance in each situation being placed on the most effective tiers – "practice makes perfect".

## The vestibular system

This consists of the labyrinth in the inner ear which detects and measures acceleration of the head, and nuclei (collections of neurones) in the brain stem which integrate this information with visual and somatosensory signals.

### Evolution and development of the labyrinths

Primitive static gravity detectors called statocysts developed more than 600 million years ago. A statolith, like a small stone, lay in a fluid filled cavity. Changes in body position altered the position of the stone and this was detected by special sensory cells lining the cavity. This principle is preserved in man's labyrinthine system.

### Structure and function (Fig. 3) (Wright, 1988)

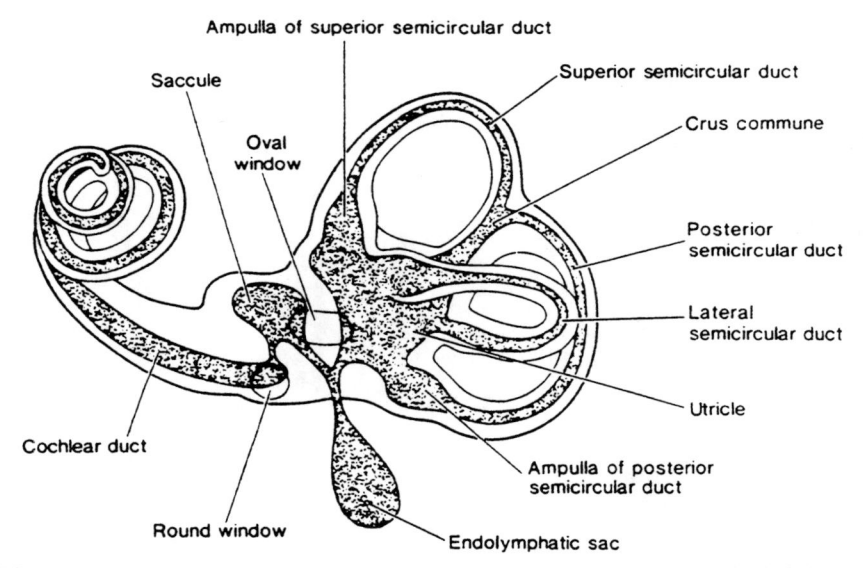

FIG. 3. Anatomy of labyrinth. The membranous labyrinth is shown by the stippled areas.

The vestibular sensory organs are enclosed in the tortuous and aptly named labyrinths. The two labyrinths are bony tunnels set in the petrous temporal bone on each side of the head. Each labyrinth consists of three chambers, the cochlea, the vestibule, and a posterior chamber in which there are openings for the three semicircular canals. The bony labyrinth is filled with fluid, perilymph, which resembles cerebrospinal fluid, the fluid which bathes the brain. Within this is suspended the delicate membranous labyrinth which contains the sensory structures of the vestibular system and the cochlea. The membranous labyrinth resembles a balloon inside the bony labyrinth, and is filled with a different, high potassium/low sodium fluid called endolymph. The two fluids do not normally mix.

The spiral shaped cochlea lies in front and deals with hearing. Behind it and adjacent to the middle ear is a small oval chamber called the vestibule (or entrance

– because it is the route taken by sound vibrations passing into the inner ear). The vestibule contains the membranous saccule and utricle, with connections to the cochlea and the posterior labyrinth, and the endolymphatic sac which is responsible for reabsorption of the fluids from the inner ear to prevent high pressures building up.

Behind the vestibule the labyrinth consists of three semicircular canals set roughly at right angles to each other, the superior, posterior and lateral (or horizontal) canals. These open into the utricle, and at one end of each canal is a dilatation called the ampulla.

The ampullae house the cristae, saddle-shaped protrusions which detect angular acceleration. The utricle and the saccule each contain a small flat patch of cells (about 1mm$^2$) called a macula or otolith organ. The maculae in the utricle and the saccule are set at right angles to each other and detect linear acceleration, especially gravity.

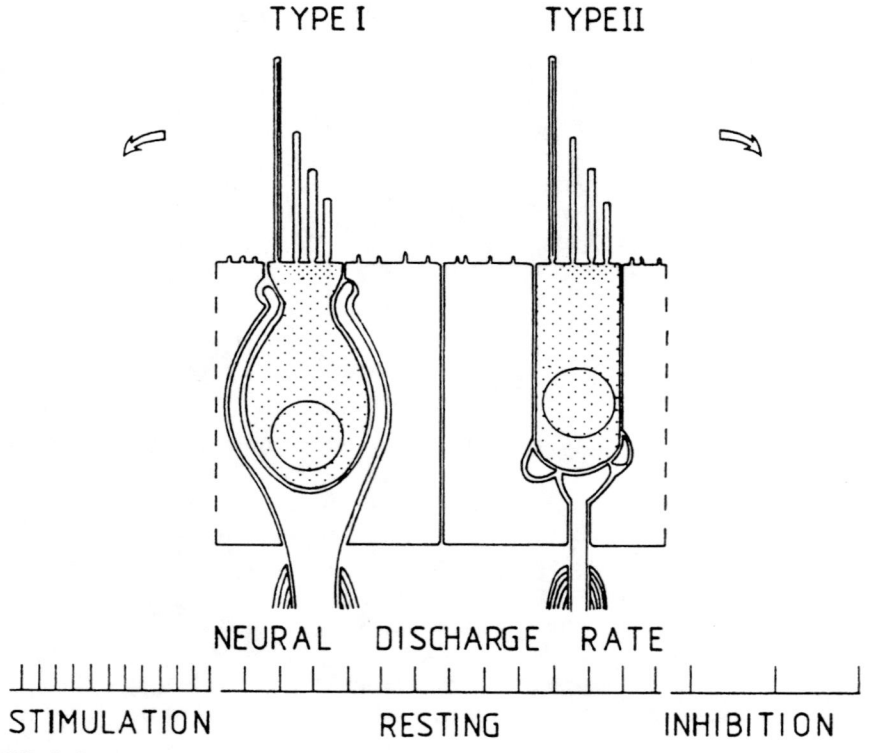

FIG. 4. Structure and function of labyrinth sensory cells. At the bottom is a representation of the firing pattern of a single nerve fibre. When the ciliary bundle is bent towards the kinocilium the nerve is stimulated and firing rate increases. As it is bent the other way the reverse occurs.

The cristae and the maculae are both collections of sensory cells and their nerves in a supporting membrane (Fig. 4). Two kinds of hair like structures (cilia) protrude in a cluster from the cell bodies. There is a single long kinocilium which can bend throughout its length, and there are multiple shorter and stiffer stereocilia which pivot about their base of insertion into the sensory cell. At rest the cell fires electrical impulses at a steady rate. When the bundle of cilia is deflected towards the kinocilium the rate of firing increases and when it is deflected away from the kinocilium the rate of firing falls. The cell can therefore detect both the movement and the direction or polarity of the movement. The sensory cells are organized in strict patterns in the cristae and the maculae, with their polarity dictated by the orientation of the kinocilia.

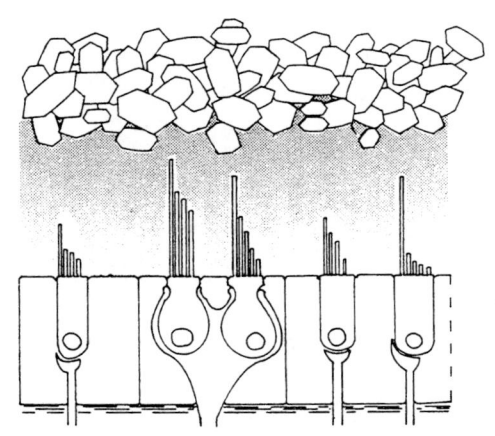

FIG. 5. Structure of macula or otolith organ. The cilia are embedded in a gelatinous membrane which also contains the otoconia on and in its upper surface.

In the utricle and saccule the maculae are arranged with the ciliary bundles projecting into a loose gelatinous substance called the otoconial membrane (Fig. 5). Embedded in the upper layer of this and on its surface are barrel-shaped crystals of calcium carbonate called otoconia, which appear suspended between the gelatinous surface and endolymph. When the head is at rest the otoconia weigh downwards and distort the cilia to enable the cells to detect gravity.

The sensory cells of the maculae move with the head, but during linear acceleration the otoconia lag behind and distort the otoconial membrane, causing the sensory cells to signal the acceleration. At a steady speed the elastic recoil of the membrane returns it and the sensory signal to their resting states. When the head and the sensory cells slow down again the otoconia continue to move through their own momentum, and distort the membrane in the opposite direction. The cells are oriented so that they signal acceleration in a variety of directions including forward and backward, side to side and up and down.

The way in which the sensory cells are activated is different in the cristae of the semicircular canals. Each saddle shaped crista protrudes into the ampulla at the end of its canal and supports rows of uniformly oriented sensory cells. These are lined up so that they are sensitive to movement of fluid through the canal. The semicircular canals and the cristae rotate together with the head. As rotation speeds up (angular acceleration) the endolymph lags behind and flows within the canal. The fluid bends the clusters of cilia and alters the firing rates of the sensory cells. When the head is rotating at a constant velocity the passage of endolymph over the crista slows and stops. When the head slows down again the momentum of the endolymph causes reverse flow and signals the deceleration.

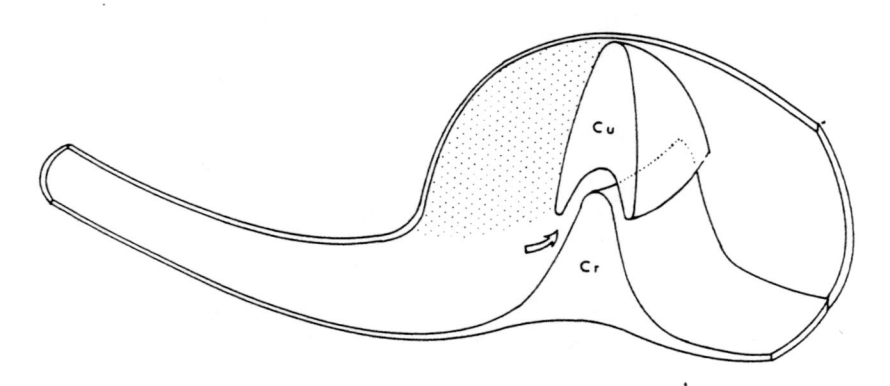

FIG. 6. The cupula (or cupola): the two theories. (a) The ampulla of the semicircular canal is seen split along its length with the crista (Cr) running along across the width of the canal. The gelatinous cupula (Cu) sits astride the crista and directs the flow of endolymph across the surface of the crista. (b) The hair cells and cilia of the sensory cells on the crista are embedded in the cupula, which acts as a "sail" catching and amplifying the effect of the flow of endolymph. The top of the sail may be free to flap about.

## Central connections

Nerve fibres from the cristae and the maculae come together with auditory fibres from the cochlea to form the eighth cranial nerve, and pass to the vestibular nuclei in the brainstem. The cells of the vestibular nuclei link the labyrinthine signals with signals from vision and proprioception and connect with five main systems.

   1   *Eye movement control centres* in the brainstem, which move the eyes to compensate for head movements – the *vestibulo-ocular reflex* or VOR. The VOR

holds the direction of gaze constant during head movements by moving the eyes in the opposite direction to the head at just the right velocity and amplitude. If it fails the retinal image slips and this is perceived as apparent motion of the visual scene.

The overall effect of the VOR can be easily observed by looking at one's own eyes in a mirror. If the gaze is fixed on one eye in the mirror while turning the head to the left the eye is seen to swivel to the right to maintain fixation. Similarly if the head is tilted to the left (anticlockwise in the mirror image) the eye rotates clockwise to minimize slippage of the visual vertical. This is called the ocular tilt reaction. The effect is most easily seen by watching the small blood vessels on the white of the eye which show up the rotation.

If the head turns a long way the eyes cannot move far enough to compensate. The slow vestibular-induced eye deviation is then interrupted by a fast movement in the opposite direction. This combination of movements in opposite directions is called nystagmus. Because nystagmus is almost always involuntary and is very difficult to fake, it is powerful evidence that real or illusory movement has been detected.

Overstimulating the semicircular canals by spinning round and round readily generates nystagmus. On stopping it is replaced by a sensation of vertigo (producing an aftersensation of vertigo when the spinning ceases).

Vision too can provoke nystagmus on its own. So called optokinetic nystagmus is generated when looking sideways out of a moving car. Vision is sharpest when the image is held stationary on the fovea, the most sensitive part of the retina. The brain detects any image slip and causes the eye to lock on to an object and track it across the field of view. This allows time to register detail before the eye can move no further, and it flicks back to choose another target. The system improves visual acuity because images that are moving over the retina are seen far less clearly.

2  *Body movement control* systems in the spinal cord and higher centres. Just as the vestibular system can directly drive eye movements, it has close and fast acting links with trunk and limb muscles, the vestibulo-spinal reflexes. These maintain posture through antigravity muscles, and compensate automatically for the destabilizing effects of movement. The pattern of response is more variable and less predictable than eye movement control.

3  *The cerebellum* which acts to smooth and coordinate movements.

4  *The autonomic nervous system* controls blood pressure, pulse, and other "vegetative" functions. When signals to the vestibular system are unexpected or do not match it is the connections with the autonomic nervous system that are responsible for the unpleasant effects of nausea, vomiting, pallor and sweating. They also contribute to fear and apprehension which may already be aroused by conscious appreciation of the mismatch. Sometimes people feel unwell even before they are aware of the cause.

5  *The parietal and temporal lobes of the cerebral cortex* which are responsible for conscious appreciation of balance, orientation and spatial perception.

## Physiological disturbances of balance

This section deals with situations which can cause normal people, with no disease, to feel off balance or become disoriented.

Our senses are designed to detect change. They are much less effective at monitoring the status quo. We have seen that the vestibular system responds to acceleration but not to constant velocity, or no movement at all. Analogous constraints apply to other sensory systems including vision.

Anaesthetists experimenting with paralyzing drugs found that if a person was completely paralyzed, the head stationary and the eyes unable to move, he/she gradually went blind. As soon as even fractional movement occurred vision returned. Individual photoreceptors in the retina may become "exhausted" if presented with an unvarying stimulus, and stop responding. Staring fixedly at objects does not normally cause them to disappear because undetected micro-movements of the eyes make the image move about slightly on the retina and avoid photoreceptor "fatigue".

The loss of one source of information, e.g. vision is not usually enough to cause loss of balance. People may feel unsteady if two sources are lost or the information becomes less reliable, such as when standing on one foot (i.e. less proprioception) with eyes closed. Single clues of sufficient quality can suffice, especially when there is no conflicting signal from another source. Equally, unusual or distorted signals from a single source can be enough to cause imbalance or vertigo.

*Proprioception*

The brain "knows" the position of limbs and trunk, and this knowledge contributes to the perception of balance and self-motion. Movement of the limbs can by itself provoke a compelling illusion of self-motion (this type of illusion is called vection), and induce nystagmus even without labyrinthine or optokinetic stimuli.

One form of this, arthrokinetic nystagmus, is illustrated in Fig. 7. Subjects sit in darkness on a rotating chair inside a cylinder. They place one hand against the inner wall of the cylinder and when the cylinder rotates the hand moves with the wall and turns the whole body and the chair. If the chair is then surreptitiously locked and prevented from rotating the brain may interpret the movement of the arm as rotation of the trunk and head in the opposite direction. The VOR generates nystagmus as if the eyes were tracking the cylinder (Brandt et al., 1977).

Similar nystagmus and illusions of self-motion can be generated by a moving sound source (Dodge, 1923), by imagining a moving visual image (Zikmund, 1966), or even by hypnotic suggestion of moving images (Brady and Levitt, 1964).

A completely different kind of illusion of self motion can be provoked by setting up false proprioceptive signals. Vibration of the tendon of a muscle such as the biceps muscle stimulates the muscle's spindle cells (powerful proprioceptors) and causes a reflex contraction of the muscle which flexes the elbow. The movement is purely a reflex set up in the spinal cord and has no associated corollary discharge

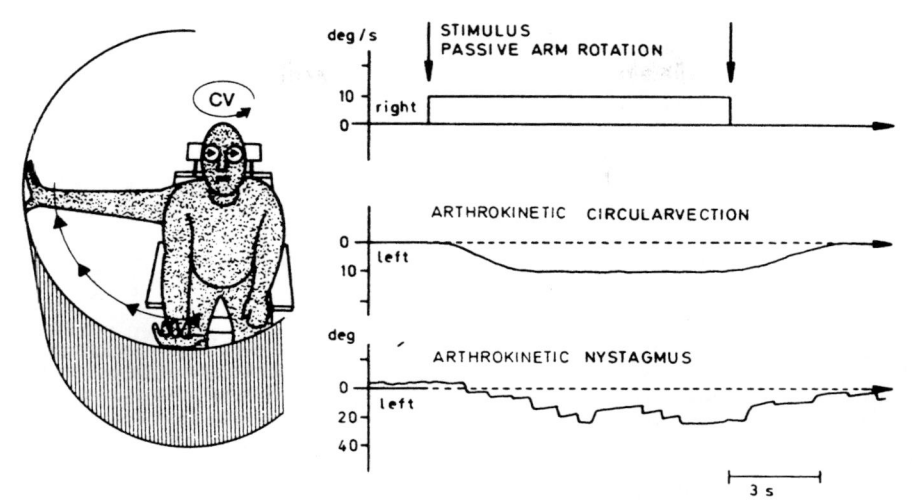

FIG. 7. Arthrokinetic circularvection and nystagmus (see also under *Moving or vection illusions*). The stationary subject sits with eyes closed inside the rotating drum. His hand is touching the wall of the rotating drum. Passive rotation of the arm to the right by the rotating drum induces nystagmus and a sensation of self motion to the right.

or efference copy within the brain, so the brain is unaware that the elbow is bending.

If the forearm is physically restrained the brain falsely senses that the muscle is being passively stretched and interprets this stretch as being due to passive extension of the elbow. The increased muscle spindle activity the brain is receiving represents re-afferent signals without a corollary discharge (see Fig. 2), and normally this happens only during a passive movement. By vibrating the appropriate muscles it is possible to provoke illusory movement of the body into almost any desired position or cause subjects to feel that joints are assuming anatomically impossible positions.

The illusions can be strong enough to overwhelm labyrinthine position sense and cause a fall. Thus, if a person standing with eyes closed has vibration applied to his achilles tendon he will sense that his calf muscle is lengthening, which should occur only if his toes and foot are lifting upwards. This would normally indicate he is about to fall forwards, and attempting to compensate for the illusion may make him fall over backwards — so care must be taken to prevent injury in this experiment.

If vibration is applied to the triceps muscle there is a strong illusion that the elbow is flexing. More curiously, if the subject sits holding his nose, the illusion is transmitted to the nose and the subject may feel that the head is tipping backwards (or sometimes that the nose is being pushed into the head) (Lackner, 1988).

These illusions carry a more general message: the brain uses all of the information supplied and decides on the "best" solution when it receives conflicting signals. Even its image of the length of a limb or part of the trunk is not fixed and may be instantly modified if that is the "best" solution. Correct information may be ignored if erroneous signals are powerful enough, and posture and balance may be impaired. Fortunately in everyday life vibration is rarely so selectively applied, and vibration of a joint stimulates muscles pulling both ways and does not move the joint or cause any illusions.

*Vision*

*Static illusions and tilt* The human eye is remarkably good at telling whether lines in a scene or a picture are "vertical" or "horizontal" relative to the scene, though it is much less efficient at judging other angles. Vertical or horizontal lines are also more easily seen than other orientations (Davidoff, 1974) and it has even been shown that infants as young as six weeks of age prefer to look at horizontal or vertical gratings than at tilted ones (Leehey *et al.*, 1975).

If there are no obvious cues such as the vertical side of a building or a horizontal water level, lines close to vertical may appear to be more vertical than they really are. This is called tilt normalization. Whole scenes tilted by as much as 4° from vertical may sometimes be perceived as vertical (Howard, 1982).

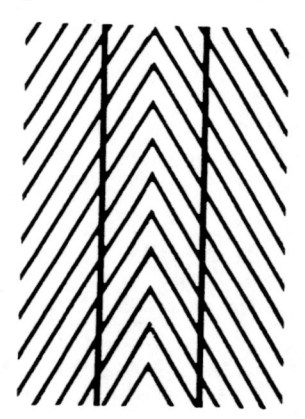

FIG. 8. Zöllner illusion.

*Tilt contrast* is another curious phenomenon well illustrated by the Zöllner illusion (Fig. 8). The two vertical lines are apparently splayed outward at the top because of the contrasting tilt of the superimposed background lines. In the tilt after-effect prolonged observation of tilted lines as in Fig. 9 can result in a brief shift of apparent vertical even in different directions at the same time in different parts of the scene (Howard, 1982).

These illusions result in simple misjudgement of orientation. Other well known but more complex visual illusions include apparently tilted rooms, tricks of perspective, distorting mirrors and ambiguous objects.

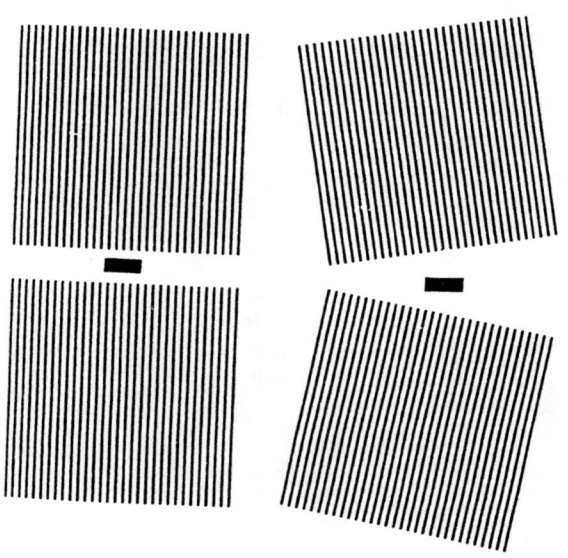

FIG. 9. Tilt after-effect. Look at the small black rectangle on the right for about half a minute and then look at the one on the left. Each of the vertical test gratings on the left should appear to tilt in the opposite direction to its corresponding inspection grating on the right.

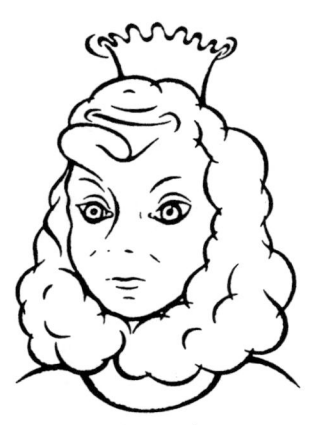

FIG. 10. Ambiguous image which changes its appearance when viewed upside down.

*Vision and gravity* These purely visual illusions can influence the body's static posture and balance in themselves, but more powerful effects are seen in visual-vestibular interactions in which visual vertical is judged against gravity. With the head held straight there is normally no conflict between visual, somatosensory and vestibular signals. When there is no visual frame of reference, such as in a dark room, normal people can set an illuminated line to vertical to within 0.5° (Howard,

1982). They detect vertical by using otolith and somatosensory clues. If the head or the whole body is tilted slightly to one side, the previously vertical line appears to tilt in the same direction. This has been called the *E-effect* (Müller, 1916). If the head is tilted beyond about 70° this illusion may reverse and the line appears tilted in the other direction, the *A-effect* (Aubert, 1861). These illusions have not been fully explained. They may be caused by countertorsion of the eyes, by changes in otolith or proprioceptive signals, or a combination of all three.

Experiments in which these various signals are excluded have shown that we use different combinations of senses according to the situation – skin pressure cannot signal up or down when the body is immersed in water, and if visual clues such as air bubbles are eliminated we rely on otolith signals to orient ourselves. These work well up to 90° of head tilt but beyond 90° they are much less accurate, and divers who are upside down may even feel their bodies are erect and swim the wrong way. Other experiments confirm that when we are only tilted a little we can use otolith signals on their own to judge gravitational vertical. As we tilt further we begin to need more and more help from somatosensory signals such as pressure on the skin.

If both labyrinths are destroyed by disease, patients can still balance and judge vertical when they can see about them. Even in darkness such patients can stand erect, balancing by detecting proprioceptive signals and the differential pressure of the ground on their feet. However, they are much less stable and more easily disoriented.

*Detection of movement and maintenance of balance*   There are several ways in which vision can detect movement. Firstly, there is the movement of the whole visual scene across the retina of one or both eyes, or the movement of the eyes needed to track the scene. Secondly there is changing perspective, movement of some objects in the scene relative to others, or change in the apparent size, shape or orientation of objects. Thirdly the focussing system of the eye can measure the distance to objects, especially if they are within grasping range. This works mainly by gauging the convergence of the eyes, the degree to which they aim inwards to enable both eyes to see close objects. Balance mechanisms use vision in several different ways. Most of this section describes systems which effectively give a continuous "servo-loop" measurement of head and eye position relative to the surroundings, producing reflex movements of the body to compensate. Vision can be used for *intermittent* adjustment or correction of errors which have crept in through other systems, and it can also act as a trigger for actions in *anticipation* of movements to come.

Anticipation becomes increasingly important when situations are familiar. Well-trained pilots know much better than trainees what vestibular, somatosensory and visual changes to expect during manoeuvres in real flight. Surprisingly, trained pilots develop motion-sickness in flight simulators more often than do learners – but perhaps this is not really surprising because flight simulators cannot provide all the real sensations of flight. Seasoned pilots are more likely to detect a mismatch of expected and actual experience, and it is the mismatch which provokes the motion sickness.

*Height vertigo* Many people suffer from fear of falling when exposed on high buildings or cliffs. It ranges from vague unease to pure panic, and is commonly held to be psychological – as indeed it can be. However, there is a simple physiological reason why normal people feel (and are) more unsteady. When standing erect we all sway slightly, and vision helps to maintain balance by monitoring the relative movement of our surroundings. If there are objects nearby we may detect that they appear larger and then smaller as we sway, or that they move relative to our eyes or to distant objects. This information matches and reinforces somatosensory and vestibular signals. Vision can reduce body sway by about 50% (Travis, 1945).

If only distant objects are visible, we effectively lose visual stabilization of posture. We would have to sway much more before vision could detect a change in either the size or relative positions of distant objects. The extra sway is dangerous, and the mismatch of reduced visual with normal vestibular and somatosensory sensitivity to sway produces vertigo and fear. This is a sensible and useful warning system which is clearly of high biological value.

Perhaps because it is a response to sway, height vertigo takes a few moments to build up and is most likely to happen when standing erect. It is often abolished by lying down as this prevents sway. Vertigo may occur as little as 3m above ground and is already maximal at 20m. It can be provoked by either downward or upward gaze because it is the distance which is critical, not the direction.

People can be trained to minimize the psychological response to height vertigo, and to avoid aggravating the physical factors. Holding on to something is an obvious and effective way to minimize sway and block vertigo. Arranging to have something nearby in line of sight is helpful, and this is most easily done by standing back a little or looking through a screen or slightly dirty window. Conversely, looking out through binoculars is very dangerous because they change vision in a novel way. They alter the magnification and exclude nearby visual clues to sway. It is also dangerous to stand watching a moving object such as an aeroplane because it does not provide a fixed visual reference point. Peripheral vision may still be able to monitor a fixed object, but it is less effective at detecting sway.

*Moving or vection illusions* A compelling illusion of self-motion called vection is commonly felt when gazing at moving clouds or when the train at the next platform moves off from the station. These two are examples of *linear vection*, with the illusory movement being in a straight line. We can normally see both active and passive movement. To the eye, however, the appearance of a moving visual scene is just the same whether it is the scene itself that is moving or the eye moving past it. The brain uses the vestibular system to decide between the two possibilities.

Unfortunately the vestibular system is not very good at distinguishing between rest and movement at a constant velocity, as shown by the common experience of passengers riding in a car with their eyes shut. They rely largely on vestibular information to judge speed, but the labyrinth can tell us only about acceleration and deceleration. Once the car reaches a constant speed the otoliths settle back to their resting position so the passengers do not know whether they are moving slowly, quickly, or sometimes whether they are moving at all. Skiers in mist or "white-out" conditions often experience the frightening realization that they cannot tell how fast they are moving, or even whether they are going uphill or downhill. The inability of the vestibular system to signal the velocity at a constant speed means that the two interpretations of a moving visual scene – self motion or movement of the surroundings – appear equally valid.

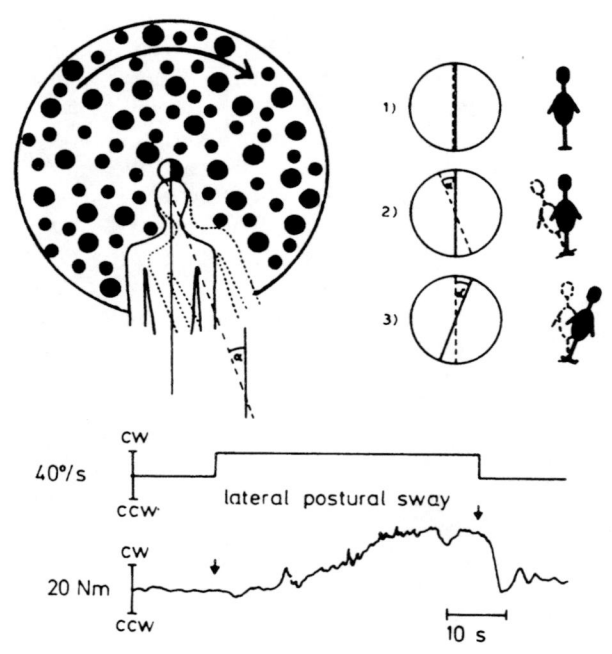

FIG. 11. Roll vection. Clockwise rotation of the patterned disc causes an anticlockwise displacement of perceived visual and body vertical (2). Visuospinal compensation for this causes body tilt in the direction of pattern motion (3). The bottom recording shows that after a few seconds delay the body tilt builds up slowly to a maximum, and returns to normal when the disc rotation stops. CW – clockwise rotation, CCW – counterclockwise rotation.

Thus if the whole visual scene moves there is an illusion of self motion just as in a real body movement. It begins after a few seconds and gradually speeds up to a maximum. It often continues for a while as an after-effect when the visual scene slows down. Movement in the peripheral visual field (corner of the eye) is more likely to produce a powerful vection illusion. Movement in the central field of view is more often interpreted correctly as object rather than self motion.

Vection illusions can profoundly affect balance because apparent self-motion in one direction evokes a reflex action to counterbalance the movement. This reflex can be strong enough to cause a change of posture or even a fall. Just as linear vection occurs with movement of the visual scene in a straight line, *circular vection* can occur if the visual surround is moving horizontally around us on a vertical axis as in a revolving restaurant, and *roll vection* with rotation around a horizontal axis, like the hands of a clock.

Roll vection can affect judgement of gravity. If a person stands watching a large visual scene rotating clockwise such as the disc in Fig. 11 he experiences a continuous sensation of self-motion, of roll in the opposite direction, and a feeling that he is tilting that way. Automatic attempts to compensate for the illusory tilt cause a real clockwise tilt.

The continuous visual vection illusion is countered by otolith and somatosensory signals that there is no real change of gravity, so despite the feeling of continuing movement the degree of apparent tilt is limited (Dichgans *et al.*, 1972), although it can still be strong enough to cause a fall. Stronger illusions of tilt occur in people who have lost labyrinthine function, or in astronauts in space where there is no gravity signal from the labyrinths.

*Vestibular*

***Static illusions*** Gravity is a special form of linear acceleration which is always acting on earth-bound mortals. We detect it and thus orient ourselves using the maculae, the otolith organs of the saccule and utricle. These sensors are at their most sensitive and efficient with the head upright, but are prone to allow a variety of illusions.

An aircraft pilot in level flight feels gravity as a purely downward force, and experiences his aircraft and himself as being level. If he accelerates he generates an apparent backward force into his seat (the "kick in the pants"). The force also acts on the otoliths and distorts the otoconial membrane. The apparent direction of gravity changes so the pilot feels he and his aircraft are pointing upwards (Fig. 12). The reverse occurs when he decelerates, and is very dangerous as this often happens when the air brakes are applied on approach to landing. The pilot senses that the aircraft is pitching down and may attempt to over-correct at a critical moment (Benson, 1988).

Signals from the "static" macular receptors interact with those from the "dynamic" receptors of the semicircular canals. The canals measure angular acceleration, or a change in speed of rotation of the head. Normally, angular acceleration of the head is registered by the cristae of the semicircular canals at the same time as the otoconia detect a change in the apparent direction of gravity. Sometimes, however, angular acceleration is so slow that the stimulus is below the threshold required to activate the semicircular canals.

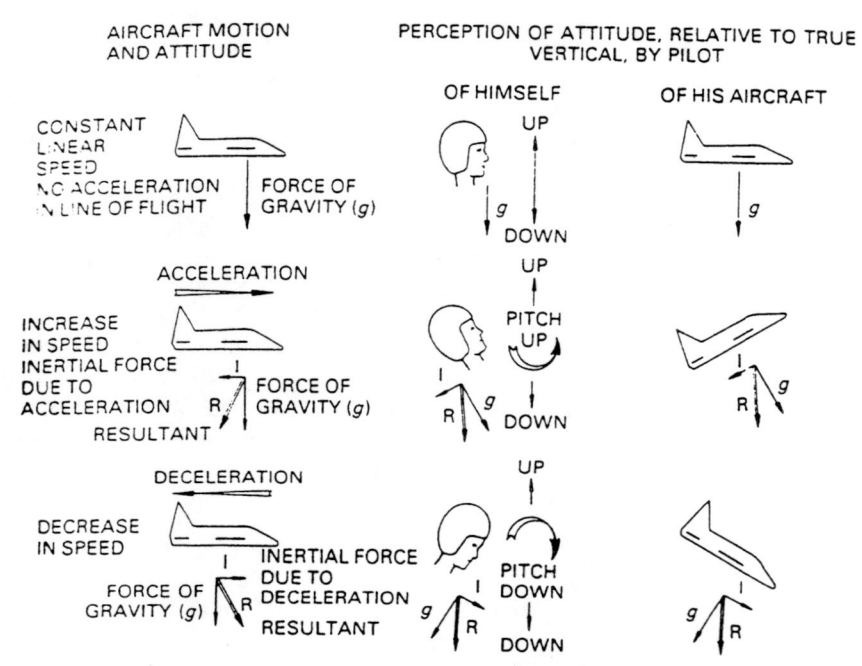

FIG. 12. Illusions of gravity and pitch during acceleration and deceleration whilst remaining in level flight.

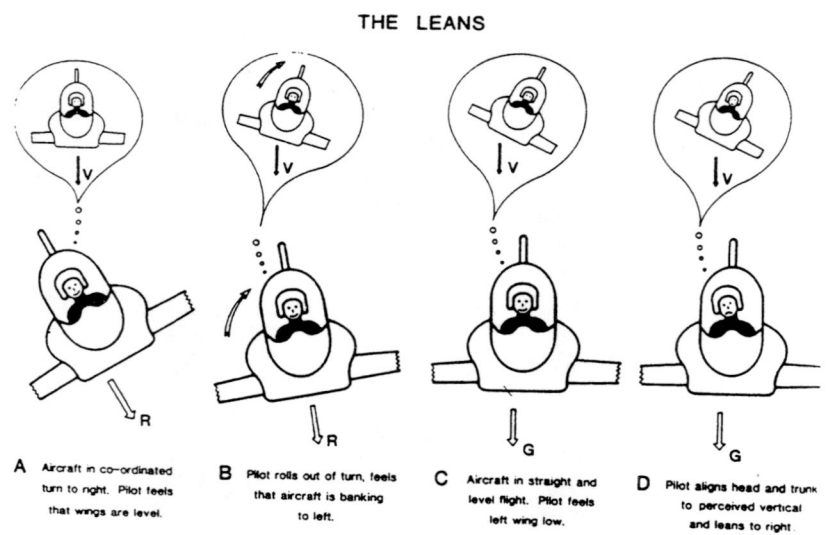

FIG. 13. Diagram showing one cause of " The Leans".

This can occur in pilots flying in cloud or at night and is illustrated in Fig. 13 as one cause of the "leans" (Benson, 1988). If the pilot cannot see the horizon considerable changes in attitude can occur without him being aware of them. A pilot flying level may gradually roll to the left, so slowly that his semicircular canals fail to register the change. Instruments tell the pilot that he is tilted and he corrects rapidly to level flight as shown by his instruments. The semicircular canals detect this more rapid change but the brain interprets it as a roll to the right from apparently level flight.

### Dynamic illusions

Everyone has experienced the brief illusion of rotation provoked by a sudden stop after spinning round a few times. As spin builds up fluid in the semicircular canals lags and stimulates the sensory cells in the cristae to signal angular acceleration. Once spinning at a constant velocity the fluid catches up and is moving at the same velocity as the head. If the spin suddenly stops the fluid's momentum causes it to flow the other way past the cristae and provokes the sensation of spinning. The perceived rotation is opposite to the recent real spin. The vestibulo-optic reflex stimulates a post-rotational nystagmus which reinforces the illusion. This parallel impairment of visual and labyrinthine stimuli is called the oculogyral illusion. Fortunately it usually resolves itself quickly.

### Coriolis effect

The semicircular canals can produce false sensations of movement when head movements are made in a car or aircraft which is turning. If the head is level the vehicle's turn causes flow of fluid mainly in the horizontal semicircular canal. If the head is tipped forward, perhaps to look at instruments or read a book, the vertical canals are brought into the plane of movement instead. Fluid moves in the vertical canal and slows in the horizontal canal. If there is no view of the outside world this complex cross-coupling can create a bizarre illusion that the head and thus the car or aircraft is pitching forwards and down. There is a direct and unresolvable mismatch of labyrinthine and somatosensory signals which is a potent cause of travel sickness, especially in passengers who are less likely to be watching the road and do not have visual signals to expose the real situation.

### Tullio phenomenon (sound induced vertigo)

Tullio originally showed that noise can induce nystagmus(1929), unsteadiness and vertigo by transmission of sound energy in the inner ear fluids. Sound waves travel from perilymph (bathing the oval window) to endolymph and stimulate the otoliths or cristae. Loud, low frequency or sudden or rapidly changing noise such as blowing the nose can cause symptoms. The Tullio phenomenon arises most often in diseases causing a hole (fistula) opening into the labyrinth, or if the chain of auditory ossicles is too rigid and transmits excessive force. It has however been reported in normal people (Ehrlich and Lawson, 1980).

## Vertigo due to pressure and temperature changes

Fliers and divers are subject to marked changes of air or water pressure which are transmitted throughout the body. The middle ear is an air filled chamber normally ventilated by the Eustachian tube passing to the back of the throat. If the tube is blocked, the air pressure in the middle ear may not equilibrate and this can cause a shift of the round and oval windows. The distortion produces painful fullness of the ear and may be transmitted to the vestibular sensory cells and provoke vertigo and nystagmus.

Swimmers who have one ear blocked by wax or have a perforated eardrum may develop vertigo. Water cools one ear and its set of semicircular canals. The cold fluid sinks and sets up a flow within the canal. The brain registers this as rotation, provoking nystagmus and often severe disorientation and vertigo. Oddly, if both ears are affected the abnormal stimuli from the two sides act in opposite directions and may cancel each other out.

## Motion sickness

Many species including man are liable to motion sickness (Money, 1970). Vertigo may occur whenever spatial orientation and perception of movement are disturbed. In boats, aircraft, cars and space vehicles there may be a conflict between senses which do not match the expected pattern. Unpleasant illusions of movement provoke a gradual build up of unease, tiredness, pallor, then nausea and vomiting. Motion sickness is a warning signal to withdraw from the provocative situation with which the body is unable to deal properly.

For motion sickness to develop the labyrinths must be functioning. If both labyrinths are destroyed or inactivated, men and animals become immune to motion sickness, and it is probably the semicircular canal function which is critical. Motion sickness may be caused by mismatched or confusing signals from the canals alone, as in the Coriolis effect (see above). In space sickness the important sensory mismatch may be between the semicircular canals (signalling angular acceleration) and the otolith gravity detectors.

Blind people can still develop motion sickness, so vision is clearly not a prerequisite (Desnoes, 1926). However, mismatch arising from visual stimuli alone can be enough to provoke motion sickness, as in vection illusions. Equally, providing a stable and reliable visual horizon can ease motion sickness. At sea, motion sickness may be reduced by standing on deck watching the horizon, in cars a front seat car passenger able to watch the road is less liable to sickness. Drivers almost never feel sick as they not only have a stable visual horizon, but they also control and can anticipate movement of the car.

Seasickness or space sickness usually subsides over a few days' voyage because the stored pattern of expectation is modified. The "land sickness" which may occur after a sea voyage long enough to cause such adaptation may be due to the need to relearn the normal pattern.

If prism spectacles are worn, the whole visual scene is inverted. Normal people quickly develop motion sickness because the visual scene moves the wrong way for their head movements. They adapt over days or weeks by inverting the vestibular-optic reflex (VOR). It is, however, possible to adapt without motion sickness as it has been shown that under stroboscopic light the VOR inversion and adaptation can still take place, but no motion sickness occurs (Melvill Jones and Mandl, 1980).

## Pathological imbalance and vertigo

This section deals briefly with some common illnesses causing unsteadiness and vertigo. There are many others, including disease of the cerebellum, of the peripheral nerves, of the supply of blood, glucose or oxygen to the brain and vestibular system.

### Drugs

Alcohol causes imbalance and vertigo partly by disabling the cerebellum and its coordinating role, partly by affecting the semicircular canals. The cupola attached to the cilia of the hair cells in the cristae normally has the same density as endolymph so it is not affected by gravity. Alcohol is lighter than endolymph, and at blood levels of more than 40mg/100ml (below the British legal limit for driving) it diffuses into the cupola more quickly than into the endolymph. The cupola becomes comparatively lighter and tends to float, bending the sensory cilia and imitating the effect of fluid flowing upwards past the crista. Drinking heavy water (deuterium oxide) has the opposite effect – perhaps we should combine the two!

There are many drugs such as streptomycin which damage the balance (and often hearing) organs, or which sedate or stimulate them. Some cause heart or circulation problems which indirectly affect balance. Others alter the metabolism of the sensory cells or the composition of the labyrinthine fluids.

### Benign paroxysmal positional vertigo (BPPV)

This is the commonest form of vertigo in the elderly. Brief attacks of vertigo and nystagmus are provoked by rapid head movement. It is thought to be caused by cupulolithiasis "stony cupula". Small particles dislodged from otoconia by spontaneous degeneration or head trauma are carried by endolymph until they lodge on the cupola, most importantly in the posterior canal. The cupola becomes heavy and oversensitive to flow of endolymph in the posterior canal when moving the head to look up. The sufferer feels he is tipping backwards and this can be dangerous – for instance, if he happens to be standing on a ladder, BPPV can produce a fall.

### Vestibular Neuronitis

There is abrupt onset of prolonged severe rotational vertigo, nystagmus, imbalance and nausea, but with no alteration of hearing (Brandt, 1990*a*). In most cases it is probably caused by a viral infection. Tests show reduced responsiveness of one horizontal semicircular canal or the vestibular nerve. During health the sensory organs of each canal generate a signal even when at rest. The sensation is of "no movement" when the signals are equal on the two sides. If signals from one side are reduced, the imbalance creates the illusion of rotation and thus vertigo. This can be a disabling and frightening condition. Fortunately it usually recovers, either because the underlying problem clears up or because the brain adapts (central compensation) to the difference in canal signals from the two sides.

## Meniere's disease

This is the fourth commonest cause of vertigo and presents a striking clinical picture. Starting in middle age, attacks occur abruptly, irregularly and unpredictably. Sufferers begin with a feeling of fullness in the ear, followed by tinnitus, deafness, vertigo, nystagmus, nausea and imbalance. Attacks can be disabling but most of the symptoms subside over days or hours. Repeated attacks eventually cause more persistent hearing loss and tinnitus. Meniere's disease is primarily caused by impaired absorption of endolymph by the endolymphatic sac. This can occur for a variety of reasons and leads to fluid overload within the membranous labyrinth (endolymphatic hydrops). The balloon-like labyrinth becomes distorted and stretched and may rupture so that endolymph periodically leaks into the perilymph in the outer labyrinth. The different chemicals in the endolymph contaminate and poison the perilymph throughout the whole labyrinth to provoke disruption of hearing and balance. Once the excess pressure starts to fall healing of the ruptured membrane may occur.

## Psychogenic vertigo: chicken or egg?

Because vertigo is an illusion of movement it is a purely subjective complaint, and may be a sympton of psychiatric illness such as neurosis, anxiety or depression. Unfortunately vertigo due to physical disease can *also* provoke anxiety and panic attacks and may cause depression if it is prolonged. It is often difficult to distinguish any underlying physical abnormality using available tests because they are rather crude, so doctors may struggle to tell whether the physical symptoms or the psychiatric problems came first. To make it even more difficult, drugs such as phenothiazines used to treat psychiatric disease may damage balance mechanisms or alter their function, and vice versa.

*Agoraphobia*, the fear of open spaces, may present as dizziness and imbalance. It is possible that it is triggered by the same mechanism as height vertigo – visual stabilization of sway is more difficult when walls or other visual cues to stability are too far away. Sufferers associate their unsteadiness with the situation and develop a fear of open spaces.

*Claustrophobia* .This is not the whole story, since crowded spaces may produce a similar effect. The constant movement of people may also affect judgement of sway by blocking stationary objects from view, or by provoking frequent but erratic visual vection illusions in the periphery of vision. The sufferer is overwhelmed by conflicting stimuli.

*Phobic postural vertigo (PPV)* is a closely related and very common condition.

It tends to occur in people with obsessive-compulsive or hysterical personalities, but may be triggered by minor physiologically induced vertigo. Attacks of anxiety, usually fleeting unsteadiness or vertigo, and fear of impending death occur often in settings specific to the sufferer. Characteristically sufferers describe their attacks as awful and terrifying, yet may be able to conceal and ignore them and continue everyday activities.

PPV may be caused by transient uncoupling of afference and efference copy (Brandt, 1990*b*) (see Fig. 2). This may occur in healthy people especially when they are exhausted or intoxicated by drugs or drink. The difference between a voluntary head movement and external movements may become blurred. Car drivers sometimes report a dream-like illusion that their car is stationary and the road is moving like a film on screen – perceived self-motion flips over to become apparent movement of the environment, and can as quickly revert back. This is akin to a vection illusion, but any of the physiological illusions decribed above could have an analogous effect. Normal people accept these illusions without worry. Phobics become more consciously aware of them and mentally patrol their state of balance. Adjustments of balance which are normally subconscious may thus be consciously perceived and trigger attacks of anxiety and PPV.

## Motor problems causing imbalance

The somatosensory, visual and vestibular sensory systems may be working perfectly, but, if the brain is unable to work out or signal the proper movements (e.g. after a stroke) or transmit the signal to muscle (perhaps because of spinal cord or peripheral nerve disease), or if the muscles themselves are weak, then appropriate corrective action will not be forthcoming and falls may result.

Sometimes diseases of one or other sensory or motor system cause undue reliance on other systems. For instance, in vestibular and cerebellar disease and in Parkinson's disease, patients may become "hooked" on vision and rely less on vestibular and somatosensory signals. This makes them prone to an excessive response to vection illusions, and causes vection induced unsteadiness and falls (Bronstein, *et al.*, 1990).

### Abnormal efference copy (corollary discharge)
Another intriguing problem arises if the brain fails to record accurate efference copy or corollary discharges (Moore, 1987) (Fig. 14, see also Fig. 2). Re-afferent signals then fail to match the efference copy and the mismatch provokes automatic but inappropriate postural readjustment. This may happen in Parkinson's disease and be partly responsible for the unsteadiness and falls which can occur. In parkinsonism there is no weakness but there is generalized slowing, reduced amplitude and poor coordination of movement. One explanation for this is that the corollary discharge is "reduced" so that when it is combined with re-afferent signals in the central processor the resultant signal suggests that any movement occurring

is more than is required. An automatic "correction" is then made to slow or reduce the amplitude of the movement (Moore, 1987).

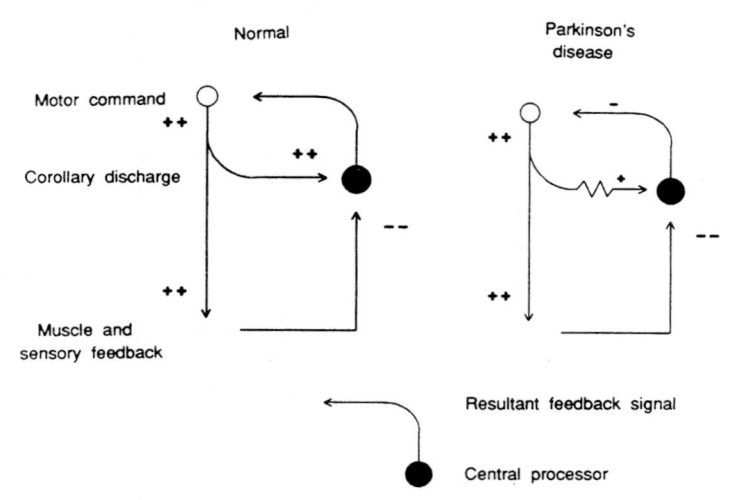

FIG. 14. The principle of corollary discharges in the control of movement. Normally the motor command passes to the muscles, simultaneously giving off a corollary discharge (efference copy) of equivalent strength. This passes to a comparator which correlates it with returning sensory (or afferent) signals, and the resultant, a kind of error signal, passes back to the motor command and is used to adjust the movement. In Parkinson's disease the corollary discharge may be diminished. The comparator perceives more effect than was required and its resultant tends to reduce the motor command (Moore, 1987).

## Conclusion

In this short chapter it is impossible to cover all the ways in which the senses can produce illusions of balance and tilt in normal people or in disease. We can appreciate the delicacy of the balancing act which Orwell's pigs were so keen to emulate whilst understanding the conflicts of sensory input which can arise.

## References

Aubert, H. (1861). Eine scheinbare dedeutende Drehung von Objekten bei Neigung des Kopfes nach rechts oder links. *Virchows Archivs,* **20**, 381-393.
Benson, A.J. (1988). Spatial disorientation – common illusions. *In* "Aviation Medicine". 2nd Edn. Chapter 21. (Eds J. Ernsting and P.F. King), Butterworth, London.
Brady, J.P. and Levitt, E.E. (1964). Nystagmus as a criterion of hypnotically induced visual hallucinations. *Science,* **146**, 85-86.
Brandt, T., Buchele, W. and Arnold, F. (1977). Arthrokinetic nystagmus and ego-motion sensation. *Experimental Brain Research,* **30**, 331-338.
Brandt, T. (1990a). Vertigo – a systematic approach. *In* "Recent Advances in Clinical

Neurology". (Ed. C. Kennard). pp.59-84. Churchill Livingstone, Edinburgh, London.
Brandt, T. (1990*b*). "Vertigo: its Multisensory Syndromes". Springer-Verlag, London.
Bronstein, A.M., Hood, J.D., Gresty, M.A. and Panagi, C. (1990). Visual control of balance in cerebellar and Parkinsonian syndromes. *Brain,* **113**, 767-779.
Davidoff, J.B. (1974). An observation concerning the preferred perception of the visual horizontal and vertical. *Perception,* **3**, 47-48.
Desnoes, P. (1926). Seasickness. *Journal of the American Medical Association,* **86**, 319-324.
Dichgans, J., Held, R., Young, L.R. and Brandt, T. (1972). Moving visual scenes influence the apparent direction of gravity. *Science,* **178**, 1217-1219.
Dodge, R. (1923). Thresholds of rotation. *Journal of Experimental Psychology,* **6**, 107-137.
Ehrlich, M.A. and Lawson, W. (1980). The incidence and significance of Tullio phenomenon in man. *Otolaryngology Head and Neck Surgery,* **88**, 630-635.
Howard, I.P. (1982). "Human Visual Orientation". Wiley, Chichester.
Kelly, J.P. (1991). The sense of balance. *In* "Principles of Neural Science". (Eds E.R. Kandel, J.F. Schwarz and T.M. Jessel). pp. 501-511. Elsevier, London.
Lackner, J.R. (1988). Some proprioceptive influences on the perceptual representation of body shape and orientation. *Brain,* **111**, 281-297.
Leehey, S.C., Moskowitz-Cook, A., Brill, S. and Held, R. (1975). Orientational anisotropy in infant vision. *Science,* **190**, 900-901.
Luxon, L.M. (1984). The anatomy and physiology of the vestibular system. *In* "Vertigo". (Eds M.R. Dix and J.D. Hood). pp. 1-36. Wiley, London.
Melvill Jones, F. and Mandl, G. (1980). "Motion" sickness due to vision reversal: its disappearance in stroboscopic light. *Annals of the New York Academy of Science,* **374**, 303-311.
Money, K.E. (1970). Motion sickness. *Physiology Review,* **50**, 1-39.
Moore, A.P. (1987). Impaired sensorimotor integration in Parkinsonism and dyskinesia: a role for corollary discharges? *Journal of Neurology, Neurosurgery and Psychiatry,* **50**, 544-552.
Müller, G.E. (1916). Uber das Aubertsche Phänomenen. *Zeitschrift für Psychologie, Physiologie und Sinnesorgie,* **49**, 109-246.
Orwell, G. (1972). "Animal Farm". New Windmill Series. Heinemann.
Travis, R.C. (1945). An experimental analysis of dynamic equilibrium. *Journal of Experimental Psychology,* **35**, 216-234.
Tullio. (1929). "Das Ohr und die Entstehung der Sprache und Schrift." Urban und Schwarzenberg, München.
Wright, A. (1988). "Dizziness: a guide to disorders of balance". Croom Helm, London.
Wright, A. (1991). The human vestibular system. *In* "Current Approaches to Vertigo". (Ed. D. Hood). Ch. 1. Henry Ling Ltd, Dorset Press.
Zikmund, V. (1966). Oculomotor activity during visual imagery of a moving stimulus pattern. *Study of Psychology (Prah),* **8**, 254-272.

# 3. Olfaction

C.H. Hawkes

Most animals depend heavily on their sense of smell for their perception of the world about them. Their emotional and behavioural reactions are closely bound to the stimulation of olfaction via the connections of the limbic system within the brain. In this respect, other special senses are more remote. Thus, whilst primates have developed vision almost to the exclusion of the older olfactory brain (rhinencephalon), subtle links remain between olfaction and its effects on emotion and behaviour.

**Anatomy**

The nose, "the Sentinel of the Senses" (Macdonald Critchley, 1986) is an intriguing anatomical structure with a double nerve supply. The trigeminal sensory nerve supplies the inner mucosal lining of the nose with perception of touch, temperature, pain, tickle and itch. The receptor area of the olfactory nerve is small and located high in the nasal cavity. Most odorous compounds stimulate both nerves to varying degrees. Vanillin is one of the few purely olfactory stimulants; whereas ammonia has powerful trigeminal and olfactory components. It has been suggested that the trigeminal nerve contributes to smell appreciation, but the issue has never been fully resolved.

The dog has approximately 4 billion ($10^9$) olfactory receptor cells: the human a mere 12 million. The axons of the bipolar olfactory cells are incredibly small at 0.2μm diameter, making them amongst the tiniest and slowest conducting in the nervous system. Groups of these non-myelinated axons are enclosed in one sleeve of a neurolemmal cell hence axons are virtually in direct contact with each other and "cross-talk" between axons is theoretically possible.

The anatomy of the bulb is complex with 20 or more known neurotransmitters. An elaborate network of axo-dendritic synapses links the olfactory cells with mitral and tufted cells to form curious clumps, or glomeruli. There are only 12 thousand glomeruli available to handle messages from 12 million olfactory axons. Impulses next pass along the olfactory tracts which lie on the undersurface of the frontal lobes. Some fibres project back to the opposite olfactory bulb. Interestingly the olfactory neurons are the only ones in the central nervous system capable of regeneration – a point that probably reflects their ancient origins – but on a more practical level explains why some people may eventually recover their sense of smell after injury.

The limbic system to which many of the central connections of olfaction project, thereby explaining the close linkage between olfaction and emotional and behavioural reactions, is formed by certain core structures – amygdaloid nucleus, hippocampus, limbic lobe and hypothalamus – developed at a "phylogenetically" early stage in the evolution of the brain. The limbic lobe is a ring of cortex encircling the fluid-filled ventricles of the brain (limbic literally means a belt or ring-like structure) and includes the cingulate gyrus, parahippocampal gyrus, uncus and primary olfactory cortex.

The central connections are complex, but basically split in three directions to: (1) *septal area* thence projecting via the stria medullaris to the habenular nucleus, thalamic intralaminar nuclei and interpeduncular nucleus and as part of the "Papez circuit" to the hippocampus; (2) *amygdaloid nucleus* with connections to neocortex and parahippocampal gyrus, dorsomedial nucleus of thalamus, preoptic and septal areas; and (3) *primary olfactory cortex* which is situated medially within the temporal lobe. Neurones from the primary olfactory cortex converge on to the orbito-frontal cortex which is probably a secondary "association" area concerned with identification and discrimination.

There are other connections to the hypothalamus and basal ganglia but what is unusual is the fact that impulses associated with olfaction reach the cerebral cortex without relaying through the thalamus unlike all other sensory modalities. This fact emphasizes the primitive origins of the rhinencephalon which evolved long before other sensory paths that relay in the thalamus. In this respect the olfactory bulb serves as the equivalent of the thalamus.

The link between olfaction and the limbic system or "visceral" brain has been recognized in myths and traditions. For a friend to say "God bless you" when a person sneezes is said to ensure that the soul does not leave the body. Snuff has been used in Indian Ayurvedic medicine to induce sneezing, thereby to restore the balance of the humours, and African traditional healers believed that their mental patients had worms in their head that could be expelled by violent sneezing. In many parts of the third world inability to sneeze has been associated with mental illness (Shukla, 1985; 1989): 2.6% of his patients complained of inability to sneeze. The majority had endogenous depression, or schizophrenia and a few had neurotic depression or hypochondriasis.

**Physiology**

The initial phase of olfactory analysis is the act of sniffing which redirects air from its usual mainly horizontal path upwards to the olfactory cleft high in the nose. The frequency with which animals and humans sniff would suggest that the manoeuvre enhances odour analysis and detection. This mechanism possibly aids the detection of certain chemicals at extremely low concentrations. For example, methoxyisobutylpyrazine (musty) may be detected in a concentration of 0.0002 parts per billion (ppb,v/v) and those not congenitally anosmic to it may detect androstenone (urinous) at 0.2 ppb.

Odours somehow interact with the mucus covering the olfactory epithelium and diffuse to the cilia and terminal processes of the olfactory receptor cells, reversibly binding to proteinaceous receptor sites located on one or both of these structures. A biochemical change involving receptor proteins induces a train of intracellular chemically-mediated events resulting in an action potential along the nerves. The process of generating such a potential is relatively slow – around 200 msec. A curious fact is that only one nostril is ever fully patent at a time in 80% of healthy people and this will vary throughout the day – the "nasal cycle". The precise reason for this apparent economy is ill understood.

**Coding of Olfactory Information**

Smell differentiation depends, according to the stereo-chemical theory (Amoore, 1977), on variations in molecular shape of the odour in question, which "lock" on to and activate specific receptor sites on olfactory neurons. There is good evidence of specific pheromone receptors located in the antennae of insects, such as the silk moth, where receptors for sex pheromones are highly tuned to particular isomers of the active compounds (Kaissling, 1971). These cells coexist with broadly tuned receptors.

In the human olfactory epithelium, receptor cells sensitive to a particular odour, respond to stimuli by increased discharge frequency rates. Variations of intensity and frequency relate to odour concentration. However, it appears that all receptor cells respond to the majority of odourants irrespective of their physico-chemical properties. It is surmised that receptor cells have varying sensitivities and that a "population" pattern is generated from many cells with similar sensitivity (Holley, 1991). Neurons which are activated by an individual smell or class of smells have not been found as yet.

A slightly different approach (Freeman, 1991$a$), posits that perception of odours depends on the simultaneous cooperative activity of millions of neurons spread throughout wide areas of the cortex. He claims that every neuron in the olfactory bulb participates in generating each olfactory perception. The information is carried by 40Hz electrical rhythms that Freeman calls $\gamma$ waves. Information is thought to be transmitted not by the wave form but by the amplitude pattern across the entire olfactory cortex. This pattern of $y$ wave activity is generated by a unique nerve cell assembly that functions according to the principles of mathematical chaos – as has also been proposed for the visual cortex.

It will be recalled that whilst there are 12m olfactory neurones in the human nose there are only 12 000 glomeruli. Such 1000:1 convergence probably serves to amplify the signal but at the same time there is bound to be some distortion or loss of information; furthermore each glomerulus is in contact with the dendrites of many mitral and tufted cells (i.e. divergence of signal). The latter cells are involved in complex reverberating circuits which allow positive and negative feedback. It is thought that reciprocal inhibition between neighbouring mitral or tufted cells causes sharpened contrast between adjacent channels, similar to that known to occur in visual and common sensory pathways.

Experiments in the rat (Pinching and Doving, 1974) suggest that there is a topographic arrangement in the bulb according to odour class. In the olfactory cortex there are small areas which receive input from large areas of the bulb; conversely large areas of olfactory cortex receive signals from small areas of the bulb.

It should be clear by now that the process of signal transmission to the brain is poorly understood, highly complex, and capable of considerable distortion *en route*. Early debates regarding receptor specificity for common sensation were resolved only through the application of electron microscopic techniques. Tuned olfactory receptors may well exist in humans as in insects – it is a matter of finding them.

A transient decrease or loss of smell perception will occur for varying periods following odour exposure due to receptor "fatigue". Thus continuous inhalation of lemon or orange vapours can result in complete loss of smell sense for up to 11 minutes in healthy people. Whilst fatigue depends primarily on the duration and concentration of odour, certain compounds are more conductive to fatigue than others, e.g. vanillin is notorious in this respect.

The ability to localize and lateralize olfactory signals is poorly developed. Unless the head is moved it appears impossible for the position of an odour to be perceived. If the signal is introduced directly into the nostril, it may be lateralized only if the odour has some coexisting trigeminal component (e.g. menthol). A pure olfactory stimulant such as vanillin cannot be lateralized at all (Koball *et al.*, 1989).

Differences occur in transmission of odours according to their hedonic properties. Kobal and Hummel (1991) found that reponses to unpleasant odours, such as menthol and hydrogen sulphide elicit a cerebral evoked response of shorter latency and smaller amplitude upon stimulating the left nostril compared with the right, and vice versa with more pleasant stimulants such as vanillin or phenyl-ethyl-alcohol (rose-like). Pleasant emotions are mainly represented in the left cerebral hemisphere and unpleasant in the right (Dimond *et al.*, 1976). Because the major projection from one nostril is unilateral it may be argued that the higher amplitude latency response on the left is the one for hedonic analysis. This would appear logical in that it allows pleasant odours to be savoured and examined at leisure. The unpleasant odours project more rapidly to the left side only – but the R/L latency differences are small suggesting that bilateral cerebral activation is occurring – perhaps as a prelude to activating a motor response.

The complex central connections of olfaction via the limbic system can lead to a wide variety of effects. Those via the Papez circuits to the amygdalo-hypothalamic pathways, if interrupted, can impair feeding and neuroendocrine function, at least in animals, affecting taste or odour aversions, odour preference learning and odour-mediated aspects of reproduction. Medial bilateral temporal lobe lesions permit odours to be detected but not identified or finely discriminated. Removal of a temporal lobe impairs discrimination from the ipsilateral nostril but the right fronto-orbital lobe appears to be "dominant" for higher olfactory analysis and its removal is accompanied by discriminatory loss affecting both nostrils.

## Specific Anosmia

Specific anosmia, or smell blindness, is a condition of reduced detection threshold for a particular odour or class of odour akin to colour blindness. The overall frequency estimates vary from 3 – 47% depending on the odour and other factors such as sex and race. Guillot (1948) claimed there were eight primary odours: isovaleric acid (sweaty); pyrroline (spermous); trimethylamine (fishy); isobutyraldehyde (malty); androstenone (urinous); pentadecalactone (musky); carvone (minty); ceneole (camphorous).

Specific anosmia is known to be associated with all these compounds especially androstenone, isobutyraldehyde and cineole. There are undoubtedly more than eight compounds to which people may be smell blind and estimates have ranged from 43- 118 classes of odour. Because of the frequency of smell blindness it is probable that very few of us have a perfect sense of smell and that we all perceive a complex multicomponent aroma such as coffee or perfume in a slightly different fashion (Amoore, 1986). There is some evidence that specific anosmia is inherited as an autosomal recessive characteristic.

## Clinical Evaluation of Olfaction

The measurement of olfactory ability is not straightforward. Simple olfactory testing is made difficult because of the dual nerve supply of the nose. The majority of commonly used test odours causes simultaneous activation of trigeminal and olfactory nerve endings within the nose (especially ammonia, menthol and camphor). In addition many ingredients found in test kits are rarely found in everyday life, and hence will be difficult to identify, e.g. camphor, eucalyptus, oil of cloves, oil of wintergreen.

If a more detailed analysis is needed one may use the University of Pennsylvania Smell Identification Test (UPSIT) (Doty *et al.*, 1984*a*). This employs the scratch and sniff principle, i.e. odour which is released on scratching an impregnated cardboard strip. For each of 40 test smells, the subject makes a forced choice from four possibilities. Normal individuals under 60 years should score at least 30/40, whilst anosmics will attain an average of 10 +/- 5. Malingerers score 0-5 as they intentionally deselect the correct answer. The UPSIT has proved a reliable procedure but at the same time assesses cognitive function, i.e. the more intelligent may not recognize the correct odour but can identify those that are wrong, thence reach a correct answer by a process of elimination.

A more refined approach is to determine the absolute level of a particular odourant that the patient can detect. Air dilution olfactometry requires complex apparatus. A more practical alternative is to use phenyl-ethyl alcohol in varying dilutions contained in small flasks or sniff bottles. However, these tests are subjective and evaluate cognitive function to varying degrees.

Olfactory evoked potentials (OEP) represent one of the more sophisticated and objective tests. Selected odours are embedded in a fast flowing airstream which enters the nostril by way of a short piece of teflon tubing thus avoiding trigeminal stimulation. By introducing a very short odour pulse (i.e. 200msec) an evoked potential is obtained after an interval of approximately 420msec. What OEP emphasize is the relatively slow rate of signal transfer to the cortex. Visually evoked responses reach the striate cortex in 100msec and somatosensory signals in 20msec.

Brain mapping is an alternative technique which allows the spatial distribution of cerebral electrical activity to be displayed in the form of a contour map. When used with evoked potential studies it has shown that pure olfactory signals such as vanillin are maximally represented in the central parietal zones whereas impure odours, i.e. those with trigeminal activity cause a response further forward, suggesting a different generator site (Kobal and Hummel, 1991). Freeman has applied this technique to the rabbit olfactory bulb and shown that the contour map changes in response to conditioning. In humans the averaged spatial EEG pattern has been shown to differ when pure odours are used in comparison to mainly trigeminal stimulants (Van Toller and Reed, 1989).

## Influences on Olfaction

Wine or perfume sampling involves deliberate smell analysis. In other situations exposure to odours is usually passive and for an odour to be remembered it probably requires arousal. However there is some evidence that sleeping new born babies (and adults) may respond to odours without waking. Several types of odour-memory have been described, i.e. long and short term memory. Another variety is "working memory" which is the continual process of environmental monitoring for changes in background odour quality.

Enhancement of olfactory memory by training is an undisputed faculty. Furthermore, training can alter smell sensitivity. Wysocki *et al.* (1986) showed that repeated exposure to androstenone over 6 weeks caused substantial improvement in threshold recognition. It is estimated that the average human can identify 2-4000 different odours but with practice the skilled perfumer may increase this repertoire to as many as 10 000. Such skill requires considerable training.

There is a shortage of descriptive language whereby the untrained person may attach words to smells. It is speculated that this may relate to the relatively poor connections between the precentral gyrus and superior temporal gyri language centres and the olfactory areas. Of the numerous endeavours to classify smell, the most bizarre stems from Piesse who (following Huysmans) believed that odours "harmonized" with the notes of a musical scale (M. Critchley, 1986). There have been more recent attempts to overcome the problem of categorization – odour profiling and multidimensional scaling. Clearly such an approach is subjective and dependent on semantic rather than sensory attributes but it has value in deciding acceptable standards, for example, for public water supplies.

Engen *et al.* (1991) proposed that smells are appreciated as a whole and that this in some way hinders analysis. It is suggested that the characterization of odour is more like describing a human face than a scene. To communicate facial appearances the easiest method is to point out resemblances to other faces rather than describing the shape of the nose or eyes. Similarly odours are perhaps best described by reference to other smells rather than by their primary qualities. Professionals, but not amateurs, are capable of recognizing the ingredients of several components in a mixture. This requires knowledge of the smells of each compound and how they are changed when mixed together. It could imply that the neural message representing a pure odour is not structured differently from that of a complex odour. Olfactory perception is intimately related to olfactory memory. Recognition memory of odours is characterized by a lack of clear distinction between long and short term (Engen *et al.*, 1991). Furthermore, recognition memory appears to be modest in the short term (as compared to visual memory) but is not affected by time and therefore good in the long term.

If someone is exposed to a novel odour which is associated with a significant event, it is stored in long term memory – apparently after only a single exposure – and with similar reliability to those odours that are deliberately learnt. The ability of smell to evoke memories from the distant past is well recognized and exemplified in the writings of Proust. In a famous passage from his novel "Remembrance of Things Past" (1954), Proust was in the bedroom of his Aunt Leonie when he detected the aroma of petit madeleines (sponge cakes) dipped in tea. This immediately brought forth a vivid memory of an old grey house with a clarity that could not be surpassed by the sight or feel of madeleine. Zola noted that olives would invariably conjure up scenes of Provence where childhood was spent. Whilst the ability of a sensory signal to evoke former memories is not unique to the olfactory system, perhaps the vividness of past recall is distinctive. A possible reason for this is the strong anatomical connections between the olfactory pathways and the limbic system which is concerned with memory and emotion. The interrelationship between memory, emotion and smell is further exemplified in the novel "Perfume" by Süskind (1987) in which a perfumer incensed by the smell of a young lady was able to track her down by following her body odours. It seems that her odour provoked feelings of extreme violence which culminated in her brutal murder. Conversely the aroma-therapist attempts to relax individuals by massage or bathing with odours thought to be soothing such as lavender or jasmine. Use of the steroid musk "Osmone 1" is claimed to have tranquillizing effects and has been proposed as a substitute for benzodiazepine drugs (Birchall, 1990).

## Odour Memory in the Elderly

With advancing years the ability to identify discriminate and remember odours declines (Doty et al., 1984b). The decrement is quite steep after the age of 70 such that a healthy 90-year-old will identify correctly only half the odours of a 20-year-old. Engen et al. (1991) asked elderly subjects to identify odours at intervals varying from 0-30 seconds. When there was no delay 80% of the odours were identified accurately but if this was increased to 30 seconds the accuracy of recognition declined to only 56%. Further experiments suggest that this decline of smell sense is not paralleled by any similar decline in visual memory.

## Demography

In 1986 a massive world wide analysis of olfaction was undertaken through the readership of the *National Geographic Magazine* (Wysocki, 1991). On the basis of approximately 1.42 million replies a wealth of data was obtained about basic demography, their subjective ability to smell, use of perfume, and subjective rating of androstenone (urinous), amyl-acetate (banana like), galaxolide (musky), eugenol (cloves), mercaptans (sulphurous), and rose. Women from the USA scored highest in their self-rating of smell sense and this aspect applied generally to females in the rest of the world. Males from Europe gave themselves the lowest ratings. Of the six test odours employed, all except androstenone and mercaptans were rated pleasant irrespective of nationality and gender. Males rated amyl-acetate, androstenone and mercaptans more pleasant than did females, whereas females rated galaxolide, eugenol and rose more pleasant than did males.

Androstenone, a gonadal steroid, is perceived (if at all) either as stale urine, musk-like or sweet. People who rated androstenone as unpleasant, gave this a high intensity rating – especially those from Europe. This observation correlates with other data which suggest that if a subject has a low threshold to the perception of androstenone it is rated unpleasant; if the threshold is high it will be rated indifferent or pleasant. Amyl-acetate was given a fairly uniform hedonic rating whereas for galaxolide there were major differences. It received lowest pleasantness rating in Asians and highest in Australians, 50% of whom said they would be prepared to wear it as a perfume. Whilst the majority thought that mercaptans were unpleasant there was one exception – those from India liked it: about 70% of Asians were not willing to eat something which smelt like eugenol whereas 30% Whites were so prepared. Other regional differences occurred probably representing cultural and environmental factors. One reason for variable hedonic responses to different odours may relate to the degree of physical contact between friends and relatives: N. European nations being mainly "non-contact" cultures; S. European primarily "contact" societies.

Four of the six odours evoked a vivid memory. Galaxolide and mercaptans were the least likely to do so. The ability to identify the six odours was fairly universal. Androstenone gave great difficulty with only 20% giving a correct response.

Galaxolide was equally difficult especially for males. These facts support the existence of specific anosmia to either androstenone or galaxolide. Androstenone anosmia was present in 33% of males and 24% females from America in contrast to 22% males and 14% females in Africa.

Many other factors influence the ability to smell, notably: gender, smoking habits, exposure to toxins, drug usage and disease. Women are generally superior in tests of identification, detection and discrimination. Tobacco smoking results in mild depression of identification ability, with a slow return to normal if the habit is abandoned (Frye et al., 1989). Environmental toxic exposure, as might be expected, will lead to temporary or permanent impairment of smell. Plastics workers, for example, show significant olfactory loss proportional to the duration of exposure (Schwartz et al., 1989). Paradoxically smokers were less affected than non-smokers.

Many drugs are claimed to interfere with the sense of smell, including nifedipine, streptomycin, carbimazole, opiates, antidepressants and amphetamine. The nasal "snorting" of proscribed drugs, especially cocaine, is associated with anosmia because of destruction of the olfactory epithelium and even the nasal septum.

Lesions, such as tumours of the tip of the temporal lobe (uncus) may give rise to "uncinate" epilepsy, in which the fit is heralded in by an olfactory aura. The hallucinatory smell is nearly always unpleasant, e.g. gas or oil.

Local nasal disease is the commonest reason for anosmia, next most common are viral illnesses including the common cold, and thirdly head injury, not necessarily involving a skull fracture. Of interest to the neurologist is the association of neuro-degenerative disease such as Alzheimer's disease, Korsakoff's psychosis and parkinsonism with disturbance of olfaction. Loss of smell may occur at an early stage of Alzheimer's disease. In patients with the alcoholic form of Korsakoff's psychosis there is difficulty in discrimination but no loss of sensitivity. To what extent this difficulty reflects cognitive dysfunction and memory is debated but the consensus is that impairment does not relate to any defect in acuity, learning or recollection.

**Disorders of Perception**

Distortion or perversion in the perception of an odour is called parosmia – or cacosmia if unpleasant. Such perversions are common with local nasal disease but may follow trauma or chemical exposure. Parosmia may occur with normal or diminished smell sensitivity, and minor degrees are not necessarily abnormal. Thus, unpleasant smells can linger for several hours and may be subsequently rekindled by other olfactory stimuli – "phantosmia".

Hyperosmia is another disorder of perception in which there may be increased sensitivity to one or more aromas. Undue sensitivity to aromas may occur with Addison's disease, head injury, neuroses and migraine.

A true olfactory hallucination, in the absence of an odour in the environment, can arise almost anywhere along the smell pathway, but may be treated neurosurgically with stereotactic lesions of the amygala. One of the earliest descriptions of olfactory hallucination was by Hughlings Jackson (1890) of a cook who experienced epileptic attacks emanating from the temporal lobe, "in the paroxysm the first thing was tremor of the hands and arms; she saw a little black woman who was always very actively engaged in cooking; the spectre did not speak. The patient had a very horrible smell (so-called subjective sensation of smell) which she could not describe. She had a feeling as if she was shut up in a box with a limited quantity of air... she would stand with her eyes fixed... and then say what a 'horrible smell' ... After leaving her kitchen work she had paroxysms with the smell sensation but no spectre."

Apart from uncinate seizures, olfactory hallucinations and delusions usually signify a psychiatric illness. There is complaint of a large variety of smells, mainly foul. A patient may mistakenly believe that a foul smell emanates from himself ("intrinsic hallucination") and he may attribute this to something wrong with the nose, etc. In others they seem to come from an external source. In a review of depressed patients, Pryse-Phillips (1975) found olfactory symptoms to be an early and predominating complaint in half his patients with typical endogenous depression and termed this an "olfactory reference syndrome". They usually suffered from intrinsic hallucinations whereas those due to schizophrenia had extrinsic hallucinations, apparently induced by someone for the purpose of upsetting the patient. Reactions to the hallucinations varied from none at all to petitioning police and neighbours or continual washing and social withdrawal.

**Conclusions**

Olfaction is the least well understood of all human sensory experience apart from taste. The rhinencephalon is phylogenetically old and transmits at a snail's pace in comparison with common sensation. It is not yet known whether specific receptors exist in the nose, nor how the signals to the brain are evaluated. Nonetheless, Freeman (1991*b*) has proposed an intriguing hypothesis and one of the few attempts to provide a unifying concept to sensory experience:

"The brain seeks information mainly by directing an individual to look, listen and sniff. The search results from self-organizing activity of the limbic system which funnels a search command to the motor systems. As the motor command is transmitted, the limbic system issues a 'reafference message'"alerting all the sensory systems to prepare a response to new information. Next, every neuron in a given region participates in a collective activity – a burst. Synchronous activity in each system is then transmited back to the limbic system where it combines with similarly generated output from other sensory systems to form a gestalt. Shortly after another search for information is demanded and the sensory systems are prepared again by reafferance".

## References

Amoore, J.E. (1977). Specific anosmia and the concept of primary odours. *Chemical Senses and Flavor*, **2**, 267-281.

Amoore, J.E. (1986). The chemistry and physiology of odor sensitivity. *Journal of American Water Works Association*, **78**, 70-76.

Birchall, A. (1990). A whiff of happiness. *New Scientist.* 25 August 44-47.

Critchley, M. (1986). The citadel of the senses: the nose as its sentinel. *In* "The Citadel of the Senses". pp. 1-14. Raven Press Books.

Dimond, S.J., Farrington, L. and Johnson, P. (1976). Differing emotional responses from right and left hemispheres. *Nature*, **261**, 690-692.

Doty, R.L. (1991). Olfactory dysfunction in neurodegenerative disorders. *In* "Smell and Taste in Health and Disease". Chapter 47 (Eds T.V. Getchell, R.L. Doty, Bartoshuk and J.B. Snow). Raven Press, New York.

Doty, R.L., Shaman, P., Kimmelman, C.P. and Dann, M.S. (1984a). University of Pennsylvania Smell Identification Test: a rapid quantitative olfactory function test for the clinic. *Laryngoscope*, **94**, 176-178.

Doty, R.L., Shaman, P. *et al.* (1984b). Smell identification ability: changes with age. *Science*, **226**, 1441-1443.

Doty, R.L., Gregor, T. and Settle, R.G. (1986). Influences of inter-trial interval and sniff bottle volume on the phenyl-ethyl-alcohol olfactory detection threshold. *Chemical Senses*, **10**, 297-300.

Engen, T., Gilmore, M.M. and Mair, R.G. (1991). Odor memory. *In* "Smell and Taste in Health and Disease". Chapter 16. (Eds T.V. Getchell, R.L. Doty, Bartoshuk and J.B. Snow). Raven Press, New York.

Freeman, W.J. (1991a). Analytic techniques used in search for the physiological basis of the EEG. *In* "Handbook of Electroencephalography and Clinical Neurophysiology". Vol. 2. Chapter 18. pp. 583-664.

Freeman, W.J. (1991b). The physiology of perception. *Scientific American*, **264**, 434-41.

Frye, R.E., Doty, R.L. and Schwartz,. B. (1989). Influence of cigarette smoking on olfaction: evidence for a dose-response relationship. *Journal of the American Medical Association*, **263**, 1233-1236.

Guillot, M. (1948). Ansomies partielles et odeurs fondamentales. *Comptes rendus de l'Academie des Sciences, Paris* **226**, 1307-1309.

Holley, A. (1991). Neural coding of olfactory information. *In* "Smell and Taste in Health and Disease". Chapter 17 (Eds T.V. Getchell, R.L. Doty, Bartoshuk and J.B. Snow). Laven Press, New York.

Jackson, J.H. (1890). Case of tumour of the right temporosphenoidal lobe bearing on the localization of the sense of smell and on the interpretation of a particular variety of epilepsy. *Brain*, **12**, 346-357.

Kaissling, K.E. (1971). Insect olfaction. *In* "Handbook of Sensory Physiology". Vol. 4. Part 1. (Ed. L.M. Beidler). pp. 351-431. Springer Verlag, New York.

Kobal, G. and Hummel, T. (1991). Olfactory evoked potentials in humans. In "Smell and Taste in Health and Disease". Chapter 13. (Eds. T.V. Getchell, R.L. Doty, Bartoshuk and J.B. Snow). pp. 269-270. Raven Press, New York.

Kobal, G., Van Toller, S. and Hummel, T. (1989). Is there directional smelling? *Experientia*, **45**, 130-132.

Pinching, A.J. and Doving, K.B. (1974). Selective degeneration in the rat olfactory bulb following exposure to different odours. *Brain Research*, **82**, 195-204.

Proust, M. (1954). "Remembrances of Things Past". Translated by C.K. Scott-Moncrieff and S. Hudson. London. 1957.

Pryse-Phillips, W. (1975). Disturbance in the sense of smell in psychiatric patients. *Proceedings of the Royal Society of Medicine*, **68**, 472-474.

Schwartz, B., Doty, R.L., Monroe, C., Frye, R.E. and Barker, S. (1989). The evaluation of olfactory function in chemical workers exposed to acrylic acid and acrylate vapors. *American Journal of Public Health*, **79**, 613-618.

Shukla, G.D. (1985). "Asneezia" a hitherto unrecognized psychiatric symptom. *British Journal of Psychiatry*, **147**, 564-65.

Shukla, G.D. (1989). "Asneezia" some further observations. *British Journal of Psychiatry*, **154**, 689-90.

Süskind, P. (1987). "Perfume". Translated by H. Hamilton. Penguin Books.

Van Toller, S. and Reed, M.K. (1989). Brain electrical activity topographical maps produced in response to olfactory and chemosensory stimulation. *Psychiatry Research*, **29**, 429-430.

Wysocki, C.J. Beauchamp, G.K., Schimdt, H. and Dorries, K.M. (1986). Change in olfactory sensitivity to androstenone with age and experience. 9th Annual Meeting of ACHemS. Sarasota, FL. Abs 172.

Wysocki, C.J., Pierce, J.D. and Gilbert, A.N. (1991). Geographic, cross-cultural and individual variation in human olfaction. *In* "Smell and Taste in Health and Disease". Chapter 15. (Eds T.V. Getchell, R.L. Doty, Bartoshuk and J.B. Snow). Raven Press, New York.

# 4. Deafness and communication

Brendan Monteiro and E.M.R. Critchley

The theme of this volume is the uncertain nature of reality and the fact that, with or without challenges to the senses, it may be difficult for people to understand the nature of their reality. Many authors have treated deafness as a disability, that brings with it a dual impairment – the so-called failure of a major sensory organ and blockade of a conventional mode of communication. The knowledge and experience of working with deaf people at a mental health centre, specifically designed for deaf people, challenge these conventional ideas and strongly support the view that deaf people form a cultural and linguistic minority. The practical problems of outlining the reality of deaf people can be appropriately addressed in specialized mental health units established to meet the needs of deaf people.

The severity of deafness – an audiological concept – can be measured accurately:

A deaf person is one whose lack of ability to hear precludes the successful processing of linguistic information through the auditory channel, with or without a hearing aid.

A hard of hearing person is one who, with the use of a hearing aid, has sufficient residual hearing to enable successful processing of linguistic information through audition.

(Report of the Ad Hoc Committee to Define Deaf and Hard of Hearing)

The other important variable is the age of onset of deafness.

## Late Onset Deafness

Acquired deafness in later life is usually insidious, neither the patient nor those with whom he is in contact are initially aware of the gradual impairment of hearing. He appears not to be paying attention, appears remote or socially dulled. He may fail to grasp part of the conversation and draw a wrong conclusion from what is said. His feelings may be hurt: or he may fail to understand the feelings of others. "Partial deafness without awareness of its source is associated with changes in cognitive, emotional, and behavioural functioning, and paranoid thinking may emerge as a cognitive attempt to overcome the difficulty in hearing. Misunderstandings may provoke frustration and anger". (Leading article; *Lancet*, 1981),

It may not be possible, in the elderly, to separate a disorder of hearing from a disorder of comprehension, and the conclusion is often made that the individual is dementing. Society is remiss in its failure to examine and differentiate between these two disorders. Hearing is essential not only to interpret words for their meaning but for the nuances, emotional inflexions, stresses, urgency, sense and manner of communication. When speaking, those with normal hearing can monitor their own speech, control the loudness, tone, and accuracy of what is said, and bar unacceptable intrusions into speech. Encroaching deafness may also bring the need to adjust to spontaneous firing from auditory neurones, both peripheral and central. This may take the form of tinnitus – usually in the form of whistling noises – other formed or unformed noises, and even hallucinatory speech and music (Chapter 13).

## Deafness in Childhood and Adolescence

Wright (1969), who became deaf when he was seven, gives a moving account of his deafness and the way it affected his life. He describes the difference between his deafness and that of someone who becomes deaf at birth or at a very early age.

What is crucial is the age at which hearing is lost. The deaf-born cannot pick up speech and language naturally like ordinary children. They have to be taught, a difficult and slow process, the slower and more difficult the later the teaching begins. That is why older children and adults find it an effort. But the born deaf and those who become deaf in early childhood have the compensation that they do not feel the loss of a faculty they never had or cannot remember.

## Early Onset Deafness

A child born without hearing presents the greatest challenge to the theories of evolution and human development, which incorporate ideas based on the concept of sound. All mammals, all birds, and some reptiles are able to hear. Reptiles and fish can appreciate vibration. The child can be presumed to have an auditory cortex, central nervous connections for hearing, and a potentially utilizable peripheral sensory organ for hearing. We normally assume that maldevelopment has affected part of the inner ear and, where possible, we seek a remediable cause. We do not know whether the central apparatus is functioning, or silent; whether, with the innate plasticity of the nervous system, parts of the auditory apparatus are put to other functions; or whether through lack of stimulation they remain undeveloped and in an immature state. Some of the causes of congenital deafness, such as rubella embryopathy, rhesus incompatibility, anoxia at birth, and prematurity, also affect other anatomical sites within the nervous system and possibly involve the auditory pathways and cortex at several levels. What is known is that central disorders of language – various forms of word deafness, development dysphasia, and idiopathic language retardation – may mimic deafness unless properly analyzed.

In every case, the essential difference between people with early profound deafness and those with onset of profound deafness in later life is the acquisition of verbal language. "Verbal" is used to mean the use of words.

Speech is an innate human function, and except in extreme instances is independent of intelligence, brain size or brain weight, and is triggered by, and dependent upon, the stimulation of others. Fry and Whetnall (1954) coined the phrase "readiness to listen" to describe the child's language position at between 6-12 months and "readiness to speak" for the second phase between 12-24 months. The vocalizations of a child of 8-9 months reflect the language sounds of its parents – mimicry without understanding. At this stage one can distinguish between the babblings of a Japanese, American or German child. The neonate, according to Spiegel (1959), is subjected to communication as an essentially passive-receptive vehicle. He receives communication from his mother, predominantly through the closeness of direct body contact and also through empathy. In mid-infancy, the mother reinforces "selected sounds from his vocalization which are in the range of her language, and appeals to his imitativeness in their affectionate interplay. She reads the first meanings into his syllables – da da, ma ma; she structures little situations to which the word is appropriate, and the learning of speech begins".

The profoundly deaf child requires a different trigger to develop language: sign language. Not surprisingly the 15% of deaf children, born to deaf parents, develop native sign language skills often superior to those of deaf children of hearing parents. The definition of deafness above involves lack of ability to hear within the linguistic range. But this does not exclude the hearing of high explosives, low flying aeroplanes, cars backfiring, motor cycles, heavy lorries, carts clattering over cobblestones, wurlitzers, pneumatic drills (Wright, 1969) or ability to dance in time to the rhythm of a band, reinforced by the vibrations of wooden floors (Mow, 1970).

Children born deaf, even if residual hearing can be reinforced by hearing aids, find the acquisition of verbal language extremely difficult. Without the foundation of auditory language on which to build an inner vocabulary of verbal language they are dependent on those sounds they can hear, often incompletely – and vision. A prerequisite of lip reading is a well developed internalized vocabulary. Lip reading is inexact and depends on a range of conditions being met: good light, a one-to-one situation and proper facial characteristics (a beard or moustache makes lip reading extremely difficult). Some sounds of speech are not accompanied by movements of the mouth or lips, and even the most accomplished lip readers only discriminate about 60% of the spoken word. Problems with the acquisition of an adequate inner verbal language may also lead to difficulties in comprehending concepts, ethics and abstract words (e.g. up, under, above, within), be they spoken or written.

In the formative period the child may be protected with the school or home environment; but, Groce (1985):

A deaf person's greatest problem is not simply that he or she cannot hear, but that the lack of hearing is socially isolating. The deaf person's knowledge and awareness of the larger society are limited because hearing people find it difficult or impossible to communicate with him or her. The difficulty in communicating [and] the ignorance and misinformation about deafness that is pervasive in most of the hearing world combined to cause difficulties in all aspects of life for deaf individuals – in education, employment, community involvement and civil rights.

She goes on to say (in her book on hereditary deafness in Martha's Vineyard), that, on the Vineyard, the hearing people are bilingual in English and Island sign language thus downing the wall that separates most deaf people from the rest of us.

Currently, many deaf people perceive themselves as part of a cultural and linguistic minority. Several factors contribute to this.

Firstly, the education of deaf children has been fraught with controversy. The educators of deaf children have, in the main, subscribed to the oral/aural approach which concentrates all efforts on the acquisition of speech and proscribes sign language believing such an approach necessary for the integration of deaf people into a hearing society (2nd International Congress on the Education of the Deaf, Milan, 1880). Even today, sign language is either not discussed or grossly undervalued in the counselling of hearing parents of deaf children.

Secondly, deafness is viewed in medical terms as a disease, and even if not genetically determined is regarded eugenically as an unacceptable trait which requires isolation and eventual elimination. A pariah syndrome is added to any inferiority complex or presumed social inadequacy.

Thirdly, deafness is invisible; it has no visual characteristic. Furthermore, 85% of deaf children are born to hearing parents. These children are thus part of the culture and race into which they are born, even though they cannot gain proper access to the shared norms and experiences of a shared culture. Their parents are encouraged to view their deafness as a disability and frequently resist their integration into the deaf community because of the misguided advice they receive. Schlesinger and Meadow (1971), described the attitudes of hearing parents to their deaf children, stating that the deaf children's parents showed some frustration and irritation with the impediments of parent-child communications while insisting that the deaf child was really no different from his hearing sibs.

Deaf children of deaf parents are a good example of people who become natural members of the deaf community. These children and their families perceive their deafness as a normal experience. They acquire sign language naturally as their mother tongue, and develop a strong deaf identity. Through sign language and finger spelling they may acquire a considerable vocabulary. They do not experience many of the difficulties faced by deaf children of hearing parents and frequently become key members of the deaf community.

Those not in the deaf community have difficulties keeping in touch with the larger hearing population. They may have few problems with integration, if they have been well taught, have adequate support at home or at work, are particularly skilful at a trade. But if for some reason integration is absent they become remote, isolated, appear to lose touch with reality: in short, they can appear psychotic. Some deaf people are referred to psychiatrists to clarify the nature of their experiences; many do not suffer a mental illness but may have encountered a variety of problems and difficulties. Those referred to mental health services include:

1   Deaf people who have been inappropriately educated

Some deaf people are educated in schools that adopt an oral/aural approach. Some schools for the deaf still shun sign language and do not provide the environment for deaf children to develop a deaf identity and pride in their language. The 1981 Education Act emphasized the integration of children with special needs into mainstream schools. On occasion deaf children were placed in "hearing" classrooms with some additional support or in partially hearing units where they were taught together for part of the day and "integrated" at other parts of the day.

A major disadvantage of such systems is that deaf children are relatively isolated. They are prone to develop a negative self-image, and are often on the periphery of both deaf and hearing groups. Deaf children in "mainstream" education are denied opportunities to develop sign language techniques, and can become isolated both in the linguistic and social dimensions. The problems are further complicated when such individuals live in rural communities, are completely engulfed by their hearing families and cannot maintain regular contact with the deaf community.

2   Deaf people with disabilities

The incidence of intellectual impairments, physical disabilities, blindness and other disabilities is higher in the deaf than in the hearing population. A multicentre study of 3000 deaf children in nine European countries (Martin, 1979) revealed that 29.3% had some disability, of which 9.9% were intellectually impaired.

Although deaf people with intellectual impairments have the potential to acquire sign language skills at a basic level, they often experience great difficulties in acquiring verbal language. Their ability to conceptualize and think in abstract terms is extremely limited. As a consequence of their difficulties and poor achievement, they often lack the knowledge, ability and social skills necessary to make an adjustment in either deaf or hearing communities. Such people may be referred because they lack the ability to communicate either verbally or by sign and gesture. It is imperative to develop a helpful relationship, then seeing what forms of communication are understood, and finally enlarge and develop some form of signing even if only mutually comprehensible between the person and his carers.

**The Boundaries of Reality**

The experience of sound for a deaf person depends upon the age of onset of deafness and the degree of deafness. Deaf people who can hear speech may have difficulties (in discriminating) and may misinterpret what is being said. Those who are born profoundly deaf form 1 in 1000 of the world's population. It is still unclear whether they live in a silent world. They do not complain of silence or of tinnitus. They are often able to hear noises and some state they can perceive certain sounds such as the banging of doors, horns of cars. They often wear hearing aids to hear environmental sounds to help awareness and safety in their surroundings.

For those deafened after acquiring speech language, the experience of noise and sound is somewhat different, and they retain an auditory memory, as do those who have become deaf at an early age who may have a subsequent progressive hearing loss. Thus Wright (1969) describes his perceptions of "sound" when others speak. He describes "phantasmal voices" that he hears when anyone speaks to him, provided he can see the movements of their lips and faces. Sacks (1989), elaborates on this phenomenon. This hearing (that is imagining) of "phantasmal voices" when lips are read is quite characteristic of the post-lingually deaf, for whom speech (and "inner speech") has become an auditory experience. This is not "imagining" in the ordinary sense; rather an instant and automatic "translation" of the visual experience into an auditory correlate (based on experience and association) – a translation that probably has a neurological basis (of experientially established visual-auditory connections). As with "photisms" which may be provoked in blind people by sound: so the deaf may experience "acuphenes" in response to visual stimuli.

Communication is important in all medical practice; in psychiatry it is of absolute and crucial importance. The process of diagnosis in psychiatry relies on the ability of the patient to give an account of his experiences and the psychiatrist's ability to understand him. The clinical interview constitutes the main tool for both assessment and treatment in psychiatry (Rutter and Cox, 1981).

The diagnosis of mental disorder poses immense difficulties if psychiatrists do not have an understanding of the cultural, sociological and linguistic aspects of deafness, and cannot communicate using sign language. Historically, it has been stated that all people with early profound deafness have communication difficulties. It is now widely acknowledged that when deaf people have good facility in sign language, the communication difficulties are those of the examiner.

Communication difficulties affect the Mental State examination of deaf patients. The examiner may have difficulties establishing rapport and understanding the patient's communication, and the patient may experience immense difficulties understanding the nature of the interview and the questions asked. The patient who experiences early profound deafness is likely to have limited verbal language and therefore the use of the written word will be misleading and could lead to misdiagnosis. Mis-spelt words, poor grammar and syntax may be regarded as evidence of intellectual impairment. Conversely, the behaviour of some deaf people (e.g. the overt expression of emotion that characterizes communication through sign language among groups of deaf people) may lead to the mistaken diagnosis of mental illness because failure to communicate effectively may lead to a lack of understanding of the causes of anger, frustration and other everyday emotions which may be mistakenly attributed to symptoms of mental illness.

Early profound deafness is, unfortunately, sometimes mistakenly equated with intellectual impairment – deaf-and-dumb. [Dumb has two meanings: inability to speak and of low IQ]. Aristotle, for example, believed that those who were born deaf were "incapable of reason"; and, if the psychologist is unaware of the clinical, psychological, cultural and linguistic implications of deafness, then verbally loaded questions may be used, and the deaf person will invariably underscore. There are also grave problems in the interpretation of results (Denmark, 1985).

The communication issues related to early profound deafness, and especially the limitations of verbal language, can make diagnosis difficult even when they are examined by experts with the requisite communication skills (Denmark and

Eldridge, 1969). A psychiatrist needs to enquire into the presence of complex symptoms: thought disorder, perceptual abnormalities, passivity phenomena, and delusional ideation representing the loss of ego boundaries. Without the requisite skills he may attribute symptoms such as withdrawal or agitation to the deafness. The difficulties of assessing the subjective experiences of deaf people who are without speech and have limited verbal language, cannot be over-estimated (Critchley *et al.*, 1981). The examiner often has to resort to leading questions. This practice then raises serious doubts about the validity of the deaf person's answer, especially as it is well-known that deaf people may agree with questions by giving a positive nod when in actual fact, they have not understood the question.

The diagnosis of psychotic conditions with impaired reality testing, such as schizophrenia, is particularly fraught with difficulty. The incidence of schizophrenia in the deaf population is the same as in the hearing population. Furthermore, relatives of deaf schizophrenics were found to manifest schizophrenia with the same frequency as relatives of hearing schizophrenics (Mendlewicz, 1980). Traditionally, psychiatrists have attached primary importance to the presence of thought disorder in the diagnosis of schizophrenia but this is particularly difficult to detect where the means of interpersonal communication are rudimentary. In clinical practice the diagnosis is more commonly based on the presence of clusters of symptoms such as Schneider's first rank symptoms (1957). In the absence of coarse brain disease, certain symptoms are considered diagnostic of schizophrenia.

Thus auditory hallucinations in the form of voices are considered strongly to support the diagnosis of schizophrenia and were reported in 74% of hearing schizophrenics (Wing *et al.*, 1974).

In practice the frequency of hallucinatory experiences among profoundly, prelingually deaf schizophrenics differs subtly from those of their hearing contemporaries (Critchley *et al.*, 1981). The frequency of haptic hallucinations, passivity phenomena and delusions often of a paranoid type was similar. Visual hallucinations, which are rare among hearing schizophrenics (2-4% see Feinberg, 1962) occurred in 10 out of 12 deaf patients; some of the experiences were classical scenic hallucinations, but others are more accurately described as visuo-verbal hallucinations as though the verbal picture had been substituted for a verbal commentary. Non-auditory modes of communication familiar to profoundly deaf people, such as writing on the wall and sign language, were described among the hallucinatory experiences of three patients but invariably in association with "auditory" experiences which were described by 10 out of 12 patients. Voiced experiences, whether presenting as a running commentary on the subject's thoughts or behaviour, as voices in discussion or as specific instructions addressed to the patient, differed widely in their clarity (Critchley, 1983). Furthermore, Evans and Elliot report that nine "primary" symptoms – loss of ego-boundaries, delusional perception, restricted affect, illogicality, abnormal explanations, hallucinations, remoteness from reality, inappropriate affect and ambivalence – are useful screening criteria in the diagnosis of schizophrenia in deaf patients.

## Can Deaf People Hear Voices?

There is clear evidence that experiences analogous to auditory hallucinations may be experienced by schizophrenics who have been profoundly deaf from birth or early infancy. The frequency of pseudo-auditory experiences among deaf schizophrenics and the wide variety of possible explanations for the apparently meaningful information received may support the concept of a nuclear form of schizophrenia and are of considerable theoretical interest in the wider context of the relationship between thought processes and language.

Accepting that the speech audiogram occupies only part of the wider range of appreciation of musical and other sounds, Critchley (1983) was impressed by the insistence of deaf patients themselves that the communicated experiences did not involve speech reading or sign language. When pressed for an explanation, only one admitted she did not know how she could hear voices, another described "queer talk – not signs", others were adamant that they had heard and not lip read the experience – finger spelling the word "heard" with great emphasis. In those who experienced both vocal and non-vocal communication there appeared to be a primacy of auditory communication; thus God spake but St Theresa signed to the same patient. However, those whose life-work has been with deaf people – Basillier, Denmark, Warren, and Wilson – continually return to the fact that it is necessary to put leading questions to patients: Is it a sound, noise or voice? Does it exist inside the head? Whose voice is it? What is the voice saying? Is there more than one voice? Such questions may in themselves be suggestive of an answer or difficult to comprehend. The following case-histories serve to illustrate both the fascination of the study of these hallucinations and the difficulties they pose in interpretation.

(a) A 41-year-old lady with early severe deafness as a result of neonatal jaundice communicated using speech and lip reading. She had no facility in sign language. Of low average intelligence, she was referred from a home for those with learning difficulties. She recounted sexual fantasies and the voices she complained of were always those of male staff at the home. She developed delusional ideas incorporating them and often declared that she was in love with them.

Comment: The case illustrates the attribution of one's own desires to hallucinatory "voices". The lady was sexually frustrated, had unfulfilled sexual wishes and projected these wishes on to male staff in the form of hearing voices. She complained of hearing voices that were ego-connected and fulfilled her wishes by making her think that the staff in question were communicating with her.

(b) A 31-year-old man with severe post lingual deafness – onset aged 6, communicated using a combination of speech, sign-supported English and finger spelling. He had been mistakenly diagnosed as intellectually impaired and had attended a school for the educationally abnormal until, at 11, he was transferred to a deaf school. In five admissions to psychiatric hospitals various diagnoses were made, including organic disorder, mental impairment, paranoid psychoses, personality disorder. He complained of "hearing voices". He had residual hearing for speech and claimed that when others spoke, he could hear voices of God and the Devil telling him to harm himself and harm others. When communicating with God, he did not use sign language, but claimed to use telepathy. He claimed that he received clear messages from God who talked to him. There was no evidence of visual hallucinations. He could not describe the quality, pitch or tone of God's voice. A detailed diagnostic assessment revealed that he was of normal intellect and suffered personality difficulties. He responded to individual and group therapy.

(c) A 50-year-old, profoundly deaf since birth, communicated using sign language and finger spelling. He was highly intelligent but developed a paranoid psychosis. He had systematized delusions and he described hallucinatory experiences; thus he informed the interviewer that Jesus came to him at night and "spoke" to him. He denied his inability to hear Jesus' voice on account of deafness. He claimed that he could see God's lips moving and could understand the message.

To most people these three case-reports support the original observation of Basilier (1973) that the auditory hallucinations found in 44% of deaf schizophrenics mean no more than "receiving meaningful information". However it could be that true auditory hallucinations occur only in those patients who at some point in their lives had experienced sound to some degree. The question still remains unresolved. Other case-reports emphasize the range of schizophrenic phenomena encountered among deaf schizophrenics; but that schizophrenia essentially involves the boundaries of communication is illustrated by a final case-report.

(d) A 60-year-old deaf lady of Irish origin was found to suffer from a paranoid schizophrenic illness. She had psychotic symptoms. She was educated at a school for the deaf in Dublin where one-handed Irish alphabet and International Sign Language (ISL) was used. She claimed to see a person in her mind's eye who was communicating with her, using the one-handed finger spelling alphabet (as used with ISL). She was examined following treatment over a period of 6 months. The nature of her hallucinatory experiences gradually changed. She could see someone communicating with her using the two-handed British alphabet. She could not explain the nature of the change, and acknowledged that it was due to her changing her own sign language.

This case describes a fascinating phenomenon of the content of hallucinations remaining the same but the language changing with experience of a "new" language. It is interesting to speculate that hearing people, who emigrate to a new country and have to learn a new language, may experience a similar change.

The direct relationship of brain activity to perceptual experiences was first clearly seen by the French scientist and philosopher Descartes. It is immaterial whether brain events are caused by stimulation of the cerebral cortex or some part of the sensory nervous pathway (Eccles, 1973). Thus, where deafness is involved, experience shows that deaf people are the subject of various auditory phenomena, some real, some illusionary, some hallucinatory. The difficulty in eliciting the exact nature of such phenomena is compounded because most professionals lack the ability to communicate effectively with deaf people.

## Summary

Deafness is a term which covers many clinical conditions. In assessing deaf people and considering the boundaries of their reality, it is vitally important to consider variables such as age of onset and degree of deafness. It is also important to recognize that deaf people form part of a cultural and linguistic minority. In order properly to access their experiences, it is important that professionals acknowledge this socio-cultural model of deafness and communicate effectively using sign language. The recently developed policy of employing deaf mental health professionals greatly enhances the ability to understand various experiences of deaf people. A question often posed is: Can deaf people hear voices? How can people, who do not have an intact auditory apparatus, experience auditory hallucinations? On the other hand, can the sensory deprivation of a hearing loss lead to the presence of hallucinations and pseudo-hallucinations. The study of these phenomena and the underlying factors is extremely fascinating and, at the same time, difficult to comprehend. There is a need for ongoing research and debate to shed light on one of psychiatry's most fascinating questions: "Do deaf people hear voices?"

## References

Basilier, T. (1973). "Horselstep og egentlig dovhet". Universitets fürlager, Oslo.
Critchley, E.M.R., Denmark, J.C., Warren, F. and Wilson, K.A. (1981). Hallucinatory experiences of prelingually profoundly deaf schizophrenics. *British Journal of Psychiatry,* **138**, 30-32.
Critchley, E.M.R. (1983). Auditory experiences of deaf schizophrenics. *Journal of the Royal Society of Medicine,* **76**, 542-544.
Denmark, J.C. (1978). Early profound deafness and mental retardation. *British Journal of Mental Subnormality,* **24**, 1-9.
Denmark, J.C. (1985). A study of 250 patients referred to a department of psychiatry for the deaf. *British Journal of Psychiatry.* **146**, 282-286.
Denmark, J.C. and Eldridge, R.W. (1969). Psychiatric services for the deaf. *Lancet,* **ii**, 259-262.
Descartes, R. (1964). "The Principles of Philosophy". Part 4, Principle 196. Translation, 1961.
Eccles, J.C. (1973). "Facing Reality". Editiones Roche, Basel.
Evans, J.W. and Elliot, H. (1981). Screening criteria for the diagnosos of schizophrenia in deaf patients. *Archives of General Psychiatry,* **38**, 787-790.
Feinberg, I. (1962). "Hallucination". Chapter 5, (Ed. L.J. West). Grune and Stratton, New York.
Fry, D.B. and Whetnall, E. (1954). Preparedness for speech. *Lancet,* **i**, 583.
Groce, N.E. (1985). "Everyone Here Spoke Sign Language – Hereditary Deafness in Martha's Vineyard". Harvard University Press.
Martin, J.A.M. (1979). "Deaf Children in 9 European Countries".
Martin, J.A.M. (1982). Aetiological factors relating to childhood deafness in the europoean community. *Audiology,* **21**, *149-158.*
Mendlewicz, J. (1980). "Handbook of Biological Psychiatry". Part III, (Ed. H.M. van Praag),

pp. 81-100. Dekker, New York.

Mow, S. (1970). How do you dance without music? *In* "Answers". (Ed. J.A. Little". Santa Fe New Mexico School for the Deaf.

Report of the Ad Hoc Committee to Define Deaf and Hard of Hearing 1975. *American Annals of the Deaf.* **120**. 509-512.

Rutter, M. and Cox, A. (1981)Psychiatric interviewing techniques/methods and means. *British Journal of Psychiatry,* **138**, 273-282.

Sacks, O. (1989). "Seeing Voices". Pan Books, University of California Press, Picador Edition.

Schlesinger, H.S. and Meadow, K.P. (1971). "Deafness and Mental Health, a Developmental Approach". Langley Porter Neuropsychiatric Institute, San Francisco.

Schneider, K. (1959). Primäre und sekundäre Symptomen bei Schizophrenie. *Fortschrift Neurolgie und Psychiatrie,* **25**, 487.

Wing, J.K. *(see* World Health Organization below).

Wright, D. (1969) "Deafness – A Personal Account". Stein and Day.

World Health Organization. (1973). "Report of International Pilot Study of Schizophrenia". Vol. 1. WHO Press, Geneva.

# 5. Sensory deprivation in hostage situations

Gordon Turnbull

**Introduction**

Man is limited in his awareness of reality by the nature of his special senses: the quality of these special senses is tempered by available information and shaped by previous experience. If this statement is true then a study of those who have endured the special experience of being hostages has a very special interest for those who wish to explore the boundaries of sensory reality.

The Diagnostic and Statistical Manual of the American Psychiatric Association (DSM-III, 1980 and 1987) attempted to categorize the reactions of normal individuals to unusually high-magnitude and often life-theatening stresses in terms of traumatic stress reactions and, in particular, to Post-Traumatic Stress Disorder (PTSD). The PTSD constellation is ubiquitous, is not culture-bound and takes its familiar form across the spectrum of race, religion, sex, age. It is also unmodified by the type of stressor, representing a "final common pathway" for the expression of the impact of the stress and, with typical biological parsimony, a bid to resolve it at the same time. Acute Post-Traumatic Stress Reactions have all the features of the chronic version but lack the enduring biological adaptations as described by Friedman (1991).

DSM-III describes the development of these inter-related constellations of symptoms within the rubric of PTSD: intrusive recollections of the traumatic incident, physiological hyperarousal, and avoidance phenomena including emotional "numbing". It is possible to see the trilogy of symptom clusters as a "cascade" from flashbacks to hyperarousal to avoidance, and also to view this sequential arrangement not only as inevitable but also as an arrangement with inherent survival value. That is to say, the re-experiences provide an opportunity to review and learn from hazardous life events; the hyperarousal provides the energy, drive and receptiveness to increase awareness and contribute to action if that is required, and the avoidance follows the old and trusted maxim for survivors "once bitten, twice shy". Human beings respond to stressful changes in their environment as individuals and by following homogeneous pathways. These apparently conflicting attitudes survive as happily contented bedfellows.

## Sensory Deprivation

History provides many examples of distortions of perception in those individuals who have become isolated either because they chose to be solitary or because they have been deprived of their freedom. There are accounts of perceptual distortions in sailors undertaking single-handed voyages, Arctic and Antarctic explorers, priests and mystics in retreat, space explorers and even long-distance lorry drivers as well as in prisoners and hostages. In extreme cases, when individuals are cut off from virtually all sensory stimulation, disordered perception almost inevitably occurs. It is also interesting to observe that, when formerly isolated individuals attempt to "re-enter" the normal world, there is often evidence of dramatic distortions of perception with visual illusions and hallucinations being most prominent. These more overt expressions of the central nervous system to "re-calibrate" are underpinned by a plethora of more subtle psychological, emotional and cognitive disturbances all of which are dedicated to the goal of "getting back".

The predominant conclusion seems to be that loss of sensory inputs leads to the liberation of the active subconscious mind to "imagine up" fantasies to fill the void. These fantasies may be dramatic and overwhelming. Fairly consistent levels of sensory stimulation appear to be required to maintain the sensory system in equilibrium. This has practical importance for sporting activities, in schools and universities and at work. Companionship and competition provide sensory awareness of others which is seen to be "healthy"; thus, space flights should be made by several crew members and not individually, and there may be isolation problems for divers and others working and living alone (Gregory, 1987). Palmai (1963) describes his year-long tour of duty with a team of Antarctic explorers in which he highlights the development of interpersonal difficulties within the group ranging from squabbles to ostracism. Those naturally isolated or intraverted were less affected than the more gregarious, and highly educated isolates were particularly unaffected. Palmai drew a favourable comparison between his observations and those of Bettelheim (1943) who found that intraverted individuals adapted better to the highly abnormal conditions of a concentration camp than did prisoners who were outgoing. The dynamics of the group almost certainly lead to different patterns of perceptual and emotional distortion from those which occur in the stimulation-deprived isolated individual. Palmai also observed that there appeared to be a direct relationship between morale and the number of daylight hours. The relationship between social isolation and the development of new perceptions even in groups needs to take into account the physical as well as the human environment. Rohrer (1959) related an increase in depression and apathy to a decrease in work load in US Naval personnel and Hebb (1930) has provided experimental evidence that work is an important human need.

"Brainwashing" and the experiences of prisoners-of-war repatriated at the end of World War II created a new high profile for the subject of sensory deprivation. William Sargent (1957) wrote his seminal work on brainwashing and sensory deprivation based upon his clinical experience with returned hostages and other war-trauma victims in "Battle for the Mind". In the same volume Robert Graves was invited to write upon the theme of brainwashing in ancient times which served to emphasize that basic human behaviour patterns do not seem to change.

Hebb et al. (1954) brought solitary confinement into the laboratory to test the hypothesis that an important element in brainwashing is prolonged exposure to sensory isolation. They demonstrated that volunteer subjects deprived of visual, auditory, and tactile stimulation for periods of up to seven days developed increased suggestibility. Some subjects also showed characteristic symptoms of the sensory deprivation state: anxiety, tension, inability to concentrate, body illusions, somatic complaints, uncomfortable and distressing moodstates, and vivid sensory imagery – usually visual and sometimes reaching the proportions of hallucinations with delusionary quality.

Heron, Doane and Scott (1956) reported remarks made by subjects on returning from the isolation laboratory to a normal environment indicating that disturbances of visual perception has occurred – those observed after six days in isolation were profound and prolonged. Visual disturbances began to appear soon after commencing the period of isolation. At first, mistiness and impressions of three-dimensionality began to appear. "Looking into a tunnel of fog" was described. Hallucinations emerged as soon as the second day in all participants. At first these were simple, taking the form of rows of dots, geometrical patterns and mosaics but later become more complex with the appearance of scenery, people and bizarre architecture. The effects, which were observed both monocularly and binocularly, took five forms:

1   apparent movement independent of movement by the observer – fluctuation, drifting, swirling of objects and surfaces in the visual field;

2   apparent movement associated with head or eye movements of the observer – the position of objects would appear to change when head or eye movements occurred;

3   distortions of shape;

4   accentuation of after images;

5   effects on perception of colour and contrast.

Again the clinical impression is that exposing a subject to a monotonous sensory environment can cause disorganization of brain function similar to, and in some respects as great as, that produced by drugs or lesions. Heron, Bexton and Hebb (1954) went on to describe lapses of attention in a monotonous task which have considerable practical significance for certain occupations, both military and civilian, such as watching a radar screen. These cognitive deficits, combined with potential perceptual disturbances, emphasize the need to take such factors into account in any human situation where isolation occurs. The hostage situation provides not only the correct ingredients for sensory deprivation, but does so spectacularly well, as is manifest in the classic texts of Schulz (1965) and Zubeck (1969).

## Distortion of Sensory Perception

Many types of distortion are experienced by those who are deprived of sensory inputs either in or out of the laboratory. These are divided into sensory deceptions and sensory distortions.

Illusions and hallucinations are examples of sensory deceptions. Illusions are misperceptions of sensory inputs. There are special types of mental images such as eidetic images which are vivid visual images with an accentuated pictorial quality. Pareidolia is the vivid perception of visual images in response to an indistinct stimulus such as seeing "faces" or other images in the flames of a fire or in wallpaper patterns. Here is evidence of the imagination "filling the void" as mentioned above. Hallucinations are false perceptions, due to sensory distortion or misinterpretation, which occur at the same time as background real perceptions. Certain types of hallucination have a special significance for an exploration of the theme of sensory deprivation. These are functional hallucinations provoked by a stimulus but experienced with the background stimulus; for example hearing voices from a running tap or from wind rattling roof tiles. Reflex hallucinations occur when a stimulus in one sensory modality produces a hallucination in another. Hypnagogic and hypnopompic hallucinations occur in normal people while falling asleep or waking up, respectively. They may be visual or auditory and often take the form of a voice calling a person's name. Dissociative hallucinations are intense feelings and knowledge of being in the presence of someone, or something, which the individual feels they can almost see and hear. This term is also applied to hallucinations occurring in two sensory modalities simultaneously such as the vision that also speaks; dissociative hallucinations are regarded as normal in grief states. These types of mental phenomena occur in sensory deprivation states and can be viewed as compensatory.

Sensory distortions or changes in the intensity of perceptions may result from changes in the physiological threshold of mental state, especially that of the emotions. Intensity of colour perception is enhanced in some drug-induced states and with elevation of mood, while a depressed individual might perceive the world as jaded and colourless. In depersonalization, the self, and in derealization, the world, seem unreal (Appleby and Foreshaw, 1990). Sensory distortions play a significant role in response to sensory deprivation and will be discussed in depth later.

## Theories of Sensory Deprivation

Psychological theories are epitomized by Freud (1950) who wrote "It is interesting to speculate what could happen to ego function if the excitations or stimuli from the external world were either drastically diminished or repetitive. Would there be an alteration in the unconscious mental processes and an effect upon the conceptualization of time?" Since normal ego functions such as maintaining perceptual contact with reality and logical thinking are suspended in states of sensory deprivation, the result will be confusion, irrationality, fantasy formation and the emergence of hallucinations. The subject of sensory deprivation becomes dependent upon the gaoler or the experimenter and must trust him for the satisfaction of such basic needs as feeding, toileting and physical safety. This dependency may extend into the psychopathological area of the "Stockholm Syndrome" *in extremis*, but there is room in this area also to suggest that a patient undergoing psychoanalysis or hypnosis is in a sensory deprivation laboratory (soundproofed room, subdued lighting, couch) in which primary-process mental activity is encouraged through free association and so may also have positive, therapeutic value.

Physiological theories maintain that optimal conscious awareness and accurate reality testing depend upon a baseline level of alertness. This alert state, in turn, depends on a constant stream of changing stimuli from the external world, mediated through the ascending reticular activating system in the brain stem. In sensory deprivation such a stream of stimuli is reduced, absent or impaired and alertness diminishes, direct contact with the outside world fades, and impulses from the inner body and the central nervous system may become the most prominent sensations and may then proceed to become the basis of the distortions which lead to the development of hallucinations.

Cognitive theories emphasize that the brain is an information-processing machine, the purpose of which is optimal adaptation to the perceived environment. If the machine lacks sufficient information it will be unable to form a cognitive map, against which incoming current information is matched. The results are disorganization and maladaptation. This interesting viewpoint maintains that, in order to monitor one's own behaviour and attain optimal responsiveness, the brain must receive continuous feedback. Without this feedback, the individual is forced to project outward idiosyncratic themes from within the self as a means of compensation for the inadequate system. These projected themes may have little relationship to reality. This situation bears a close resemblance to the cognitive hypotheses of the development of psychoses (Kaplan and Sadock, 1991).

The common element in all theoretical approaches to the phenomena of sensory deprivation is the mobilization of internally stored mental material to fill the void when sensory stimuli from the external environment are reduced. The resultant psychological and physiological state was recognized in ancient Greece and can be successfully replicated in the laboratory.

**Dissociation**

Recent experiences in the psychological debriefing of released prisoners-of-war and released hostages (Mitchell, 1988; Dyregov, 1989; Turnbull and Busuttil, 1993) have reaffirmed that dissociative defence mechanisms are of fundamental importance in survival.

Dissociation implies that mental processes are coexistent or alternate without becoming connected. They also do not influence one another. Before Freud described the Unconscious, dissociation was a term much used in psychiatry to explain many neurotic symptoms such as "repression" or "splitting". The historical postulate was that dissociation represented a constitutional weakness of the integrative function, as a result of which performing actions, thinking thoughts, dreaming by day and night became disconnected from the real personality. Freud suggested that dissociation consists of a collection of phenomena through which the subject maintains a course of action in which he appears not to be motivated by his usual self; or, alternatively, his usual self appears not to have access to recent memories that he would normally be expected to have. Examples would be sleep-walking, trances, fugues (in which the subject wanders off, not knowing who or where he is), loss of memory for a definite, recent period of time and multiple personality in which the subject appears to change from one person to an alternative one. These mental mechanisms are activated at the unconscious level (Gregory, 1987) and are protective against anxiety.

Dissociation may represent the fundamental psychobiological mechanism underlying a wide variety of altered forms of consciousness, trance, multiple personality, fugue states and spirit possession states. This mechanism has great individual and species survival value. Under certain conditions, it serves to facilitate at least seven major functions (Ludwig, 1983):

1  automatization of certain behaviours;
2  efficiency and economy of effort;
3  resolution of irreconcilable conflicts;
4  escape from the constraints of reality;
5  isolation of catastrophic experiences;
6  cathartic discharge of emotions;
7  enhancement of "herd sense", e.g. submersion of the individual ego for the group identity or greater suggestibility.

Dissociation may therefore be an extreme point on a continuum of awareness that also includes repression, denial, suppression, and full awareness, which is compatible with the Freudian concept. These altered ego states are characterized by difficulty in assessing and evaluating perceptions of the external world, and by disturbances of the sense of self; they include such conditions as depersonalization and derealization; disturbances of the sense of time, such as timelessness and deja vu phenomena; fugue states; multiple personality disorders; and the sense of the uncanny. Such conditions are not clinical entities in themselves. They occur as symptoms of many conditions and even occur in everyday life (Arlow, 1992).

Although unconscious mental mechanisms may be ultimately responsible for the deployment of such phenomena, it remains possible that chemical substances might also precipitate them. This possibility always exists in the case of hostages, whose captors control the supply of food and drink. Haltresht (1976) has epitomized this conundrum by exploring Thomas de Quincey's pre-Freudian dream, "Dream-Fugue Founded on the Preceding Theme of Sudden Death" found in the English Mail Coach. The dream is examined on several levels, and its content and symbolism are related to facts of de Quincey's life. The collision of his mail coach with a gig carrying a young couple provided the raw material, but on other levels the dream is seen to represent for de Quincey a paradigm for human helplessness in the face of a disaster and suffering and his own ambivalent and guilt-ridden relationship with women. Elements related to de Quincey's addiction to opium, and to his feelings towards his mother and sister, are discussed. Opium caused his deepest wishes and anxieties to emerge in dream form as he struggled with his misery, fears and desires for forgiveness for his sins, real or imagined.

McKinney and Lange (1983) postulated a genetic factor in the development of fugue states, although there may also be a learned aspect. They described a fugue involving a 24-year-old, whose father had also experienced fugue states. The subject was hospitalized and interviewed while under the influence of sodium amytal, during which he discussed his overwhelming desire to run away. He was treated successfully with assertiveness training and brief group and individual psychotherapy.

Steingard and Frankel (1985) suggested that some highly hypnotizable subjects may experience transient but severe psychotic states. Thus Keller and Shaywitz (1986) describe a 16-year-old male with total retrograde amnesia. No evidence was found for organic causes, toxic-metabolic derangements, epilepsy, encephalitis, vasculitis, trauma or central nervous system tumour. He had experienced a psychogenic fugue state with spontaneous recovery in memory over several days.

That emergent dissociative material can have all of the qualities of real experience is confirmed by Haberman (1986) in the case of a 37-year-old Vietnam veteran who developed flashbacks 10 months after returning from duty. When he heard dogs barking, he would suddenly feel as if he were back in Vietnam. During one of these episodes, he took a gun and was chased in the woods by the police, who were using dogs to find him. Upon hearing the dogs approach, he felt as if he were about to be captured by the Viet Cong and shot himself.

Cancio (1991) studied the stress of freefall parachuting in US Army trainees, finding that about 35% of 59 subjects (aged 18-63 years) who completed a survey indicated that they had experienced either a trance-like state or an episode of altered consciousness before, during, or after a jump. The respondents agreed that skydiving is a stressful sport, but only at times. A majority of subjects used mental imagery or another mental or physical technique to prepare for jumps. Results supported the notion that stress facilitates the development of an hypnotic trance. Such a trance, when unconsciously evoked during emergencies (spontaneous dissociation), may account for some parachuting accidents: alternatively self-hypnosis may provide the jumper with a way to control his level of arousal and facilitate cognitive rehearsal, thus enhancing performance (Cancio, 1991).

Crip (1983) described multiple personality as a dissociative condition in which there are two or more autonomous personalities. Fugue states, amnesia, fainting spells and feelings of strangeness and unfamiliarity usually occur. Somnambulistic states are often reported to have been present in childhood. The most important diagnostic criterion of multiple personality is that each personality exists in the body of an individual and has a highly developed form of its own. These personalities can alternate (although one becomes dominant at any one time) may be co-conscious when one functions consciously while the other functions unconsciously, or be intra-conscious when one personality knows the thoughts of the other.

**The Hostage Situation**

Released hostages and prisoners-of-war will inevitably have been affected by the experience. This need not be a detrimental influence in their lives but the re-entry phase into normal life will require adjustments. The term "survivor" for such a person is therefore preferred to one much used, "victim", simply because there is real opportunity in the re-adjustment for personal growth and maturation. The foregoing material suggests the profound potential for altered perception, sensitivity, thinking and mood when hitherto normal people re-emerge from periods of sensory deprivation, especially after prolonged periods of captivity during which the new modes of perception and thinking have moved on from the initial bewilderment phase to a novel, stable "modus vivendi".

It is impossible to exclude a mention of psychological debriefing when discussing this subject but full description is beyond the scope of this chapter. Psychological debriefing is a process of making a detailed, progressive review of the events since the identified critical incident – in this case being captured – with a systematic review of the feelings and emotions associated with these events. This has to be approached flexibly, non-judgementally and at the pace dictated by the survivor. The aims are reconstruction of the memories of the traumatic events without distortions, assimilation of the resultant, clarified material, integration of meaning, and emotional ventilation without the encouragement of catharsis. The overall goal is to restore normal function (RAF Psychiatric Division, 1993).

From the moment of capture the victim is held in a state of "torture" by his captors. The World Medical Assembly has defined torture in the Declaration of Tokyo of 1975 as "the deliberate or wanton infliction of physical or mental suffering by one or more persons acting alone or on the orders of any authority, to force another person to yield information, to make a confession or for any other reason." Both physical and psychological means of torture are used. It is important to realize that physical torture also has a psychological impact. Psychological tortures are described by Somnier and Genefke (1986). They categorize methods into "weakening techniques" and "personality destroying techniques". The former is designed to induce helplessness in the victim and the latter to induce guilt, fear and loss of self-esteem. Delivery is by adoption of three main strategies, which are described as Deprivation, Constraint, and Communication.

Deprivation, (of especial relevance to this chapter) means the reduction of environmental stimulation. Schultz (1965) lists visual deprivations as taking the form of poor lighting, contrast and colour and the use of blindfolds; auditory stimulation is limited to whispers within the group of hostages, threatening commands from the guards, and deliberately muted sounds from the external environment. Sensations of smell and taste are limited by monotonous diet and a stale atmosphere. Touch may be limited by the confines of a small cell and few, if any, personal possessions. Kinaesthetic deprivation results from constraint of limbs with ties or chains with consequent impairment of movement, physical discomfort and pain (Zubeck, 1969).

Constraint forcibly submits victims to experiences and stimuli alien to them in respect of their accustomed codes of conduct and personality. Victims are commanded to obey regulations in a setting of close supervision and over which they have no control. Violation of the rules results in punishment. Dignity and identity are violated by humiliation and further degraded by inadequate sanitation and hygiene. Making impossible choices and mock executions also come under this rubric. Hostages are deprived of their own emotionality since aggressive drives must be repressed if survival remains a goal.

Communication strategies utilize exposure to ambiguous and contradictory messages designed to induce confusion. Turner and Gorst-Unsworth (1990) reviewed the literature and described psychological reactions to torture as being tri-dimensional. First, the traumatic stress reaction characterized by the familiar core features of post-traumatic stress disorder described at the beginning of this chapter, re-experiencing, hyperarousal and avoidance phenomena. Second, the "Existential Dilemma" which fundamentally addresses the dilemma of having to return to a world which they now know from first-hand experience contains such horrors as torture and feeling guilty about behaviour during incarceration. Third, the development of depression: mainly the result of loss events including the loss of parts of the body, health, family, friends, freedom and social status.

Symonds (1980) recognized that victim responses follow a set and sequential pattern regardless of the type of insult to the individual. He drew his conclusions from extensive studies of hostage-takings, kidnappings, robberies and rape. He described four phases, the duration and intensity of each being influenced by the nature and quality of contact with the perpetrator. Symonds found that victims of sudden, unexpected violent crime initially respond with shock and disbelief – a denial mechanism. The second phase follows close on the first and is characterized by emotional reactions including rage, apathy, resignation, irritability, tension and also by recollection of the trauma through dreams and fantasies. Self-recrimination is also a frequent facet of the second phase. In the third phase, Symonds suggests that previous personality traits begin to exert their influence. Those with high dependency traits appear to become depressed and introspective. Phobic behaviours tend to grow from this development and risk the formation of hostile dependent relationships with family and friends after the ordeal. Others with more "freedom-orientated, detached, power-orientated and aggressive" personalities tend to show intensified trait behaviours leading to social withdrawal and reclusive, paranoid irritability. Phase three is seen only in traumatic events of short duration and long-term hostages tend to remain in phase two because of the torture. Phase four is reached as the individual attempts to integrate the traumatic experience, comes to terms with it and moves into the future. This phase of resolution and integration is characterized by the development of sharpened psychological barriers such as defensiveness and increased vigilance. Revision of values and also attitudes towards other people are often profound.

In the case of hostages held for long periods, these phases cannot be processed until after release; they are in suspension until the fear reaction has subsided. In the case of hostages, exposure to torture, solitary and group confinement will inevitably lead to the emergence of complex patterns of adaptive behaviour during captivity, the resolution of which after release result in a challenging prospect for those involved in rehabilitation (Busuttil and Turnbull, 1993).

## Solitary and Group Confinement

Solitary confinement is the extreme form of isolation. It may be experienced as a kind of special punishment, a part of a psychological torture, or may be inevitable if the victim is the only hostage taken. The effects of isolation have been recognized for many years and were described by Allers (1920) and Eitinger (1961). Both authors reported acute psychotic disturbances among prisoners-of-war who were unable to communicate effectively because of language barriers. Early studies of voluntary immigrants revealed an increased incidence of psychosis, a similar phenomenon (Oodegaard, 1932). Eitinger's later study of voluntary immigrants and refugees (1959) revealed an incidence of psychosis five times higher than expected in a control Norwegian population.

The deprivation strategy already mentioned and used by captors in their torture of hostages can result in the development of the "Concentration Camp Syndrome" and "risk annihilation as a person" (Solomon and Keelman, 1985). At face value, group confinement appears a preferable option, compared with solitary confinement. Zubeck (1969) has summarized the particular difficulties which arise out of group confinement under three headings: Interpersonal Stresses: Group Interactions, and Relationships with the Outside World.

Interpersonal stresses are the result of overt and covert interpersonal frictions leading to irritability and hostility. Group interactions in a confined group depend on the members' interdependence for purposes of survival; in effect, individuals cannot alienate the remainder of the group and overt expressions of the problems provoked by the confinement are blocked. Communication and other interactive activities are seen to decline with time. Territoriality and privacy needs become steadily pre-eminent and the end result is withdrawal from group activities. Zubeck (1969) has described the apparent paradox of loneliness despite sharing confinement with others. In some cases this can take the form of diurnal inversion, sleeping by day and being awake and by oneself at night. An interesting example can be the development of the ability to dissociate at will. This affords a "comfort zone", always attainable provided that distractions are kept to a minimum, and an unbroken thread of "escape" and "release" to be woven into the otherwise flimsy and ragged fabric of an existence filled with wretchedness, despair and pessimism. The meaningfulness and influence of the outside world is downgraded in hostage groups, and can provide a useful point of attack at which the group can project outwards its frustrations. People and objects outside the group are attacked. Politicians, governments and even friends or relatives are frequent targets for vicious criticism.

A special situation is the difficulty encountered by an established group of hostages in its bid to integrate another hostage who has previously been held in solitary confinement. Here the two different styles of adaptation clash in an extreme and incompatible way. Busuttil and Turnbull (1993) report the remarkable supremacy in strength of the repressive defence mechanisms when compared with the expressive. Only later, following release, were the conflicts revealed during confidential debriefing sessions. In the case of hostages, much anger will inevitably be directed against the captors, although transference and counter-transference issues including the development of the "Stockhom Syndrome" (Symonds, 1980), cannot be ignored.

## Coping with Confinement

Schultz (1965) has described a variety of coping techniques used by hostages and others in confinement. The most frequently described method is some form of mental exercise ranging from counting actual to complex intellectual diversions, keeping a diary or log is another frequently used technique, as is some form of work (Peters and Nichol, 1992, and Mann, 1991).

Another common factor found in survivors of confinement was the conviction that they would inevitably survive. A striking example of this phenomenon is described by Cohen (1954) who emphasizes that, despite the high death rates in the Nazi concentration camps, the optimism for ultimate survival increased the longer the imprisonment lasted. Moreover, survival by any means became the dominant motivating factor in such cases.

There are considerably fewer descriptions of emotional distress producing problems in confined groups than in studies of individual isolation. This may be the result of the effectiveness of the repressive defence mechanisms described above, blocking expression of distress. Certainly descriptions of illusions, hallucinations and other psychotic symptoms are rare. More characteristic are insomnia, depression, compulsive behaviour and psychosomatic disorders (Zubeck, 1969).

Studies which compare the effects of both types of isolation are rare. In one such study, however, Ursano et al. (1981a) observe that the development of psychiatric symptoms, mainly those of PTSD, were less likely to develop in US Air Force Vietnam veterans who were captured after 1969, when solitary confinement fell out of favour as a means of holding prisoners-of-war. Another study by Ursano *et al.* (1981*b*) suggests that the "group" exerts a strongly protective effect for confined prisoners. Despite the development of an increased sense of "territoriality" and "need for privacy" and their influence towards social withdrawal, prisoners in group confinement are still likely to talk, at least informally, together about their predicament (McCarthy and Morrell, 1993; Keenan, 1992). Indeed, strong bonds of friendship may develop which persist after release. The facts of their situation, resultant emotions and feelings, and their sensory perceptions or lack of them can, at least, be shared and contrasted. These are the basic elements of Critical Incident Stress Debriefing (Mitchell, 1988) and Psychological Debriefing (Dyregov, 1989) which are thought to be protective against the development of PTSD. Those confined in a group may, therefore, instinctively "debrief" each other as the predicament unfolds. In the case of the British hostages released from Beirut in 1991 the improvement in living conditions, including the provision of a radio which permitted not only contact with the outside world but also with their own culture, further optimized "re-entry".

## The Psychological Impact of being a Hostage

As described, the experience of being held hostage is multi-faceted and exposes victims to a wide variety of stressors. This raises the question as to whether the resultant psychological impact is similarly multi-faceted. Our closer look at the nature of the stressors reveals many common threads. There appear to be four distinct categories of significant psychiatric sequelae to exposure to the extremely stressful circumstances of being held hostage:

1   Stress disorder: mainly PTSD as a result of the initial trauma of capture, subjection to torture, solitary and group confinement experiences and the positive relationship between PTSD and weight loss (Sutker *et al.*, 1990).

2   Depressive disorders: most strongly correlated with torture, loss events and being held hostage.

3   Cognitive defect states: related to weight loss, head injury and central nervous system infections.

4   Psychosis: strongly associated with solitary confinement and sensory deprivation.

Any attempt at rehabilitation after release of hostages must therefore take into account that all or some of these clinical states might be present. The work of reconstruction can commence only after careful initial assessment, essential to exclude the development and severity of any of the above potential clinical states.

## Concluding Thoughts

This chapter has been written to introduce the reader to the types of stress which hostages have to endure, and to explain the psychological impact of such stresses and the ways in which hostages cope with their unenviable situation. The experimental work on sensory deprivation is very helpful in enhancing the understanding of the effect of solitary confinement on, in particular, human beings.

"No man is an island", wrote Donne and this is never more true than for the hostage, despite the closest possible approximation to that state of stark isolation and removal from others.

Re-entry of the released hostage will, inevitably, involve reunion with family and friends. In order to promote the optimal reunion, reintegration and rehabilitation of the family unit, it is essential that an understanding is sought, and gained, of the psychological consequences for the family members left behind. The enforced separation has made them into hostages too.

## References

Allers, R. (1920). Uber psychogene storungen in sprachfremder unbetung (der verfolungswahnder sprachlich isolierten. *Zeitschrift für gesamte Neurolgie und Psychiatrie,* **60**, 281-289.
American Psychiatric Association (1980). "Diagnostic and Statistical Manual of Mental Disorders III". American Psychiatric Association, Washington.
Appleby, L. and Foreshaw, D. (1990). "Postgraduate Psychiatry". Butterworth-Heinemann, Oxford.
Arlow, J.A. (1992). Altered ego states. *Israel Journal of Psychiatry and Related Sciences,* **29**, 65-76.
Bettelheim, B. (1943). *Journal of Abnormal Social Psychology,* **38**, 417.
Busuttil, W. (1993). Prolonged incarceration: effects on prisoners of war and hostages of terrorism (awaiting publication – refer to author).
Cancio, L.C. (1991). Stress and trance in freefall parachuting: a pilot study. *American Journal of Clinical Hypnosis,* **33**, 225-234.
Cohen, E.A. (1954). "Human Behaviour in the Concentration Camp". Jonathan Cape, London.
Crip, P. (1983). Object relations and multiple personality: an exploration of the literature. *Psychoanalytical Review,* **70**, 221-234.
Dyregov, A. (1989). Psychological debriefing. Paper presented at the survival seminar at the Tavistock Institute of Human Relations, March 1989, Proceedings.
Eitinger, L. (1961). Pathology of the concentration camp syndrome. *Archives of General Psychiatry,* **5**, 371-379.
Eitenger, L. (1980). The concentration camp syndrome and its late sequelae in survivors, victims, and perpetrators. "Essays on the Nazi Holocaust". (Ed. J.E. Dimsdale), Hemisphere, Washington.
Freud, S. (1922). Group psychology and the analysis of the ego. Trans. Strachey, J. (1955). *In* "Complete Psychological Works" Vol. xviii, London.
Friedman, M.J. (1991). Biological approaches to the diagnosis and treatment of post-traumatic stress disorder. *Journal of Traumatic Stress,* **4**, 67-92.
Gregory, R.L. (1987). "The Oxford Companion to the Mind". Oxford University Press, Oxford, New York.

Haberman, M.A. (1986). Spontaneous trance or dissociation: a suicide attempt in a schizophrenic Vietnam veteran. *American Journal of Clinical Hypnosis*, **28**, 177-182.

Haltresht, M. (1976). The meaning of de Quincey's "Dream-Fugue on sudden death". *Literature and Psychology*, **26**, 31-36.

Hebb, D.O. (1930). *Teachers Magazine (Montreal)*, **12**, 23.

Heron, W., Bexton, W.H. and Hebb, D.O. (1953). Cognitive effects of decreased variation in the sensory environment. *The American Psychologist*, **8**, 366.

Heron, W., Doane, B.K. and Scott, T.H. (1956). Visual disturbances after prolonged perceptual isolation. *Canadian Journal of Psychology*, **10**, 13-16.

Kaplan, H.I. and Sadock, B.I. (1991). "Synopsis of Psychiatry". 6th Edn. Williams and Wilkins, Baltimore.

Keenan, B. (1992). "An Evil Cradling". Hutchinson, London.

Keller, R. and Shaywitz, B.A. (1986). Amnesia or fugue state: a diagnostic dilemma. *Journal of Developmental and Behavioural Pediatrics*, **7**, 131-132.

Ludwig, A.M. (1983). The psychobiological functions of dissociation. *American Journal of Clinical Hypnosis*, **26**, 93-99.

Mann, J. and Mann, S. (1992). "Yours Till The End". W.H. Publishing, London.

McCarthy, J. and Morrell, J. (1993). "Some Other Rainbow". Bantam Press, Transworld Publishers, London.

McKinney, K.A. and Lange, M.M. (1983). Familial fugue: a case report. *Canadian Journal of Psychiatry*, **28**, 654-656.

Mitchell, J. (1988). The history, status and future of critical incident stress debriefing. *Journal of Emergency Medical Services*, Nov. 1988.

Oodegard, O. (1932). "Emigration and Insanity". Copenhagen.

Palmai, G. (1963). Psychological observations on an isolated group in Antarctica. *British Journal of Psychiatry*, **109**, 364-370.

Peters, J. and Nichol, J. (1992). "Tornado Down". Michael Joseph, Penguin Books, London.

Rohrer, J.H. (1959). *US Naval Reserve Review*.

Royal Air Force Psychiatric Division, (1993). The debriefing of released British hostages from Beirut. *British Journal of Psychiatry*, (Bulletin) January 1993.

Sargant, W. (1957). "Battle for the Mind: a Physiology of Conversion and Brain-washing". Heinemann, London.

Schultz, D.P. (1965). "Sensory Restriction: Effects on Behaviour". Academic Press, New York.

Solomon, P. and Kleeman, S.T. (1985). Sensory deprivation. *In* "Comprehensive Textbook of Psychiatry". 4th Edn. (Eds H. Kaplan and B.J. Sadock). pp. 321-326. Baltimore.

Somnier, F.E. and Genefke, I.K. (1986). Psychotherapy for victims of torture. *British Journal of Psychiatry*, **149**, 323-329.

Steingard, S. and Frankel, F.H. (1985). Dissociation and psychotic symptoms. *American Journal of Psychiatry*, **142**, 953-955.

Symonds, M. (1980). Victim responses to terror. *Annals of New York Academy of Sciences*, **347**, 129-136.

Turnbull, G.J. (1992). Debriefing British POWs after the Gulf War and released hostages from Lebanon. *Wismic Newsletter*, **4**, 4-6.

Turner, S. and Gorst-Unsworth, C. (1990). Psychological sequelae: a descriptive model. *British Journal of Psychiatry*, **157**, 475-480.

Ursano, R.J. (1981a). The Vietnam era prisoner of war: pre-captivity personality and the development of psychiatric illness. *American Journal of Psychiatry*, **138**, 315-318.

Ursano, R.J. (1981b). Psychiatric illness in US Air Force Vietnam prisoners of war: a five year follow up. *American Journal of Psychiatry*, **138**, 310-315.
Zubeck, J.P. (1969). "Sensory Deprivation: Fifteen Years of Research". Appleton-Century-Crofts, New York.

# 6. Recognition and reality

Andrew W. Young

## Introduction

All of us know that if we are very ill, or under the influence of drink or drugs, we may lose our grip on reality and start to misperceive or imagine things, and even to act on them. Conversely, we know, too, that we can daydream when awake, or have "lucid" dreams whilst asleep, without mistaking these imaginings as real.

How can we so easily see one group of phenomena as unreal, yet accept other imaginings as real? Wherein lies the difference? The question is seldom raised, because we so much take for granted our experience of the reality of the external world. Yet it is central to everyday conceptions of insanity, in which loss of touch with reality is a central feature. Moreover, the discoveries of modern science do not reveal that the world is exactly as it is presented to us by our senses.

Striking examples of failures of reality discrimination arise in hallucinations. Slade and Bentall (1988) have marshalled impressive evidence pointing to the conclusion that hallucinators mistake internally generated phenomena for external events, and have shown that they suffer more widespread difficulties in distinguishing between internal and external states. Much the same point arises in confabulation, which can also be seen as a disturbance of reality testing (Benson and Stuss, 1990). Some patients can provide vivid accounts of memories and events which are entirely fictitious, yet they do not seem to be deliberately lying. These confabulations occur in people who have suffered damage to the frontal lobes (Stuss *et al.*, 1978). In the absence of any easy way of distinguishing fantasy from reality, the confabulator may take her or his imaginings as real.

One of the ways in which we establish the "reality" of things and events is by recognizing them as meaningful and appropriate to the context in which we are located. If you saw a herd of elephants enter your living room, you might well be disconcerted if you did not recognize the source of the image as a television screen. In fact, studies of mental illness have shown that some patients will treat television images as real (Förstl *et al.*, 1991*b*) or, conversely, react to everyday events as if they were part of an elaborate film production (Shubsachs and Young, 1988; Vié, 1944).

More specific misidentifications can also be caused by brain disease, where they may arise as part of a confusional state or in an otherwise clear sensorium

(Geschwind, 1982). Like confabulations, these delusional misidentifications imply a failure of reality testing (Benson and Stuss, 1990), and they can lead to extraordinary statements about the misidentified objects, such as that relatives have been replaced by impostors, or that the patient is in a hospital which is an exact duplicate of the original but in a different geographical location.

This chapter examines how visual recognition mechanisms support our experience of reality by looking at some of the consequences of recognition impairments, and especially those caused by brain injury. This will involve considering our emotional reactions to visual stimuli relate to our ability to recognize them, and examining preserved non-conscious aspects of recognition in cases of face recognition impairment after brain injury (prosopagnosia), everyday recognition errors, and delusional misidentifications in psychiatric and neuropsychiatric patients.

## Preference and Overt Recognition

It is tempting to equate recognition with the ability to recognize things overtly and make an explicit identification. However, evidence suggests that overt recognition is only part of a much more complex process. In particular, studies following from the seminal work of Zajonc and colleagues have found that certain types of affective reaction to familiar visual stimuli need not depend on overt recognition (Bornstein, 1989; Kunst-Wilson and Zajonc, 1980; Zajonc, 1980).

In a now famous experiment, Kunst-Wilson and Zajonc (1980) showed people some eight-sided random shapes. Five exposures of each shape were given, but these were all for only 1 msec so that the shapes could not be consciously seen. Afterwards, each of the shapes was paired with a new (unseen) shape, and subjects were asked which they had seen before, which they preferred, and how certain they were of each judgement. Although recognition of previously seen shapes was at chance level, people did tend to prefer them.

In experiments on preference, people often prefer things that are familiar to things that are novel. However, Kunst-Wilson and Zajonc's (1980) findings show that this preference for familiarity can extend to stimuli the familiarity of which need not be consciously recognized at all. It is therefore clear that preference need not depend on overt recognition. As Zajonc (1980) explains, such findings contradict the commonly held assumption that affect is postcognitive. Instead, he suggests that "affective judgements may be fairly independent of, and precede in time, the sorts of perceptual and cognitive operations commonly assumed to be the basis of these affective judgements. Affective reactions to stimuli are often the very first reactions of the organism, and for lower organisms they are the dominant reactions." (Zajonc, 1980, p. 151).

Surprising though they may be, similar findings have been reported in other studies (Bornstein, 1989). Of course, there is a sense in which the familiarity of the briefly presented stimuli must have been registered somewhere in the visual system in order for subjects to show any preference. But the important point is that this is independent of consciously experienced recognition that the preferred stimuli have been seen before. Some form of non-conscious recognition is involved.

## Covert Recognition in Prosopagnosia

A dramatic demonstration that recognition mechanisms can operate automatically and non-consciously has come from studies of prosopagnosia, a neurological impairment characterized by an apparent inability to recognize familiar faces (Meadows, 1974).

Prosopagnosic patients usually fail all tests of overt recognition of familiar faces. They cannot name the face, give the person's occupation or other biographical details, or even state whether or not a face belongs to a familiar person. Even the most well-known faces may not be recognized, including famous people, friends, family, and the patient's own face when looking in a mirror. The patients know when they are looking at a face, and can often describe and identify facial features, or even use facial information to determine age, sex, and expression, but appear not to experience any sense of recognizing to whom the face might belong. In order to recognize familiar people, they must thus rely on non-facial cues, such as voice, name, and sometimes even clothing or gait.

The brain lesions that cause prosopagnosia involve inferior and mesial occipitotemporal cortex and underlying white matter, especially in the region of the lingual, fusiform and parahippocampal gyri (Damasio et al., 1982; Meadows, 1974). Often, the cerebral damage is more extensive, or, macroscopically confined to the right cerebral hemisphere (De Renzi, 1986; Landis et al., 1986; Meadows, 1974; Sergent and Villemure, 1989).

Although prosopagnosic patients no longer recognize familiar faces overtly, there is substantial evidence of covert, non-conscious recognition from physiological and behavioural measures (Bruyer, 1991; Young and de Haan, 1992).

Bauer (1984) used the Guilty Knowledge Test, a technique sometimes used in criminal investigations, which is based on the view that a guilty person will show some involuntary physiological response to stimuli related to the crime. He measured skin conductance whilst a prosopagnosic patient, LF, viewed a familiar face and listened to a list of names. When the name belonged to the face LF was looking at, there was a greater skin conductance change than when someone else's name was read out. Yet if LF was asked to choose which name in the list was correct for the face, his performance was at chance level. Comparable findings have been reported with a different technique in which the patients simply looked at a series of familiar and unfamiliar faces (Tranel and Damasio, 1985; 1988). Skin conductance changes were greater to familiar than unfamiliar faces, even though the patients experienced no sense of familiarity.

Behavioural indices of covert recognition complement these electrophysiological measures. Eye movement scan-paths differ to familiar and unfamiliar faces, despite the absence of overt recognition (Rizzo et al., 1987). The patients are better at matching photographs of familiar faces than photographs of unfamiliar faces across transformations of orientation or age (de Haan et al., 1987; Sergent and Poncet, 1990). In name classification tasks, they show interference from simultaneously presented face distractors (de Haan et al., 1987) and priming from previously presented face primes (Young et al., 1988). When looking at a face, they are better at learning correct information than incorrect information about that person (de Haan et al., 1987; de Haan et al., 1991a; Sergent and Poncet, 1990). This superior learning of correct over incorrect information is found even for faces of people who have been known only since the patient's illness (de Haan et al., 1987). All of these findings imply that faces can be recognized to some degree, even though the patient is not aware of this.

A question which naturally arises concerns whether or not such findings will hold for all patients with severely impaired overt face recognition ability. In fact, although covert recognition has been demonstrated for some patients with a number of techniques, several patients who failed to show covert recognition have also been reported in the literature (see Young and de Haan, 1992, for a review). As clinicians have long suspected, there is more than one form of prosopagnosia (De Renzi et al., 1991; Meadows, 1974); the presence or absence of covert recognition may thus provide an important pointer to the nature of the functional impairment in each case.

For cases with covert recognition, what seem to be preserved are those aspects of recognition the operation of which is relatively automatic and does not require conscious initiation (Young, 1988). We might therefore expect that the Zajonc "preference" effect would be among those shown by such patients, and this has been demonstrated by Greve and Bauer (1990). They showed faces to the prosopagnosic patient LF for 500 msec each, and then paired each of these faces with a completely novel face. LF tended to choose the faces shown to him previously as being "more likeable" than the faces he had not seen before, whereas, when he was, told that he had seen one of the faces before and asked which it was he performed at chance level. This is equivalent to the findings of preference without overt recognition in normal subjects.

Such findings profoundly alter our conception of the nature of prosopagnosia, since they show that it is inadequate to think of it as simply involving loss of recognition mechanisms. Instead, at least some degree of recognition does take place; what the patient has lost is *awareness of recognition*.

Bauer (1984; 1986) offered an intriguing hypothesis concerning the neuroanatomical pathways involved in this phenomenon. He suggested that overt recognition depends on a ventral visual system-limbic system pathway involving ventromedial occipitotemporal cortex, whereas a more dorsal visual-limbic pathway through the superior temporal sulcus and the inferior parietal lobule subserves processes of emotional arousal. In prosopagnosia, the ventral pathway is impaired, whereas the dorsal pathway may remain intact, leading to covert recognition of familiar faces that cannot be recognized overtly.

It is worth spending a little more time on the properties Bauer attributed to the dorsal pathway. He suggested that it "subserves processes of selective attention and tonic emotional arousal, and is implicated in the process whereby 'relevance' is attached to an attended object" (Bauer, 1984, p.466). Thus it has multiple functions encompassing automatic emotional responses to stimuli which have personal relevance; these have been widely implicated as putative specialized functions of the right cerebral hemisphere (Bear, 1983; Van Lancker, 1991).

**Everyday Errors**

Prosopagnosia involves a dense and often permanent impairment of overt recognition, but there are also transitory errors which all of us make from time to time. Studies of these everyday difficulties and errors show that many of them reflect breakdown at different levels of overt recognition (Young et al., 1985). For example:

1  We may completely fail to recognize a familiar face, and mistakenly think that the person is unfamiliar.

2  We may recognize the face as familiar, but be unable to bring to mind any other details about the person, such as her or his occupation or name.

3  We may recognize the face as familiar and remember appropriate semantic information about the person, whilst failing to remember her or his name.

The orderliness of these types of everyday error suggests that overt recognition involves some form of sequential access to different types of information, in the order familiarity then semantics then name retrieval, and other studies of normal subjects have given strong support to this suggestion (Ellis, 1992).

Each of these types of error can also arise after neurological impairment. In such cases, a brain-injured patient will make her or his characteristic error to many or almost all seen faces. In prosopagnosia, for example, known faces seen unfamiliar, which corresponds to error type 1. My colleagues and I have recently reported a case in which known faces were familiar only (de Haan et al., 1991b), corresponding to error type 2. In anomia (a defect in the ability to name objects), name retrieval to known faces may become problematic even though semantic information can be properly accessed (Flude et al., 1989), as in error type 3.

We thus have converging evidence from studies of normal people and people with brain injuries indicating that the functional organization of the face recognition system involves sequential access to different types of information. Recent work has therefore concentrated on how this might be achieved, and Burton and his colleagues have offered plausible computer simulations (Bruce et al., 1990; 1992).

The basic structure of Burton et al.'s (1990) model consists of of active units connected to each other by modifiable links which can be excitatory or inhibitory. Their model is able to simulate known properties of the face recognitions system derived from experimental studies and, surprisingly, it provides a simple account of some aspects of covert recognition in prosopagnosia. This is because preserved priming and interference effects without explicit classification of face inputs, which are functionally equivalent to effects found in cases of prosopagnosic, can be demonstrated with the Burton et al. (1990) model by halving the connection strengths between two of its pools of units (Burton et al., 1991). This makes the finding of this pattern in some cases of prosopagnosia much less mysterious, though it does not provide a complete account of covert recognition effects; for example, the simulation does not offer any detailed explanation of the skin conductance findings, for which a neurological model such as Bauer's (1984; 1986) may well be more useful.

Bauer's (1984) model is also important in that it highlights the interplay of cognitive and affective aspects of recognition. This interplay may be important in generating anomalous experiences that all of us have from time to time, and which can also arise in pathological states, such as déjà vu (Fleminger, 1991; Sno and Linszen, 1990).

**Delusional Misidentification**

Delusional misidentification is a problem which used to be considered to be purely "psychodynamic", but modern neuro-imaging techniques have revealed evidence of brain injury in many cases. Recent reviews have therefore emphasized the importance of organic factors in delusional misidentification (Cutting, 1991; Förstl et al., 1991a), and modern psychiatric opinion is that a thorough search for organic factors should always be made when such delusions are present (Collins et al., 1990).

Different types of delusional misidentification have been identified by clinicians (Vié, 1944). Joseph (1986) gives a list of 11 specific variants, which are usually considered as distinct syndromes, but we can question the wider appropriateness of the syndrome concept since each of the types of delusional misidentification is really only defined by a single symptom (the delusion itself) and they can quite often occur in combination with each other (Cutting, 1991; Förstl et al., 1991a).

Here, I will concentrate on two of the most widely discussed forms of delusional misidentification; the Capgras delusion (Capgras and Reboul-Lachaux, 1923), in which patients claim that relatives have been replaced by "doubles" or impostors, and reduplicative paramnesia (Pick, 1903), in which patients claim to be in a "duplicate" hospital.

## The Capgras delusion

The Capgras delusion used to be considered very rare, perhaps because it is often unrecognized, and its prevalence is probably rather higher than was once thought (Förstl et al., 1991a,b). The patient's belief that relatives (and sometimes non-relatives) have been replaced by impostors usually seems to be genuinely and strongly held, but can have some curious features. The impostors are usually considered to be almost exact replicas of the originals, but the patients tend to claim that they differ in some way which is difficult to put into words. A case we investigated, ML, expressed it like this: "There's been someone like my son's double which isn't my son... I can tell my son because my son is different... but you have got to be quick to notice it." (Young *et al.*, in press).

Most Capgras patients do not show too much concern about what has happened to their "real" relatives, and some of them accept the substitutes with a compliant equanimity; Wallis (1986) pointed out that a substantial proportion (around 30%) were friendly toward the duplicates. However, there are also cases where there is verbal abuse of the "impostor"; for example, Vogel's (1974) case 1 commented that "I call him Earl but he answers to ass-hole too", and there is an appreciable overall risk of (sometimes extreme) physical violence (de Pauw and Szulecka, 1988). A review of 260 cases of delusional misidentification by Förstl *et al.* (1991b) found that physical violence had been noted in 46 cases (18%).

There can be insight into the absurdity of the delusion, even when it is subjectively convincing. The following dialogue comes from a case reported by Alexander *et al.* (1979):

E. Isn't that [duplicate families] unusual?
S. It was unbelievable!
E. How do you account for it?
S. I don't know. I try to understand it myself, and it was virtually impossible.

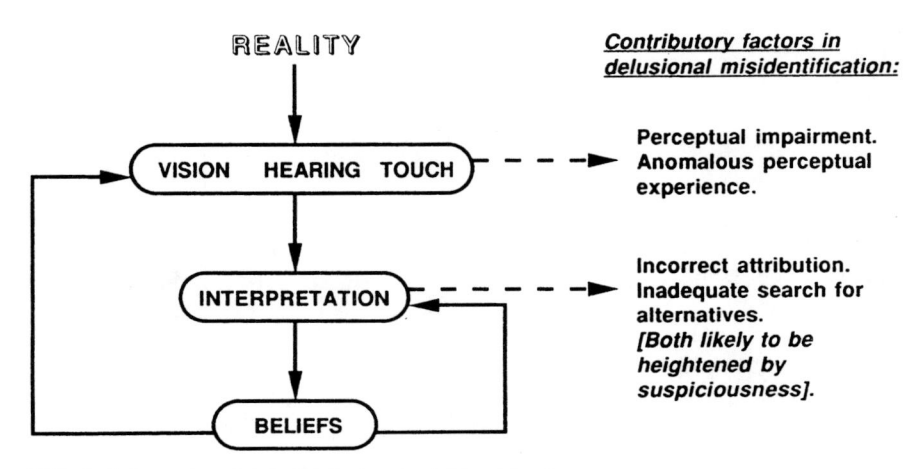

FIG. 1. Schematic model of delusional misidentification.

Work on the Capgras delusion was initially dominated by psychodynamic accounts (Berson, 1983; Capgras and Carrette, 1924; Vogel, 1974), most of which proposed that conflicting or ambivalent feelings of love and hate are resolved by the delusion, so that the double can be hated without guilt. However, psychodynamic hypotheses do not imply a direct role for brain disease, and hence have difficulty in accommodating the now frequent finding of an organic contribution. Furthermore, we have noted that Capgras patients' attitudes to the doubles often fail to show the overt hostility which would be expected on the psychodynamic view (Wallis, 1986). In making these points I am not trying to deny that *psychological* factors may play a role in some or all cases of reduplication; only that the psychodynamic account is insufficient as a sole explanation.

In Capgras cases with clear neurological damage, there are usually occipitotemporal or temporoparietal lesions, often of the right hemisphere only, and frontal lesions which can be bilateral (Alexander *et al.*, 1979; Feinberg and Shapiro, 1989; Förstl *et al.*, 1991a,b; Joseph, 1986; Lewis, 1987). However, although such observations of brain disease in patients who experience the Capgras delusion are obviously important, they do not in themselves explain the peculiar content of the delusion. One needs a theory that can link the observed brain disease to the disturbed psychological functions that create the delusion. Our studies of cases of Capgras delusion have convinced us that a principled account can be achieved by integrating neuropsychological investigations with recent findings on delusions derived from work in clinical psychology and psychiatry.

Our working hypothesis is that the Capgras delusion may be due in part to impairment of the visual system. In effect, the patient's beliefs change because the evidence on which they are based has altered. If correct, this emphasizes the fundamental importance of vision as a source of evidence about the world.

To examine this further, a simple schematic model of how delusional misidentifications might arise is shown in Fig. 1. This proposes that we can only know the world through our senses, but beliefs are created through (among other things) the interpretation of sense data. Once formed, beliefs will affect both how we interpret the data available and what kind of information we seek; we become predisposed to see what we expect, and Fleminger (1992) has given a compelling analysis of how such expectations contribute to delusional misidentification.

In the model shown in Fig. 1, delusional misidentification is taken to reflect an interaction of impairments at two levels. One set of contributory factors involves perceptual impairment, or anomalous perceptual experience, and the other factors lead to an incorrect interpretation of this. Incorrect interpretation might happen for various reasons. In Fig. 1, I have drawn attention to two of these; incorrect attribution of the perceptual changes, and an inadequate search for alternatives to the delusional explanation. The influence of both of these factors would be heightened by the suspiciousness which is often noted in Capgras patients.

The suggestion of an inadequate search for alternatives to the delusional explanation is based on the work of Huq *et al.* (1988), who found that people with delusions were more confident and requested less information than non-deluded people before reaching a decision in a probability judgement task. This is an important finding because, superficially, probability judgements would seem to have nothing to do with the patients' delusions. The other factor favouring misinterpretation, incorrect attributions, has been noted in suspicious patients by Kaney and Bentall (1989) and Candido and Romney (1990), who found that people with persecutory delusions were inclined to attribute hypothetical negative events to *external* causes, whereas depressed people attributed them to *internal* causes. The persecutory delusions and suspiciousness that are often noted in Capgras cases may therefore contribute to the fundamental misinterpretation in which the patients mistake a change in themselves for a change in others.

It is thus plausible that the Capgras delusion is caused by the misinterpretation of unusual perceptual experiences. But what kind of unusual experiences? The presence of right occipito-temporal lesions in Capgras cases is reminiscent of the brain lesions that cause prosopagnosia, and the possibility of a link between prosopagnosia and the Capgras delusion is strengthened by observations that Capgras patients perform poorly on face processing tests (Morrison and Tarter, 1984; Shraberg and Weitzel, 1979; Tzavaras *et al.*, 1986; Wilcox and Waziri, 1983; Young *et al.*, 1993). However, it is necessary to treat this possible link carefully (Ellis and Young, 1990; Lewis, 1987). It seems unlikely that there is any direct and sufficient causal connection. Prosopagnosic patients do not usually experience the Capgras delusion and, conversely, although their ability to recognize familiar faces may be impaired (Young *et al.*, 1993), Capgras patients still can recognize a number of highly familiar people; for example, they still recognize that the "double" looks like their husband, wife or whoever. Hence any link to prosopagnosia must be more subtle.

Lewis (1987) and Ellis and Young (1990) have suggested that the basis of the Capgras delusion lies in damage to neuro-anatomical pathways responsible for appropriate emotional reactions to familiar visual stimuli, such as Bauer's (1984) dorsal visual-limbic route. The delusion would then represent the patient's attempt to make sense of this puzzling change; it typically involves close relatives because these would normally produce the strongest reactions, and hence suffer the greatest discrepancy. On this hypothesis, the Capgras delusion represents a mirror-image of prosopagnosia, in which Bauer's (1984) dorsal route is more severely affected than the ventral route. Since substantial parts of the pathways which imbue visual stimuli with affective significance are in close proximity to those involved in visual recognition, one would expect that few brain lesions will compromise emotional reactions to visual stimuli without also affecting other visual functions involved in recognition to some extent. Most Capgras patients will thus show defective face processing abilities because these are, for neuro-anatomical reasons, likely to co-occur with the fundamental problem in affective reactions.

The proposal that defective emotional reactions to familiar visual stimuli are implicated in the Capgras delusion was one which often found favour in early descriptions (Brochado, 1936), but other accounts of the impairment that underlies the Capgras delusion have also been suggested. Joseph (1986) proposed a cerebral hemisphere disconnection hypothesis, in which each cerebral hemisphere independently processes facial information, and the Capgras delusion arises when the two processes fail to integrate. Cutting (1991) argued against a perceptual account, and thought that the delusion is due to a breakdown of the normal structure of semantic categories, leading to a disturbance in the judgement of identity or uniqueness. Staton et al. (1982) drew attention to the possibility of a memory deficit, in which the Capgras patient compares a present percept with an old representation of the face, and notes the mismatch. Feinberg and Shapiro (1989) noted a failure to register familiarity, and suggested that the Capgras delusion resembles a state of selective persisting jamais vu.

Some of these hypotheses are clearly incompatible with the model presented here, whereas others can be regarded as variants with a different emphasis; for example, Feinberg and Shapiro's (1989) proposal can be accommodated by suggesting that the pervasive sense of strangeness resulting from the malfunction of the dorsal visual-limbic route is described by the patient as a lack of familiarity. The important point, however, is that all of the accounts lead to testable predictions which can be investigated in future cases.

The Capgras delusion is one of the most striking neuropsychiatric problems, but the use of tests to determine whether or not measurable cognitive deficits play any role in the creation and maintenance of the delusion is still at an early stage. However, it is clear that this approach has promise for uncovering the basis of this bizarre phenomenon.

## Capgras and Cotard Delusions

In the 1880s, Cotard described a syndrome of nihilistic delusions (le délire de négation) in which everything seems so unreal that the patient thinks she or he has died (Cotard, 1880; 1882). This was recognized as of sufficient importance to justify a monograph by Seglas (1897), who adopted Regis's suggestion that it should be known by the eponym Cotard's syndrome. Although a key feature of this syndrome was the delusion of being dead, Cotard had noted that there could be differing and fluctuating degrees of severity. Other florid symptoms associated with the Cotard syndrome included thinking that the entire world had ceased to exist, feelings of putrefaction of internal bodily organs, self-mutilating or (paradoxically) suicidal urges, and beliefs in the absence or (conversely) enormity of parts of the body. However, the 11 patients reported in Cotard's (1882) key paper did not invariably display all of these accompanying features, which again brings into question the utility of the syndrome concept in cases presenting with the delusion of being dead, if by syndrome is meant a pattern of symptoms which will inevitably co-occur. For this reason, we have preferred to refer to the specific symptom of believing that you are dead as the Cotard delusion.

At first sight, the Cotard and Capgras delusions would seem to have little to do with each other, except that they both involve bizarre claims about existence (for self or others). On closer examination, however, there are other parallels. Both delusions can be produced by broadly similar types of brain injury (Drake, 1988; Young et al., 1992). For example, in a case we investigated, WI, the Cotard delusion followed contusions affecting temporoparietal areas of the right cerebral hemisphere and some bilateral frontal lobe damage (Young et al., 1992). Moreover, there are similarities in the cognitive impairments. WI not only became convinced that he was dead, but he also experienced difficulties in recognizing familiar faces, buildings and places, as well as feelings of derealization; all of which are often noted in Capgras cases. In fact, people suffering the Cotard delusion commonly report that they must be dead because they "feel nothing inside", which presses the parallel with the hypothesized lack of affective reactions in Capgras cases still further. Young et al. (1992) therefore suggested that the underlying pathophysiology and neuropsychology of the Cotard and Capgras delusions may be related. We think that, although these delusions are phenomenally distinct, they may represent the patients' attempts to make sense of fundamentally similar experiences.

Young et al. (1992) noted that this suggestion of a link between the Capgras and Cotard delusions is strengthened by the fact that cases of coexistent or sequential Capgras and Cotard delusions have been described in the literature. The underlying basis of both delusions could therefore lie in a delusional interpretation of altered perception (especially loss of affective familiarity).

A clue to how this could happen comes from the studies which have shown that people with persecutory delusions tend to attribute negative events to external rather than internal causes, whereas depressed people tend to attribute them to internal causes (Candido and Romney, 1990; Kaney and Bentall, 1989). The relevance of these findings is that it is quite common for the Cotard delusion to arise in the setting of a depressive illness and for the Capgras delusion to be accompanied by persecutory delusions and suspiciousness (Enoch and Trethowan, 1991; Wright et al. in press). Hence, whilst the persecutory delusions and suspiciousness that are often noted in Capgras cases contribute to the patients mistaking a change in themselves for a change in others ("they must be impostors"), people who are depressed might exaggerate the negative effects of a similar change whilst correctly attributing it to themselves ("I must be dead").

These points were in fact made or anticipated by Cotard, but many of them seem to have got lost in the intervening century. Cotard's 1882 paper ends with a very thorough Table listing the parallels and differences between delusions of negation and delusions of persecution. This Table gives a version of the attribution hypothesis, in which Cotard points out that in delusions of persecution "Le malade s'en prend au monde extérieur", whereas in delusions of negation "Le malade s'accuse lui-même". Even the combination of the specific delusions of being dead oneself and having one's relatives replaced by impostors is hinted at in this report; as well as experiencing nihilistic delusions, case 4 in Cotard's (1882) series had claimed that her daughter was a devil in disguise, and did not recognize her husband and children when they visited (though Cotard implied that she may not have recognized her husband and children because she no longer believed in their existence). Moreover, in his 1880 paper, Cotard commented that there was a kind of logic to the delusions, and in 1884 he noted the presence of a loss of visual imagery in his patients (Cotard, 1884). Loss of visual imagery is a frequent concomitant of visual recognition impairments, and Cotard's mentor, Charcot, had recently described such a case (Charcot and Bernard, 1883; Young and van de Wal, in press). Considering this to be more than a coincidence, Cotard (1884) suggested that the delusions reflected a misinterpretation of this change. Plus ça change...

## Reduplicative Paramnesias

Patients with reduplicative paramnesias assert "the presence of two or more places with nearly identical attributes, while only one exists in reality" (Patterson and Mack, 1985). The term comes from Pick (1903), who described two cases; patient 1 "asserted that there were two clinics exactly alike in which he had been, two professors of the same name were at the head of these clinics, &c", whereas patient 2, who was in a clinic in Prague, "imagined she was in K., and in reply to the assistant's question how it was that he was in K. also, she said that she was very pleased to see him *here too*". Both of Pick's cases were similar in that they thought there were duplicate hospitals; they differed in that for patient 1 the hospital staff and patients had been duplicated as well, whilst when patient 2 was asked how the same staff and patients would be in both clinics she replied that "They come from one place to the other".

The parallels between reduplicative paramnesia and the Capgras delusion have been widely recognized (Alexander *et al.*, 1979; Feinberg and Shapiro, 1989; Stanton *et al.*, 1982; Weinstein and Burnham, 1991). Not only is there a parallel in the phenomenon of reduplication itself, but the brain lesions responsible for reduplicative paramnesias often involve bilateral frontal atrophy and a more discrete lesion in the region of the temporo-parieto-occipital junction of the right hemisphere (Benson *et al.*, 1976; Hakim *et al.*, 1988; Staton *et al.*, 1982). In addition, as is suggested by Pick's (1903) patient 1, the Capgras delusion and reduplicative paramnesia can be found together (Alexander *et al.*, 1979; Staton *et al.*, 1982). For example, Staton *et al.*'s (1982) patient stated that "everything is so different" [from before the accident]. Friends and relatives, including his parents and siblings, were not "real" – but were slightly different "look-alikes", or doubles – not the real people he had known before the accident. This was also true of places, including the family farm and the city where he was hospitalized." (Staton *et al.*, 1982, p.24). In a particularly expansive case, a patient thought that there were eight entire duplicate cities, each an exact replica of his home city, and each peopled with duplicates of his family members; he knew these were impostors "because they did not 'feel'like the real people to him" (Thompson *et al.*, 1980).

If reduplicative paramnesia involves fundamentally similar mechanisms to those which create the Capgras delusion, and if the Cotard and Capgras delusions are also closely related, we might expect to find cases showing the Cotard delusion and reduplicative paramnesia; yet there seems to have been only one historic report to date (Förstl and Beats, 1992). The rarity of this combination of delusions may, however, be in part explained by suggesting that reduplicative paramnesias would be masked in cases where the Cotard delusion led the patient to question the reality of his or her surroundings.

Recently, a further variant of delusional misidentification has been recognized, involving the duplication of inanimate objects (Anderson, 1988). Anderson's 1988 patient, Mr B, was a 74-year-old man with a pituitary tumour. He believed that his wife and nephew had been plotting across 10 years to ruin him by stealing his belongings, and had kept a typewritten record of over 300 items they had "stolen"; these were predominantly household items (screws, nails, paint brushes, screwdrivers) or personal belongings (shirts, underpants, wellingtons, electric razor). According to Mr B, some of these items had been replaced by inferior doubles identical in size, shape, colour and manufacturer's name. Mr B agreed that this story was incredible and would be difficult to believe, but he sincerely believed it himself, and he made his wife sleep on the kitchen floor because of his persecutory delusions.

Anderson (1988) suggested that this is a variant of the Capgras delusion, and that "the reason why Mr B presented the delusion of doubles for objects rather than people lies in understanding his character and interests. Mr B was a private and solitary man who made few friends, and obtained pleasure in life from his pastimes of repairing and using his tools, areas in which he had developed some expertise and spent many hours." (Anderson, 1988, p. 698). Anderson went on to propose an account of such delusions which is very similar to that given here, suggesting that they are due to "lesions of the pathway for visual recognition at a stage where visual images are imbued with affective familiarity. This results in familiar images evoking unfamiliar and incongruous affective responses and such inconsistency is then rationalized by the interpretation that the image cannot be that which it physically resembles." (Anderson, 1988, p.698).

## Conclusions

Studies of recognition impairments offer an interesting insight into one facet of the complex neurological mechanisms that sustain our experience of the world as real. The Capgras and Cotard delusions seem to contravene quite basic assumptions we generally make about our own existence and that of other people. Both delusions may hinge on powerful perceptual experiences in which things do not seem to be the way they should; even when recognized, they feel strange and unfamiliar. Yet more severe recognition impairments, such as prosopagnosia, are not generally linked to delusions. This points to the idea that delusional misidentifications result from interactions between different impairments, but it also underlines the complexity of the processes involved in recognition. In particular, I have emphasized the interplay of cognitive and emotional aspects in normal recognition, and shown how the breakdown of this interplay may provide a pointer to understanding how brain injuries can sometimes lead to bizarre delusions.

Investigations of these issues have also served to highlight areas in which our models of recognition need refinement. One of these is the notion of "familiarity". As we have noted, a striking form of recognition error, which occurs both in everyday life and after certain types of brain injury, involves knowing that a face is familiar but having no idea *who* it is, and such observations have led us to model familiarity as if it were a relatively basic piece of cognitive information (Young *et al.*, 1985; Bruce and Young, 1986). This has been a useful tactic, but studies of the Capgras delusion and related conditions show that familiarity is more complex. We will now need to pay more attention to distinguishing different kinds of familiarity (Critchley, 1989; Mandler, 1980), and integrating these into an overall model which can encompass cognitive and affective reactions to people, things and events which have personal relevance (Van Lancker, 1991).

## References

Alexander, M.P., Stuss, D.T. and Benson, D.F. (1979). Capgras syndrome: a reduplicative phenomenon. *Neurology*, **29**, 334-339.

Anderson, D.N. (1988). The delusion of inanimate doubles. *British Journal of Psychiatry*, **153**, 694-699.

Bauer, R.M. (1984). Autonomic recognition of names and faces in prosopagnosia: a neuropsychological application of the guilty knowledge test. *Neuropsychologia*, **22**, 457-469.

Bauer, R.M. (1986). The cognitive psychophysiology of prosopagnosia. *In* "Aspects of Face Processing" (Eds H.D. Ellis, M.A. Jeeves, F. Newcombe and A. Young). pp. 253-267. Martinus Nijhoff, Dordrecht.

Bear, D.M. (1983). Hemispheric specialization and the neurology of emotion. *Archives of Neurology*, **40**, 195-202.

Benson, D.F. and Stuss, D.T. (1990). Frontal lobe influences on delusions: a clinical perspective. *Schizophrenia Bulletin*, **16**, 403-411.

Benson, D.F., Gardner, H. and Meadows, J.C. (1976). Reduplicative paramnesia. *Neurology*, **26**, 147-151.

Benson, R.J. (1983). Capgras' syndrome. *American Journal of Psychiatry*, **140**, 969-978.

Bornstein, R.F. (1989). Exposure and affect: overview and meta-analysis of research, 1968-1987. *Psychological Bulletin*, **106**, 265-289.

Brochado, A. (1936). Le syndrome de Capgras. *Annales Médico-Psychologiques*, **15**, 706-717.

Bruce, V. and Young, A. (1986). Understanding face recognition. *British Journal of Psychology*, **77**, 305-327.

Bruce, V., Burton, A.M. and Craw, I. (1992). Modelling face recognition. *Philosophical Transactions of the Royal Society, London*, **B335**, 121-128.

Bruyer, R. (1991). Covert face recognition in prosopagnosia: a review. *Brain and Cognition*, **15**, 223-235.

Burton, A.M., Bruce, V. and Johnston, R.A. (1990). Understanding face recognition with an interactive activation model. *British Journal of Psychology*, **81**, 361-380.
Burton, A.M., Young, A.W., Bruce, V., Johnston, R. and Ellis, A.W. (1991). Understanding covert recognition. *Cognition*, **39**, 129-166.
Candido, C.L. and Romney, D.M. (1990). Attributional style in paranoid vs. depressed patients. *British Journal of Medical Psychology*, **63**, 355-363.
Capgras, J. and Carrette, P. (1924). l'Illusion des sosies et complexe d'Oedipe. *Annales Médico-Psychologiques*, **82**, 48-68.
Capgras, J. and Reboul-Lachaux, J. (1923). l'Illusion des "sosies" dans un délire systématisé chronique. *Bulletin de la Société Clinique de Médicine Mentale*, **11**, 6-16.
Charcot, J.-M. and Bernard, D. (1883). Un cas de suppression brusque et isolée de la vision mentale des signes et des objets (formes et couleurs). *Le Progrès Médical*, **11**, 568-571.
Collins, M.N., Hawthorne, M.E., Gribbin, N. and Jacobson, R. (1990). Capgras' syndrome with organic disorders. *Postgraduate Medical Journal*, **66**, 1064-1067.
Cotard, J. (1880). Du délire hypocondriaque dans une forme grave de la mélancolie anxieuse. *Annales Médico-Psychologiques*, **4**.
Cotard, J. (1882). Du délire des négations. *Archives de Neurologie,* **4**, 150-170, 282-295.
Cotard, J. (1884). Perte de la vision mentale dans la mélancolie anxieuse. *Archives de Neurologie*, **7**, 289-295.
Critchley, E.M.R. (1989). The neurology of familiarity. *Behavioural Neurology*, **2**, 195-200.
Cutting, J. (1991). Delusional misidentification and the role of the right hemisphere in the appreciation of identity. *British Journal of Psychiatry*, **159**, 70-75.
Damasio, A.R., Damasio, H. and Van Hoesen, G.W. (1982). Prosopagnosia: anatomic basis and behavioral mechanisms. *Neurology*, **32**, 331-341.
de Haan, E.H.F., Young, A. and Newcombe, F. (1987). Face recognition without awareness. *Cognitive Neuropsychology*, **4**, 385-415.
de Haan, E.H.F., Young, A.W. and Newcombe, F. (1991a). Covert and overt recognition in prosopagnosia. *Brain*, **114**, 2575-2591.
de Haan, E.H.F., Young, A.W. and Newcombe, F. (1991b). A dissociation between the sense of familiarity and access to semantic information concerning familiar people. *European Journal of Cognitive Psychology*, **3**, 51-67.
de Pauw, K.W. and Szulecka, T.K. (1988). Dangerous delusions: violence and the misidentification syndromes. *British Journal of Psychiatry*, **152**, 91-97.
De Renzi, E. (1986). Prosopagnosia in two patients with CT scan evidence of damage confined to the right hemisphere. *Neuropsychologia*, **24**, 385-389.
De Renzi, E., Faglioni, P., Grossi, D. and Nichelli, P. (1991). Apperceptive and associative forms of prosopagnosia. *Cortex*, **27**, 213-221.
Drake, M.E.J. (1988). Cotard's syndrome and temporal lobe epilepsy. *Psychiatric Journal of the University of Ottawa*, **13**, 36-39.
Ellis, A.W. (1992). Cognitive mechanisms of face processing. *Philosophical Transactions of the Royal Society, London*, **B335**, 113-119.
Ellis, H.D. and Young, A.W. (1990). Accounting for delusional misidentifications. *British Journal of Psychiatry*, **157**, 239-248.
Enoch, M.D. and Trethowan, W.H. (1991). "Uncommon Psychiatric Syndromes". 3rd Edn. John Wright, Bristol.
Feinberg, T.E. and Shapiro, R.M. (1989). Misidentification-reduplication and the right hemisphere. *Neuropsychiatry, Neuropsychology, and Behavioral Neurology*, **2**, 39-48.
Fleminger, S. (1991). Déjà vu phenomena. *American Journal of Psychiatry*, **148**, 1418-1419.
Fleminger, S. (1992). Seeing is believing: the role of "preconscious" perceptual processing in delusional misidentification. *British Journal of Psychiatry*, **160**, 293-303.

Flude, B.M., Ellis, A.W. and Kay, J. (1989). Face processing and name retrieval in an anomic aphasic: names are stored separately from semantic information about familiar people. *Brain and Cognition*, **11**, 60-72.

Förstl, H. and Beats, B. (1992). Charles Bonnet's description of Cotard's delusion and reduplicative paramnesia in an elderly patient (1788). *British Journal of Psychiatry*, **160**, 416-418.

Förstl, H., Almeida, O.P., Owen, A.M., Burns, A. and Howard, R. (1991a). Psychiatric, neurological and medical aspects of misidentification syndromes: a review of 260 cases. *Psychological Medicine*, **21**, 905-910.

Förstl, H., Burns, A., Jacoby, R. and Levy, R. (1991b). Neuroanatomical correlates of clinical misidentification and misperception in senile dementia of the Alzheimer type. *Journal of Clinical Psychiatry*, **52**, 268-271.

Geschwind, N. (1982). Disorders of attention: a frontier in neuropsychology. *Philosophical Transactions of the Royal Society, London*, **B298**, 173-185.

Greve, K.W. and Bauer, R.M. (1990). Implicit learning of new faces in prosopagnosia: an application of the mere-exposure paradigm. *Neuropsychologia*, **28**, 1035-1041.

Hakim, H., Verma, N.P. and Greiffenstein, M.F. (1988). Pathogenesis of reduplicative paramnesia. *Journal of Neurology, Neurosurgery, and Psychiatry*, **51**, 839-841.

Huq, S.F., Garety, P.A. and Hemsley, D.R. (1988). Probabilistic judgements in deluded and non-deluded subjects. *Quarterly Journal of Experimental Psychology*, **40A**, 801-812.

Joseph, A.B. (1986). Focal central nervous system abnormalities in patients with misidentification syndromes. *Bibliotheca Psychiatrica*, **164**, 68-79.

Kaney, S. and Bentall, R.P. (1989). Persecutory delusions and attributional style. *British Journal of Medical Psychology*, **62**, 191-198.

Kunst-Wilson, W.R. and Zajonc, R.B. (1980). Affective discrimination of stimuli that cannot be recognized. *Science*, **207**, 557-558.

Landis, T., Cummings, J.L., Christen, L., Bogen, J.E. and Imhof, H.-G. (1986). Are unilateral right posterior cerebral lesions sufficient to cause prosopagnosia? Clinical and radiological findings in six additional patients. *Cortex*, **22**, 243-252.

Lewis, S.W. (1987). Brain imaging in a case of Capgras' syndrome. *British Journal of Psychiatry*, **150**, 117-121.

Mandler, G. (1980). Recognizing: the judgement of previous occurrence. *Psychological Review*, **87**, 252-271.

Meadows, J.C. (1974). The anatomical basis of prosopagnosia. *Journal of Neurology, Neurosurgery, and Psychiatry*, **37**, 489-501.

Morrison, R.L. and Tarter, R.E. (1984). Neuropsychological findings relating to Capgras syndrome. *Biological Psychiatry*, **19**, 1119-1128.

Patterson, M.B. and Mack, J.L. (1985). Neuropsychological analysis of a case of reduplicative paramnesia. *Journal of Clinical and Experimental Neuropsychology*, **7**, 111-121.

Pick, A. (1903). Clinical studies: III. On reduplicative paramnesia. *Brain*, **26**, 260-267.

Rizzo, M., Hurtig, R. and Damasio, A.R. (1987). The role of scanpaths in facial recognition and learning. *Annals of Neurology*, **22**, 41-45.

Séglas, J. (1897). "Le Délire des Négations: Séméiologie et Diagnostic". Masson, Gauthier-Villars, Paris.

Sergent, J. and Poncet, M. (1990). From covert to overt recognition of faces in a prosopagnosic patient. *Brain*, **113**, 989-1004.

Sergent, J. and Villemure, J.-G. (1989). Prosopagnosia in a right hemispherectomized patient. *Brain*, **112**, 975-995.

Shraberg, D. and Weitzel, W.D. (1979). Prosopagnosia and the Capgras syndrome. *Journal of Clinical Psychiatry*, **40**, 313-316.

Shubsachs, A.P.W. and Young, A. (1988). Dangerous delusions: the "Hollywood" phenomenon. *British Journal of Psychiatry*, **152**, 722.
Slade, P. and Bentall, R.P. (1988). "Sensory Deception: a Scientific Analysis of Hallucinations". Croom-Helm, London.
Sno, H.N. and Linszen, D.H. (1990). The déjà vu experience: remembrance of things past? *American Journal of Psychiatry*, **147**, 1587-1595.
Staton, R.D., Brumback, R.A. and Wilson, H. (1982). Reduplicative paramnesia: a disconnection syndrome of memory. *Cortex*, **18**, 23-26.
Stuss, D.T., Alexander, M.P., Lieberman, A. and Levine, H. (1978). An extraordinary form of confabulation. *Neurology*, **28**, 1166-1172.
Thompson, M.I., Silk, K.R. and Hover, G.L. (1980). Misidentification of a city: delimiting criteria for Capgras syndrome. *American Journal of Psychiatry*, **137**, 1270-1272.
Tranel, D. and Damasio, A.R. (1985). Knowledge without awareness: an autonomic index of facial recognition by prosopagnosics. *Science*, **228**, 1453-1454.
Tranel, D. and Damasio, A.R. (1988). Non-conscious face recognition in patients with face agnosia. *Behavioural Brain Research*, **30**, 235-249.
Tzavaras, A., Luauté, J.P. and Bidault, E. (1986). Face recognition dysfunction and delusional misidentification syndromes (DMS). *In* "Aspects of Face Processing" (Eds H.D. Ellis, M.A. Jeeves, F. Newcombe and A. Young), pp. 310-316. Martinus Nijhoff, Dordrecht.
Van Lancker, D. (1991). Personal relevance and the human right hemisphere. *Brain and Cognition*, **17**, 64-92.
Vié, J. (1944). Les méconnaissances systèmatiques: étude séméiologique. *Annales Médico-Psychologiques*, **102**, 229-252.
Vogel, B.F. (1974). The Capgras syndrome and its psychopathology. *American Journal of Psychiatry*, **131**, 922-924.
Wallis, G. (1986). Nature of the misidentified in the Capgras syndrome. *Bibliotheca Psychiatrica*, **164**, 40-48.
Weinstein, E.A. and Burnham, D.L. (1991). Reduplication and the syndrome of Capgras. *Psychiatry*, **54**, 78-88.
Wilcox, J. and Waziri, R. (1983). The Capgras symptom and nondominant cerebral dysfunction. *Journal of Clinical Psychiatry*, **44**, 70-72.
Wright, S., Young, A.W. and Hellawell, D.J. (in press). Sequential Cotard and Capgras delusions. *British Journal of Clinical Psychology*.
Young, A.W. and van de Wal, C. (in press). Charcot's case of impaired imagery. *In* "Classic Cases in Neuropsychology". (Eds C. Code, C.-W. Wallesch, A.R. Lecours and Y. Joanette). Lawrence Erlbaum, London.
Young, A.W. (1988). Functional organization of visual recognition. *In* "Thought without Language" (Ed. L. Weiskrantz). pp. 78-107. Oxford University Press.
Young, A.W. and de Haan, E.H.F. (1992). Face recognition and awareness after brain injury. *In* "The Neuropsychology of Consciousness" (Eds A.D. Milner and M.D. Rugg), pp.69-90. Academic Press, London.
Young, A.W., Hay, D.C. and Ellis, A.W. (1985). The faces that launched a thousand slips: everyday difficulties and errors in recognizing people. *British Journal of Psychology*, **76**, 495-523.
Young, A.W., Hellawell, D. and de Haan, E.H.F. (1988). Cross-domain semantic priming in normal subjects and a prosopagnosic patient. *Quarterly Journal of Experimental Psychology*, **40A**, 561-580.
Young, A.W., Reid, I., Wright, S. and Hellawell, D. (1993). Face processing impairments and the Capgras delusion. *British Journal of Psychiatry*, **162**, 695-698.

Young, A.W., Robertson, I.H., Hellawell, D.J., de Pauw, K.W. and Pentland, B. (1992). Cotard delusion after brain injury. *Psychological Medicine*, **22**, 799-804.

Zajonc, R.B. (1980). Feeling and thinking: preferences need no inferences. *American Psychologist,* **35**, 151-175.

# 7. The neurological boundaries of visual reality

John Harrison and Christopher Kennard

---

## Introduction

Ludwig, the "brain-in-a-vat" thought experiment (see chapter 10) requires the student to consider the frailty of the epistemological status of our outside world, in recognition of the fact that the fundamental coinage of the nervous system is electrochemical in nature, but more importantly one in which the component units communicate in a binary code. This *gedankenexperiment* is designed to illustrate the questionable status of knowledge gleaned from the world via the senses and achieves this by suggesting that we may all be brains-in-vats and that we are stimulated to believe in the existence of tables, sunsets and experiments by receiving the appropriate stimulation to our nerve fibres. Sipping a sundowner at sunset whilst listening to Strauss' *Im Abendrot* might simply be the manipulation of input to our brain by a mad, alien scientist.

The nature of reality is thus a debatable point, though for the purposes of this discussion we will forego the luxury of invoking the viewpoint of the epistemological sceptic. However, it is as well to bear in mind that the interpretation of our environment is anything but an unsullied piece of pure data analysis. It is more likely a momentary icon upon which our prejudiced minds place an interpretation. We shall explore the nature of human interpretation of "visual" information by examining the unusual abilities of exceptional individuals, both those who have been denied normal functioning through loss as well as those who appear to have additional capacity.

An early theory of memory (Atkinson and Schiffrin, 1971), based on Sperling (1960), posits that incoming information is held in an extremely short-lived memory register, which for visual information has been termed "iconic memory". This constitutes the only stage in the process of perception where the perceiver deals with pure sense data. Thereafter the brain seeks to interpret this iconic information by imposing a structure upon it. For example, Bugelski and Alampay (1961) showed pictures of animals to one group of individuals whereas a second group received no pretraining. Both groups were then shown the same figure (Fig. 1, below) and asked to describe what they saw. The figure was deliberately ambiguous, resembling the face of an elderly, bespectacled man, or a rat.

The experimenters demonstrated that the figure tended to be interpreted as a rat by those who had been exposed to pictures of animals and as a man's face by those who had received no pretraining. This experiment strongly supports the idea that subjects had been perceptually set to interpret the figure according to recent experience. It also provides evidence of the brain's capacity to engage in "top-down processing" by superimposing an interpretation on incoming stimuli.

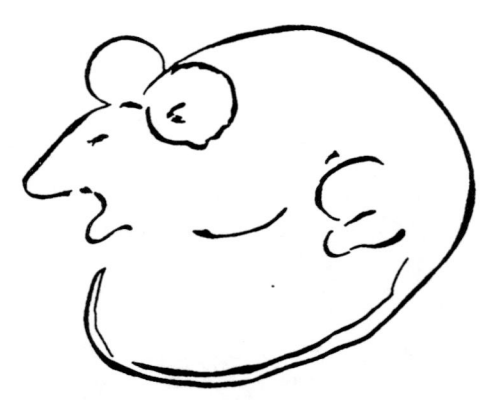

FIG. 1. The ambiguous stimuli used by Bugelski and Alampay (1961).

**Colour Constancy**

Information received at the eye about objects and our perception of them, is a function not just of the spectral reference of the object, but also of the spectral power distribution of the illuminating light. The normally specific relationship between the perceived colour of an object and the light it reflects does not hold true when the object is a part of a complex scene. The human brain seems capable of perceiving a stable colour despite variation in the amount of illumination the scene receives.

Colour constancy is the ability of the normal human visual system to maintain consistency of the colour of perceived objects in spite of variability in the amount of light absorption by the cone receptors in the retina. Cones are divided into three groups on the basis of the frequency of light to which they preferentially respond. Consequently, there are "blue" cones which preferentially respond to light of 440nm, "green" cones at 530nm and "red" cones which react most strongly to light of about 600nm. Given that colour constancy is maintained even across variations in receptoral light absorption, the mechanism by which we perceive constancy must be an interpretation of reality. The mechanism must therefore be a form of visual adaptation in response to changes in illumination. Yet in spite of this knowledge, no single comprehensive theory of colour constancy has emerged. For our purposes it is enough to observe that in normal individuals the brain performs some act of adjustment that ensures we see a stably-maintained coloured scene. Thus we possess a brain, which, in principle, is capable of veridically representing the visual world, but at the same time may override a literal representation and instead provide us with an interpretation.

**Out of Body Experiences (OOBEs)**

Occult practitioners and prophets have for some time predicted a renaissance in the esoteric arts. Many have suggested that interest in "new age" techniques and practices are merely the heralds of the Aquarian age, due to begin at the close of this millennium. Certainly, many individuals seem to attribute credibility to "magical" practices, even those as obviously mundane as the "stars" in their daily papers. An example of just a "magical" phenomenon is so-called "out of body experiences" (OOBEs), which are frequently recounted by subjects who have suffered "near death experiences" (NDEs). Interest in these NDEs has been a feature of the medical literature from the 1960s, though Bhowmick (1991) credits a Swiss geologist Heim as being the first to collect accounts of NDEs just over a century ago.

Researchers including Moody (1975) have examined accounts given by patients who have suffered respiratory and/or cardiac arrest before being resuscitated. Recently, a British psychologist, Susan Blackmore (1988) has examined accounts of "astral travel" and NDEs and reports being impressed by the apparent consistency of the accounts given by individuals from disparate geographical locations and different cultural backgrounds. With the release of films such as "Poltergeist" and "Flatliners", both of which deal with NDE, caution should be exercised in interpreting recent accounts. However, the survey of individuals experiencing NDEs carried out by Ring (1980) shows a certain amount of similarity. Ring has characterized NDEs as having five stages, beginning with a feeling of peace followed by body separation, the entering of a tunnel or darkness, followed by "seeing the light" and then finally, entering the light. Interestingly, in the accounts given these stages tended to unfold in this order, and perhaps more interestingly, the first stage is reported to be the most commonly experienced whereas the fifth stage the least common.

This consistency is indeed remarkable, and there has been no shortage of theory, be it scientific, exotic or esoteric to explain such impressive correspondence. Probably the most interesting and scientifically credible account is that given by Blackmore (1988) who suggests that NDE, whilst not telling us much about an afterlife, does tell us a great deal about globally disordered brain function. Her explanation is highly theoretical, but then the very nature of NDE makes predictive experimentation difficult to engage in. The element of her explanation that is of most interest to us in the context of vision is that regarding the illusion of passing down the tunnel towards the light. This, Blackmore proposes, is one manifestation of a relatively restricted set of four possible types of iatrogenically induced visual hallucinations described by Kluver (1935). He noted that these experiences tended to take forms which he characterized as being either like a cobweb, a tunnel, a spiral or a lattice. Blackmore points out that hallucinations of an apparently similar sort can occur in migraine and epilepsy, as well as being the consequence of meditation or pressure on both eyeballs. She goes on to point out that hallucinatory states appear to be the consequence of the disruption caused by agents such as LSD and mescaline to raphe cells which regulate visual cortical activity. Whatever the cause, this disruption of raphe cells can lead to a highly excitable state which upsets normal cortical functioning.

Based on a theory proposed by Cowan (1982), that a possible consequence of this excitability is the propagation of stripes of activity in the visual cortex, she quotes Cowan as proposing that this pattern of striped activation in cortex would cause the outside world to look as though it possessed concentric rings, tunnels or spirals. Movement of the stripes would suggest an expansion or reduction in the apparent size of the visual environment. By analogy with the other causes of this effect, Blackmore suggests that just such a breakdown in normal function might occur due to a loss of bloodflow in the brains of NDE subjects. The bright light, she argues, is the consequence of having a greater number of neurons in the cortical representation of the central area of the visual field due to the cortical magnification factor which is high for the central field.

This would seem to provide a plausible account of NDE, though as Blackmore admits, it does not constitute a complete account. A fundamental issue here is why is it that NDE subjects seem to be persuaded by the reality of their experience? Blackmore tackles this issue and suggests that our knowledge of reality is gleaned from our everyday existence and our capacity for establishing what is normal and expected, and what is not. She suggests that a brain suffering hypoxia hangs on to the best version of events it can obtain from the available data, which in the case of these subjects is that derived from the misleading "visual " information.

The issue of the nature of reality is tackled again later in the context of synaesthesic percepts, but other "states of brain" experienced by most individuals at one time or another can give rise to unusual hallucinatory experiences. John Keats in his wonderful poem *Ode to a Nightingale* recounts lying in bed listening to a nightingale; he comments on his uncertainty of the nature of the experience by concluding:

> Was it a vision, or a waking dream?
> Fled is that music – Do I wake or sleep?

Here Keats appears to be alluding to what has come to be known as hypnagogic and hypnopompic imagery, states which are sometimes experienced as occurring either on the cusp of sleep (hypnagogia) or on the cusp of wakefulness (hypnopompia). His account appears to be multisensory but most often the experience is recounted as being purely visual. The images reported by subjects in these two states are often similar in fundamental form to those described by Kluver's subjects, except that they appear to be rather more transitory, typically lasting only moments. The initiation of sleep is still little understood, but we have known since Jouvet's (1967) experiments that non-REM sleep appears to require changes in the activity of the raphe centre. It might be thought plausible then, that the changes which accompany the onset of sleep and wakefulness may also involve changes in the usually inhibitory role of the raphe upon the visual cortex.

Similarly, little is known about the nature of dreaming, though we can be reasonably sure that REM sleep is punctuated by bursts of activity which originate in the pons and then proceed to the occipital cortex via the lateral geniculate nucleus. These PGO (Pons Geniculate Occipital) spikes provide electrochemical stimulation to the visual cortex which may give rise to visual images. We know from EEG records that REM sleep occurs on the ascent from the deepest stage of sleep (stage 4) to wakefulness on the cusp from stage 2 to stage 1. Not surprisingly therefore we often wake from our last period of REM sleep, a testament to which is the capacity we have for recalling our last dream as well as the sympathetic autonomic arousal we experience on waking.

## Synaesthesia

In her explanation of NDEs, Blackmore suggests that we come to understand what is normal and real from the accumulation of our experience. This experience is derived from our capacity to sense and interpret the environment, "reality" is determined for us by our sensory systems. For this reason it is interesting to look at a condition called synaesthesia as individuals with this capacity experience the world in a subtly different way from the average, "normal" person. Synaesthesia (from the Greek; syn = union, aisthesis = sensation), appears to have been recognized as a condition as early as 1710 when Thomas Woolhouse (1650-1734) reported on a blind subject who reported perceiving sound-induced coloured experiences. We have few details of this individual, but it is indeed intriguing that a subject deprived of normal visual experience should report "visual" phenomena. Reports of this condition have been described since the time of Woolhouse, though caution must be exercised regarding the nature of these accounts as the principal source of data is from the subjective accounts of those individuals who report synaesthetic experiences. Caution is required because if we wish to posit the idea that synaesthesia is perceptual and brain-based then we must exclude at least two other explanations.

Firstly, there is the possibility that synaesthetic percepts may be the product of either deliberate or unconscious associative memory processes. The second possibility to exclude is related to the first, but involves our being able to decide between metaphor and genuine synaesthesia. Metaphor has, of course, a very rich history in both art and science and allows for the description of what we shall term pseudo-synaesthesic ideas. For instance, an individual may report an experience of "greenness" whilst listening to Dvorak's "New World" symphony or "purpleness" when reading Keats, but these would constitute metaphorical accounts rather than genuine synaesthesia.

Marks (1975) lists some articles and points to the possibility that for some writers synaesthesia is merely a contrived correspondence between a letter and a colour. An example of this appears to be Rimbaud's (1871) *Le Sonnet Des Voyelles* in which the poet attributes a colour to each of the vowels where A in black, E is white, I is red, O is blue and U is green. Marks points out that Rimbaud later describes these correspondences as his "invention", indicating a contrived correspondence. In a similar vein is Cilla McQueen's (1987) poem synaesthesia, which begins;

> the lines the eye can see the mind can hear
> the sounds the eye has found the ear can see
> the landscape sings inside my inner ear
> invisibly its silent harmony.

Again, this seems to indicate a form of metaphor rather than genuine synaesthesia, in spite of the poem's title. Cytowic (1987) makes much of the synaesthesia reported by the writer Vladimir Nabokov who appears to have shared his condition with his mother (Nabokov, 1949). Historical accounts of the condition are of course very hard to verify as we have no objective or empirical tests of the genuineness of synaesthesia. However, factors seem to be validated across studies which suggest that synaesthetes can be diagnosed by the possession of certain characteristics.

One of the most interesting of these is the finding that in all the studies carried out in recent years, substantially more women than men have been found to be synaesthetes. This has been found in both the United States (Cytowic, 1989, 1991) and in the UK (Baron-Cohen *et al.*, 1993). Cytowic reports a ratio of 2.5 to 1 whereas the UK ratio is put at about 4:1, reproduced on two separate occasions. Caution must be exercised with regard to these estimates as in both our respondent sets subjects were self-selecting. On the first occasion (1988), following an appearance on the radio by Dr Baron-Cohen, individuals who believed themselves to be synaesthetes were invited to write in to "Science on Four", a programme which the producers believe has an equal distribution of male and female listeners. Later publicity for our work in the form of a newspaper article elicited a similar response distribution, and yet again the likely readership was held to be approximately evenly split between the genders. This consistency is interesting and suggests that synaesthesia is a predominantly female trait.

Many of the respondents show a similar historical pattern to their condition. Subjects will often report having mentioned their synaesthesia at an early age and being looked at very oddly and treated as slightly weird. Consequently many subjects are found to have said no more about their synaesthesia until having heard or read about the condition. Other consistencies are apparent, especially regarding the quality and nature of the synaesthetic percepts and the words or letters that elicit the colour. Typically synaesthetes will report that for as long as they can remember the percept will have remained the same. In many cases this will have been since the age of 4 or even earlier, as all subjects have a strong conviction that they have synaesthesia for quite literally as long as they can remember. These comments appear to be true for all the cases of synaesthesia we have observed and appear also to be true for the subjects reported by Cytowic (1987). On the basis of his observations Cytowic has come up with a set of diagnostic criteria for the condition.

1   Synaesthesia is involuntary but elicited. By this Cytowic means that the phenomenon is unsuppressable and occurs only in response to an objective stimulus. This "automatic" elicitation is reported by all the subjects seen in our study.

2   Synaesthesia is projected. Cytowic proposes that synaesthesic percepts are experienced as being external rather than in the "mind's eye". He later says that subjects who lack this projection usually have restricted forms such as coloured numbers and letters. The vast majority of our subjects lacked this projection and those that did all had their synaesthesia restricted to letters and numbers.

3   Synaesthetic percepts are durable and discrete. This is a criterion derived from observation with which we would definitely concur. All of our subjects firmly stated that the colours they perceived for stimuli had unwaveringly remained the same over the whole of their lives.

4   Synaesthesia is memorable. Cytowic suggests that a strong relationship exists between synaesthesia and hypermnesis, a consequence of which is that synaesthetic percepts are vividly remembered. This is echoed in the anecdotes supplied both by our subjects and also by Luria's (1968) account of a mnemonist whose memory was substantially aided by the synaesthesiae that accompanied events and objects. Of course, what is difficult to determine is whether the synaesthesia causes the hypermnesis or vice versa.

5   Synaesthesia is emotional. According to Cytowic synaesthetes possess an unshakeable conviction that their perceptions are real. This is again echoed by our subjects who conveyed a strong belief that what they perceived was undoubtedly real.

In order to choose between the competing theories of learnt association and brain based percept, a methodology needed to be devised. Such a test was devised by Baron-Cohen *et al.* (1987) who created an empirical test of synaesthesia, which has come to be known as "the Test of Genuineness" (TOG). This test requires subjects to give their colour percept descriptions to more than 100 lexical items. Later after a specified interval the subject is again tested on the list and the two sets of responses compared in order to test their consistency. In the Baron-Cohen *et al.* study the synaesthesic subject EP achieved 100% concordance across a period of 10 weeks, as compared with 17% accuracy for a control subject who was prewarned that she would be retested.

A consequence of the reporting of the above experiment is that a large number of putative synaesthetic individuals contacted our group. We decided to test a group of 10 chromatic-lexical synaesthetes using an extended version of the TOG, this time including 130 items including letters and homophones. All subjects were tested for IQ (NART) and memory (Wechsler Logical Memory) and were matched with controls for age and gender. On this occasion controls were tested 1 week later and synaesthetes 18 months later and whilst the synaesthetes did not perform perfectly they were at least three times more accurate than controls (Baron-Cohen et al., 1993). An interesting difference emerged between the responses of the original subject EP. Whereas for EP each word had a very detailed and idiosyncratic colour, for the synaesthetes tested in the above experiment it seemed to be the case that the colour of the word was dictated by the colour of the dominant letter, usually the first. Consequently, if "Penny" was found to be blue, so too was "Pound", "Pig" and any other word where "P" is the dominant letter.

The results thus far obtained appear to show that these individuals do indeed enjoy some kind of colour experience in connection with words. Quite what the nature of their ability is remains unexplained. Aghajanian (1983) found that hallucinogenic compounds appear to stimulate the locus caeruleus, a part of the brain where fibres from the sensory modalities meet. He points to this as being the cause of synaesthesia and proposes that it is possible that in synaesthetic individuals fibres from different modalities synapse onto one another. Consequently the subject may have visual experiences that co-occur with hearing words. This unusual linkage may be a hereditary brain state which, as we have mentioned, appears to be passed predominantly to female offspring. In a bid to uncover the nature of synaesthesic percepts we have recently tested synaesthetes and controls using positron emission tomography (PET) (Paulesu et al., in prep). Subjects in two groups were deprived of visual input and played tapes of either pure tones, which would elicit no colour experience in either group, or words which elicit colours for the synaesthetic group only. The full results of this experiment are not yet available but preliminary analysis has shown differences in brain activation between the two groups in the visual cortex, especially in those areas held to be responsible for dealing with colour, the lingual and fusiform gyri (Lueck et al., 1989).

Our synaesthetic subjects, who were all of "sound mind", appear to have an experience of reality that differs from that of individuals without the condition. Every synaesthete we have seen has stated their firm belief that to them these synaesthesic percepts are undoubtedly "real". Bertrand Russell said that the nature of reality issue is the one that causes the most trouble in philosophy and as with most problematic areas of philosophy, truth or even consensus, has been extremely hard to come by. The core of the debate seems to focus on whether objects exist only in the sense that we perceive them or whether they enjoy an existence independent of our perceptions. Those who subscribe to the philosophy of Realism adopt the intuitive, common sense viewpoint that physical objects exist independently of our perceptions. Others such as Berkeley, have been puzzled by this and have maintained that what is required for an object to exist is for it to be perceived. Realists, such as G.E. Moore, maintain that this Idealist view is subject to refutation in that Idealists appear to confuse the mind-dependent act of seeing a colour with its object which is the colour itself. However, the Idealists retort that if we are not currently perceiving an object then how can we know that it exists? Realists maintain that universals, or properties, have a real existence and are represented mentally by being compared with a mental concept. Consequently a car is red by virtue of our matching the colour of the car with our concept of redness. This echoes J.S. Mill's view that material objects were possessed of "permanent possibilities of sensation and thus an object is perceived when some or all of these possibilities are realized". An idealist, however, would maintain that objects exist only by virtue of the fact that their universals have a real existence. Problematic for the Idealist view of reality were phenomena such as after-images and phantom limb pain for which percepts existed for the individual but did so in the absence of environmental stimuli and could not therefore be considered to be "real" qualities of the world.

A new philosophy emerged which took account of these phenomena and came to be known as Critical Realism. Critical realists held that we can gain knowledge of the world by virtue of a reliable correspondence between internal data and external objects. Critical Realism therefore retained a belief in the independence of physical objects but held that these are not always directly presented to us and in these instances require different explanations.

It therefore seems that any conclusion we may reach concerning whether or not we are prepared to grant synaesthetic percepts the status of reality, is dependent on the paradigm we adopt. This situation appears to be an extension of the argument concerning the status of phantom limb pain and after image. Patients suffering with phantom limb pain appear to be in no doubt as to the reality status of their pain; for them it is a real experience. The experience of pain is a consequence of our biology in much the same way as other aspects of our perceptual experience. We may argue that if phantom limb pain is experienced by its sufferers then we may consequently accord it the status of reality. This situation does not seem to accord with either the idealist or realist view of reality. It is difficult to imagine that realists would want to accept that synaesthetic percepts are a quality of the world in much the same way as they would have problems accepting that after-images exist independently of our perceptions. The idealists would presumably regard this as problematic in that they claim that the reality of objects can only be known by their universals. Consequently, in order to accept synaesthetic percepts as being real we would have to accept that words do possess the quality of synaesthetic word colour. As we have seen, the colour experienced by each synaesthete for each word whilst being consistent is also idiosyncratic. This view that we can know objects by virtue of there being a consensus of opinion regarding the nature of the object, would thus seem to preclude synaesthetic percepts from being accorded the status of reality.

As a psychological, rather than philosophical, perspective on the reality status of percepts, Still (1979) reports that psychology since Descartes has taken a constructionist view of the world. He quotes Douglas (1970) who proposes that "In a chaos of shifting impressions, each of us constructs a stable world". Still considers another theory of perception which he labels a form of realism, the substance of which echoes much of the philosophy of realism rehearsed above in which he concludes that to make a choice between constructionism (idealism) and realism is impossible, as we cannot provide logical or empirical refutation of either theory.

difficult to accept that synaesthetic word colour is a "real" property of the world in that it exists independently or our perceptions, a conclusion that would seem to preclude a "realistic" acceptance of synaesthetic percepts. However, if we accept an "idealistic" explanation of reality then it is possible to consider these percepts as real in the sense that they are part of the construction of reality made by synaesthetes. This construction of the world would run contrary to the experience of non-synaesthetes, and if we define reality as being the view of the majority then we would be forced to conclude that synaesthetic percepts are not real qualities of the world. However, we cannot claim any logical justification for this definition.

## References

Atkinson, R.C. and Shiffrin, R.M. (1971). The control of short term memory. *Scientific American*, **225**, (2) 82-90.

Baron-Cohen, S., Wyke, M. and Binnie, C. (1987). Hearing words and seeing colours: an experimental investigation of a case of synaesthesia. *Perception*, **16**, 761-767.

Baron-Cohen, S., Harrison, J., Goldstein, M. and Wyke, M. (in press). Coloured speech perception: Is synaestheias what happens when modularity breaks down?

Bernard, J.W. (1986). Messiaen's synaesthesia, the correspondence between colour and sound structure in his music. *Music Perception*, **4**, (1) 41-68.

Bhowmick, B.K. (1991). Recurrent near death experience with postvagotomy syndrome. *Journal of the Royal Society of Medicine*, **84**, (5) 311.

Blackmore, S.J. (1988). Visions from the dying brain. *New Scientist*, **118**, 1611, 43-46.

Bugelski, B.R. and Alampay, D.A. (1961). The role frequency in developing perceptual sets. *Canadian Journal of Psychology*, **15**, 205-211.

Cytowic, R. (1989). "Synesthesia: a Union of the Senses". Springer-Verlag, New York.

Galton, F. (1883). "Enquiries into Human Faculty and its Development". Dent and Sons, London.

Jouvet, M. (1967). The states of sleep. *Scientific American*, **216**, 62-72.

Lueck, C. (1989). The colour centre in the cerebral cortex of man. *Nature*, **340**, 6232 386-9.

Marks, L. (1975). On coloured-hearing synaesthesia: Cross-modal translations of sensory dimensions. *Psychological Bulletin*, **82**, (3) 303-394.

McQueen, C. (1987). Synaesthesia. *Landfall*, **41**, (3) 324-325.

Moody, R. (1975). "Life after Life". Mockingbird, Covington, Georgia.

Nabokov, V. (1949). "A Voyage Round my Mother".

Paulesu, E., Baron-Cohen, S., Harrison, J. and Frith, C.D. (in prep). "The Anatomy of Coloured Hearing".

Rimbaud, A. (1871). "Le Sonnet Des Voyelles". Trans. by W. Rees (1992). *In* "The Penguin book of french Poetry". 1820-95. Penguin

Ring, K. (1980). "Life at Death: a scientific investigation of the near death experience". Coward, McGann and Geoghegan. New York.

Samuel, C. (1976). "Conversations with Oliver Messiaen". Trans. F. Apprahamian Stainer & Bell.

Sergent, J. (1984). An investigation into component and configural processes underlying face perception. *British Journal of Psychology*, **75**, 221-242.

Sperling, G. (1960). The information available in brief visual presentation. *Psychological Monographs*, **74**, 11.

Young, A. (1987). Finding the mind's construction in the face. *Cognitive Neuropsychology*, **4**, (1) 45-53.

# 8. Synaesthesia

E.M.R. Critchley

---

The most neutral definition of synaesthesia is as a phenomenon whereby a stimulus presented in one mode seems to call up imagery of another mode as readily as its own. Many of the alternative definitions can be faulted in that they imply unproven underlying mechanisms which may not be appropriate to all varieties of synaesthesia. Thus synaesthesia is said to represent a "subjective" or "involuntary" joining of the senses, or an "overspill" of sensory information which develops as the strength of a modality of sensation increases to produce an emotional response stimulating a reverberation or echo among the other sensations. An accurate but dramatic definition by the art critic, E.H. Gombrich, is of a splashing over of impressions from one sensory modality to another, and it is in literature, art and music that this phenomenon is seen at its most sophisticated. Could it represent an uncanny intellectual attainment as the deliberate yet instantaneous replacement of orthodox associations by others which are arresting, unexpected and even impudent – the awakening among those of superior ability of a whole range of mental imagery?

Let us first examine the fundamental principles involved in synaesthesia. Sensation requires the recognition of an external stimulus. It is then transmitted centrally reaching awareness as a perception. If the sensation, its transmission and its perception are all within the same modality, the reality of the sensation is considered to be readily verifiable. If however there is a change of modality, either from an overspill into a second mode or by a "knight's move" with loss of the primary modality, the reality of the percept is frequently questioned. If the primary sensation is taken over or "contaminated" by a different input at a higher sensory level, for example from memory, clang associations (made between two words because they sound similar – such associations are often made by schizophrenics) or thought processes, the outcome may appear artificial and totally lacking any real basis.

It is possible to analyze synaesthesia as a purely cultural phenomenon in literary or semantic terms; and it would be wise to do this because the use of synaesthesia underlies so much creativity in all forms of art, from music to architecture. Many people throughout the world strive to achieve through synaesthesia an aesthetic harmony essential for a deeper ecstatic or religious experience. High flown phrases, intimating a state of sensory interfusion by a consciousness in which body and soul are realized as one, often permeate philosophical thought. William Blake had a vision of man's natural condition, and the condition man shall return to following the apocalyptic disclosure of the present era, as that of a psychosensory unity in which each sense is not a "narrow chink" walled off from the other senses but in a state of free communication with them. And Ogden, Richards and Wood in "The Foundations of Aesthetics" (1934) put forward a synaesthetic theory of aesthetic experience to describe the appreciation of beauty as a coming together, an equilibrium, or harmony of impulses incited in contemplation once an object is sensed to be beautiful.

If indeed synaesthesia is a harmonization or a break out from the confines of the recognized modalities of sensory perception, a scientific or psychological explanation is needed. There are, in essence, two potential neurophysiological hypotheses: aberrant neural transmission across collateral or converging sensory pathways somewhere between the sense organs and the cortex, leading to an illusionary misinterpretation of sensory data; or an ability to form cross-modal associations perhaps at a higher functional level in the absence of abnormalities of neural transmission. Thus the initial sensory experience, which may later become embroidered or elaborated as an art form, may represent a special kind of hallucinatory activity. Those with the gift may receive a sensory impression, translate it into a sensory percept within the same sensory modality, and then, in the course of extracting from it an emotional appeal or some equivalent higher sensory recognition, invoke other sensory percepts involving unrelated and apparently disparate modalities of sensation; for example, the blast of a trumpet may awaken waves of golden sound. These additional percepts are internal, unconnected to the stimulus in terms of neural mechanisms or pathways, and thus hallucinatory. Somehow those subject to such synaesthetic sensitivity are able to conjure forth a variety of secondarily associated memory traces – imagery and sensation – which belong to different sense modes. There will be situations in which the additional, unusual sensory experience will be felt either as a true sensation, or be imagined, or come to awareness in a person's thoughts in association with the primary stimulus.

In the process of an intellectual awakening of a whole range of mental imagery, or a skilful orchestration of a chain of mental associations, many of the intermediate links will be lost and drop out of awareness. Such a happening may be all too apparent in literary phrases that have become hackneyed with time: e.g. loud, perfumed colours; the scarlet blast of a trumpet; the red smell of danger; a dry, flinty, robust wine; sickly green; or darkness, winged and stinking.

Although the Founder Members of the Royal Society spoke of the harmony of the spheres as a form of celestial synaesthesia, credit for the modern concept of synaesthesia must lie with the publication of Charles Henry's "Cercle Chromatique" (1888). The Impressionists were the first group to achieve artistic freedom and talk about the personal uniqueness of their vision. Henry's psychophysical theories provided the transcendental consciousness for the Neo-Impressionists in which art is a mental abstraction visually represented by lines. He held that not only could the different arts be integrated but they could be blended to bring about in the human organization a corresponding harmonizing and transcendental experience or ecstasy: synaesthesia. In quasi-biological language, he claimed that the social function of art is to *dynamogenize* consciousness and to create a sense of continuity of behaviour. His primary impact was upon the art of Georges Seraut and Paul Signac and later upon the more maverick art of Odilon Redon, who described himself as the peintre symphonique.

The earliest scientific reports date back to the 17th century when John Locke, in his "Essay Concerning Human Understanding", and John Thomas Woolhouse independently described blind people who perceived colours whilst listening to musical sounds. In 1881 Bleuler and Lehmann in Switzerland, and in 1883 Sir Francis Galton in Britain, interviewed large groups of people to determine whether they experienced colour associations. Galton coined the word "eidetic" to explain strong visualizers with specifically exteriorized imagery (i.e. those with exact photographic memories) and explored the schematized patterns of colour and other associations whereby individuals recollect the days of the week, seasons of the year, numerals and other visual material. Pattern analyses, diagram and number forms provide useful memory aids. Such is undoubtedly the case with Luria's famous mneumonist "S" (1968) who possessed an outstandingly vivid, detailed and persistent visual memory, almost certainly eidetic, with an unusual degree of synaesthesia. Among artists van Gogh, Kandinsky, Klee and Chagall were intrigued by theoretical colour associations; and Blake retained an eidetic imagery characterized by sharpness of definition, optical reality and involuntary appearance, often under conditions of intense nervous excitement, with an explosion of auto-suggestion in which a new image would impose itself upon another.

The pooling of the senses supplying a creative energy is found in many religions. Lama Govinda in "The Psychological Attitude of Early Buddhist Philsopy" (1961) seems to suggest that the Buddhist approach anticipates that of Kant: "the Buddhist does not inquire into the essence of matter, but only into the essence of the sense perceptions which create in us the idea of matter". Hindu philosophy equates *Nada Brahman,* the primordial sound, with the Absolute, the Creator. It is significant that *shakti,* the energy of the creative power of Brahman, is also called *nada* (sound) or *sabda* (word). *Anahata nada,* or unstruck sound, is not a matter of sense perception but a mystic experience in which sound and light are fused together in a direct perception of the Absolute. *Raga* is a Sanskrit term central to all Indian music. It portends a passion, colour and attachment, something that has the effect of colouring the hearts of men. Hindustani music in particular does not isolate individual notes but glides over the intervals which separate them. Each note in the scale, when heard along with the tonic, yields, as a word does in language, a colour and emotional charge. For instance (to quote Sheila Dhar, 1988), one might say arbitrarily that the perfect fifth is red, positive, strong; that the third is sky blue, tranquil, lucid; and that the flat third or sixth is grey, introspective, plaintive, and so on. This sense of the inherent emotional content of intervals is a common language understood in general terms by all who share the regional culture of which this system of music is a product. The skilled musician uses these colours, leading his audiences into delicately shaded areas, carrying them all through the creative process, line by line, stroke by stroke, colour by colour.

R.E. Cytowic in his study of a selected group of "synesthetes", "Synesthesia: A Union of the Senses" (1989), differentiates spontaneous, or idiopathic, synaesthesia from acquired synaesthesia associated with drugs, eplilepsy or pathological states of the central nervous system. Others suggest that the evoked colours can range in strength from visual imagery or fantasy to architectural shapes and true hallucinations. Thus Colman (1894) describes four "degrees" of secondary sensations evoked by music:

1   flashes of light (photisms) located internally behind the eyes or within the skull;
2   colours appearing in the background behind actual objects in the environment, though not obscuring them;
3   photisms projected spatially towards the source of the auditory stimulus; and
4   brilliant visual impressions which obliterate all about them or blend with the colours of the environment to engender a totally different hue.

**Types of Synaesthesia**

Most synaesthetic experience is a cross-modal association between two sensory systems. Polymodal synaesthesia is rarer by comparison. Almost any combination can occur. Schultze (1912) described a patient for whom coloured music was associated with gustatory sensations. Pain can conjure forth geometric sounds, sounds smells, colours sounds, and sounds colours. Most common, as the enormous variety of synonyms suggests, is sonogenic synaesthesia giving rise to colours: oratio colorata, Farbenhoren, Farbighoren, audition colorée, colour hearing or psycho-chromaesthesia. Sir Isaac Newton even tried to devise mathematical formulae which would approximate frequencies of sound to appropriate wavelengths of light. The sound stimulus may be non-melodic or melodic. Some normal individuals see flashes of light, recognizable as sharp activity on the electro-encephalogram, if aroused from a dreamy state by a sharp noise. Such sound-induced hynagogic photisms are called *Schrekblitz* and *Weckblitz* in the German literature where they were first described.

Many musicians describe an uncommonly powerful or compulsory evocation of colours following the presentation of sounds. Colour theories have stimulated much creativity, though the strength of the synaesthetic stimulus is by no means uniform. Olivier Messiaen combined religious mysticism with highly personal theories of composition which he explained in two volumes entitled "Technique de Mon Langage Musicale" (1947): "I try to convey colours through music; certain combinations of tones and certain sonorities are bound by certain colour combinations and I employ them to this end." Liszt when Kapellmeister at Weimar bewildered his players at rehearsals by urging... "more pink here, if you please", or by declaring "that is too black", or, "here I want it all azure". There are several comprehensive studies of synaesthesia and music. P.A. Scholes' "Oxford Companion to Music" devotes eight pages to the subject of colour and music and Macdonald Critchley in "Music and the Brain" (1977) has a chapter entitled Ecstatic and Synaesthetic Experiences during Musical Perception.

As in Walt Disney's film "Fantasia", musical instruments, notes, tunes and compositions elicit particular colours. Voices may be a rich brown, or primrose yellow. Compositions such as *Der Fliegende Holländer* may appear as a mysterious green. Ireland wrote his *Scarlet Ceremonies* and Bliss his *Colour Symphony* in which he labelled the movements, I Purple, II Red, III Blue, and IV Green. Even composers have been recognized by distinctive colours. Skriabin, Rimsky-Korsakof and many others have attributed colours to keys, and this may be an aid to memory just as colouring of letters can help the dyslexic. Some of those who have sought to project synaesthetic relationships have been regarded as eccentric personalities and showmen. Louis Bertrand Castel (1688-1757) published a book, "La Musique en Couleurs", and constructed a harpsichord for the eyes in which each key also played light on coloured tapes. A. Wallace Rimington (1854-1918), with his colour organ, focused on a screen of changing colours. Thomas Wilfred's clavilux used vibrations to project fantastic figures moving rhythmically, changing their shapes and hues incessantly. Laszlo invented a colour piano. More especially, Schönberg's *Die glückliche Hand* and Skriabin's *Prometheus* or "Poem of Fire" notated the details of an actual play of colours to be projected on to a screen during the performances of the musical work.

Chromatogenic synaesthesia has likewise stimulated many abstract painters. One of the earliest was a Lithuanian, M.K. Cuirlionis, a musical prodigy who suddenly turned to painting. His aim was to paint music. His colour compositions were conceived as symphonic movements with such titles as *Ocean Sonata, Sun Sonata, Snake Sonata*. Luigi Russolo (1885-1947) was a musician who took to painting as a member of the Futurist movement. He became obsessed with the development of Brutish musical instruments inventing many and producing a manifesto, "The Art of Noises" (1913). Some of his paintings *Music* (1911) and *Fog*, (1912) clearly have a synaesthetic appeal. The Belgium painter, Antoine Wiertz (1806-1865), was yet more bizarre. He painted portraits for bread and huge apocalyptic religious and historical canvases for honour. He refused to sell the latter, believing that they surpassed the masterpieces of Rubens, Raphael and Michelangelo. These fantastic, macabre and often erotic compositions were designed to be viewed to the accompaniment of a concealed choir. The combination of painting and music is by no means original: El Greco (aping the modern teenager with his Walkman) used to obtain inspiration when painting from the playing of a hidden orchestra close by. Wassily Kandinsky (1866-1944), a serious artist and theoretician with a musical background, who was one of the leading members of the Blaue Reiter movement and the Bauhaus, provided many synaesthetic paintings with such titles as *Dreamy Improvisation, Yellow Accompaniment, Compositions V, and VII,* and *Green Sounds*. Kandinsky wrote that painting can develop the same energies as music. Forms and colours should penetrate the beholder, reverberate in him and move him in his depths, as music does the listener. Each modality possesses an energy or vibration; it is only as a step towards the spiritual vibration that the physical impression is important. His pictures are often a dazzling constellation of moving, thrilling and nervous forms. Mondrian's painting *Broadway Bougie Woogie* is an excellent example of synaesthesia. Klee, Kubin, Arp all shared the same vision and van Gogh prophesied that painting promised to become more subtle, "more music and less sculpture".

To attribute synaesthesia to writers is often less certain. It is too easy for them to adopt a successful genre. However, Baudelaire (1860), "Les Paradis Artificiels", and J-K Huysmans (1889), "A Rebours", are undoubtedly genuine. Huysmans describes the unusual sensory experiences of his hero, Des Esseintes. Each liqueur corresponded in taste with the sound of a particular instrument and the music of the liqueurs had its specific scheme of interrelated tones. Others such as Gautier (1843) experimented with hashish ("Le Club des Haschischiens") to achieve a synaesthetic state: "J'entendais le bruit des couleurs. Des sons verts, rouges, bleus, jaunes, m'arrivaient par ondes parfaitement distinctes". This is not an inevitable result of hallucinatory drugs, even among so-called synaesthetes. It has been suggested that synaesthesia is a special aptitude or ability akin to mathematical, musical or artistic talent. The visions conjured up are intensely personal, and apply to less than 10% of the population. As a result works claiming a specific synaesthetic appeal may fail to convince. Thus few performances of Skriabin's *tastiera per luce* have succeeded outside Russia. Those not gifted with colour-hearing were left cold or puzzled. Audiences were equally perplexed when Dame Edith Sitwell used the expression, "Emily coloured primulas". She explained that she meant pink: others conceived "Emily" as a white pepper colour, or yellow, or even mauve.

## The Physiological Basis of Synaesthesia

The simplest physiological hypotheses imply a mixing of sensory information either because the sensory systems are primitive and undifferentiated or because there is some defect permitting aberrant neural transmission. The activation of a secondary sensory mode is thus illusory. Many would argue that synaesthesia and similar phenomena such as eidetic vision are more likely to be met with in childhood and tend to disappear as the nervous system becomes more mature with greater insulation or myelination of nerve fibres. Thus Bleuler regarded synaesthesia as a physiological condition, present in everyone but available for conscious experience to only a minority of adults.

There is much evidence from acquired synaesthesia to suggest that impaired transmission can cause synaesthetic sensations. Touch and pain synaesthesia has already been described in an earlier chapter when trauma to the spinal cord or phantom limb phenomena result in aberrant sensations at a secondary site remote from the stimulus. With concussion we can become dazed or "see stars". Pressure on the eyeball can elicit photisms of light. Movement of the eyes can produce flick phosphenes in healthy individuals and flashes of light if the optic tract loses insulation from demyelination as with retrobulbar neuritis or multiple sclerosis. Scintillations may occur with retinal arterial vasoconstriction in migraine, and "lightening streaks of Moore", vertical curved streaks of brilliant white or sluggish bluish light, sometimes slightly zig-zag, may appear in the temporal visual field in the presence of vitreous detachment. A clear example of synaesthesia of epileptic origin is presented by Jacome and Gummitt (1979). Their patient had episodic seizures characterized by sudden pain over the right side of the face; simultaneously he heard the word "five" and saw the number "5" on a grey background before both eyes. These episodes occurred about ten times a month.

Some ephaptic spread or blending occurs physiologically within adjacent sensory channels. Sophisticated sensory information from the periphery ascends mainly in the limbic system and Cytowic and others believe that this system offers the possibility for a degree of anatomical and physiological mingling of sensory information. Although the main concentrations of auditory or other stimuli may be projected onto specific areas of the cortex, there is, in addition, a more random cortical distribution of sensory information as is evident from examination of the cerebral hemispheres by dichotic listening techniques and somatosensory action potentials. With strokes and other catastrophes, apparently unconnected parts of the brain may be impaired through diaschiasis or spreading depression. Presumably similar mechanisms have some role in healthy states. The cortex may be divided into primary, receptive or motor areas and secondary, association areas where information from memory sources, intuitive urges, and sensory receptors is correlated. Within these association areas, synaesthesia maybe induced by means of an abnormal loosening of information processing, which in turn allows undue diffusion or "seepage" from one input channel to another. A loosening of the boundaries between modalities of sensation can be expected in drug-induced states and in schizophrenia, and, indeed, synaesthetic phenomena due to intoxication from hallucinatory drugs or as psychotic experiences in delirious states are well recognized. By way of contrast, agnosia can be regarded as the restriction of processing, which prevents interaction between a damaged channel and those which remain undamaged. Thus in agnosia the assessment, and ultimate expression, of information received in one channel cannot be augmented by other impressions.

Psychological theories of synaesthesia abound. Characteristically Hug-Hellmuth declared that synaesthesia resulted from early childhood experiences where the memory associations are later repressed. Infantile sexual experiences, by stirring up pleasurable and painful emotions, can heighten synaesthesia and cause them to become fixed in memories or fantasies. A more modern hypothesis is that of Reichard, Jakobson and Werth (1949) who interpret the frequent occurrence of synaesthesia among children as an important stage in the development of memory and the learning of language. Other psychological theories (e.g. Goldstone, 1962) differ from psychological explanations in that they place the element of sensory interaction in synaesthesia at a conceptual level. The neural mechanisms for making intersensory distinctions may be "built in" but the experience or perception of these distinctions is more probably of a learned, conceptual nature. I would like to think that synaesthesia, even if it has arisen as part of the learning process or is due to prolonged fetalization wherein cells retain into adult life a pluripotency or undifferentiated state, is an example of man's ability to rise above or control the normal restraints of his environment or the framework in which he is encased: that it is a stimulus to creativity which owes much to man himself.

## References

Arguelles, J.A. (1975). "The Transformative Vision". Shambhala, London.
Baudelaire, C. (1860). "Les Paradis Artificiels". Gallimard, Paris.
Bleuler, E. and Lehmenn, K. (1881). "Zwangsmaessige Lichtempfundungen durch Schall und verwandte Erscheinungen auf der Gebiete der anderen Sinnesemmpfindungen". Fues S. Verlag, Leipzig.
Bleuler, E. (1913). Zur Theorie der Sekundarempfindungen. *Zeitschrift für Psychologie und Physiologie, Sinnesorg*, **65**, 1-39.
Castell, L.B. (1920). "La Musique des Couleurs".
Colman, W.S. (1894). Hallucinations in the sane associated with local organic disease of the sensory organs. *British Medical Journal*, **i**, 1015-1017.
Colman, W.S. (1984). Further remarks on colour hearing. *Lancet*, **i**, 22-4.
Colman, W.S. (1898). On so-called colour hearing. *Lancet*, **i**, 786-8.
Critchley, E.M.R. (1987). "Hallucinations and Their Impact on Art". Carnegie Press, Preston.
Critchley, M. (1977). Ecstatic and synaesthetic experiences during musical perception. *In* "Music and the Brain". (Eds M. Critchley and R.A. Henson). pp. 217-232. Heinemann, London.
Cytowic, R.E. (1989). "Synesthesia: a Union of the Senses". Springer Verlag, London.
Dhar, S. (1988). Hindustani music. *In* "India". pp. 140-147. Specially published for the Festival of India.
Fraser-Harris, D. (1905). On psychochromaesthesia and certain synaesthesiae. *Edinburgh Medicine Journal*, **18**, 529.
Galton, F. (1883). "Enquiries into Human Faculty". Dent and Dutton, London.
Goldstone, S. (1962). Psychophysics, reality and hallucinations. *In* "Hallucinations". (Ed. L.J. West). Grune and Stratton, New York.
Gomrich, E.A. (1960). "Art and Illusion". Phaidon Press, London.
Govinda, L.A. (1961). "The Psychological Attitudes of Early Buddhist Philosophy". London.
Henry, C. (1888). "Cercle Chromatique". Charles Verdin, Paris.
Hug-Hellmuth, H. (1912). Ueber Farbenhoeren. *Imago*, **1**, 228-264.
Huysmans, J-K. (1889). "Against the Grain (A. Rébours), Paris and Illustrated Editions Co., New York, 1931.
Jacome, D.E. and Gummit, R.J. (1979). Synaesthetic seizures. *Neurology*, **29**, 1050-1053.

Luria, A.R. (1968). "The Mind of a Mneumonist". Basic Books, New York.
Messiaen, O. (1956). "Technique de Mon Langage Musicale". Alphonse Leduc, Paris.
Moore, R.F. (1935). Subjective lightening streaks. *British Journal of Ophthalmology*, **19**, 545-547.
Ogden, C.K., Richards, L.A. Wood, J. (1934). "The Foundations of Aesthetics". London.
Reichard, G., Jakobson, R. and Werth, E. (1949). Language and synaesthesia. *Word*, **5**, 224-233.
Rizzo, M. and Eslinger, P.J. (1989). Colored hearing synesthesia. *Neurology*, **39**, 781-784.
Scholes, P.A. (1977). "The Oxford Companion to Music". 10th edn. Oxford University Press. Oxford.
Zaret, B.S. (1985). Lightening streaks of Moore. *Neurology*, **35**, 1078-.

# 9. Alterations in conscious awareness

Peter Fenwick

## Introduction

Our view of the world is conditioned by the functioning of the brain. In this scientific era there is little to support the view that mind is more than neural nets and neurological processes. Science demands a neurocognitive explanation for all subjective experience. But here is the difficulty. For, as yet, we have no comprehensive scientific explanation of subjectivity. As Sherrington said, when using the energy scheme to trace the light from a star to the eye, retina, optic nerve, pathways and cortex: "At this point the scheme puts its finger to its lips and is silent." There is no explanation of how the star comes into subjective experience.

### Models of the World

Western science is based on the rationalism of Descartes, Galileo, Locke and Newton. Galileo defined a two-stuff universe: matter and energy, with primary and secondary qualities. The primary qualities were those aspects of nature that could be measured, such as velocity, acceleration, weight, mass, etc. The secondary qualities were those of subjective experience, such as smell, vision, truth, beauty, love, etc. Galileo maintained that the domain of science was the domain of primary qualities. Secondary qualities were non-scientific. Science has held this view ever since and has consequently not taken account of secondary qualities or subjective experience. Descartes had a similar world view. He too argued for the existence of two substances: that of the physical world, the res extensor, and that of the mental world, the res cogitans. Science, he claimed, acted in the domain of the res extensor.

Einstein's recognition, that mass and energy could be precisely equated, changed Galileo's two-stuff universe into a one-stuff universe. And that is the universe we have today. The other major advance of the early part of the 20th century was the discovery of quantum mechanics and Bell's theorem. This theorem postulated the non-locality of matter, and gave an explanation for the wave particle duality theory of Schrödinger. In its simplest form this principle states that the wave function which defines each particle is spread throughout space. At the moment of trying to measure a particle, the wave function collapses and the position of the particle can then be measured within the rules of quantum mechanics.

## Mind models

The view that matter is distributed throughout space does not easily accord with the view that mind is only a function of the brain. It is important to understand the two major philosophical schools which currently attempt to explain mind. Dennett's neuro-philosophy characterizes one extreme. He argues that consciousness and subjective experience are just the functions of neural nets. Explain neural nets in detail and you will also have explained subjective experience and personal consciousness; nothing else is required. This is clearly a reductionist approach, equating subjective experience entirely with neural mechanisms.

The other extreme is characterized by the philosophy of Nagel, who argues that it is never possible to know the quality of another first person experience. Subjective experience is not available to the scientific method, and cannot be validated in the public domain. Nagel argues that however much we understand about the neurophysiology of the functioning of a bat's brain, we will never know what it is like to be a bat. This view suggests that the explanation of subjective experience requires a new principle which is beyond neural nets.

Searle argues from an intermediate position. He regards subjective experience as being a property of neural nets, but he does not agree with Dennett that our current understanding of neural net functioning is sufficient to explain subjective experience. Recently he has expressed the opinion that we need an entirely new principle – an Einstein of neurophysiology – to produce a synthesis between first and third person experience.

Until there is a satisfactory scientific explanation of the nature of mind, it will not be possible to answer questions about the nature of subjective experience, religious experience and the possibility of extrasensory perception. This field is by definition still beyond the confines of science. At present, any scientific theory of mind must explain everything in terms of brain function. However, I expect there are many people who, like Schrödinger, feel claustrophobic when asked to accept that the broad sweep of the soul is contained only within the grey porridge of the brain. "Now our skulls are not empty. But what we find there, in spite of the keen interest it arises, is truly nothing when held against the life and the emotions of the soul." (Schrödinger, "Mind and Matter").

## Objective versus subjective experience

The gold standard of science is the repeatability of a third person phenomenon. When considering the significance of subjective experience one must always ask whether or not the experience has any objective validity or is entirely subjective, as, for example, the passivity phenomena of schizophrenia, where the schizophrenic patient feels that he is able to read the minds of others. Experiences arising from disorders of the temporal lobe, such as premonitions or déjà vu feelings, fall directly into this category of non-veridical subjective experience.

## The Physiology of the Religious Experience

Religious experience is very common in the population. Although very little evidence exists concerning wide mystical states, there are many studies of mystical or religious experience. Hay in his book "Exploring Inner Space" (1982), reviews the early literature on religious experience. Early studies of religious experience by Gloch and Stark (1965) showed that over 45% of Protestants, and 43% of Roman Catholics had had "a feeling that you are somehow in the presence of God." Gallup surveys in the United States by Back and Bourque in 1963, 1966 and 1967, showed that 20.5%, 32% and 44% respectively had had a "religious or mystical" experience. The percentage increased as the decade advanced, perhaps because the Hippie movement allowed people to express their mystical experiences more freely. However, a survey by the Princeton Religious Research Center in 1978 found a positive response of only 35% to a similar question, possibly a reflection of a waning of popular interest in the mystical. In Britain, Hay's NOP survey of 1976, found a similar rate of reply: about 36% gave positive responses. Of interest is the finding that although about a third of all people have had the experience, only 18% have had it more than twice and only 8% "often" and more. There was no correlation with age, but positive replies were commonest in those whose education continued beyond 20 years of age, e.g. the more articulate university graduates. There was also, interestingly, a sex difference: 41% of women gave positive replies, only 31% of men. Duration varied; 51% said it lasted between seconds and minutes, 74% that it lasted less than a day.

Wider mystical states, in which the subject describes a feeling of universal love, are much less common. These ecstatic states occur spontaneously, but they, or fragments of them, may also occur in near death experiences, very occasionally in temporal lobe epilepsy, in certain drug experiences, and frequently in psychosis, when they are usually associated with an elevation of mood. It is thus likely that the ability to experience an ecstatic state is part of normal brain function. This would be supported by the training processes carried out in many Eastern religions which lead directly to the experience of feelings of universal love.

Buck, a Canadian psychiatrist who lived at the turn of the century, was one of the first Western scientists to attempt to define (in his book "Cosmic Consciousness") mystical experience. He quotes, among many, the experience of a nun:

> Now came a period of rapture so intense that the Universe stood still as if amazed at the unutterable majesty of the spectacle: only one in all the infinite universe. The all-caring, perfect one, perfect wisdom, truth, love and purity: and with rapture came insight. In that same wonderful moment of what might be called supernal bliss came illumination... what joy when I saw that there was no break in the chain – not a link left out – everything in its place and

time. Worlds, systems, all blended in one harmonious world, universal, synonymous with universal love.

Buck lists nine features which have been used as a basis by subsequent authors to categorize the elements of the experience. Pahnke and Richards (1966) give a comprehensive account of the features of drug-induced mystical experience: this is essentially comparable with Buck's list.

1   Unity. The feeling that the panorama of life is underpinned by a unifying and eternal principle.

2   Objectivity and reality. Shown by (a) insightful knowledge or illumination and b) authoritativeness, or the certainty from the experiences that such knowledge is truly or ultimately real, in contrast to subjective feelings which are a delusion.

3   Transcendence of space and time. Space and time are generally meaningless concepts although one can look back in a transcendent way on the totality of history.

4   The sense of sacredness. A non-rational intuitive hushed palpitant response in the presence of inspiring realities. It has a special value and is capable of being profaned.

5   Deeply felt positive mood. Feelings of joy, blessedness, peace, and bliss.

6   Paradoxicality. Mystical consciousness is often felt to be true in spite of violating Aristotelian logic. The ego is transcended and the experience is universal. They are still clearly personal experiences.

7   Ineffability. The subject claims that language is inadequate to contain or even adequately to reflect such experiences.

8   Transiency. Unless the subject becomes spiritually "realized" the duration of the mystical consciousness is temporary.

9   Positive change in attitude or behaviour. The person is said to be marked by his experience and frequently has positive changes in attitude towards himself, others, life and mystical consciousness itself.

All the features described above are quoted widely in mystical literature, but what is clear is that they are not in any way limited to spontaneous mystical experience, but are part of everyday experience. Elements of the mystical state are also included in pathological experiences such as psychoses.

If mystical experience is so common, then it is logical to assume that there must be a brain mechanism which underpins the experience. The question then is, what mechanism? Much of the evidence we have about the brain mechanisms which mediate such states has been acquired through the study of pathologically induced mystical experiences. Epileptic states are one such example.

## Temporal Lobe Epilepsy (TLE) and mystical experience

The prime example of a mystical experience associated with an epileptic seizure is that of Prince Mishkin in Dostoevsky's "The Idiot".

> He was thinking... there was a moment or two in his epileptic condition...
> when suddenly amid the sadness, spiritual darkness, and depression, his brain
> seemed to catch fire at brief moments... all his agitation, all his doubts and

worries seemed composed in a twinkling, culminating in a great calm, full of serene and harmonious joy and hope, full of understanding and knowledge of the final cause.

Dostoevsky was known to have epilepsy and so it seems reasonable to assume that he was describing his own experience. Others have suggested that it was his literary genius that ascribed this experience to the epilepsy, and that it did not occur in his aura but independently of a seizure.

In any event, positive experiences as part of the temporal lobe aura are extremely rare. In Gower's 1881 study of 505 epileptic auras only 3% were said to be emotional, and none positive. In the Lennox (1960) study of 1017 auras, only 9 were said to be pleasant (0.9%) and of these, "only a few showed positive pleasure." Penfield and Kristiansen (1951) cite only one case of an aura with a pleasant sensation, followed by an epigastic feeling of discomfort. However, in 1982 Cirignotta published an account of a patient who had just such an aura as that described by Dostoevsky before a temporal lobe seizure arising in his right temporal lobe. There is thus undoubted scientific evidence that such auras do exist prior to a seizure and that they are likely to be associated with the right side of the brain. It is not uncommon to find fragments of this experience in the epileptic aura. They often occur in patients who have had a psychotic episode and are associated with seizures arising usually but not exclusively in the left temporal lobe. A standard question to ask a patient is whether, during their auras, they have spoken to God. It is surprising how often the answer is yes. These findings suggest again a common link between psychosis and temporal lobe function and between temporal lobe function and mystical experience.

Dewhurst and Beard (1970) look specifically at those cases of TLE collected from the Maudsley and Queen Square Hospitals which showed religious conversion. The conversion usually came suddenly and was not always related to a mystical aura; of more interest, the majority of their cases had previously had a psychotic illness. It was thus difficult to know whether their experience was related to their epilepsy or their psychosis. It is worth noting that both the Slater and Beard studies, and the Dewhurst and Beard studies had several patients in common and so were not totally independent.

**TLE, Mystics and Saints**

Many authors have drawn attention to the relationship between the mystical experience of some of the saints and reported alterations in their consciousness and behaviour. Often changes in behaviour are accompanied by an alteration in consciousness which could be interpreted as being epileptic in nature. Dewhurst and Beard mentioned that St Catherine de Ricci (1522-1590) had frequent hallucinations and stigmata. She lost consciousness regularly, at weekly intervals, being "out" from noon on Thursday till 4.00 p.m. the next day. These could have been epileptic although they are rather too long; some were possibly hysterical.

St Theresa of Lisieux (1873-1897) had a series of mystical experiences when she was 9 years old. They started with attacks of violent trembling, such that she thought she was going to die. Later, she had frightening hallucinations leading to a mystical experience and complete conversion. These experiences could possibly be attributed to TLE. Dewhurst and Beard quote Leuba (1925):

> These other Christian mystics also suffered from abnormal mental states which he tentatively diagnosed as hysteria, although their symptoms equally well suggest temporal lobe epilepsy. They were St Catherine of Genoa (1447-1510), Mme. Guyon (1648-1717) and St Margaret Marie (1647-1690). These mystics had periodic attacks which include the following symptoms: sensations of extremes of heat and cold, trembling of the whole body, transient aphasia, automatisms passivity feelings, hyperaesthesie, childish regression, dissociation, somnambulism, transient paresis, increased suggestibility, and inability to open the eyes.

Bryant (1953) suggest that St Paul's "thorn in the flesh" could have been epilepsy and he quotes in support of this his sudden religious conversion on the road to Damascus, with photism, paralysis, transient blindness and confusion. Bryant is also an enthusiast about genius and epilepsy. In his book he quotes the following people as having genius, epilepsy and mystical experience: Buddha, Socrates, St Cecilia, Caligula, Bohme, Pascall, Napoleon, George Fox, Caesar, Alexander, St Paul, Mahomet, Van Gogh, Peter the First (the Great), Paul 1st of Russia, Swedenborg, William Pitt, Byron and Swinburne. But not everyone agrees. It is important to keep in mind that, despite the wide ranging of epileptologists throughout the world's mystical literature, very few true examples of the ecstatic aura and the temporal lobe seizure had been reported prior to 1980. It is likely that the earlier accounts of TLE and temporal lobe pathology and the relation to mystic and religious states owes more to the enthusiasm of their authors than to a true scientific understanding of the nature of temporal lobe functioning.

It thus seems clear that the temporal lobe is to some extent involved in the normal synthesis of mystical feelings and states, but it is also clear that these states are associated equally with normal brain function and psychotic illness. A parsimonious view would be that mystical experiences are normal and that temporal lobe structures are involved with their synthesis but that their expression in fragmented form is frequently associated with pathology.

## The Maudsley Hospital Population

Sensky and Fenwick (1982) attempted to reproduce American findings relating to TLE and religious experience. Subjects were taken from the Maudsley Hospital Epilepsy Clinics and compared with national samples of the general population.

In this area confusion with regard to terminology rages unchecked through the literature. Religiosity, religious interest, mystical states and ecstatic states, have been frequently used as synonyms or left undefined. Sensky and Fenwick took this into account by using standard questions to assess mystical states. The questions included: "Did your faith come gradually or was there a point at which you suddenly 'saw the light'"? and "Have you ever felt at one with the Universe and in touch with the Universal.?" If the responses were thought to occur as part of a psychotic illness they were discounted. There was a 76% response rate to the questionnaire. Of the 55 responders, 28 were male and 27 female. Fourteen patients had generalized epilepsy (26%) and 30 (56%) had a diagnosis of TLE. Of the TLE, 16 had dominant foci, 7 non-dominant, and 7 bilateral. The results are shown in Table 1.

These results show that people with TLE are not more inclined towards religion than those with generalized epilepsy. Nor did they report more frequently a belief in, or an experience of, mystical or psychic states. Of more importance, the epileptics under-report mystical and psychic states compared to the general population. This finding would seem to be at variance with that of the American workers who find "religiosity" over-represented in their temporal lobe epileptics. It does suggest that the term "religiosity" may not be travelling across the Atlantic very well and that part of the confusion is one of terminology.

TABLE 1. *Reported belief in, and experience of, mystical and other psychic phenomena in temporal lobe and generalized epilepsy.*

|  | TLE (n = 30) | Generalized epilepsy (n = 16) | Controls* (n = 1865) |
|---|---|---|---|
| Religious | 56% | 72% | 57% |
| *Mystical experience* | | | |
| Sudden gaining of faith | 40% | 62% | 42% |
| In touch with the universe | 12% | 33% | 19% |
| *Other psychic states* | | | |
| Belief in | 54% | 100% | 65% |
| Experience of | 4% | 36% | 20% |

*data from Hay and Morisy 1978, based on a specified sample of the UK population.

## Psychic Gifts and the Mystical Experience

Many anecdotal accounts from the psychic literature have linked head injury with the onset of psychic powers. There is a frequently quoted case of a Dutchman who fell off a ladder, and on regaining consciousness in hospital, it is said that he could read the minds telepathically of his doctors and nurses. Nelson (1970) found temporal lobe EEG abnormalities in 10 out of 12 mediums, suggesting an abnormality of temporal lobe function. Neppe (1980) describes a significant similarity between temporal lobe epileptic symptoms and subjective paranormal experiences. Andrew (1975), Broad and Broad (1975) and Broughton (1975) have suggested that there is a definite hemisphere functional asymmetry in psychic experiences; the non-dominant hemisphere is more important.

Fenwick *et al.* (1985) asked psychic "sensitives" about the occurrence of psychic gifts and mystical experiences. The study was set up to see how psychic sensitivity related to brain function. Twenty psychic sensitives were allocated to the study by the College of Psychic Studies, although only 17 took part. Seventeen age and sex matched controls were obtained from local church congregations: they had to have attended church weekly throughout the preceding year. Each subject was given a long interview enquiring about medical data, head injuries, periods of unconsciousness, mystical and psychic experiences. Each subject was then given the shortened Weschler Adult Intelligence Scale test, the Wechsler Logical Memory Test (test of left temporal functioning) and Benton's Visual Retention Test (right hemisphere and right temporal functioning).

TABLE 2. *The medical history of the sensitives and the control group is shown with the significance of the differences between them using a chi-test.*

|  | Sensitives | Controls | Significance chi square |
|---|---|---|---|
| Normal birth | 100% | 94% | NS |
| Serious operations | 47% | 47% | NS |
| Serious illnesses | 47% | 6% | 0.05 |
| Serious head injury | 59% | 12% | 0.01 |
| Knocked out | 47% | 12% | 0.05 |
| Blackouts | 41% | 6% | 0.04 |
| Epilepsy | 0% | 0% | NS |
| Migraine | 53% | 24% | NS |
| Prolonged medication | 35% | 12% | NS |
| Consulted psychiatrist | 41% | 6% | 0.04 |
| Right handed | 94% | 88% | NS |

The relationship between the medical history, psychic gifts and mystical experiences is shown in Tables 2 and 3. The experiences of precognition and clairaudience were significantly associated with right hemisphere damage, as was the experience of the presence of a psychic helper or psychic guide. Telepathy showed a trend towards being significantly correlated with head injury. Significant mystical experience was statistically more common among the sensitives, 88%, but it was also surprisingly common among the controls (47%). Note that the control rate is little different from general population surveys. Other differences were also seen between the groups, the sensitives being rather more fragile than the controls. The sensitives were single significantly more often. They had more serious illnesses, head injuries, episodes of being knocked unconscious, having had blackouts. And had consulted a psychiatrist more frequently. The psychological tests showed a significant difference in verbal IQ between the groups – 129 for the sensitives and 139 for the controls. There was no difference in performance IQ – this was 118 in both groups. No significant differences were found for any of the other tests, so that groups were then combined. There were no left hemisphere abnormalities for either group, although both right hemisphere and right temporal abnormalities were found.

TABLE 3. *Significant associations with right temporal lobe impairment.*

| $n = 34$ | With Significance | Without Significance | chi square |
|---|---|---|---|
| Precognition | 27% | 12% | 0.04 |
| Clairaudience | 24% | 9% | 0.05 |
| Telepathy | 33% | 21% | 0.07 trend |
| Have psychic guide | 33% | 16% | 0.05 |
| Work with psychic helper ($n = 18$) | 39% | 22% | 0.01 Fisher's test |
| Right hemisphere impairment | | | 0.04 |

In the combined groups, there is a clear relationship between the previously significant psychic gifts, clairvoyance, and mystical experience, all with right hemisphere damage. But it must be recognized that there was no correlation between tests of right temporal lobe impairment and right hemisphere impairment.

TABLE 4. *The relationship in the combined group of sensitives and controls between different psychic gifts and those with and without head injuries.*

| Combined groups ($n = 34$) | With (12) head injury | Without (22) head injury | Significance chi square |
|---|---|---|---|
| Has psychic guide | 32% | 3% | 0.002 |
| Precognition | 24% | 15% | 0.03 |
| Clairaudience | 21% | 12% | 0.04 |
| Sense guide in physical space | 27% | 9% | 0.04 |
| Clairvoyance | 29% | 27% | 0.04 |
| Mystical experience | 11% | 35% | 0.06 (trend) |
| Telepathy | 24% | 12% | NS |
| Clairsentience | 24% | 12% | NS |
| Healing | 15% | 21% | NS |
| Mediumship | 15% | 50% | NS |

In our study two subjects, one control and one sensitive, who had moderately severe head injuries with right temporal memory scores of nearly zero, had very wide mystical experiences after their head injuries. This adds support to other studies which suggest that the right hemisphere and particularly the right temporal lobe may be impaired in some subjects who have mystical experience. But it also suggests that mystical experience can occur in subjects *without* any right hemisphere impairment.

## Implications

The studies discussed above have several implications. It is reasonable to assume that there is a relationship between the right temporal lobe, mystical experience, and psychic gifts. However this is not an absolute relationship as many subjects in the control group who were clearly not brain damaged and did not have temporal lobe lesions, also had mystical experiences. So many people do claim to have had mystical experiences that it is difficult to ascribe the occurrence of such experiences to pathological events. A much better hypothesis is that disfunction affecting the right hemisphere represents only one of many possible mechanisms; that these experiences may require a large right temporal input in their genesis, but that they also involve many different brain areas which can be triggered in different ways.

The implications for epilepsy are also clear. There is certainly evidence that discharges in the right medial temporal structures can lead to an aura with some features of the mystical experience. It is not clear that there is any other direct relationship. In our survey it was the patients with generalized seizures who more often reported belief in and experience of mystical phenomena.

Psychic phenomena are more difficult to explain and clearly have a multiple causation. In our survey, the mediums were more fragile people, who had had more serious illnesses, more blackouts, and had consulted psychiatrists more frequently. Neither the controls or the psychics suffered from epilepsy and yet there was a significantly greater number of blackouts in the psychic groups. Both groups certainly showed a relationship between psychic gifts and head injury. The interpretation of this is difficult. The mediums who had an unusually sensitive personality may have seen connections and interpreted bodily sensations in a way that their more down-to-earth brethren did not. The relationship with head injury is only preliminary and needs further studies to validate it. It could be argued that the appearance of psychic gifts is due to a release of a natural capability after a head injury, or it could be that the head injury itself distorts brain function and that the faults in cognitive processing are interpreted as psychic gifts. We shall have to wait for more evidence.

## Other Mystical Experiences

We have discussed both spontaneous mystical experiences and, in a more limited way, those experiences that may arise with pathology. The nature of the pathology has suggested that the right hemisphere and right temporal lobe may be preferentially involved. There is, however, a set of experiences which are linked with either extreme anxiety or with the approach of death. Elements of these experiences may also occur spontaneously for no apparent reason and with no accompanying pathology. These experiences, because they appear to be common, have given us further insights into the phenomena of the mystical experience.

## Near Death Experiences

Questions about the nature of consciousness and the structure of the world are raised by the phenomena of near death experiences. In his book "Life After Life" (1972) Moody describes the experiences reported by people who come close to death. He called these "near death experiences" (NDEs) and has always been careful to argue that they were not an extension of consciousness beyond death.

NDEs have been reported from many cultures at different times throughout history. Lorimer (1990) relates the experience of Professor Albert Heim, a Swiss geologist who published a monograph "Notes on Deaths from Falls" in 1891. His interest in this subject stemmed from his own fall from a mountain:

I saw my whole past take place in many images, as though on a stage at some distance from me. I saw myself as the chief character in the performance. Everything was transfigured as though by a heavenly light, and everything was beautiful without grief or anxiety, or without pain. The memory of very tragic experiences I had had was clear, but not saddening. I felt no conflict or strife: conflict had been transmuted into love. Elevated and harmonious thoughts dominated and united the individual images, and like magnificent music a divine calm swept through my soul.

Heim found that other people who had come near to death in accidents had experienced many of these same phenomena. What is of interest is that the experience was generated by the anxiety of falling and not by any change in brain function due to the process of dying.

In the near death experiences described by Moody and numerous workers since, these same features of a life review, heavenly light and an understanding of the universal significance of life recur. The main workers in the field, Moody (1975), Grayson (1984), and Ring (1980), have formalized data on NDEs into a sequence. This sequence is theoretical; not all people who have NDEs will experience every feature. The experiences described below are from Moody's book "Life after Life".

1    The first stage occurs at the onset of the event. It will accompany the pain of a myocardial infarct and the realization that death is inevitable, or it would accompany the realization that a car accident is imminent. The subject moves from a position of panic and fear to one of calm and detachment. They see the events unfolding both within themselves and around them, but are not affected by them. All is warmth and calm.

I began to experience the most wonderful feelings. I couldn't feel a thing in the world except peace, comfort, ease – just quietness. I felt that all my troubles were gone and I thought to myself, well how quiet and peaceful and I don't hurt at all. (p. 29).

2   In the second stage consciousness separates from the body and comes to be located on the ceiling, so that the experiencer looks down on his own unconscious body, perhaps being worked on by the resuscitation team. In the case of a car accident they may wander around the scene of the accident and watch what is happening.

> I became very seriously ill... and I left my body. I had a floating sensation as I felt myself get out of my body and I looked back and I could see myself on my bed below and there was no fear.(p. 38).

3   If the experience deepens, in the third phase the subject goes down a dark tunnel. This has the characteristics of movement and is described as not unlike flying. The subject becomes aware that there is a small point of light, nearly always described as white or gold, at the end of the tunnel and that they move progressively nearer to it. Only 5% of subjects in a survey which we carried out saw lights of any other colour. The light is always associated with love and peace. They may recognize that they are dying. The experience may terminate here or it may continue to the fourth stage.

> I heard the doctors say that I was dead, and that's when I began to feel as though I were tumbling actually kind of floating through this blackness...
> Everything was very black except that way off from me, I could see this light. It was a very, very brilliant light, but not too large at first. It grew larger as I came nearer and nearer to it. I was trying to get to that light at the end because I felt that it was Christ and I was trying to reach that point. (p.62)

4   In stage 4 the person enters the light, which is experienced as bliss consciousness, total love, universal being. It is supportive, all-embracing, all-good. The person becomes aware of their own limitations and negativity, but in the presence of total supportive love they can tolerate their own imperfections. They may enter into a dialogue with a being whom they sense within the light. Communication is usually through the mind, no actual words are spoken. The being, if seen at all, tends to be culturally determined, with Christians seeing Christ or a saint, and other religions the appropriate deity. What is common to the experience is the intensity and purity of the light and the total love in the experience. It seems that the clothing of the emotion is cultural.

At this point the experience branches. It can either go straight to decision, or there can be a life review.

> It was a bright yellowish white – more white. it was tremendously bright; I just can't describe it. It seemed that it covered everything, yet it didn't prevent me from seeing everything around me – the operating room, the doctors and nurses, everything. I could see clearly, and it wasn't blinding.
> At first, when the light came, I wasn't sure what was happening, but then, it asked, it kind of asked me if I was ready to die. It was like talking to a person, but a person wasn't there... The love that came from it is just unimaginable, indescribable. (p. 63).

5   The life review is one of the most interesting features of the NDE. Firstly, it links in to popular anecdotal accounts of people drowning, who report that their

whole life flashes past their eyes. In the life review the subject is shown his whole life in a panoramic fashion. This is done within the all-loving enfoldment of the light. The actions of the individual are frequently seen as shabby and self-interested. This experience of guilt, however, can be tolerated by the supportive quality of the surrounding love. Often the subject will experience the results of the action as they were perceived by the recipient. They may experience the pain of a physical blow that they gave in a fight, or the psychological pain they inflicted. The consequence of the life review is a feeling that they have learned from this and therefore they determine to do better and change.

> When the light appeared, the first thing he said to me was "What do you have to show me that you've done with your life?" or something to this effect. And that's when these flashbacks started... it was like I was walking from the time of my very early life, on through each year of my life, right up to the present. (p. 65).

6  Decision is the final stage before returning from the experience. It may be preceded by leaving the light and walking in a heavenly countryside where there may be brilliantly coloured birds and flowers, heavenly music, and dead friends or relatives (and in the case of children, living friends as well). The experiencer may "talk" (though again, actual words are not used) to a relative or to the Being of Light, or they may just come to realise that they have to return. There is a realization that if they continue their progress then they will leave their bodies and die. Once the realization has occurred that they wish to return, then they find themselves back in their body and experiencing pain.

> I wondered whether I should stay there, but as I did I remembered my family, my three children and my husband. Now, this is the part that is hard to get across. When I had this wonderful feeling, there in the presence of the light, I really didn't want to come back. But I... knew I has a duty to my family. So I decided to try to come back. (p.78).

Following the experiences there is frequently a subjective change in the individual which is directed towards a greater awareness of spiritual values. Frequently they change their lifestyle in a significant way, setting out to be more altruistic and conscious of the community.

There is a debate as to whether or not these experiences tell us anything about the process of dying and the continuation of personal consciousness after death, or whether they are the distortions of a dying brain. The arguments for the dying brain hypothesis are as follows:

Science defines consciousness in the terms of neural nets and cognitive structures, and thus any experiences must be due to an alteration of brain function. The early part of the NDE, the feelings of calm, are said to be due to a dissociated state. Dissociated states are known to occur in response to anxiety and in such states calmness and tranquillity are commonly experienced as a protection against overwhelming anxiety or physical pain.

The separation of consciousness from the body is described by science as "autoscopy" and this can occur spontaneously, in response to stress, or during the auras of temporal lobe epilepsy. It can also be induced by brain stimulation with implanted electrodes in the temporal lobe. It is thus postulated that as body image and consciousness of self is synthesized within the brain and usually placed just behind the eyes, it is possible for the brain in unusual circumstances to use different spatial coordinates and project this feeling from its usual position behind the eyes to a corner of the ceiling or to any other location outside the body.

The tunnel and the approach of the light are formulated as a disintegration of function within the visual cortex and its attempt to model a failing reality. In these circumstances it is these that are experienced as the tunnel.

The very strong feelings of emotion are thought to be due to a failure in the medial temporal structures which synthesize emotion. It is known that these structures are particularly sensitive to anoxia and thus it is argued that with cardiac failure and the appearance of severe cerebral anoxia these structures respond by generating wide mystical experiences.

The populating of the heavenly experiences with culturally appropriate religious figures and dead friends/relatives is part of wish fulfilment for a continuation of personal consciousness in the presence of overwheming anxiety, fear and brain failure.

There are, however, several major objections to elements of the above explanation. Firstly, full NDEs can be experienced in the face of overwhelming anxiety such as falling off mountains, when cerebral anoxia will not occur. Thus a further explanation is required for the generation of the emotion of universal love. Secondly, the experiences are described as vivid, true and real. They always carry the tag of absolute reality and are described as being more real than everyday life. A failing brain, by definition, produces experiences which are limited, confused and disorganized. The very opposite is true of the NDE. Thirdly, there are anecdotal accounts of information being gathered away from the site of where the NDE is occurring, e.g. patients will wander down hospital corridors and see their loved ones arriving and hear their discussions with their doctors. In the case of accidents patients are able to describe what occurred throughout the accident site, quite remote from where their bodies were lying. As yet these are only anecdotal accounts and there is only one scientific study in the literature which confirms their authenticity (Sabom, 1982). Further studies are needed but if they reach the same conclusion then science will need to reformulate its understanding of consciousness and mind.

Nothing occurs singly in nature and it seems unreasonable to dissociate NDEs with their view of the universe as consisting of universal harmony and love from those of the mystical experience which contain very similar features. It would seem more logical to see one as the subset of the other. The similarity and persuasiveness of the accounts and the realness of the experience must lead one to ask whether the true nature of reality is being seen. Once that question is proposed then evidence from different areas can be used to support it as it maps directly onto both religious and esoteric experiences. In all religions there are specific esoteric methods which, when practised, lead to the experiencing of a transcendent reality. There is little doubt that these methods act neurophysiologically and modify brain action. Meditation is one such method and, although the scientific literature detailing the effects of meditation on the brain is at the moment rudimentary, it does allow the possibility for scientific study of brain changes which may underpin the transcendent.

The religious view of man as transcendant and containing within himself a spark of the divine, is echoed in the NDE . Could it be that our current concept of religious man is itself based on these experiences? If so, then could it be that many religious concepts (our notion of heaven for example) are based on the altered physiology of the brain? This view would be exactly in concordance with that of Dennet. It is all in the neural nets and we need look no further. However our science is not yet sufficiently complete to answer this question, as we do not know the nature of subjective experience. It could be that these experiences allow us to see through into the structure of nature, and that man, as the experiences suggest, is a reflection of the divine.

If this is so, might it not be that the one stuff of the universe is not energy as suggested by science but love as suggested by the mystics? Or perhaps these may be simply different views of the same stuff?

**Sleep, Dreams, Hypnagogic States**

Night time consciousness or dream states have always been thought of as essentially different from daytime or waking states. In biblical and Shamanic literature dreams are seen as either a privileged road to God or to some elemental force that can foretell or influence the future. Is there evidence that this is so?

Our present understanding of sleep stems from Dement's key experiments of early 1954, when he and his co-workers applied the then infant science of electroencephalography to the sleeping brain. He measured the EEG changes that accompanied a night's sleep and he was able to divide the sleeping period into two major phases; slow wave sleep and rapid eye movement (REM) sleep. Slow wave sleep is divided into four stages, according to the frequency of the EEG, which slows, from stage 1 to stage 4, with the increasing depth of sleep (Dement, 1957).

Dement showed that as you go to sleep the electrical brain rhythms gradually decrease in frequency, pulse and respiration rates decrease and muscle tone relaxes. This continues for about 90 min, when the deepest level of sleep is reached. There is then a switch and the brain rhythms accelerate. This is accompanied by rapid eye movements from side to side. After a short period of REM sleep, slow wave sleep again reestablishes itself, but for a shorter period, and at a lighter stage. These 90 min cycles of slow wave sleep and REM sleep continue throughout the night, with REM sleep occurring in progressively longer periods towards the end of the night, and the level of slow wave sleep becoming progressively lighter towards morning.

There are three distinct physiological states of sleep. The first is sleep onset, stages 1 and 2, the lightest phase of sleep, and is equivalent to deep relaxation. The second is stage 3 and 4 sleep, when the physiology of the brain changes. Growth hormone is secreted in this phase of sleep, which is thought to be associated with physical repair to the body. Puberty also takes place in this phase of sleep; initially it is during the night that the sex stimulating hormones are secreted from the pituitary. The third state is REM sleep: Dement's major contribution to our understanding of sleep was that he showed that people awoken from this level of sleep appeared to be dreaming.

## Hypnagogic states

Dreaming occurs throughout the sleeping state but the nature of dreams differs according to the phase of sleep. Hypnagogic dreams are those which occur at sleep onset as reality starts to fade and the dream world arises. They contain a mixture of external and internal phenomenology. Some people experience very strong imagery which may be highly structured and colourful, while in others the transition into sleep appears to be consciousness-free. This phase of sleep has been used creatively by many people. Eddington is reported to have held steel balls in his hands when thinking about a problem. As he drifted into the hypnagogic state the muscles of his arm would relax, allowing the steel balls to drop from his grasp onto a metal saucer below. The sound they made would wake him, and he would hope to find that a solution to the problem would have spontaneously arisen. Charles Dickens used hypnagogic imagery to create scenes later incorporated into his stories. The chemist Kekule is said to have discovered the structure of the benzene ring while half asleep in front of the fire watching the chains of atoms dance in front of his eyes, and seeing one chain seize its own tail to form a ring.

## Slow wave sleep dreams

Dreams occur throughout the night, but their character depends on the phase of sleep that you are in. Dreams in slow wave sleep have different characteristics from those of REM sleep. The dreams of slow wave sleep are usually described as kinaesthetic and verbal. This means they are feelings of body movements or body sensations combined with words and thoughts. Recent work has however suggested that visual imagery is much more common in slow wave sleep dreams than was previously acknowledged. REM dreams are what we normally think of as dreams. They are visuo-spatial, narrative, and highly structured. There is some evidence from recent studies that the qualities of experience in slow wave dreaming and relaxed waking life are very similar, thus arguing for a common cerebral mechanism for both dreaming and daytime consciousness.

## Night terrors and sleepwalking

For many centuries sleepwalking has been described. There are accounts from as far back as Greek and Roman times of crimes having been carried out during sleep

It has always been felt that behaviour during sleep is not the responsibility of the sleeper and thus sleepwalkers have been protected by law.

Sleepwalking is described as a state-transition disorder, and it occurs between slow wave sleep and REM sleep. The sleepwalker starts to change into dreaming sleep but the process becomes interrupted and, over some minutes he may alert into full consciousness. During this time he may arise from bed and carry out either simple or complex behaviour. Sleepwalkers commonly get dressed, urinate in cupboards, open bedroom doors and walk about the house. If woken they seldom have any dreaming imagery although they may have access to dream thoughts. One sleepwalker awoke kneeling in her bedroom, and claimed she was looking for roses to be potted. Sleepwalking should never be taken lightly: sleepwalkers have climbed out of windows and fallen to their death, and injured themselves in falls from fire escapes and stairs. Memory function is impaired in stage 4 sleep and this contributes to the lack of dream recall on awakening after a sleepwalking episode.

Night terrors are the same as sleepwalking in their timing. The sleeper awakes in a state of severe fear, anxiety and panic. He will sit up with a piercing cry and scream and scream. He may then get up and rush through the house as if fleeing in terror. On awakening some sleepers will describe a nameless terror without form; others may have some imagery and very occasionally detailed imagery does occur but it tends to be simple. One sleeper described a large round ball from which sparks were coming and which was about to engulf him in nameless destruction.

Sleepwalking and night terrors run in families. Episodes may be precipitated by stressful life events, excessive tiredness, alcohol and drugs. The law in the UK has recently been changed regarding crimes committed during a sleepwalking episode. The sleepwalking episode begins on the arousal from stage 4 sleep. Thus the law regards sleepwalking as arising from an internal abnormality of the sleeper and as such it is legally classified as insane automatism. That means that there is now no automatic acquittal and that the sleeper may be sent to hospital if the judge feels this is necessary. In Canada the law is, however, different, as the sleepwalking episode is deemed to have started at the moment that the sleeper goes to sleep. Going to sleep is a normal function and thus sleepwalking is part of a normal (sane) automatism. Canadian sleepwalkers go free (Fenwick, 1991).

What is the sleepwalker doing when he is sleepwalking? The current view is that there is a dissociation between the automatic activity of the sleepwalker and his consciousness. The question then arises as to whether this dissociation may incorporate motivated wishes. It has been suggested that many sleepwalkers are people who are able to dissociate easily, and that sleepwalking episodes do have a meaning for the sleepwalker.

### REM dreams

Current concepts of the mental phenomena that occur during sleep are derived from cognitive psychology. These concepts find considerable support from animal experimental work. Cognitive psychological theory predicts the presence in the cortex of neuronal net systems which underpin each cognitive ability. There is thus a specific system of neuronal cells which are responsible for the recognition of faces or the synthesis of body image, etc. It is the activation of these cognitive structures within the cortex which is thought to give rise to our subjective experience of the functions they subserve.

Llinas and Pare (1991) have proposed the most radical and the most attractive current theory of dreaming. They argue that the onset of dreaming is triggered by cholinergic cells (cell populations whose neurotransmitter is acetylcholine) in the brainstem reticular formation.

These cells activate the cognitive structures within the cortex and allow them to process information. At the same time as the cholinergic system is activated, a noradrenergic system in cell populations close to those of the cholinergic system (locus coerulius) switch off a noradrenergic drive to the cortex. The effect of this is to reduce the input of externally derived signals from the body surface to the thalamus and so to the cortex. The result of this changeover is that the cognitive neural structures during dreaming sleep are activated more by internal activity with a reduction of messages from the external body surface.

Llinas's insight is to suggest that the brain makes cognitive models at all times and does so on the data that are available. Thus the dreaming state, where the brain is dependent on internal signals, is the basic state of the brain. The waking state is a modification of the dreaming process. "We sleep, perchance to dream" could be rewritten "We dream, perchance to wake." Dreams will thus contain daytime residues from memory, as well as spontaneous excitation from internal sources of cortical cognitive units. Brain damage can be expected to lead to dream damage.

Hobson in a review (1990), like Llinas, argues that the experiences of dreaming sleep are due to brain-stem stimulation of those cortical cognitive structures which are normally used in our analysis of the external world. This is an attractive hypothesis as it has consequences which can be tested by dream researchers. The first consequence is that damage to these cortical cognitive structures will lead to an alteration in specific dream imagery. There is some evidence to support this. Llinas and Pare (1991) report dreams of faceless subjects in a patient who had damage to the structures involved in facial recognition. There is also evidence that unilateral neglect of the body following right parietal damage leads to similar neglect within dreams. There is also some evidence that damage to verbal structures in the dominant left hemisphere may prevent dreaming, or certainly dream reports. Further work on the correlation between damaged cognitive abilities in the waking state and their reflection in the dreaming state still needs to be carried out. Antrobus in a review paper (1991) takes these ideas further and involves the concept of neural nets in his theory. The argument is essentially the same as Hobson's, but more detailed, and suggests again the activation in REM sleep of cortical cognitive structures. Both Jones (1991) and Antrobus describe the current understanding of the neurophysiological mechanisms which underpin dreaming sleep.

It has been known for some years that during dreaming (REM) sleep the body is paralysed. Animal experiments have shown that a group of cells in the brainstem reduces the activity of spinal motor neurones so that the drive from the motor cortex no longer activates movements. If these cells are destroyed so that the dreaming animal is no longer paralysed, then the animals appear to act out their dreams. This again suggests that the same cognitive structures are used in waking and dreaming. Dramatic support for this has recently come from two fields. One is neurological damage to similar structures in the brain in man, and the other is from the effects of old age on the inhibitory mechanism. In both these cases, when the paralysis is not sufficient to inhibit motor movements in sleep, subjects will get out of bed and act out their dreams. A typical account is that of a man, dreaming of playing rugger and tackling an opponent, who awoke to find blood streaming from his head as he had tackled a chest of drawers in his bedroom.

Further evidence comes from the work of Fenwick *et al.*, who have studied lucid dreaming. This is thought to be a stage of dreaming which occurs when the subject is physiologically more alert in his/her dreams than is usual. These are the dreams during which the dreamer "wakes", and, it has been found, can then direct the content of the dream. In a series of experiments a lucid dreamer was able to show that movements of his "dream eyes" resulted in equivalent movements of his real eyes. The dream body was also identical to the real body. Dream memory and dream time were directly equivalent to real memory and real time.

Thus the dream world and the real world appear from the point of view of physiology to be very similar. Both seem to use the same brain structures and an analysis of their features shows them to be similar. Is the dream then a royal road to God? Without a scientific explanation of subjective experience it is impossible to say, but certainly there does not seem to be any brain function or structure involved in dreaming that is significantly different from that of the waking state.

**Meaning in Dreams**

The Russian philosopher Ouspensky divided dreams into three different types. There were dreams that were "rubbish", our day to day dreaming; those that contained clear meaning, provided an answer to a current problem, and initiated a new line of behaviour in the dreamer. Finally there were those that occur only once or twice during a lifetime and provide deep insights about the dreamer and his life. The first two types of dreams can easily be explained by science. Those that have a wider meaning or warn of future events are outside the realms of science. There are numerous anecdotal accounts of such prophetic dreams from as far back as Old Testament times – Joseph was certainly one of the most notable dreamers in history.

To test whether or not dreams do have meaning, Schatzman gave some of his friends problems to solve during their dreams. Once he knew that it was possible to solve problems from the waking state in dreams, he published some such problems and asked readers not to solve them while awake, but to aim to solve them during sleep, and to send their dream solutions to him. He repeated this experiment with a radio audience. The first problem given was to find an English word which began in HE and ended in HE. One dream solution was as follows: The dreamer was in a lecture and became aware of a pain in her chest. The lecturer suggested that she should leave the lecture. As she went out she became aware that the pain had spread to her head. She had to rush out of the lecture hall in case she should forget something. She then awoke feeling that she had the answer to the problem. On recalling her dream she was quickly able to see the answer to the problem – heartache and headache. Awareness that problems could be solved in dreams came from another caller who reported that he had lost a marble for which he had searched everywhere. While taking off his jeans to go to bed he remembered the dream programme and was determined to find the marble in his dreams. He dreamed that he was asleep in bed and that he couldn't go to sleep because the bed was very uncomfortable. He was better if he turned on his side, but on his back, just above his buttock, was a large mound which kept him awake. He awoke to realize that he had remembered where his marble was – in the back pocket of his jeans.

These experiments are an excellent demonstration of the relationship between the waking and sleeping brain. Information is available to the dreamer from his ordinary daytime state, and this information can be made use of in the dream narrative. The dream seems to be able to make connections which are not always available to the waking subject. There thus seems to be scientific evidence that the advice to sleep on a problem is good advice.

## Conclusion

Science has not yet provided an explanation for the nature of subjective experience. Without this, as scientists, we are forced to understand our subjective world as a mechanical distillation of brain function. The genetic programme produces, in the brain, an organ of majestic complexity, but nothing more. Our current science thus dooms us to an existence in which the only meaning is biological, and is in the relationships between humans, and between humans and their environment. The possibility of meaning beyond this is denied, as subjective experience is seen to arise simply from the programming of neuronal nets within the brain. Science certainly accepts the presence of subjective experience, and thus of a personal consciousness. Schrödinger comments that without consciousness the activities of creation would be "played out on empty beaches". Consciousness as formulated by science cannot take this any further forward. Science, as yet, has no means of dealing with creativity and subjective experience. Thus science can only analyse those "qualities of the world" that appear as third party experience.

When an explanation for subjective experience is found, then the relationship of conscious experience to the universe as a whole will be better understood. This might then validate the non-materialistic "empathic" meaning of mystical experience."

## References

Andrew, K. (1975). Psychokinetic influences on an electromechanical random number generator during evocation of "Left hemispheric" VS "Right hemispheric" function. *In* "Research in Parapsychology". (Eds J. Maurice, W. Roll and R. Mauric). Scarecrow Press, Metuchen, N.J.

Antrobus, J. (1991). Dreaming: cognitive processes during cortical activation and high afferent thresholds. *Psychological Review,* **98**, 96-121.

Bear, D.M. and Fedio, P. (1977). Quantitative analysis of interictal behaviour in temporal lobe epilepsy. *Archives of Neurology,* **34**, 454-467.

Bear, D.M., Levin, K., Blumer, D., Chetham, D. and Ryder, J. (1982). Interictal behaviour in hospitalized temporal lobe epileptics: relationship to idiopathic psychiatric syndromes. *Journal of Neurology, Neurosurgery and Psychiatry,* **45**, 481-488.

Broad, W.G. and Broad, L.W. (1975). The Psi-conducive Syndrome: 3-response GESP performance following evocation of "left-hemispheric" v "right-hemispheric" functioning. *In* "Research in Parapsychology". (Eds J. Maurice, W. Roll and R. Mauric). Scarecrow Press, Metuchen, N.J.

Broughton, R.S. (1975). Brain hemisphere specialization and its possible effects on ESP performance. *In* "Research in Parapsychology". (Eds J. Maurice, W. Roll and R. Mauric). Scarecrow Press, Metuchen, N.J

Bryant, J.E. (1953). "Genius and Epilepsy. Brief Sketches of Great Men who had Both". Ye Olde Depot Press, Concorde, Mass.

Cirignotta, F., Todesco, C. and Lugaresi, E. (1980). Temporal lobe epilepsy with ecstatic seizures (so-called Dostoevsky epilepsy). *Epilepsia,* **21**, 705-710.

Dement, W. and Kleitman, N. (1957). Cyclic variations in EEG curing sleep and their relation to eye movements, body motility, and dreaming. *Electroencephalopathy and Clinical Neurophysiology,* **9**, 673-690.

Dewhurst, K. and Beard, A.W. (1970). Sudden religious conversions in temporal lobe epilepsy. *British Journal of Psychiatry,* **117**, 497-570.

Fenwick, P. (1991). Automatism and medicine, the law. *Psychological Medicine,* Monograph supple. 17.

Fenwick, P., Galliano, S., Coate, M., Rippere, V. and Brown, D. (1985). Sensitives, "Psychic gifts", psychic sensitivity and brain pathology. *British Journal of Medical Psychology,* **58**, 35-44.

Fenwick, P., Schatzman, M., Worsley, A., Adams, J., Stone, S. and Baker, A. (1984). Lucid dreaming: correspondence between dreamed and actual events in one subject during REM sleep. *Biological Psychology,* **18**, 243-252.

Geschwind, N. (1979). Behavioural changes in temporal lobe epilepsy. *Psychological Medicine,* **9**, 217-219.

Gloch, C. and Stark, R. (1965). "Religion and Society in Tension". Rand McNally, Chicago.

Gowers, W.R. (1881). "Epilepsy and other Chronic Convulsive Diseases". Churchill, London.

Grayson, B. and Flynn, C. (1984). "The Near Death Experience". Charles C. Thomas, Springfield, Ill.

Hay, D. (1982). "Exploring Inner Space. Is God Still Possible in the 20th Century"? Penguin, Harmondsworth.

Hobson, J.A. (1990). Sleeping and dreaming. *Neuroscience,* **10**, 371-382.

Lennox, W. (1960). "Epilepsy and Related Disorders". Vol. 1. Churchill, London.
Llinas, R.R. and Pare D. (1991). Commentary of dreaming and wakefulness. *Neuroscience*, **44**, 521-535.
Lorimer, D. (1990). "Whole in One the Near Death Experience and the Ethic of Interconnectedness". Arcana, London.
Moody, R. (1975). "Life After Life". Mockingbird Books, New York.
Mungus, D. (1982). Interictal behaviour abnormality in temporal lobe epilepsy. A specific syndrome or non-specific psychopathology. *Archives of General Psychiatry*, **39**, 108-111.
Nagel, T. (1993). What is the mind-body problem? *In* "Experimental and Theoretical Studies of Consciousness". Ciba Foundation Syposium 174. John Wiley, Chichester, 1-13.
Nelson, G.K. (1970). Preliminary study of the electroencephalographs of mediums. *Parapsychologia*, **1b**, 9, 30-35.
Neppe, V.H. (1980). Subjective paranormal experience and temporal lobe symptomatology. *Parapsychological Journal of South Africa*, **1**, 2, 78-98.
Penfield, W. and Kristiansen, K. (1951). "Epileptic Seizure Patterns". Charles C. Thomas, Springfield, Ill.
Ring, K. (1980). "Life at Death". Coward, McCann and Goghagan, New York.
Sabom, M. (1982). "Recollections of Death". Harper and Row, London.
Searle, T.R. (1992). "The Rediscovery of the Mind". MIT Press.
Sensky, T. and Fenwick, P. (1982). Religiosity, mystical experience and epilepsy. *In* "Progress in Epilepsy". (Ed. F. Clifford Rose).
Waxman, S.G. and Geschwind, N. (1975). The interictal behaviour syndrome of temporal lobe epilepsy. *Archive of General Psychiatry*, **32**, 1580-1586.

# 10. On the nature of consciousness and the unconscious from the point of view of neuroscience and neurophilosophy

J. R. Smythies

Over the last few years there has been a vast increase in our knowledge of how brain functions are related to many aspects of "mentality" as investigated by cognitive neuroscientists. This includes "lower" functions such as raw sensation and motor activity, as well as "higher" functions such as attention, memory, planning, foresight, programme evaluation, spatial analysis, social relevance, emotional responses, etc. Some 100 years ago Freud divided the mind into his famous triumvirate – Ego, Id and Super-Ego. In his hands these subdivisions of mental *functions* became mental quasi *entities* interacting with each other as people or organizations do. Of course Freud did not discover these entities. Plato gave a wonderful description of how the Id manifests itself in dreams. The Super-Ego appears extensively in medieval religious literature as man's conscience, and the description of the Ego, as man's rational humane mind, forms much of the substance of the writings of the great philosophers of the Enlightenment such as Locke, Berkeley and Hume. Freud codified the system and filled in a vast amount of detail from his studies of the dreams, thoughts and actions of his psychoneurotic patients. Maclean and Koestler (1969) have described an anatomical basis for the triumvirate: a Super-Ego based in the frontal lobes and the Id based in the hypothalamus and limbic system. The efforts of the Super-Ego and the Ego to control the baser instincts of the Id can be seen in the context of Hughlings Jackson's Doctrine of Levels, with the higher cortex, programmed to respond to learned psychosocial imperatives, continually in conflict with the Id which mediates the gratification of baser instincts and emotions.

To give an account, in the terms of modern of neuroscience, of the problems that Freud dealt with in terms of the psychology of his day requires some definitions.

## Consciousness

It seems hardly likely that we can understand the unconscious unless we first give a clear idea of the nature of consciousness itself. It is notorious that there is currently much confusion over the use of this term and we must distinguish clearly between at least three quite different usages: (i) the medico-behavioural sense as "the patient lost consciousness at 4.30" (ii) the attentional-attitudinal sense as "Emily became conscious that George was looking strangely at her"; and (iii) the phenomenal sense, as the collection of all sensations, images and thoughts available to introspection at any moment. Consciousness in this sense is the field of investigation by introspectionist psychologists such as Gregory (1984), Vernon (1962), Ramachandran (1986) and many others including myself (1959, 1960).

## Mental occurrents and mental features

In 1970 Rorty made a key distinction between mental *occurrents* (such as pains and sensations) and mental *features* (such as beliefs, desires, hopes). Psychoanalysis deals mainly with mental features, whereas the phenomenology of consciousness deals mainly with mental occurrents. The key distinction must be kept in mind when we are trying to relate psychoanalytical terms and theories to the terms and theories of modern neuroscience and introspectionist psychology.

## The Ego

In phenomenology the "Ego" is usually used to denote the observing, experiencing Self, or "Pure Ego" – the central entity of consciousness – in Berkeley's words:
> How often must I repeat, that I know or am conscious of my own being, and that
> *I myself* am not my ideas, but somewhat else, a thinking active principle that
> perceives, knows, wills and operates about ideas. I know that... I am therefore one
> individual principle, distinct from colour and sound; and, for the same reason,
> free from all other sensible things and inert ideas.

Others, David Hume in particular, have found it difficult to believe in the existence of the Ego as the entity that Berkeley describes so vividly. Hume complained that whenever he searched around in his mind all he could find were his own sensations, images and thoughts – and never an Ego. However, we can use Hume's argument to *define* the Ego: as that which in Hume's mind was doing the searching. Descartes confused the Ego and its thoughts with the total mind.

## The Unconscious

This has two somewhat different meanings in cognitive science.

(i) If we assume for the moment that the theory of psychoneural identity (IT) is true, then all the events in phenomenal consciousness must be held to be identical with certain specifiable neuronal events in the brain that lie at the *apex* of a most complex series of parallel distributed processors that perform a multitude of computations in their neural nets on the incoming sensory inflow including the visceral inflow channelled via the amygdala. Below this apex, composed of neurones whose activities are identical with the events that we experience in consciousness, there exists a subconscious mind composed of the computational activities of all the nerve nets, in both cortical and subcortical areas, that lie outside, or below, the select apical consciousness neurones. The orderly arrival in consciousness of our train of perceptions, thoughts, images and feelings of our impulses, purposes, ideals, loyalties, ambitions, etc., all depend on a vast array of these subconscious mechanisms to which we have no direct access or experience, any more than the TV viewer has direct access to the complex machinery inside the set that actually constructs the TV picture. Likewise on the motor side many of our actions, e.g. in driving a car or playing a piano sonata, are effected by subconscious motor mechanisms into whose workings we have no direct conscious access and of the existence of which we have no direct knowledge.

(ii) The second meaning of "consciousness", used in psychoanalysis, is somewhat wider and includes the Self as well as the rational aspects of mental function in the Heideggerian sense – that is, all mental functions that do not derive from our conscience (Superego) or from the Id. The latter form the Unconscious.

But there are two aspects of this subconscious mind that seem to go beyond the functioning of these subsidiary servo-mechanisms no matter how complex. These are (i) when unconscious motivations, from noxious conditioning regimes, take over the control of our activities in complex situations leading to "irrational" behaviour or to unwanted memories; and (ii) when we consider how the "royal road" to the unconscious – dreams – is organized. To consider these in turn:

(i) One of the most fruitful concepts in contemporary neuroscience is that of the neuronal cell assembly (NCA) (Freeman, 1990). In this the computations that lie at the basis of the brain's activity are carried out by collections of neurones connected into nerve nets based on Hebbian synapses (synapses whose loading is a function of how often these synapses fire when the target cell does). Brains do not function as do digital computers with their binary "on-off" codes and algorithms, but as analogue computers in which very many neurones take part in individual computations, and in which one neurone may take part in several different computations. The computations themselves are functions of the connectivity of the nerve net. At lower levels, e.g. the visual system, each group of NCAs scattered throughout the more than 24 different retinotopic cortical visual areas, responds to a specific feature of the visual input (e.g. colour, radial movement flow, shape from shading, etc.). From the higher sensory cortex major pathways lead to (a) the inferior temporal lobe (and thence to the entorhinal area and the hippocampus); (b) to the frontal lobe where many aspects of socially relevant behaviour are organized; and (c) to subcortical areas, for example the pulvinar nucleus of the thalamus where attention is organized.

Freeman has described in the olfactory bulb how each specific incoming olfactory stimulus triggers a specific NCA or pattern of excited neurones evidenced by unit recordings and by a unique pattern of amplitude of a field potential ($\approx 40$ Hz) he calls gamma waves. A completed NCA discharges *en masse* to the olfactory cortex. This powerful signal conveys the information "Olfactory stimulus X present and has been identified as such." The olfactory cortex repeats the same process with its own NCAs and signals the results to other higher cortical centres. NCAs scattered throughout the great limbic circuits linking the temporal and frontal cortices as well as the hippocampus and amygdala with each other and other limbic centres could signal messages like "Situation X present needing response Y" or "Strategy A will gain love object B and thwart hated rival C." The limbic generators of these strategies may be supposed to act merely on logical and computational principles without regard to learned social and ethical conventions. So strategy A may read "Bump off hated rival C". This message reaching the frontal cortex would clash with the ethical imperative stored therein reading "People are not to be killed in these circumstances". The different regions of the higher cortex normally co-operate in an harmonious way to engineer the phenomenology of consciousness and to organize a coherent and relevant programme of behaviour.

However, if negative emotional feelings (e.g. hatred for C) are intense enough, and particularly if the conditioning of emotional reactions and psycho-social responses were faulty, then a powerful NCA might be set up that would be blocked from its normal access to the consciousness neurones and premotor cortex. But it could still influence emotional responses and behaviour by other neuronal pathways short-circuiting, as it were, the consciousness centres. If actual behaviour depends on (1) sensory information (e.g. "C is present") plus (2) motivation (e.g. "C threatens my interests and must be thwarted by strategy A") plus frontal lobe endorsement (e.g. "Strategy A is O.K."), then, if (1) and (2) are present and (3) is missing, a type of retrograde activation of a primitive limbic fear centre may result and lead to a phobia of sharp knives.

Many phobias and obsessions, in which aberrant or mismatched NCAs may generate unwanted and painful thoughts, emotions and impulses, may result from the activity of quasi-autonomous and pathological NCAs. Such systems of autonomous NCAs may be set up by other means – post-hypnotic suggestion, for example. There is evidence to support the suggestion that behaviour is determined, in part, by information circling in the great limbic circuits linking the hippocampus, amygdala, hypothalamus and reticular formation with the limbic and higher cortex, acting as a sort of tape directing behaviour (Smythies, 1973). In modern terms, this would appear as an interlocked series of NCAs in these various cortical and subcortical centres continually influencing each other in vastly complex patterns, whose final output to the premotor cortex directs behaviour. For example, Alheid and Heimer (1988) present evidence that the corpus striatum plays an important role in motor planning, motor learning and species-specific motor programmes; and the extended amygdala (which includes the sublenticular nucleus, substantia innominata, the bed nucleus of the stria terminata and possibly the nucleus accumbens) organize basic drives and emotions.

The concept of autonomous pathological NCAs can be used to explain other psychiatric phenomena – the auditory hallucinations of schizophrenia, for example. Normally the activity of the consciousness neurones at the apex of the auditory set of PDPs is determined by the auditory inflow. The schizophrenic commonly hears derogatory voices abusing and threatening him. The biochemical lesion(s) thought to underlie the disease (Smythies and Corbett, 1981) may well result in the formation of "rogue" NCAs in the auditory cortex deriving from origins in limbic centres mediating the influence of strong negative emotions in the retrograde manner described above. Another model for this process is that of the programme "viruses" that can invade digital computers and cause devastating malfunction. Perhaps some psychiatric disorders are due to the activity of such programme "viruses".

In this theory the Unconscious in the Freudian sense is not the subconscious – precursor mechanisms that build up normal consciousness – but centres of abnormal NCAs that compete with the consciousness neuronal NCAs for control of the premotor cortex or thought mechanisms under particular circumstances.

(ii) The second aspect of the Unconscious that seems to go beyond a mere subconscious is the entity or programme, whatever it is, that scripts and performs the bizarre and complex plays that we participate in when we dream. Recent evidence indicates that the hippocampus plays an important role in dreaming and that dreams represent "rehearsals" or "replays" of psychologically important material relevant to the basic strategies of the brain. Dreams must represent the interplay of NCAs widely spread throughout the visual, auditory, somatic, spatial, language, motivational and emotional areas of the brain. Dream activity must obey different laws from those that determine activity in these centres when we are awake with an active sensory inflow. One can imagine the internal limbic "tape" directing overall brain function taking different forms when activity is driven by deeper structures such as the pons and hippocampus instead of the sensory cortex. The same consciousness neurones must act as the apical system in each case; only the scripts are different.

An intermediate situation is found in sensory deprivation experiments in which the sensory inflow is cut off from the waking brain. In this case disorders of perception such as hallucinations soon result. Another instance, that reveals something of the inner workings of the computational brain, is provided by Klüver's "form constants" of hallucinations. Widely different conditions, such as hallucinogenic drugs, stroboscopic retinal stimulation, and sensory deprivation, nevertheless induce very similar forms – commonly simple geometrical patterns such as checker boards, grids, spirals, concentric circles, mazes, etc. (Smythies 1959, 1960). These form constants may derive from scanning mechanisms, or pattern recognition mechanisms, or the production of chaotic reactions in NCAs (these patterns show a remarkable similarity to the spiral geometrical patterns produced by the Belousov-Zhabotinsky chaotic chemical reactions. Klüver's "form constants" offer a new way of determining certain basic features of brain mechanisms, but no one has yet given a wholly satisfactory explanation for them. Further research is needed.

Thus we seem to have several unknown inner "playwrights" – I have mentioned the one responsible for dreams. Another, much more artistically gifted, choreographs the flow of wonderful visual hallucinations characteristic of the psychedelic state induced by hallucinogenic drugs such as mescaline and LSD (Smythies, 1953a). Many sober and reliable observers, such as Havelock Ellis, Weir Mitchell, Klüver, and Macdonald Critchley, have stated that the complex hallucinations witnessed under the influence of a drug such as mescaline are simply inherently more beautiful than any creation by any terrestrial artist. This is not a matter of mere inebriation, or distortion of aesthetic judgement, since experiments have shown that this remains intact in the mescalinized subject — ugly objects presented are still judged to be "ugly".

These drugs act as mixed agonists/antagonists at serotonin receptors in the brain. Layer IV of the primary visual cortex VI has a heavy innervation by serotoninergic neurones of the raphe nucleus. Activity in these cuts down the signal/noise ratio in the visual input leading to the experience of super-saturated colours and presumably to the subtle changes in form and outline that bestow beauty. But such a simple mechanism could hardly be responsible for the complex scenarios of the visions — such things as "thick, glorious fields of jewels that constantly spring up into new flower-like shapes before my gaze", or wonderful landscapes, or the vision of a fleet of galleys sailing silently across a violet sea, or a monk leading a young girl out of a church, described by the subject as a moving, living sculpture of ineffable beauty. One subject reported that she had received an experience of unimaginable art of an intensity that it was necessary to experience for oneself to understand. These visions have little to do with the personal memories of the subject and everything to do with myth, fable and transcendental art. Jung (1952) has agreed with my suggestion that the visions originate from the Mundus Archetypus or Jungian collective unconscious. But it is difficult to translate that into the terms of nerve net activity. Why should the brain belonging to someone of little or no artistic talent yet be capable of producing masterpiece after masterpiece — works of art of unimaginable splendour, integrity and truth? Dream images are not works of art, so why should the mescaline images be? These visions would seem to require the presence in the brain of a most elaborate computational mechanism to construct each and every detail of each and every vision. Yet what possible evolutionary benefit could such a system confer? One can only suppose that normally this system is doing something else; but what? One possibility is presented by a new theory of the cerebral basis of the aesthetic sense that I have presented elsewhere (Smythies, 1992). This is that the feeling or judgement that a particular scene, person or picture is "beautiful" must be mediated by specific nerve nets that connect the sensory cortices with the "pleasure" areas of the brain such as the septal nuclei. Mozart's ability to write music of an ethereal quality is unlikely to have arisen from some privileged access to a Platonic external world of beautiful auditory images outwith the brain. It is more likely to be due to the fact that he had unique connectivity patterns in the nerve nets connecting the auditory cortex with the pleasure or aesthetic centres. There is no reason why the mere reverberation of neuronal patterns set up only in the auditory cortex by a Mozart sonata should lead to an aesthetic response. The pleasure areas must also be involved, and how else except by the specificity of detailed nerve nets such that certain highly specific activities in the auditory cortex, certain combinations of pitch, tone and the temporal succession of these, will trigger these specific net work connections because the nets are there. Since we have an aesthetic reaction to Mozart's music the first time we hear it, these nets must be present in us too, but not activated until we hear that particular music. So, if these nets possessed a significant serotoninergic innervation, a psychedelic drug could activate this specific net to its maximum capacity. The resulting NCAs would then carry the message "Most beautiful X is present and has been identified as such." Since the drug does not provide any particular details, in fact no details, of the pattern, the brain has to improvise. It does this at first by producing Klüver's "form constants" but always in a more complex and aesthetically pleasing form than do the other means of inducing these patterns.

## On the relation of phenomenal consciousness to its brain

In the account of mind-brain relations developed so far I have adhered to the Identity Theory that states that all mental events, including phenomenal consciousness, are identical with a limited subset of brain events – the consciousness neurones described above. If we want to discover what sort of beings we are, it will be essential to arrive at the correct and true theory of brain-consciousness relations. Yet this whole debate has been obscured for centuries by three major sources of confusion, namely (1) Descartes' mistake in claiming that extension in space is *the* important criterion for distinguishing between mental events and physical events; (2) the wide spread confusion between the "body-image" of neurology and physical body; and (3) the universal confusion between phenomenal space and physical space. To take these in turn:

## (1) Descartes' mistake

Descartes divided everything into two mutually exclusive realms – *res extensa,* physical objects extended in space – and *res cogitans,* the thinking mind lacking any extension in space. Many people have identified consciousness with *res cogitans* (mistakenly as we will see) and this led to the denial that consciousness itself has any extension in any kind of space. Yet one moment's reflection reveals this to be an absurd doctrine (1). Phenomenal consciousness contains as integral parts our various sensory and image fields, as "objective" consciousness, and it is certain that visual and somatic sensations and images possess the inherent property of extension in space. Other parts of the complex that constitutes phenomenal consciousness, such as the Ego ("subjective" consciousness) and its thoughts certainly lack any obvious extension in space. A thought does not have a spatial boundary and a spatial location in a field like a visual sensation or a visual after-image does. But this shows only that consciousness is not the single, indivisible *res cogitans* that Descartes described, but, whereas it *includes* this, it also consists of a great deal more, in particular of visual and somatic fields extended in (internal, private) phenomenal space. All this has been obscured because most people in their everyday lives unwittingly, and most philosophers when they theorize about perception knowingly, adhere to the pre-scientific theory of perception known as Direct Realism (DR). This theory mirrors the commonsense notions of the ordinary person that the coloured extended sensations, that he experiences when he sees objects, simply are direct views of the external objects themselves. That is, we look out of our eyes, *there* are the external objects arrayed before us directly in our conscious visual grasp. Sadly, modern neuroscience and neurophilosophy show that this theory is just plainly wrong – a piece of "folk psychology" inherited from our cave-man ancestors. There is a vast amount of evidence to show, in fact, that sensations are constructions of the representative mechanisms of perception. In other words vision works like television not like a telescope (2). This important fact has been obscured in turn by the second major confusion common today – that between the body-image and the physical body. Visual sensations appear to the naive observer to be located outside the experienced body. But if DR is false for vision, it is also false for somatic sensation, and the somatic sensory field (body-image) cannot be identical with the physical body as common-sense assumes, but must also be a construction of the representative mechanisms of perception.

## (2) The "body-image"

This term is used widely in neurology but unfortunately in a confused way since it has two very different meanings – the somatic sensory field and the body concept (Smythies, 1953*b*). The former is composed of all sensations that we experience in consciousness *from* (not in) the physical body; and the body concept, which is the system of beliefs and attitudes that we all have about the structure, form, function and value of our own body and its parts, in particular about such things as whether we are thin or fat, ugly or attractive, etc. So we must take care to separate these two meanings. It is best to replace the term "body-image" with the more specific terms "somatic sensory field" and "body concept". The key understanding that must be reached if a person is really to grasp the nature of his own mind and consciousness and their relation to his/her own body, is the absolute and categorical ontological distinction between the somatic sensory field and the actual physical body. This was emphasized by Paul Schilder (1950):

... the empirical method leads immediately to a deep insight that even our own body is beyond our immediate reach, that even our own body justifies Prospero's words "We are such stuff as dreams are made on, and our little life is rounded with a sleep."

Wolfgang Köhler (1947), one of the founders of Gestalt psychology, puts it very clearly:

My body [referring to the somatic sensory field] is the outcome of certain processes in my physical organism, processes which start in the eyes, muscles, skin and so forth, exactly as the chair before me is the final product of other processes in the same organism. If the chair is seen "before me", the "me" of this phrase means my body as an experience, of course, not my body as an organism in the physical world.

The philosopher J.O. Wisdom (1953) has also speculated that the problem of mind-body dualism centres around the relation of the body image and the physical body.

In spite of all this, I suggest that few living neurologists or neuroscientists actually apply what Schilder and Köhler said all those years ago to his (her) own experience of his (her) own body: in this area DR still reigns supreme. To make the required conceptual change is very difficult and induces what Harrison (1989) has called "mental vertigo". For it amounts to admitting that the object that we have experienced in our consciousness all our lives – this "body" we experience and that we have always taken merely to *be* our physical body – is actually not so and, if neuroscience and the Representative Theory (RT) are correct, as they undoubtedly are, it is actually *identical* with the activity of a number of neurones in a circumscribed area of our somato-sensory cortex (3). Visual perceptions certainly appear to be located outside "us", but, as Köhler makes plain, this "outside" is only outside relative to the somatic sensory field and not outside relative to the physical body (organism). Both visual sensations and somatic sensations are literally *inside* a part of the physical organism, the brain. So the pain that we feel when we stub a toe, is not literally located in the physical toe (as naive opinion has it) but in the toe of the somatic sensory field. We naively imagine that the processes of our *awareness* of the pain in the toe are mediated by processes in the sciatic nerve, spinal tracts, thalamus, and cortex: whereas, in fact, all this goes on before consciousness is reached and merely serves to locate the appropriate type of pain sensation in the appropriate part of the somatic sensory field. Most people think that, in considering the mind-body problem, all the difficulty arises in the mind half of the equation; whereas the main problem centres around our deep-rooted but utterly mistaken ideas of how we experience our own bodies.

This point may be driven home by reading Harrison's (1985) delightful tale about Ludwig, the brain-in-a-vat. The story is set in the far distant future when neurosurgery and neuroscience had progressed to a level unimaginable today. Ludwig was born with a magnificently developed brain but a hideously malformed body. Dr Smythson, the leading neurosurgeon and neuroscientist of the day, decided to help Ludwig by removing his brain and putting it in a life-support system. In addition to perfusing Ludwig's brain with blood, Dr Smythson connected up the cut ends of the cranial nerves and spinal cord to neurocybernetic computers and stimulators of staggering complexity. In this way he was able to deliver to the brain a sensory inflow the same as that which Ludwig would have received if he had still had his sense organs. In addition Dr Smythson connected up the cut ends of the motor nerves to the computer so that movements willed by Ludwig were also felt. Dr

Smythson programmed his computers to give Ludwig all the experiences of a perfectly normal life, indistinguishable, as far as Ludwig was concerned, from the sort of life he would have lived had his brain remained in a normal body. Ludwig was able to experience going to school and University, where Dr Smythson saw to it that he studied philosophy, going to work, getting married, etc. etc. Ludwig had absolutely no way of telling that he was not a perfectly normal young man instead of a brain-in-a-vat. His only problem was that he was totally dependent on Dr Smythson's benignity in giving him a happy life rather than a sad one. Among Ludwig's perfectly real experiences was that of having a perfectly normal body. He felt all his bodily sensations just like we do. In other words he had a normal somatic sensory field (body image) without having any body other than his brain. Of course, common sense dictates that each of us can be confident that we ourselves are no mere brains-in-vats. But, if we were ever to be subjected to Dr Smythson's procedures without our knowing it, we would never detect any phenomenal differences in our experiences and, if Dr Smythson had been skilful enough, we would never know that we had been turned into a brain-in-a-vat. This underlines the fact that it is a gross mistake to identify, as we all unwittingly do, the body that we *experience* with the total physical organism itself.

## (3) Phenomenal space and physical space

Phenomenal space is the private spatio-(temporal) system in which our visual and somatic sense fields (with their constituent sensations) are extended and located. These, as we have seen, form an integral part of phenomenal consciousness. Physical space-(time) is the public spatio-(temporal) system in which commonsense physical objects such as atoms, brains and stars are extended and located. Under the unfortunate influence of Direct Realism it has been widely assumed that these two spaces were one and the same geographical space. But, of course, if the arguments above are correct, this is not the case as Russell (1948) has pointed out. At best, under IT the phenomenal space of one person can be identical only with a localized region of physical space, namely a small region of that person's brain.

Indow (1991) has recently reviewed the topic of "visual space" (his name for visual phenomenal space). As he says:
> Visual space (VS) is the final product of the long series of processes from retina to brain, and phenomenologically it is articulated into individual objects, backgrounds and the self... VS is the most comprehensive percept that includes all visual objects appearing in front of the perceived self.

Thus VS is a product of, and indeed an integral part of, the complex representative mechanisms of perception and cannot be identified with physical space and the stimulus field which contains the physical objects whose *representations* appear in the visual field in consciousness (VS) anymore than the pictures on the TV screen can be identical with the objects and events in the TV studio that they *represent*.

Indow reviews different opinions as to what the geometry of VS might be –

whether it is Euclidean or Riemannian. However there are two different meanings of VS that we must disentangle. Any real space must have a geometry; for example, real physical space-time has the geometry described by general relativity. Psychologists have investigated this problem by psychophysical experiments. In these the stimuli are spots of light arranged in lines of different shapes and aligned in different directions in external space. The subject's task is to line up these points of light into phenomenal straight line or "geodesics". Indow comments:

> What is meant by saying that VS is hyperbolic, for example, is that perceived straight lines and angles behave in the same way as geodesics and angles of that geometry behave. The assertion implies nothing less and nothing more.
>
> Specifically the geometry of VS is a step in the level of phenomenology, not the ultimate answer. The real question is why and how the brain generates VS as we see it.

There are three aspects of "VS" that need to be differentiated here. In these psychophysical experiments what is being investigated are the geometrical relations between the points of light in the stimulus field in physical space and the geometrical relations between the resulting phenomenal percepts in the visual field in VS. If the physical points of light arranged in a hyperbola yield percepts judged to be on a straight line, then the experimenter concludes that VS is hyperbolic.

The second sense of the "geometry of VS" is based on the requirement that any real space must have its own *intrinsic* geometry over and above its extrinsic geometry just described. The problem may be stated thus. The simplest (most primitive) visual fields are (i) the uniform black visual field that we experience in total darkness and (ii) the diffuse misty white field we experience in the Ganzfeld situation in which the S is a uniform featureless field of white light. We can ask the question "Is the geodesic (shortest path) between any two points in the black field, or in the Ganzfeld, a straight line (yielding an Enclidean geometry) or on a curved line (yielding a non-Euclidean geometry)?" Although it is difficult to think of any way of tackling this experimentally, at least the concept itself is intelligible.

But the topology of VS may be more important than its metrics. VS has a topological structure, for example, one visual sensation may be "inside" another (e.g. the sensations set up by the yolk and the white of a fried egg). Or two sensations may be "outside" each other (e.g. the sensations related to different grapes on a bunch). Visual sensations also possess other intrinsic topological relations to each other such as "above", "below", "to one side of", "between", as detailed by the great French logician Jean Nicod (1969). We can also observe that the edge of a visual sensation (e.g. an after-image) forms a Jordan curve, in that it uniquely divides the whole of VS into one "inside" and one "outside".

If we use this approach we can give a topological distinction between direct realism (DR) and RT. In the former a geodesic between two phenomenal visual objects in VS is identical with the geodesic between the two corresponding physical objects. In the Representative Theory (RT), in contrast, a geodesic in VS is identical with a geodesic in the brain. Moreover, this approach gives us a new way to express the ancient puzzle of the relation between consciousness (and VS) and its brain by asking "What are the topological relations between VS and physical space?" – that I have dealt with elsewhere (Smythies, 1994).

The last and most fundamental question raised by Indow is "... how the brain generates VS as we see it." The current approach in cognitive neuroscience to answering this question is to examine how neurones, particularly in the parietal cortex and the hippocampus, (see Selemon and Goldman-Rakic, 1988; Farah *et al.*, 1989; O'Keefe and Nadel, 1978; Quirk *et al.*, 1990; Muller and Kubie, 1989; and Rolls *et al.*, 1989) code, in their Hebbian and Hubel-and-Wiesel nerve nets and NCAs, the spatial features of the environment and of the organization's position in the environment. This answers the question "How does the brain process information about the spatial properties and locations of external objects and its own organism?" but it does not necessarily address the problem of "...how does the brain generate the VS *as we see it?*" (my italics). The problem is that the mechanical construction of the visual field is partly independent of the process of obtaining information about the external world. These two are processed by two different mechanisms. In apperceptive agnosia the patient has no difficulty in seeing the object but he is unable to recognize it, know what it is for and in general gain cognitive knowledge about it. Yet we have no doubt that the patient's visual field contains normal sensations. In contrast in blind-sight the patient cannot see the object and his visual field will lack any representation of the object, yet he can obtain veridical information about the object by a process he calls "guessing" that turns out to be right.

If we believe in realism and accept the sound principle that there cannot be function without structure, we can ask what structures or mechanisms in the brain actually mechanically construct the visual field, as we experience this, in terms that a communication engineer could understand. In television this function is carried out by the raster of the set. So what is the equivalent in the brain of such a raster mechanism? Vernon (1962) in her review of introspectionist psychology puts the same point in another way:

> It is now valuable to consider more closely the details of the process by which, when the sensory impressions have reached the receptive areas of the cortex, a fully developed percept is attained... This cannot be studied objectively but only by introspection (p. 19)... The fundamental quality of the perceived field [is] its extraordinary unlikeness, so commonly overlooked in every life, to the stimulus field... The sensory impulses which arise from the stimulation of the sense organs and peripheral nervous systems are but the raw material from which the final percepts are constructed (p. 2)... The phenomenal percept, then, is never an accurate photographic reproduction of the external stimulus field (p. 46)."

The "perceived field" in consciousness is "extraordinarily unlike the stimulus field", not because the latter is spatial and the former is not, but because, whereas *both* are spatial, the details of shape, size, colour, etc. are very different in each owing to the way that the constructive (representative) mechanisms work developing all the Gestalt and constancy phenomena reviewed in detail in Vernon's book. The phenomenal percept is "never an accurate photographic reproduction of the external stimulus field", not because it is *not a pictorial reproduction* but because it is not an *accurate* pictorial reproduction.

Support for the TV model of visual perception comes from Charlesworth (1979) from a philosophical view point. The same problem has recently surfaced in neuroscience in the form of the "binding problem" (see Anderson and Palca (1988) and Churchland (1986)). This follows from the discovery that the brain processes information about the colour, shape and movement of objects in the stimulus field in three widely separated visual areas in the cortex: and in fact the full processing of visual information requires, in the primate, more than 24 different retinotopic visual areas scattered throughout the higher cortex mainly in the temporal and parietal lobes. The problem then is how does all this get together in consciousness to form the "integrated image of the visual field that we see with the mind's eye"? (Anderson and Palca, 1988).

It may be that the reconstruction of the image built up by the brain by separating various aspects of the visual input into its component parts, e.g. shading, transparencies, perspective, overlap, and then reconstituting them into a cortical picture helps in the identification of an object (say a predator like a cheetah) from the camouflage of leaves, twigs, etc. (Albright, 1991). Gray *et al.* (1989) suggest that this is achieved by synchronized oscillations at 40Hz between groups of neurones stimulated by movement or some other characteristic of the object of interest against a more diffuse and non-oscillating background. The other question is how do anatomically arranged brain mechanisms dynamically reapply colour within shape so that both move together avoiding the phenomenon of space-colour or visual illusory spread. We know that selective cortical lesions can lead to this phenomenon; it can occur in migraine attacks, and is well illustrated by the two paintings by Matisse – *Madame Matisse: The Green Line,* where a vertical green line is central to the portrait, and in *Woman with the Hat,* where one side of her hair appears red, the other green and the face is streaked with lilac, green and blue. In a similar way the separate mechanisms mediating shape and movement can become divorced. For example, illusory movement occurs in the phi phenomenon, in which two adjacent lights blinking asynchronously are seen as one light hopping to and fro. Also psychedelic drugs can lead to a phenomenon where (for example) a lighted cigarette twirled round in a circle at arm's length is seen as a series of stationary glowing balls strung along the pathway followed by the cigarette.

Several authors (including Descartes (1965), Ryle (1966), Gregory (1984) and Dennett (1969)) have objected to the TV model of perception on the grounds that it leads to an infinite regress – because when we ask what is looking at these inner pictures, we have to posit an inner "little green man" or homunculus as the subject of consciousness. Then, they claim, we have to posit another little green man inside the head of the first to look at his inner pictures, and so on *ad infinitum.* However Fodor (1981) refutes this argument "This is, however, a bad argument. It assumes, quite without justification that, if receiving information from the environment requires having an image, recovering information from an image also requires having an image too. But why should we assume that?" I have answered this argument at length elsewhere (Smythies, 1994). Briefly, if we ask "What is looking at the inner pictures?" we are prejudicing the answer by using the word "looking". We should ask instead "What is observing the inner pictures?" And the answer is "the Ego" or "the O" referred to in innumerable experiments in introspectionist psychology. Further the Rylean argument confuses "perceiving" (how we see external objects) with "sensing" (how we experience our own sensations and how psychologists observe their own sensations in their experiments; it also covers how we experience our own hallucinations and such phenomena as eidetic images). The real "homunculus" is of course the body-image (somatic sensory field) in the "head" of which the Ego is located. The "I" does not have an eye nor does the body-image have a brain. So no vicious regress is generated and the argument for a TV model of perception stands.

There are also certain grave difficulties with IT as it stands. The events in the nerve nets of the brain consist of spatio-temporal patterns of nerve impulses located in public physical space-time. The events in a visual field in consciousness also consist of spatio-temporal patterns (i.e. sensations) located in private phenomenal space-time, and with a quite different geometry. Both contain the same *information* but in quite different forms. When formulated properly in terms of RT rather than DR it claims the identity of these two sets of spatio-temporal events that are geometrically totally incongruent with each other. No spatio-temporal series of events with structure A can be identical with a series of spatio-temporal events with structure B. Brain (1960) has pointed out that the nerve nets of the brain contain only *coded* information, whereas the visual field in consciousness contains *uncoded* representations of external objects in the form of our extended and coloured sensations. These resemble the uncoded images on the TV screen much more than they do the precursor coded events deep inside the TV set. It is axiomatic that $x$ and $x^1$ (a coded version of $x$) cannot be identical. $X^1$ represents $x$ and contains all the information that is in $x$, but $x = x^1$.

The conclusions we can draw from all this is that consciousness is the product – the mechanical TV-like product – of a vastly complex mechanism that combines the functions of mechanical computation and mechanical representation (TV-like communication). The *input* to the system consists of a variety of physical events that stimulate the external and internal sensory organs. There are two outputs (i) behaviour and (ii) phenomenal "objective" consciousness with its sensation fields and images. The Unconscious also divides into two (i) a subconscious consisting of all the above mechanisms in the brain that do not belong to the consciousness neurone system and (ii) a Freudian Unconscious that consists of (a) quasi-autonomous aberrant NCAs outside the consciousness neurone system that compete with the normal NCAs in the latter system for control of behaviour and of ideation; (these can influence consciousness neurones by roundabout routes resulting, e.g. in the production of a phobia of sharp knives in place of an attack on the hated person): and (b) the complex neuronal circuits that choreograph our dreams and the hallucinations of the psychedelic state.

These hypotheses are based on the assumption that the theory of psychoneural identity (IT) is true. However, there is no direct evidence that it is true (Smythies, 1993). It is certainly simple, plausible, Occam-friendly and is accepted by the vast majority of neuroscientists and by most philosophers. If modern physics is complete, then IT must be true, since all other theories are either trivial (like epiphenomenalism), or so general as to apply to almost anything (like functionalism) or plainly false (like Cartesian Dualism). So, in the immortal words of Sherlock Holmes "When we have eliminated the impossible, whatever remains, however improbable, must be the truth." But, recently two leading physicists, Roger Penrose (1989) and Andrei Linde (1990) have cautioned us against making the assumption that physics in 1992 is (nearly) complete. It will be remembered that physicists in 1892 were claiming with equal confidence that physics was then complete. Penrose states that physics may yet be due for further revolutions, possibly concerning the nature of time, of an importance on a par with relativity and quantum theory. Linde has suggested that matter, space-time and consciousness may have a more complex relationship than is currently supposed. He says it was at one time thought that space was merely a passive container for the really real, which was matter. Now, he says, we know that this is not so and that space-time has a reality of its own independent of matter and has its own attributes in the form of gravity waves. In a similar vein he suggests that consciousness may not be a mere by-product of matter, as is currently believed, but that it may have "its own degrees of freedom" [possibly manifest as phenomenal space-time]. In this case matter, space-time and the non-Cartesian consciousness might form an over-riding physical reality. As Indow says: "VS is dynamic, not a solid empty container into which various percepts are put without affecting the contours and intrinsic structure." Thus phenomenal space-time (and its contents) may form a part of physical reality with its own degrees of freedom from both ordinary matter and physical space-time. The philosophers Broad (1923), Price (1953), Russell (1948) and Bradley (1930) have made similar suggestions.

## Notes

(1) "The boundary between inner (non-extended) events and outer (extended) events, therefore does not divide that which is 'in consciousness' from that which is not. This inclusion of extended objects and events within the contents of consciousness runs directly counter to the fundamental bifurcation of the universe proposed by Descartes into *res extensa*... and *res cogitans*." (Velmans, 1990).

(2) "Objects of visual sensation, things seen, stand at the beginning of visual processing. Phenomenal individuals, by contrast, are constructed in the course of visual processing. Think, for example, of the question in fundamental neuropsychology of how the surprisingly many retinotopic maps in primate visual cortex are 'unified' into a single visual representation." (Kobes, 1991).

(3) What I have called the "consciousness neurones", that are identical with conscious experience, is termed "the bridge locus" as "the immediate substratum of visual perception", by Teller and Pugh (1983).

## Acknowledgements

I am most grateful to Michael Trimble, Ted Bullock and V.S. Ramachandran for their support of this work and to Paul and Patricia Churchland and Michael Shepherd for the benefit of many interesting discussions.

## References

Albright, T. (1991). Motion perception and the body-mind problem. *Current Biology*, 1, 391-393.
Alheid, G.F. and Heimer, L. (1988). New perspectives in basic forebrain organization of special relevance for psychiatric disorders: the striatopallidal, amygdaloid and corticopetal components of the substantia innominata. *Experimental Brain Research*, 27, 1-40.
Anderson, A. and Palca, J. (1988). Who knows how the brain works? *Nature*, 335, 489-491.
Bradley, F.H. (1930). "Appearance and Reality". Clarendon Press, Oxford.
Brain, Lord. (1960). Space and sense-data. *British Journal of the Philosophy of Science*, 11, 177-191.
Broad, C.D. (1923). "Scientific Thought". Routledge and Kegan Paul, London.
Charlesworth, M. (1979). Sense-impressions: a new model. *Mind*, 88, 24-44.
Churchland, P.S. (1986). "Neurophilosophy. Toward a Unified Science of the Mind-Brain". M.I.T. Press, Cambridge, Mass.
Dennett, D.C. (1969). "Content and Consciousness". Humanities Press, New York.
Descartes, R. (1965, Trans. P.J. Olscamp) "Discourse on Method, Optics, Geometry, Meteorology". Bobbs-Merrill, Indianapolis; and see 1970 edition, Cambridge University Press, Vol. 1. p. 151.
Farah, M.J., Wong, A.B., Monheit, M.A. and Morrow, L.A. (1989). Parietal lobe mechanisms of spatial attention: modality specific or supramodal? *Neuropsychologia*, 27, 461-470.
Fodor, J.A. (1981). Imagistic representation. *In* "Imagery". (Ed. N. Block). Bradford, New York.
Freeman, W.J. (1990). The physiology of perception. *Scientific American*, 264, (2), 78-87.
Gray, C.M., Konig, P., Engel, A.K. and Singer, W. (1989). Oscillatory responses in the cat visual cortex exhibit inter-columar synchronization which reflects global stimulus properties. *Nature*, 338, 334.
Gregory, R.L. (1984). "Mind in Science". Penguin, Harmondsworth.
Harrison, J. (1985). "The Philosopher's Nightmare". Nottingham University Press, Nottingham.
Harrison, S. (1989). A new visualisation of the mind-brain relation. Naive realism transcended. *In* "The Case for Dualism". (Eds J. Smythies and J. Beloff). University Press of Virginia, Charlottesville.
Indow, T. (1991). A critical review of Luneberg's model with regard to global structure of visual space. *Psychological Review*, 98, 430-453.
Jung, C.G. (1952). Personal communication.

Kobes, B.W. (1991). Sensory qualities and "homunctionalism": a review essay of W.G. Lycan's "Consciousness". *Philosophical Psychology*, 4, 147-158.
Koestler, A. (1969). *In* "Beyond Reductionism". (Eds A. Koestler and J. Smythies). Macmillan, London.
Köhler, W. (1947). "Gestalt Psychology". Liveright, New York.
Linde, A. (1990). "Particle Physics and Inflationary Cosmology". Harwood, New York.
Maclean, P. *vide* Koestler.
Muller, R.W. and Kubie, J.L. (1989). The firing of hippocampal place cells predicts the future position of the freely moving rats. *Journal of Neuroscience*, 9, 4101-4110.
Nicod, J. (1969). "The Foundations of Geometry and Induction". Routledge and Kegan Paul, London.
O'Keefe, J. and Nadel, L. (1978). "The Hippocampus as a Cognitive Map". Clarendon Press, Oxford.
Penrose, R. (1989). "The Emperor's New Mind". Oxford University Press.
Price, H. H. (1953). Survival and the idea of another world. *Proceedings of the Society for Psychical Research*, 50, 1-25.
Quirk, G.J., Muller, R.U. and Kubie, J.L. (1990). The firing of hippocampal cells in the dark depends on the rat's recent experience. *Journal of Neuroscience*, 10, 2008-2017.
Ramachandran, V.S. (1988). The perception of shape from shading. *Scientific American*, 254, 76-83.
Rolls, E.T., Miyashita, Y., Cahusac, P.B.M., Kenser, R.P., Niki, H., Feigenbaum, J.D. and Bach, L. (1989). Hippocampal neurons in the monkey with activity related to the place in which a stimulus is shown. *Journal of Neuroscience*, 9, 1835-1845.
Rorty, R. (1970). Incorrigibility as a mark of the mental. *Journal of Philosophy*, 67, 399-424.
Russell, B. (1948). "Human Knowledge. Its Scope and Limits". pp. 45 &581-593. Allen and Unwin, London.
Ryle, G. (1966). "The Concept of Mind". Penguin, Harmondsworth.
Schilder, P. (1950). "The Image and Appearance of the Human Body". International Universities Press, New York.
Selemon, L.D. and Goldman-Rakic, P.S. (1988). Common cortical and subcortical targets of the dorsolateral prefrontal and posterior parietal cortices in the Rhesus monkey: evidence for a distributed neural network subserving spatially guided behaviour. *Journal of Neuroscience*, 8, 4049-4068.
Smythies, J.R. (1953*a*). The mescaline phenomena. *British Journal of the Philosophy of Science*, 3, 339-346.
Smythies, J.R. (1953*b*). The experience and description of the human body. *Brain*, 76, 132-145.
Smythies, J.R. (1959/1960). The stroboscopic patterns. *British Journal of Psychology*, 50, 106-116 and 305-325; 51, 247-255.
Smythies, J.R. (1973). "Brain Mechanisms and Behaviour". Blackwell, Oxford.
Smythies, J.R. (1992). "The Cognitive Brain". Review of A. Trehub, "The Cognitive Brain" M.I.T. Press, Cambridge (Mass), (1991). In *"Psychological Medicine, in press.*
Smythies, J.R. (1993). Editorial: Neurophilosophy. *Psychological Medicine*, 23, 805-807.
Smythies, J.R. "The Walls of Plato's Cave", in press, (1994).
Smythies, J.R. and Corbett, L.C. (1981). "Psychiatry for Students of Medicine". Heinemann, London.
Teller, D.Y. and Pugh, E.N. Jr. (1983). Linking propositions in colour vision. *In* "Colour Vision and Psychophysics". (Eds J.D. Mollen and L.T. Sharpe). Academic Press, London.

Velmans, M. (1990). *Philosophy and Psychology*, **3**, 76-99.
Vernon, M.D. (1962). "A Further Study of Visual Perception". Cambridge University Press.
Wisdom, J.O. (1953). The concept of the phantom body. *Proceedings of the XIII International Congress of Philosophy*, **7**, 175-179.

# 11. A view of the world from a split-brain perspective

Dahlia W. Zaidel

## Introduction

Patients who have undergone brain surgery with complete division of the interconnecting fibres between the two hemispheres – commissurotomy – are commonly described as having "split-brains", a term which presupposes emotional overtones and dramatic personality changes. They have been subject to intense scientific research and represent some of the most fascinating phenomena in neurology. Understanding their performance in the laboratory has provided a challenge to students of neuropsychology, neuroscience and even philosophy. However most of the observed changes are subtle and require special laboratory testing to be elicited. The daily life of "split-brain" patients stands in sharp contrast with their behaviour and defies some of the previous concepts of how mind and brain are organized.

Normally the left and right hemispheres of the brain (the neurocortex) are connected to each other by several bundles of fibres. These rich fibre systems are severed surgically, for reasons which will be explained, thus separating the two hemispheres. The result is two halves of the brain, originally designed by millions of years of evolution to be anatomically connected, now processing information nearly independently from each other while having different functional specializations. The different hemispheric functions have come to be considered complementary and as such to represent the ideal for normal human behaviour. And yet, in daily life, the patients appear to behave as if there were no evolutionary purpose to this major forebrain neuronal connection between the hemispheres. Some functions, considered by some to be specialized in the left hemisphere, such as speech and language comprehension appear unimpaired. Previously learned functions which require bilateral interaction such as cooking, cycling, swimming or piano playing appear unchanged, and have remained so until now, as long as 30 years post-surgery in some cases. Neither have there been major changes in personality or mannerisms, or in general intelligence. There are no psychiatric symptoms such as hallucinations, delusions, fugue states, or multiple personalitites. Each patient behaves as one with a single personality and unified consciousness.

We must look at what is amiss in order to distinguish between the apparent and the real. Clues to the paradox were revealed in laboratory studies and those are discussed in the following sections of this chapter.

## Boundaries of Reality and Conscious Awareness

Boundaries of consciousness and of reality are recognized through deviation from that which is accepted and considered normal. What is normal in the split-brain patients' behaviour will be described first.

Some of the many dimensions of conscious awareness include orientation to space and time, knowledge of human biological and sociological context, intentionality, and so on. In split-brain patients, as a group, all these dimensions of awareness seem intact. Orientation with respect to where they are located at any given moment is fully acknowledged and known as is time of day, month, or year. Memory for past personal events that occurred before surgery appears intact and knowledge of national or international historical events is at a level that would be expected given their educational background. Knowledge of current events is faulty and is most likely due to their poor recent memory and the lack of interest in reading following surgery. Knowledge of sociological good or evil and, depending on the personality and intelligence level of the patient, "taking sides" all appear normal. Moreover, intentions are executed normally. Thus, if they want to touch a person or a table, they do so and they feel the difference in their sensation. If they wish to listen to music, they turn the radio on and respond appropriately to the sounds. These are only a few examples.

In laboratory tests where information is lateralized to only one hemisphere and a lateralized motor response is required, either hand can do so, even when the left hand's response is controlled by the right, non-speaking hemisphere. This is demonstrated in specially designed tests where the answer is hidden from view and the response is nevertheless provided by either hand. For instance, the examiner may request, "after feeling all the choices behind the screen, decide on the correct answer, and tap on it with your finger" (see D. Zaidel, 1990a). In daily life, either the left or the right hand reachs out to touch or to pick things appropriately. In other words, intentionality is not restricted to the dominant, speaking hemisphere and can be initiated/controlled by either hemisphere.

## Unity of Consciousness

Recently, Searle (1992) summarized the essence of unity of conscious experience: "It is characteristic of nonpathological conscious states that they come to us as part of a unified sequence. I do not just have an experience of a toothache and also a visual experience of the couch that is situated a few feet from me and of roses that are sticking out from the vase on my right, in the way that I happen to have on a striped shirt at the same time as I have dark blue socks. The crucial difference is this: I have my experiences of the rose, the couch, and the toothache all as experiences that are part of one and the same conscious event. Unity exists in at least two dimensions, which, continuing the spatial metaphors, I will call "horizontal" and "vertical". Horizontal unity is the organization of conscious experiences through short stretches of time. For example, when I speak or think a sentence, even a long one, my awareness of the beginning of what I said or thought continues even when that part is no longer being thought or spoken. Iconic memory of this sort is essential to the unity of consciousness, and perhaps even short-term memory is essential. Vertical unity is a matter of the simultaneous awareness of all the diverse features of any conscious state, as illustrated by my example of the couch, the toothache, and the rose. We have little understanding of how the brain achieves this unity." (Searle, 1992, pp. 129-130).

As far as we can tell from ordinary behaviour, there is little to indicate that the type of unity described above is absent or is disrupted in a serious way in split-brain patients, both in daily life or under special testing conditions that lateralize the information to one or the other hemisphere. However, the clue to what is involved in achieving such unity may yet be revealed in the study of these patients.

## Some Clinical Background

The split-brain patients under discussion here suffered from frequent generalized epileptic convulsions which were life threatening and could not be controlled by drugs alone (Bogen and Vogel, 1962). Surgical intervention was a last resort. The logic behind the procedure was that sectioning the forebrain commissures (hemisphere-connecting fibers) would limit or abolish transfer of abnormal epileptic discharges from one hemisphere to the other, restricting them to only one side, which would then make it possible to have greater pharmacological control over them. Indeed the surgery was successful in the majority of cases (Bogen, 1990; Bogen, 1992; Bogen et al., 1988; Bogen and Vogel, 1975).

Anatomically, the forebrain commissures are made up of three distinct structures which connect matched and non-matched areas in the left and right hemispheres: the corpus callosum has received most attention in scientific investigations. It is assumed to have more than 200 million neuronal fibers, the largest tract of fibers in the brain. It is present only in mammals and reaches its largest size in humans. And it is humans who have hemispheric functional specialization, that is, the lateralization of certain aspects of perception, memory, cognition, or emotion to one or the other hemisphere. Consequently, it has been suggested that the growth in size of the corpus callosum is intimately related to phylogenetic brain development leading to hemispheric functional separation and specialization in humans. The purpose of this extensive callosal development is to maintain easy communication between the left and right hemispheres.

## Basic Facts about Left and Right in the Central Nervous System

Human sensory and motor pathways function on the basis of contralateral innervation. Thus, sensations from the left limbs are received and processed predominantly in the right hemisphere while sensations from the right limbs are received and processed predominantly in the left hemisphere. Similarly, motor control of the right limbs is in the left hemisphere and the opposite is true for left limbs. With vision, information falling in the left visual half-field of either eye is projected initially to the right hemisphere, and the information falling in the right visual half-field is projected initially to the left hemisphere. In order for humans to interact with the physical world, sensory information from both halves of the body must be completely available to both hemispheres, and this is achieved principally, though not exclusively, through the forebrain commissures. In laboratory conditions, information is restricted to only one hemisphere at a time based on the principle of contralateral innervation.

## Neurological Pathology and Hemispheric Specialization in Split-brain Patient

In the majority of right- and left-handers, the left hemisphere is the main language and speech processor while the right is the main processor of visuo-spatial functions such as topographical orientation, facial recognition, and spatial relations. This functional separation and hemispheric specialization in high mental functions is seen only in humans (although very special laboratory training procedures have shown the precursors of functional separation in the brains of monkeys). The present group of split-brain patients is right-handed and the normal pattern of hemispheric specialization for right-handers is observed.

It is important to stress that early onset of habitual epilepsy was present in only some of the patients in the Bogen-Vogel series. A few had a later onset (e.g. ages 17 or 18). One could have predicted that at least in those in whom there was an early onset, the pattern of hemispheric specialization would have changed due to "plasticity" and functional reorganization. On empirical grounds, one could not make this prediction since there are no available data to support it. Any data that are available regarding epilepsy and functional development consist predominantly of cases suffering from temporal lobe epilepsy, and in those cases there is evidence that early onset of habitual epilepsy could lead to reorganization of speech and language (Milner, 1975). However, in the absence of convincing data on patients with generalized convulsions, the pattern of observed functional asymmetries and symmetries in split-brain patients must be assumed to be attributable to normal development.

Yet, age at time of surgery did appear to affect the extent of interhemispheric communication that developed, possibly via subcortical centres (Johnson, 1984; Teng and Sperry, 1973; D. Zaidel, 1988). Patients operated on when young (ages 12-14) showed signs of such transfer to a greater extent than older patients (ages 25-40). However, even in young patients the pattern of hemispheric specialization remained the same with no convincing reasons to believe that new functions, e.g. language, developed abnormally in the right hemisphere (D. Zaidel, 1988).

## Elements of the Paradox and Some Clues

Much of what is known now about functional complementarity in the left and right hemispheres came originally from studies of patients with unilateral focal brain damage. Some of those findings received convergent evidence from split-brain studies: but not all. There are several examples of such discrepancies. We will focus on two that concern right hemisphere specialization, prosopagnosia and hemi-neglect. In prosopagnosia, a patient with unilateral damage loses the ability to recognize previously known people by their faces alone, including the patient's own face, following damage to posterior regions of the right hemisphere (though some would attribute the syndrome to bilateral damage).

Herein lies a piece of the puzzle: if the right hemisphere specializes in facial recognition, why does the disconnected left hemisphere not show symptoms of prosopagnosia? Similarly, a patient showing hemi-neglect most likely shows the neglect for the left-half of external or personal space (severe neglect of the right half is rarely seen clinically). The right hemisphere in its normal, intact state is said to be responsible for events or actions in the contralateral half space. By logical inference, then, the left half has more biological significance than the right half of space. Otherwise, damage to the left hemisphere would result in equally frequent right neglect of space. All of this would make sense if the right hemisphere were crucial for spatial orientation, on personal or extra-personal space.

Yet, in split-brain patients, the disconnected left hemisphere does not show hemi-neglect of contralateral space (Plourde and Sperry, 1984). Nor does the disconnected right hemisphere, for the right half of space. Each disconnected hemisphere has full knowledge and awareness of both left and right halves of space. (It might be interesting to add that, in right hemispherectomy patients, prosopagnosia or hemi-neglect are rarely observed as well.) Thus, hemi-neglect or hemi-inattention may be only tangentially related to knowledge of spatial relations or of topographical orientation, for these two functions appear to be intact in the disconnected right hemisphere. Hemi-neglect, then, must be related to some other hard-to-define higher mental function.

In light of the above, should we conclude that data from hemisphere-damaged patients reflect the inhibiting effects of the diseased tissue over healthy tissue rather than of the effects of the hemispheric damage itself? Should we infer that hemi-neglect is but an epi-phenomenon resulting from an abnormal brain-behaviour interaction rather than a hemispherically specialized function? And here is the important clue to resolution of the paradox under discussion. Should we infer that the absence of such symptoms in split-brain patients reflects subcortical integration of sensory and motor information? Or, is there sufficient redundancy in functional representation for one hemisphere alone to control a wide range of behaviours? And, are the mechanisms involved in the interhemispheric interaction normal and present in the intact brain?

## Relevant Early Animal Work

The functions of the corpus callosum and of the other forebrain commissures were initially gleaned from experimental work on cats and monkeys (Glickstein and Sperry, 1960; Myers and Sperry, 1958; Stamm and Sperry, 1957). Researchers found that an animal with intact commissures can perform a particular task which it was trained to do very well with either hemisphere, when each hemisphere was tested separately. On the other hand, if another animal with sectioned commissures is trained to perform a particular task with only one hemisphere is then exposed to the same task with the untrained hemisphere, it shows initially no signs of knowing the task. This was taken to demonstrate absence of transfer of information between the hemispheres.

On the whole, the human studies provided convergent evidence regarding the role of the forebrain commissures in interhemispheric communication. However, in some isolated split-brain animal experiments, researches reported that animals learned the task with the untrained hemisphere faster than one would expect from the initial learning level of the originally trained hemisphere (see Hamilton, 1982, for review). How? The most plausible answer is that this occurred through certain sub-cortical structures which normally provide integration for direct or crossed connections to the left and right hemispheres. These sub-cortical relay stations could conceivably have allowed some minimal memory in the trained hemisphere to be tapped by the untrained hemisphere. Yet they did not provide a perfect substitute for the forebrain commissures since the animal continued to behave as if it had essentially two separated hemispheres, and, in any case, savings by the untrained hemisphere were observed rarely. Nevertheless, subcortical relay stations were hypothesized to transmit only rudimentary information.

Indeed, subsequent work on the human split-brain patients by Trevarthen and Sperry (1973) revealed that, at least for vision, there are one or two subcortical relay stations which permit uncrossed information to be integrated and then transmitted to the ipsilateral hemisphere. It was hypothesized that a "secondary visual system" in humans is a vestige of a phylogenetically older mammalian visual system and that it becomes functional when certain types of brain damage occur (possibly in "blind sight" as well). In the absence of direct communication via the forebrain commissures, the secondary visual system would provide some minimal visual integration.

## One Person Despite a Split-brain

As maintained, daily behaviour of the Bogen-Vogel group of patients' appears to show unified consciousness. Their walk is co-ordinated, their stride is purposeful, they perform old unilateral and bimanual skills, converse fluently and to the point, remember long-term events occurring before surgery, are friendly, kind, generous, and thoughtful to the people they know, have a sense of humor, and so on down a whole gamut of what it takes to be human. How is that possible given hemispheric disconnection? There are two logical possibilities: First, there is more subcortical integration of behaviour than was realized, so that in the end both hemispheres receive much the same sensory input, and the output is somehow integrated subcortically as well. Second, only one hemisphere controls the observed behaviour. Each of the possibilities poses problems to biological reality. If either possibility is true, why do we have the forebrain commissures, or two hemispheres for that matter? Is it that they are important only in the initial sorting of information, relegating it into left and right hemispheres but not afterwards?

## 1 One hemisphere in control

There are several sources of evidence that suggest that one hemisphere controls ordinary behaviour in split-brain patients, namely, the left hemisphere. First, all verbal communication is produced by the left hemisphere since this is the hemisphere dominant for speech and language comprehension in these patients. There is some language comprehension in the disconnected right hemisphere, more for auditory than for written vocabulary, and more for single words than for phrases (E. Zaidel, 1976; 1985). But the mental age-level of the vocabulary is lower than the chronological age of the patient. Given hemispheric disconnection, it is unlikely that substantial right hemisphere linguistic contribution is made in the course of a normal conversation. Similarly, the contents of the conversation, including concepts, thinking, problem solving, memory – short- and long-term, must all be controlled by the disconnected left hemisphere. Topographical orientation and memory are impaired and they represent nonverbal behaviour, indicating that nonverbal aspects of behaviour are not expressed. Indeed, what components are missing in verbal conversation or in nonverbal behaviour are very likely those components which normally are contributed by the hemisphere. The degree to which one disconnected hemisphere can support a wide range of behaviours may depend on individual differences including intelligence, sex, or genetic factors (see D. Zaidel and Sperry, 1974, for discussion).

## 2 The case for subcortical integration

In the following discussion I shall use motor control as an illustration of subcortical integration. (The case for vision was described above). I start with the following question: how is it possible that the patients under discussion walk normally and have normal bimanual co-ordination for previously learned movements and skills if cortical motor control is contralaterally innervated and the major cortical fibers allowing interhemispheric communication regarding the control are cut? Some likely possibilities include unified cerebellar control in conjunction with other subcortical structures.

After disconnection, when patients try to learn new bimanual movements, certain kinds are learned with exceptional difficulty and never reach normal levels (Preilowski, 1972; D. Zaidel and Sperry, 1977). These are skills which consist of interdependent bimanual movements such as those involved in using a children's toy called "etch-a-sketch". Other bimanual movements, such as those consisting of parallel or alternate control, are not impaired. How can we be sure that the observed manual co-ordination is not in fact controlled by only one hemisphere, namely the left? We can be reasonably sure for the following reasons: separate tests for ideomotor apraxia (the ability to carry out spoken commands) were administered in free vision and hearing, first with the request to execute the commands with the left hand and later with the right hand (D. Zaidel and Sperry, 1977). The results showed some ideomotor apraxia on the left side only. If the left hemisphere were "in charge" of motor control on both sides, we would not have observed unilateral apraxia but rather no apraxia at all. Thus, judged from this perspective, we may infer that habitual ordinary behaviours are integrated in subcortical structures while certain types of newly learned skills depend crucially on normal interhemispheric communication.

### Sense of Humour

Based on informal observations, the split-brain patients appear to have a good sense of humor. They tell funny stories designed to make the listener laugh. They use appropriate and relevant punch lines as well as dramatic pauses. They themselves laugh appropriately upon hearing others' stories. Many jokes are spontaneous and original. Some are idiomatic or are tongue-in-cheek. Their humor appears to consist of wit, puns, and some metaphors and to include references to the self, and to others. One patient repeats. "I told my husband I am a lot smarter than him; I have two brains and he has only one."

### Sex

This is a sensitive topic to raise with patients and not much is known about matters related to it. However, informal observations have revealed that their interest in the opposite sex is appropriate. Both the men and the women make socially appropriate remarks regarding physical attractiveness and flirtation. I have never heard interest expressed in the same sex. To the best of my knowledge, inappropriate touching or reference to the anatomy of experimenters have not occurred. Similarly, unlike some patients with frontal lobe pathology, lewd or sexually inappropriate remarks are not known to have been made. An interesting observation, however, is that some of the women patients enjoy telling "dirty" jokes. One in particular, wrote a few limericks with veiled, strong, albeit sexual undertones which she did show to men and women experimenters.

## Telling Personal Stories and Anecdotes

The patients relate personal anecdotes that occurred preoperatively with a beginning, a middle, and an end. They are always to the point and appear nearly always to be relevant in the conversational context. Their stories seem complete with many if not all of the facts included. Because of their poor recent memory, they repeat the same stories and anecdotes to the same audience several times in the course of a year (though rarely if ever in the course of one visit to the laboratory).

There has never been any indication that these patients confabulate in ordinary conversation. Confabulations and guessing do occur under special testing conditions in which stimuli are lateralized to the right hemisphere and the task is to name the stimuli. Stimuli cannot be named because the control for speech is in the left hemisphere and yet, since a request for a verbal answer was received in both hemispheres, the left, dominant hemisphere provides the verbal response. It is the wrong response because sensory and perceptual information of the stimulus is lateralized only to the right hemisphere. The confabulations or "guesses", then reflect an attempt to "make sense" of the world, to "fill in" so to speak, by the left hemisphere. In sum, right hemisphere removal from conscious experiences of the left hemisphere leads to left hemispheric verbal attempts to minimize the removal.

## What is Not Normal

### Memory

Clues to hemispheric involvement in daily life might be gleaned from what is not quite normal in split-brain patients' behaviour. Generally, it is assumed that their verbal output reflects left hemisphere functioning and whatever is missing in the output is the right hemisphere component or the normal interaction between left and right. Now, what appears to have suffered dramatically after surgery is recent memory (though the severity level is not comparable to anterograde amnesia) (Huppert, 1981; D. Zaidel and Sperry, 1974; D. Zaidel, 1990b). Indeed, the type of nonverbal memory usually associated with right hemisphere specialization, topographical memory, is particularly poor in everyday life. Thus, they have exceptional difficulties in relocating a parked car or in locating items around the house, or in finding their way in a highly familiar laboratory. Some verbal memory, especially newly learned material, is also not up to the level preceding surgery, as determined by family members. This is confirmed in laboratory tests as well. Even in the case of verbal material, it is assumed that what is missing in the performance is the normal right hemisphere imagerial component.

Because memory is poor they have no interest in reading novels, newspapers, and so on. Similarly, watching TV or films poses apparently insurmountable integration problems which are probably due to poor memory.

## Emotional reactions

*In daily life*
Events such as divorce or death of a close relative do not appear to produce typical reactions such as bitterness, sadness, hatred, anger, violence, or related negative emotions (Hoppe and Bogen, 1977). In over 25 years I have never heard patients speak of revenge or of violent acts. In fact, reactions to such situations are, by and large, factual. A definite dissatisfaction is expressed but there is a touch of bemusement, the degree of which varies from patient to patient. Infidelity of a spouse (they themselves are not known to be disloyal) is related simply, in the absence of what might be considered deep insight. To the listener it appears that there is no sense that death or disloyalty or infidelity are forgiven or are understood benevolently. Instead, the listener gains the impression that an account is given of yet another daily event but this time one describing an injustice. Could this be a case of denial? Hardly, since the facts are always provided. All of this is not to say that they do not feel sadness, infidelity, loss, or anger. We simply do not know if they do since no formal assessment has been undertaken beyond informal conversation.

An example: a 50-year-old patient complained after he moved his residence from one caretaker to another that he was repeatedly not offered the food he was used to eating. Instead he was offered food peculiar to the ethnic background of the caretaker and after meals he still felt some hunger. He voiced his complaint to the caretaker, he says, but to no avail. A family member subsequently intervened and the food situation improved. There was no anger or resentment as he related the story. His tone of voice merely reflected the opinion of someone treated unfairly.

*Facial expressions*
Their faces are generally expressive. Based on casual observations, these appear just as symmetrical or asymmetrical as in normal subjects. However, anecdotes about personal injustice do not often appear to be accompanied with what one would normally expect to see. Hardly ever, if at all, did I observe a sad facial expression, for instance. But I did observe facial expressions denoting disgust or dissatisfaction (with food, say, or with unusually long waiting periods).

On the whole, the general personality characteristic is "positive" rather than "negative", and this is expressed both verbally or through facial expressions.

*In the laboratory*
One young male patient was tested with the hemi-field tachistoscopic technique which allows visual presentation of stimuli to only one visual half-field at a time. With his gaze focused on a central fixation point on the screen, different simple configurations were flashed quickly one at a time either to the left or to the right side of the point and the task was to name them. He had no difficulty in naming those flashed on the right side of the fixation point (the information was transmitted to the left, speaking hemisphere) but he was unable to name simple geometrical configurations on the left (information was transmitted only to the right, mute

hemisphere). He attempted guesses or simply said he was unable to name the image. One of the configurations that was projected on the left was that of a swastika. Unlike any of the previous reactions in earlier trials, he immediately sat back in his chair exclaiming. "What was this that you just showed me!" What do you think it was, asked the experimenter. He replied, "A terrible thing, an awful thing." You did not like it, stated the experimenter. "No, I didn't", he replied, shaking his head. Was it a good thing or a bad one, probed the experimenter (who did not anticipate strong reactions to any of the items in the set). "Bad, very bad", replied the patient. He was never able to name it nor to guess what it was.

In a separate, extensive series of trials which used the Z-lens, a technique which allows prolonged presentations of visual stimuli to one hemisphere at a time, social awareness and historical knowledge in the disconnected left and right hemispheres were measured (Sperry *et al.*, 1979). Faces of well known historical figures such as Churchill, John Kennedy, Stalin, and so on, as well as faces of the patients themselves, family members, or familiar situations, were presented. The task was to indicate "thumbs up" for good and "thumbs down" for bad. The results showed that the level of social awareness and historical knowledge was the same in both hemispheres. Thus, Churchill was "thumbs up" and Stalin "thumbs down" in either the left or the right hemispheres.

## Dreams

Before surgery patients reported dreaming at night. After surgery, most reported that they stopped dreaming. It has been difficult to verify their assertions without rigorous scientific observation and this project has never been undertaken. At the same time, there have never been reports by family members that patients wake up tired or that they have spent sleepless nights.

It is uncertain whether or not dreaming did not take place at all, or that dream content was inaccessible to verbal communication or that whatever was dreamed was forgotten. In the past, in some scientific circles, there was a controversy regarding the lateralization of dreaming in the brain. That is, does dreaming take place in the right hemisphere alone. The fact that split-brain patients were unable to report their dreams was taken as support for this hypothesis. The bottom line is that there is no conclusive evidence as of now on what role hemispheric specialization plays in dreaming.

## Attitude towards the left hand

Neither the left nor the right hands are paralyzed or deprived of sensations. Yet, in some cases, remarks that appeared to personify the left hand were noted soon after surgery, and in a few cases this attitude remained for some years. These verbally expressed attitudes may fall under the rubric of "the strange hand syndrome." In traditional neurology, the syndrome is usually observed following strokes in different parts of the cortex, including in parts of the corpus callosum. There is no easy or clear explanation for the phenomenon. With the split-brain cases, one would hear the left hand described as "she won't do what I tell it", "it has a mind of its own", "my left hand takes my cigarette out of my mouth while I'm smoking", or "I turn on the water tap with my right hand and the left comes and turns it off". Such remarks about the left hand were reported in the first few months after surgery but milder aspects of the motor conflict can last longer, in some cases several years (Bogen, 1992). For example, under specific laboratory conditions, one patient often slapped her left hand lightly with her right hand when she could not come up with the correct name of a blindly palpated object, saying something such as, "Bad, bad hand this one". Since sensory input from the left hand reached only the right hemisphere, the patient was unable to name the object. In other words, she was frustrated with her left-hand anomia. Whether the "frustration" was a manifestation of left or right hemisphere mental processes is hard to tell. However, since it was the right hand that slapped, we must assume that left hemisphere mental processes were dominant.

## Quality of Life

Most people would agree that "normal" is a relative term. Similarly, a "full life" could be considered relative. One could conceive of low quality of life if memory were a serious problem (although some would argue that having a poor memory is a blessing). Poor memory could pose a serious problem for the patients if they did not make notes of impending appointments or other specific schedules. In fact, they do take notes and since they are cared for by dedicated family members, their poor memory is probably not a serious handicap. Only one patient in this group has been gainfully employed for a substantial period of time, albeit in a specially funded civic program. What may be difficult or unusual in split-brain patients' lives is their secondary limitations, namely, inability to drive due to the epilepsy and/or medication as well as their lack of interest in reading or keeping up with the last movies or TV shows. The stimulation of such activities is missing from their daily life, leaving them dependent to a certain extent on others. But since they are friendly and enjoy a good conversation they do receive some enrichment. Consequently, they are involved and aware of crucial events that could have impact on their lives.

We do not really know how often, if at all, they generate an intention, a desire, or a wish in the right hemisphere, but are unable to carry it out. Such hypothetical situations in daily life are difficult to assess, let alone judging how much they would interfere with "quality of life". There is no doubt that the surgery alleviated or eliminated the epilepsy and all acknowledge that they gained freedom from recurrent, debilitating seizures is the best thing to have happened to them.

## Conclusion: resolution of the paradox

So much can be done without the forebrain commissures and yet other things are not quite normal. What conclusions can we then draw regarding the role that these commissures play in the organization of the mind in the brain, from cognition to personality to emotions? The likely answer is that they play a crucial role in learning new things, in the initial sorting of incoming information, and the relegation of this information to specialized regions within or between the hemispheres. This would also explain why skills learned before surgery are retained and only a few have been learned afterwards, or acquired with difficulty. This might explain why personality traits and mannerisms which were all established before surgery, did not change afterwards. Indeed, learning involves memory and memory functions are impaired with damage to the forebrain commissures (even when the commissurotomy is only partial (D. Zaidel, 1990*b*)).

The extent to which observed behaviour in the complete commissurotomy patients is supported by only one hemisphere would depend on individual differences interacting with a variety of factors such as genetics, intelligence, and so on. The lesson imparted here is that there is sufficient functional redundancy in the neocortex so that the capacity to maintain a wide range of abilities is within the control of one hemisphere. And, yet, as seen in what is missing in the patients' behaviour, one hemisphere is not quite enough. Nature seems to have intended that the two hemispheres complement each other, that the full range of human behaviour be best accomplished through interaction between the left and right hemispheres.

## References

Bogen, J.E. (1990). Partial hemispheric independence with the neocommissures intact. *In* "Brain Circuits and Functions of the Mind" (Ed. C. Trevarthen). pp. 215-230. Cambridge University Press, New York.

Bogen, J.E. (1992). The callosal syndromes. *In* "Clinical Neuropsychology". (Eds K.M. Heilman and E. Valenstein). Oxford University Press, New York.

Bogen, J.E. and Vogel, P.J. (1962). Cerebral commissurotomy in man. Preliminary case report. *Bulletin of the Los Angeles Neurological Society*, 27, 169-172.

Bogen, J.E. and Vogel, P.J. (1975). Neurologic status in the long term following complete cerebral commissurotomy. *In* "Les Syndromes de Disconnexion Calleuse chez l'Homme", (Eds F. Michel and B. Schott). Hospital Neurologie, Lyon.

Bogen, J.E., D.H. Schult, and P.J. Vogel. (1988). Completeness of callosotomy shown by magnetic resonance imaging in the long term. *Archives of Neurology*, 45, 1203-1205.

Glickstein, M. and Sperry, R.W. (1960). Intermanual somesthetic transfer in split brain Rhesus monkeys. *Journal of Comparative Physiology*, 53, 322-327.

Hamilton, C.R. (1982). Mechanisms of interocular equivalence. *In* "Analysis of Visual Behavior", (Eds D. Ingle, M, Goodale and R. Mansfield). MIT Press, Cambridge, Massachusetts.

Hoppe, K.D. and Bogen, J.E. (1977). Alexithymia in 12 commissurotomized patients. *Psychotherapy and Psychosomatics*, 28, 148-155.

Huppert, F.A. (1981). Memory in split-brain patients: a comparison with organic amnesic syndromes. *Cortex*, 17, 303-311.

Johnson, L. E. (1984). Bilateral visual cross-integration following forebrain commissurotomy. *Neuropsychologia*, 22, 167-175.

Milner, B. (1975). Psychological aspects of focal epilepsy and its neurosurgical management. *In* "Advances in Neurology", (Eds J.K. Purpura., R.D. Penry and R.D. Walters). Raven, New York.

Myers, R.E. and Sperry, R.W. (1958). Interhemispheric communication through the corpus callosum. *Archives of Neurology and Psychology,* **80**, 298-303.

Plourde, G. and Sperry, R.W. (1984). Left hemisphere involvement in left spatial neglect from right-sided lesions: A commissurotomy study. *Brain,* **107**, 95-106.

Preilowski, B. (1972). Possible contribution of the anterior forebrain commissures to bilateral co-ordination. *Neuropsychologia,* **10**, 267-277.

Searle, J.R. (1992). "The Rediscovery of the Mind". MIT Press, Cambridge, Massachusetts.

Sperry, R.W., Zaidel, E. and Zaidel, D. (1979). Self-recognition and social awareness in the deconnected minor hemisphere. *Neuropsychologia,* **17**, 153-166.

Stamm, J.S. and Sperry, R.W. (1957). Function of the corpus callosum in contralateral transfer of somesthetic discrimination of cats. *Journal of Comparative Physiology and Psychology,* **50**, 138-143.

Teng, E.L. and Sperry, R.W. (1973). Interhemispheric interaction during simultaneous bilateral presentation of letters or digits in commissurotomized patients. *Neuropsychologia,* **11**, 415-425.

Trevarthen, C.B. and Sperry, R.W. (1973). Perceptual unity in the ambient visual field in human commissurotomy patients. *Brain,* **96**, 547-570.

Zaidel, D. and Sperry, R.W. (1974). Memory impairment after commissurotomy in man. *Brain,* **97**, 263-272.

Zaidel, D. and Sperry, R.W. (1977). Some long-term motor effects of cerebral commissurotomy in man. *Neuropsychologia,* **15**, 193-204.

Zaidel, D.W. (1988). Observations on right hemisphere language function. *In* "Aphasia", (Eds C.F. Rose, R. Whurr and M.A. Wyke). Whurr Publishers, London.

Zaidel, D. W. (1990*a*). Longterm semantic memory in the two cerebral hemispheres. *In* "Brain Circuits and Functions of the Mind", (Ed. C. Trevarthen). Cambridge University Press, New York.

Zaidel, D.W. (1990*b*). Memory and spatial cognition following commissurotomy. *In* "Handbook of Neuropsychology", (Eds F. Boller and J. Grafman). Elsevier, Amsterdam.

Zaidel, E. (1976). Auditory vocabulary of the right hemisphere following brain bisection or hemidecortication. *Cortex,* **12**, 191-211.

Zaidel, E. (1985). Language in the right hemisphere. *In* "The Dual Brain", (Eds D.F. Benson and E. Zaidel). Guilford, New York.

# 12. Art and reality

> Art is ruled uniquely by the imagination. Images are its only wealth, it does not classify objects, it does not pronounce them real or imaginery, does not qualify them, does not define them, it feels and presents them – nothing more.
>
> *Benedetto Croce (1909)*

E.M.R. Critchley

---

To the archaeologist, painting, sculpture and ornaments are non-utilitarian artefacts worthy of study because they yield an insight into the dreams and aspirations of those who made them – of the society as a whole rather than of individual craftsmen. For in such works (to paraphrase John Boyle O'Reilly) a dreamer lives for ever, a toiler dies in a day. By contrast, more serviceable artefacts merely tell us what was eaten or traded, what work was done and how battles were fought. The motivation, and indeed the trepidations, of a society can only be conjectured from the non-vital trappings with which a people surrounds itself. From these we can surmise their hierarchical structure, their religions, and, through their talismen, their fears.

Works in stone, paint, silver or gold were demanded by the Lords of Society to glorify themselves in the eyes of their gods or of society, or to provoke envy. The craftsmen were also required on occasion to undergo a form of ritual purification, as with a witch-doctor, in suitable preparation for the undertaking. If circumstances were ideal an additional factor would be taken into consideration – the religious fervour of the artist, on the assumption that this would enhance his commitment and strengthen the power of his imagination. The choice of artist to depict a religious subject, though made partly on the artist's reputation and the school of his apprenticeship, took into account his religious rectitude, depth of feeling and the sincerity which he was able to project into his work. Inferior work which offended the devotees of the shrine was often rejected and the artist's future suffered accordingly. Ruskin was merely reflecting previous dicta by declaring that the Dominican Fra Angelico was not an artist properly so-called but an inspired saint. A similar commitment in the manufacture of holy works survived in the production of icons in Old Russia (Massie, 1978).

> The Orthodox believed that it is possible to recognize the presence of the Holy Spirit in a man and to convey it to others by artistic means. Therefore, the

function of the icon painter had much in common with that of a priest, and although it was important for the icon painter to be a good artist, it was essential for him to be a good Christian. Those who painted icons had to prepare themselves spiritually: fast, pray, read religious texts, for it was a true test, not a pictorial work in the usual sense.

Before we read too much into art it is necessary to be aware of certain caveats lest we over-interpret a particular artist or subject.

1   Early art, and indeed primitive art, often has another function: to depict, as a pictogram for the illiterate, an event or message. The murals of Egyptian temples or medieval churches are a form of literature for the masses and based upon rote handed from generation to generation. Much of the symbolism we recognize in the visions of the early saints amounts to little more than the application of conventional signs by which each particular saint was recognized.

2   Similarly, much of the complexity of the pictorial language of modern art is contrived, furnished from an astonishing familiarity with psychiatry, orthodox and otherwise (Dali), mythology (Masson), and the traditional signs of magic (Brauner, Seligman). It can be incredibly difficult to distinguish between the imagination of the artist and the sophistication of his technique.

3   We should be forewarned that all pictures owe more to other pictures than they do to nature (Gombrich, 1972). If an established genre succeeds (i.e. sells), it will be copied. Disaster pictures, for example of shipwrecks, may have been born of the experiences of the hallucinatory imaginings of Vernet and others; but once they had achieved a popularity they found continued favour as part of the stock in trade of Romantic art, exploited and vulgarized by the market. However, we should not decry all copying as the absence of art. Who but Francis Bacon could "paraphrase" Velasquez' portrait of Pope Innocent X with such horrific brilliance? How was van Gogh able to copy in exact detail and perspective Millet's *The Cornfield* and yet add something of his own style? The perception behind such works is undoubtedly present in heightened form but its interpretation defies description.

## Perception

What exactly "perception" is, whether it is reality or deduction, cannot be overlooked in deciding the boundaries of reality. The eye of an artist is truly remarkable: "He perceives more than sense (tho' ever so acute) can discover" (Blake). The greatest sophistication in art is to be found in portraiture, displaying a caricature or the personality of the sitter. Portraits are among the hardest things to fake or reproduce. As Ruskin pronounced:

> The best pictures that exist of the great schools are all portraits. Their real strength is tried to the utmost; it is never elsewhere brought out so thoroughly as in painting one man or woman, and the soul that was in them.

Perception and perspective are allied in landscape painting. Read (1931) regards landscape painting as essentially a romantic art, an art invented by a lowland people who had no landscape of their own, a deliberate creation of atmosphere for its own sake rather than a revelation of a precise experience. The doyen of the Romantic movement, the French landscape painter, Casper David Friedreich (1774-1840), declared that "the painter must not only paint what he sees before him, but also what he sees within him. If however he sees nothing within him, then he should omit to paint what he sees before him."

As stated by Gauguin (1923):

Do not copy too much from nature, take from nature by drawing about it, always search for the absolute. Dream and then just go ahead and paint. I dream of tremendous harmonies in the midst of natural fragrances which intoxicate me. My dream cannot be formulated, admits of no allegory; a musical poem, it needs no libretto.

**Obsession**

Van Gogh was one of the most brilliant, but certainly the most obsessional artist of all time, whose art was akin to madness. As described by the art critic, Albert Aurier:

Matter and nature are frantically twisted in a wild paroxysm of distortion; form has become a nightmare, colour is flames of hot spilling lava and precious stones; light is fire, and life itself is feverish and hectic. What particularizes his entire work is the excess, excess in strength, excess in nervousness, in violence of expression. He reveals a powerful being, a male, a bold man, often brutal and sometimes ingenuously delicate. This can be seen in the almost organistic excesses of everything he had painted: he is a fanatic, a kind of drunken giant, better able to move mountains than to handle bibelots, an ebullient brain which irresistibly pours its lava into all the ravines of art, a terrible and high strung genius, often sublime, sometimes grotesque, almost always on the edge of the pathological.

Chagall openly declared that his pictures are painted arrangements of inner images that obsessed him. Ensor was obsessed with masks, Turner with sunsets, Seraphine de Senlis, before she succumbed to neurosyphilis, was obsessed by the Tree of Life caparisoned with erotic leaves and flowers. Andre Masson was noted for the violence and fury of his painting, using support words to work himself up into a rage of activity. Obsession is a key to the personality and expression of many artists, many of whom border on the pathological and are affected by pathological states with a neurotic, and sometimes even psychotic, grasp on reality. "The artist, like the neurotic, has withdrawn from an unsatisfying reality into the world of imagination, but, unlike the neurotic, he knows how to find a way back from it and once more get a firm foothold on reality" (Freud – and again): "The motive forces of artists are the same conflicts which drive other people into neuroses and have encouraged society to construct its institutions."

## Hallucinatory States

Hallucinations provoked naturally or artificially have often provided the inspiration for art, as with Munch's *The Scream*. In this respect there is a paradox whereby passive or real experiences from nightmares, deliria, neuroses, psychoses and intoxications can be reproduced artistically as exact replicas of the form in which they appeared whereas experiences actively evoked by the fertile mind, artificially created from thoughts, fantasies or crystal gazing, need heightened expression involving the full use of all the artist's sophisticated techniques. We should not dismiss hallucinations as inevitably linked with insanity: for, as de Chirico has argued:

> Such abnormal moments can be found in everyone, and it is all the more fortunate that they occur in individuals with creative talents. Art is the fatal net which catches these strange moments on the wing like mysterious butterflies, fleeing the innocence and distraction of common man.

De Chirico developed his metaphysical art, which relied upon unusual ambiguities of objects and strange architectural perspectives to create an atmosphere of mystery and hallucination, raising them to a magnificent realism of visual dreams. His memoires and other writings, such as his metaphysical novel, "Hebdomeros", are notable for the variety and apparent authenticity of his visual experiences:

1 recurrent dreams from childhood;
2 Lilliputian dreams – Lilliputian hallucinations almost certainly account for the art form of Callot (1592-1635), Van Laer *(Il Bamboccio)* 1592-1642, and Magnasco *(Il Lissandrino)* 1667-1749 who peppered their scenes with hundreds of miniscule figures;
3 the dual identity of certain objects: the real appearance and a spectral appearance, which may have a migrainous basis;
4 a changed appearance was evident with jamais vu or déjà vu phenomena;
5 telepathic experiences;
6 oneiristic experiences of twilight and drug induced scenes;
7 an excessive use of dream symbolism.

So much of his imagery suggests a mass hallucination:

> Minds haunted by visions: in public squares shadows lengthen their mathematical enigmas, over walls rise nonsensical towers, infinitude is everywhere and everywhere is mystery. Inside a ruined temple the broken statue of a god spoke a mysterious language. For me, this vision is *always accompanied by a feeling of cold* as if I had been touched by a winter wind from a distant unknown country.

Illusions, the conscious or unconscious misinterpretations of the form of external stimuli, provide much of the unexpected in art. The conjuring of visions from natural objects (*Pareidolia*) to stimulate conscious imagery has long been an acceptable and recognized device. Story-tellers have found themes by gazing upon a burning fire, artists have seen visions in clouds and soothsayers in tea leaves. Leonardo advised painters to seek chance inspiration from puddles or stars.

The use of deceit in art, *trompe l' oeil* has been recognized as a stylized art-form through the ages. Liotard (1781) declared that "painting is the most astonishing sorceress; she can persuade us through the most evident falsehoods that it is pure truth." Caravaggio (1573-1610) developed the art of chiaroscuro wherein the exaggerated contrast of light and dark to all effects abolishes the middle distance. Leonardo used sfumato in which the clarity of the boundaries is lost and edges become hazy and indefinite. Michelangelo's painting of the ceiling of the Sistine Chapel, suggesting additional architectural features, is an example of quadratura. Other artists have unwittingly used illusions. Thus Munch at the age of 69 developed a small haemorrhage within the vitreous of one eye causing a small clot shaped like a bird with a long beak. This shape was consequently to intrude into several of his paintings. Klein (1917) and Horowitz (1964) have abstracted the entoptic visions into a series of simple elements and argued that the images from anatomical structures such as the retinal ganglionic network and from luminous dust which are normally filtered out from conscious perception can impinge on the minds of schizophrenics and appear in their paintings.

The unequivocal use of hallucinatory stimuli is best displayed by Goya. At the height of his powers he was struck down with giddiness, sickness, total deafness and partial but transitory blindness and was left with episodes of depression and paranoia and a ceaseless stream of morbid, black hallucinations which he overcame by committing them to paint. By this means he kept sane and, between 62 and 73 years of age, produced 700 paintings. He described his own illness:

> When the brain is beset by an accident, or the mind disordered by dreams or sickness, the fancy is overrun with wild, dismal ideas and terrified with a thousand monsters of its own framing.... Fantasy abandoned by reason produces impossible monsters; united with it, she is the mother of the arts and origin of its marvels.

A lesser painter, John Martin (1789-1854), was noted for his apocalyptic, even oneiristic, visions: *Sadak in Search of the Waters of Oblivion, The Destruction of Pompeii and Herculaneum,* the *Seventh Plague of Egypt.* He earned the epithet "Mad" and his paintings were likened to an opium dream. In that era not only painters like Bresdin "a brain clouded with opium" and possibly Moreau, but writers such as De Quincey, Byron and Coleridge indulged in opium. But overall the impact of drugs on Western Art, though tried by every generation, has been small and usually unrewarding in inspiration. Ernest Messonier (1815-91), arch rival of Courbet, hoped for splendid hallucinations when he took hashish but to his great disappointment he saw nothing but regular symmetrical designs. The effects can be variable. Hartley (1791) wrote that a person who has taken opium sees either gay scenes or ghastly ones, according as the opium excites pleasant or painful vibrations in the stomach. Picasso said that "opium has the most intelligent of all odours" (Penrose, 1958), but it was not only the suicide of his friend Wiegels that put a stop to its use. Whilst under the influence of the drug, Picasso found that his imagination and vision became acute but his desire to paint what he saw diminished seriously. This threat of blissful sterility influenced him most.

The Symbolist movement, which took many forms, was closely allied to literature and poetry. Victor Hugo, William Blake and Dante Gabriel Rossetti were among its practitioners. Schopenhauer's dictum, "The world is my representation" provided the philosophical background of the new insight that the universe is a creation of our ideas, and Bergson and Schelling stressed the importance of intuition. Society and many of the practitioners of Symbolism were also obsessed by spiritualism and mythology. Symbolism sought to evoke the creative spirit in art; to clothe the idea in a sensuous form, and to break new paths by resolving the contradictions between the sensory world and the spiritual world (Achille Delaroche).

Examples include Hugo's The Dream – a hand raised in horror from the abyss; Fuseli's *Nightmare* full of sexual symbolism, as are the flying figures of Purvis de Chavannes; Moreau's paintings based on Wagnerian themes, Odilon Redon "powerless to paint anything which is not representative of a state of soul, which does not express some depth of emotion, which does not translate an interior vision"; Beardsley's *Salome,* and John Singer Sargeant's *Astarte.*

If Schopenhauer can be said to have provided the archetypal inspiration for Symbolism, Freud's scientific exploration of dreams, culminating in "The Interpretation of Dreams" (1900), was a godsend to the Surrealist movement, pledged to inventing a new art embracing the abnormal, the illogical and the accidental. At last they could turn from the nihilism of the Dada movement to open up the "superreality" obtained from a combination of logical reality, fantasy, dream and imagination. According to André Breton, the acknowledged founder of Surrealism, the essential premise of their movement is that absolute realism, organized and mastered in logical terms, covers only a comparatively narrow segment of our experience, yet is mistaken for the whole of reality. Opposed to this rational universe is another no less real world of images rooted in fantasy, through which imagination and intuition strive to come into existence. They wished to liberate experience from its cage of immediate utility and commonsense, where it is governed by logic and reason.

In their Manifesto, "La Révolution Surréaliste" (1924) Boiffard, Eluard and Vtrac claim that:

> Surrealism opens the doors of the dream. Surrealism is the crossroads of the enchantments of sleep, alcohol, tobacco, ether, opium, cocaine, morphine... we dream, and the speed of the lamp's needles introduces to our minds the marvellous deflowered sponge of gold.

The surrealists developed techniques and methods for opening up the store of images preserved in the unconscious. Floods of unconscious imagery could be released: by dreams and the spontaneous caprices of the imagination – hallucinations; by exploring the primordial realm of psychic improvization – psychic automatism; and by the magical expression of things freed by chance association. Modes of psychic expression included automatic poetry, "Beautiful as the accidental encounter of a sewing machine with an umbrella on an operating table" (Lautremont), and surrealist games, the most famous of which was *Le Cadavre*

*Equis,* a variation of the game of consequences which derived its name from the first sentence so created. Each individual wrote one word, folded the paper and passed it on to the next person. Typical examples are: "The winged vapour seduces the locked bird" or "The strike of the stars corrects the house without sugar".

Dali conceived the early surrealist experiments as a nocturnal phase, characterized by a descent into the subterranean labyrinths of the psyche. In the next phase, characterized by Breton's dream objects, natural objects such as stones were assembled to produced a *trompe l'oeil* effect with the objects assuming a false or suggestive substantiality, dependent essentially upon the deceptive powers of the experimenter. Although dream imagery is repeatedly used by the surrealists, there are few examples of what appear to be true dreams. Max Ernst's *Two Children Threatened by a Nightingale* starts from one of those instances of irrational panic which we suppress in our waking lives. Only in dreams could a diminutive songbird scare the living daylights out of us. The third phase of surrealism, according to Dali, consisted of those, like Dali, Miró and Magritte, who did not wait on the passivity of the dream but used the gift of clairvoyance to appraise the objects of every day and release from within them a mysterious and ominous element which normally passes unnoticed (de Chirico).

Although dreams have been interpreted from Biblical times, their value as a stimulus to art tends to be overestimated. Gerard de Nerval described the dream as a second life and Jorge Luis Borges said that "while we are asleep in this world, we are awake in another one; in this way everyman has two lives". Of the classical psychologists, C.G. Jung is closer to the surrealists than Freud, believing that the dream is "a little hidden door into the innermost and most secret recesses of the psyche". Freud described the dream state as a mental experience, predominantly visual and often vivid, with bizarre elements due to spatio-temporal distortions and a delusional acceptance of these phenomena as real at the time they occur. Modern sleep research emphasizes not the clarity of dream-thought but the frequency in sleep of semi-schizophrenic, dereistic thinking – broken, unreal and replete with neologisms. The vicarious nature of dreams – moving, fleeting and shadowy – makes their recall particularly difficult and repeated awakenings are required for their scientific study. Reasonable recital occurs immediately after awakenings but most dreams, unless the emotional content is strong, quickly fade from our minds.

There is little to suggest that pathological disturbances of sleep (encephalitis, delirium, alcoholic stupor, narcolepsy or sleep apnoea) have contributed to the furtherance of art. A possible exception is de Chirico's experience of awakening from a typhoid vigil. Delira and oneiristic experiences are recognized but occur infrequently among the non-psychotic. Most well-known examples come from literature, e.g. Coleridge's *Kubla Khan,* under the influence of opium, and Horace Walpole's "The Castle of Otranto" visualized in a dream in which he found himself on the great staircase of an ancient castle and saw on the topmost banister a gigantic hand in armour.

We cannot by any means dismiss all visionary imaginings by artists as unlikely

– very much to the contrary. Klee spoke of art as a sample of creation, a unity of conscious and unconsciousness, and "wholly embedded in them is a third factor, myself". Oskar Kokoschka, writing "On the Nature of Visions" (1912), advises that we must harken closely to our inner voice:

> The state of awareness of visions is not one in which we are either remembering or perceiving. It is rather a level of consciousness at which we experience visions within ourselves. This experience cannot be fixed for the vision is moving, an impression growing and becoming visual, imparting a power to the mind. It can be evoked but never defined. Yet the awareness of such imagery is a part of life. It is life selecting from the forms which flow towards it.

Rather than selecting the dream as the most frequent cause of visionary imagery we should concentrate on "hypnagogic" imagery which is the word most commonly applied to visual musing on waking or falling asleep. Hypnagogic images are often geometric forms, nature scenes, and noises – all experiences when falling asleep. Hypnopompic images occur on waking, though the term has also been invoked to describe the perseveration of images as can happen after driving through fog all day. Both hypnagogic and hypnopompic imagery are similar in type and take the form of microdreams like a rapidly flickering lantern show rather than a continuous cine film. Klee's description of such imagery in his "Creative Credo" (1920) is sufficient to explain the appeal of such imagery to innumerable artists:

> Before falling asleep we recall a number of things, lines of the most varied kinds, spots, dabs, smooth planes, dotted planes, wavy lines, obstructed and articulated movement, counter movement, plaitings, weavings, bricklike elements, scalelike elements, simple and polyphonic motifs, lines that fade and lines that gain strength (dynamism), the joyful harmony of the first stretch, followed by inhibitions, nervousness.

Similar imagery in children often reflects their fantasy world of monsters such as King Kong and Frankenstein and can be so frightening that they fear falling asleep, fight against sleep or waken in the middle of the night with night terrors. Advice by psychologists on how to conquer these disturbing images can help the survivors from disasters, as these images and other hallucinations in the sleep-deprived and hypersomnic can persist after wakening with a dramatic effect, so much so that they may question their own sanity. Guilleminault (1975) even states that the continued interaction of the altered state of consciousness with the surrounding world can eventually lead to marked secondary psychological disorganization. Max Ernst is said to have cultivated visions of the half-sleeping, half-waking state and gives more than one example of a person (e.g. a transparent woman with a red robe and the skeleton showing through the filigree work) standing at the foot of his bed.

Such hypnagogic hallucinations can occur in normal people but are medically associated as part of the tetrad of narcolepsy (daytime sleepiness), cataplexy (when a sudden piece of humour causes weakness of the knees), and sleep paralysis (immobility of part of the body on waking). These experiences merge into the pathological. With mountain sickness the thin atmosphere, and lack of oxygen and carbon dioxide, lessens a person's respiratory drive at altitude accounting for frequent wakenings accompanied by various hallucinations which have entered into the mythology of mountains. That people choke in their sleep – a frequent subject of nightmares, and occasionally their cause – certainly happens with the condition of obstructive sleep apnoea. The fat boy in "Pickwick Papers" with hypersomnia and daytime somnolence could fall asleep with a fist full of aces and wake with a start and an expression of fear. The dreams and sudden wakenings of the alcoholic may resemble the night terrors of childhood. Agitated slaps and kicks may endanger their spouse. They may try to get out of bed, stand up, try to walk and fall to the floor, spending the rest of the night on the carpet, bruised and in a very abnormal posture.

**Pathological States**

There are other forms of twilight happenings. In pathological delirium and confusional states there is a dissolution of consciousness; and just as normal sleep contains dreams, so the state of confusion contains oneirism, twilight states and various forms of depersonalization. In psychotic states the subject may be distressed by imaginary happenings, fight snakes under the bed, turn pictures face to the wall to stop the portraits watching and ordering his actions, break mirrors, bolt doors against imaginary assailants. Oneirism is a prolonged psychotic experience persisting for days or months. Although oneirism is often drug induced, there may be a confluence of schizophrenic psychosis and a recognizable genetic tendency. Consciousness is deeply disorganized. The dream is all the more vivid because the subject participates (sometimes with considerable motor activity), living through multiple scenic hallucinations, intense emotions and disordered perceptions. He is held prisoner by his dream as if hypnotized and unable to free himself by waking. Just occasionally this can happen quite dramatically to an apparently normal person, but schizophrenics such as the artist Adolf Wolfli can remain in a hallucinatory delirium for months at a time.

The frequency of night terrors, somnambulism and nightmares in children is related to the greater ease with which consciousness can disintegrate during sleep. If the thoughts are disturbing, nightmares can occur tormenting the victim. The symbolism of Bosch strikes many as possessing a nightmarish quality and we know that Dürer was haunted by apparitions and dreams from the depths of a soul torn by religious experience. "How often" he wrote, "do I see great art in my sleep, but waking cannot recall it; as soon as I awake, my memory forgets it." Nonetheless his dream wherein a winged devil with a pair of bellows is blowing into the ear of a man seated before a stove, *The Apocalypse, Melancholia, Agony of the Garden,* and *The Flood* could only emanate as products of a disturbed, melancholic, sleep.

Creative imaginations give way to fantasy and these can be embellished by auto-erotic musings in the sleep-wake state. Such activity may account for Dali's masturbatory works and for pornographic art – which has rarely been lacking through the centuries. Auto-erotically induced scenes vary from Hieronymous Bosch's *The Garden of Earthly Delights,* to rape scenes, orgies, and Freudian imagery of snakes, flying through the air, entering caves, etc. A continuation of this, based not just on a deep knowledge of the works of Freud but of psycho-pathology as in the writings of Krafft-Ebing (*Psychopathia Sexualis*, 1899), led to the development of Dali's paranoic-critical art.

Reality is reality even to those with impaired sensation. Not all artists have had 50:50 vision and their view of life can be made yet more visionary by misinterpretations, illusions and delusions induced by impairment. Partially sighted people may be less prepared or able to follow conventions, e.g. that shadows are either brown or dark. Lloyd Mills (1936) examines peripheral vision in art and argues that without artists with poor central vision Impressionism would not have been born. (Max Nordau, a critic much quoted by the Nazis, infatuated by the belief that all writers and artists were degenerate, attributed the revolutionary technique of the Impressionists to the depravity of their "flickering eyeballs"). Lloyd Mills' attention was drawn to the problem in the 1920s when he examined ophthalmologically an artist who had a sprightly sense of colour and contour but who created curious distortions of detail, such as too long hands and enlarged knuckles. Corrective glasses were supplied. The new spectacles made him aware of the distortions of his painting and led him to complain that the unaccustomed clarity of detail and colour made him lose the effects of masses of colour and of the essential lines of contours and form which are more marked when the vision is blurred. He was quite unable to paint in his established style when wearing glasses. Similarly Cezanne had poor, myopic sight, made worse by diabetes. J.K. Huysmans proclaimed that Cezanne was "an artist with diseased retinae who, exasperated by faulty vision, has discovered the prodromes of a new art".

Short-sightedness has a prismatic effect on light and it is scarcely surprising that many artists such as Kandinsky who were myopic were also especially interested in colour theory. With flair, distortions and even imperfections of vision, can be turned to advantage. Besides Kandinsky, Bonnard, Braque, Derain, Grosz, Matisse, Mondrian and Vlaminck were all myopic. The myope focuses minutely. Where clarity is achieved by glasses, outlines remain indistinct and blurred. A halo of luminosity may surround the object upon which attention is concentrated. Colours therefore appear with greater intensity compared with form or substance. He is more likely to be alerted to certain properties of colours which rarely impinge on the awareness of his normal (emmentropic) or hypermetropic contemporaries; one such is the Purkinje effect whereby in reduced light, as at dusk, blues and greens tend to glow brighter than reds or yellows. Thus the American romantic painter, Albert Pinkham Ryder, suffered from myopia and was noted for his broody, nocturnal moonlight scenes and in his later period for seascapes, limited to the basic elements of boat, sky, moon, cloud and sea. His example foreshadowed the "luminism" of the Hudson River Group of American painters.

Clarity of memory depends upon inner vision, not upon sharpness of sight and

Kandinsky, like Dickens or Blake, possessed an eidietic memory with total recall of a street scene, etc.

Monet, the founder of Impressionism, rarely if ever used the normal central area of maximal visual clarity and it is likely that he had a moderate degree of myopia. He depicted: "the expression of light, of air, of movement and of unceasing changes", aspects of experience which are continually taking place in the realm of side vision. In later life he also had cataracts. Cataracts will exclude all but the red end of the spectrum and following cataract extraction a person's sight becomes bathed in a surplus of blue light. These changes are well seen in the work of Sir Matthew Smith (1879-1957). Until 1952 he showed a preoccupation with greens, yellows and browns – earthy and sunny, cool and warm – against his reds which suddenly began to appear on his palette. After cataract extraction his old colours including purples, puces and violets returned. Thereafter his work sounds a quieter, serener strain with white and even blacks more evident.

Sir Joshua Reynolds who lost sight in his left eye and then developed a cataract in his right eye, becoming blind in 1789, also exhibits another phenomenon.

> Whilst there was yet some remainder of sight, I no sooner lay down in my bed and turned on my side, but a copious light dazzled out of my shut eyes, and, as my sight diminished, everyday colours gradually more obscure flashed out with a vehemence.

Berrios and Brook (1982, 1984) described the Charles Bonnet syndrome of philosophers' visions occurring in the elderly with preserved intellect but vivid, elaborate and dynamic recurrent visual pseudo-hallucinations of a pleasant nature. Visual impairment is not necessarily an obvious factor but theoretically such visions could stimulate an otherwise elderly artist and call forth a new burst of activity. Bissiere (1888-1964), whose late paintings of large tapestry-like creations in warm, rich shades of gold, brown, purple and pale green, quite suddenly achieved considerable fame and commanded high prices.

Physical or mental illness may likewise affect one's appreciation of reality and artistic endeavour. Hunger and sleeplessness can heighten visual perceptions, thus Miró claimed that his painting *Le Carnaval d'Arlequin* originated from hallucinations he experienced when starving. The visions induced by fasting as an instrument for divination and purification have inspired primitive and early religious painters. Illness, fever, intoxication after abstinence from food and a serious drug habit together provide an unstable state of affairs which marked the existence of Modigliani, Scipione, Soutine and many other artists in their early years. The incitement for many of Piranesi's drawings of imaginary prisons is said to have arisen whilst suffering from bouts of malaria. Illness can "colour" a person's outlook on life. With depression the colours are invariably sombre as with van Gogh's black crows. With hysteria, bright primary colours predominate, used childishly with lack of control. Tuberculous patients have an affinity for reds: red skies, like blood vessels. Modigliani's use of red is as remarkable as the reds with which Titian crowned his masterpieces. A superabundance of the colour red is not an invariable accompaniment of an artist who happens to be suffering from tuberculosis; rather it is the sudden appearance of splashes of red suggesting a cataclysmic stage in the disease. This was the experience of a physician who described hallucinations when trying mescaline coincidentally with the development of a tuberculous pleural effusion:

> Red is now the most prominent colour; the rectangles, dark red, salmon pink, blue, golden, and so on. Larger white specks dart rapidly in from the periphery on to the carpet like bright silver coins pouring into the centre – or like white streaks of lightning. Everything is now moving; the carpet design is breaking up and gives place to a mass of bright spangles dancing rapidly all over the picture.

Epileptic artists such as van Gogh, Edward Lear and Alfred Kubin were respected for their visionary skills. Reitman (1950) describes the art of epileptics as showing great gusto for pedantic detail. Certainly there are many epileptics who will set about a given task at a frenzied pace often ending exhausted. Also epileptics may have especially large handwriting (macrographia), but there is no uniform type of epileptic art. The three epileptic artists quoted could not be more different from each other. There are indeed many types of epilepsy and many types of hallucinatory experiences related to epilepsy.

The curiosity and interest of the populace in artists who have experienced mental illness is two fold. Have the events shaped the artistic experience with a radical departure in style related to a breakdown or change of personality (Stilwandel)? And, secondly, is there inherent in that artist's output identifiable features which suggest a particular psychotic trait? An artist, especially, must be interesting, and interest so often stems from the paranormal, whether that experience be external or internal. We can indulge in generalizations. Unsually, unless there is some positive drive as from hallucinations, the art suffers. Attempts have been made to relate increasing madness with increasing artistic merit as in the examples of Louis Wain's cat drawings and Richard Dadd's art. In fact in neither case is this correlation substantiated by facts. There is a positive correlation between realistic art and extroversion, and, contrariwise, between abstract art and introversion.

Psychopaths are said to show a subconscious identification of self in the subject matter which is often performed with skilled draughtsmanship. Simon states that there are four fundamental styles in psychopathic art: archaic massive similar to the art form of Henry Moore's sculptures, archaic line after Matisse, traditional massive after Raphael and Leonardo, and traditional linear after Dürer. The neurotic or reactive depressive will use sombre colours with a poverty of ideas but symbolic language may be inherent in the painting as a means of expressing emotions. Spatial difficulties are often apparent early on in relation to dementia. However of most interest is the art of schizophrenics.

Whereas the output of most people in the course of psychiatric illness is reduced, a schizophrenic may find it easier to use pictorial expression than language. Early visual experiences tend to break through into the patient's conscious life and they often accept the opportunity to work out their problems through the medium of drawings, paintings and sculptures. There is an innate compulsion among certain schizophrenics to use the visual medium to express their thoughts; and this tendency also surfaces in others generally regarded as more balanced but who nonetheless possess schizoid traits. It is true to say that many artists are introverted, attracted by the abstract and possess schizoid traits: but it has also to be said that a gifted artist can use any material, likely or unlikely, and derived from whatever source he chooses, provided he can create an aesthetically convincing work of art as a whole.

Two Swedish painters, Carl Fredik Hill, who belongs to the Barbizon school, and Josephson, a leading Expressionist painter, produced literally thousands of paintings after becoming insane. Josephson's themes, previously landscape art and portraiture, changed to myths, fairy tales, poems and historical narratives. Gentle lyrical motifs expressing passivity alternated with motifs of volcanic ferocity. During the acute phase of his psychoses he believed that he was guided by great artists of the past, thus two drawings from the Karolinska Institute bear the signatures of Rafael Sanzio and Velasquez through Ernst Josephson.

The mentally deranged artist who attracted most attention from the surrealists, proving that even the least cultured can possess genius, once it had abandoned itself to the promptings of the unconscious mind, was a Swiss patient Adolf Wolfli (1864-1930) (Arguelles, 1975). He was a poorly educated farm labourer. His illness began insidiously, punctuated by a downward progression of sexual perversity, until it reached fever pitch. From 1895-1899 uncontrollable chaos reigned, marked by sexual fantasies, obsessions, hysterical outbursts, oneiristic states, catatonic depressions lasting for months and violent attacks upon the guards and other inmates. A profound metamorphosis occurred in 1900. Calm prevailed and gave way to an intensively creative state of affairs which lasted until his death. Without any formal training, he produced colourful, intricately designed symmetrical forms of high merit. In the same psychic frenzy he composed music, manufacturing crude trumpets for the purpose, and wrote a cosmically endless autobiography.

**Childhood Art**

Primitive art is best described as the high art of low cultures. Often succeeding because the conventions of Western cultures are not followed and a new dimension is introduced. It is a traditional culture rather than spontaneous, emotional, mystical or intuitive. The beauty of childhood art to the artist lies in its freedom and disinhibitions. It also reflects an immature approach to body image giving a stylization of square houses and rounded faces, so much so that the intellectual age of the child can be determined by the number of buttons, or of fingers, in the drawings. Give a two year-old a pencil and it will scribble; a set of crayons and it will crayon, often preferring the more garish colours. Given a brush it will paint. But the scribbling, the crayoning and the painting will be indecipherable. Such a child is not preoccupied with meaning, form or colour but with the materials it is using and their physical manipulation. Interest lies in the act of painting. The child would prefer to paint with the finger tips but, told to hold and use a brush, makes a less certain thrust upon the paper. A four year-old may make a crude box-like drawing, but when asked what he has painted he will produce an involved dramatic story with non-sequiturs so that one may hunt in vain to connect the account with what appears on the paper. He strives after communication and the parallel with the confabulatory drawings of adult schizophrenics who will add, for example, snakes to every orifice to explain certain forms of possession, will be seen in the manner whereby a drawn object makes free a stream of disconnected thoughts. At a later age stylization becomes an obsession. Arms stick out. Fingers resemble sausages. The child steps into the picture – Me – driving an aeroplane, a train or a boat. Fantasy may dictate the choice of subject – rockets, speed, machines. Children under stress may introduce features which underlie their preoccupations and a painting may provide evidence of family conflicts (see Chapter 22). By deft questioning one may come to understand what is reality to such a child.

## Summary

A cynic might say that what we have been discussing is an inward search for the soul of an artist rather than looking outwards at the boundaries of reality. Art, no less than every other aspect of human endeavour, is hedged by conventions. Kandinsky may be quoted in this context (1911): "Every epoch is given its own measure of artistic freedom and even the most creative genius may not leap over the boundary of that freedom." Likewise every generation has its obsessions and taboos. Guilt feeling may be concentrated on religion, sex, drugs or homosexuality. Each age has its "great dragon" which it seeks to slay.

Artists are important in that they have always been permitted a greater freedom from conventional restraints than others in society. If rulers, clerics, politicians, members of the professions or even musicians break society's conventions it is news. An artist can break conventions with impunity. It might even be said that if he fails to do so he is not interesting. An artist's way of life, as seen from the outside, is expected to tell us much about the character of his creativity. Arthur Koestler in "The Sleepwalker" said that every creative art involves a new innocence of perception, liberated from a cataract of accepted belief. An artist is allowed to be mad, or, at any rate, to be outrageous.

It was not only in Stalinist Russia that those who defied conventions were regarded as mad: it is true of every age as a means of coping with the unconventional. The modern world, including primitive peoples of today such as Eskimos and the forest dwellers of Laos regard hallucinatory experiences as aspects of insanity. However hallucinations were not an essential part of the medieval concept of insanity; and the experience of possession (passivity phenomenon) is not described as occurring concurrently with or as an integral of a visionary state. In Western Europe from A.D. 500-1500, people who heard voices or saw visions considered themselves, and were conceived by their contemporaries, to have had an actual perceptual experience of either divine or satanic inspiration. They were not presumed mad or dealt with as such. Hallucinations (fantasmata) were only likened to madness when combined with trickery (prestigiae) (Kroll and Bachrach, 1982). Non-psychotic religious fervour could be expressed by visions, social withdrawal (hermits, recluses, incluses), scourgings, starvation, and even self-mutilation or destruction. Several of the medieval visions show angels or saints chastising a person for sins of commission or of omission.

There is a possible explanation why hallucinations were excluded from the criteria of madness in the Middle Ages, namely the universality of hallucinatory encounters at that time. Fevers (such as malaria), starvation, poisonous berries, adulteration of drinks and foods as with wormwood, probably meant that few could travel far from their homes without such experience. It would appear from medieval manuscripts that certain excesses were respected and applauded in the Middle Ages. Future actions depended upon establishing a visionary, and often religious, *raison d'être* – just as today in certain strata of the United States of America it is necessary to have had a cataclysmic experience and to have been born again. Religious rectitude among the revivalists of the Victorian era could be established by evidence of a soul torn by religious experience. If a non-conformist minister at the end of the 19th century declared from the pulpit that he always felt he had an angel on his shoulder to guide him, he would have evoked no more than a few Amens from the High Seat. The artist, like the priest, is also permitted to have similar visions. Salvador Dali gained the respect of his audience when describing how he came to paint *The Christ of St John of the Cross*:

> I had a "cosmic dream" in which I saw in colour this image which in my dream represented the Nucleus of the Atom. This nucleus afterwards took on a metaphysical meaning. I consider it to be the very unity of the Universe – Christ. I saw Christ drawn by St John of the Cross. I worked out geometrically a triangle and a circle, which aesthetically summarized all my previous experiments and I drew my Christ in this triangle.

In summary, the boundaries, which society through convention does not allow itself to break, may be broken on its behalf by its artists.

## References

Arguelles, J.A. (1975). "The Transformative Vision". Shambhala, Berkeley.
Aurier, A. (1891). "Mercure de France", Paris.
Berrios, G.E. and Brook, P. (1982). The Charles Bonnet syndrome and the problem of visual perceptual disorders in the elderly. *Age and Ageing*, **11**, 17-23.
Berrios, G.E. and Brook, P. (1984). Visual hallucinations and sensory delusions in the elderly. *British Journal of Psychiatry*, **144**, 662-4.
Blake, W. (1969). "Complete Writings" Ed. G. Keynes. Oxford University Press.
Boiffard, J.A., Eluard, P. and Vitrac, R. (1924) "Le révolution surréalist"e. Tract.
Breton, A. (1934). "Qu'est ce que le Surréalisme?" Trans. D. Gascoigne. What is Surrealism? 1936.
de Chirico, G. (1919). On Metaphysical Art. *In* "Memories". (1971) Trans. M. Crossland. Owen, London.

Critchley, E.M.R. (1987). "Hallucinations and their Impact on Art". Carnegie Press, Preston.
Croce, B. (1909). "Aesthetic: Science of Expression and General Linguistics". London.
Freud, S. (1901). On dreams. *In* "(1953-1974). Complete Psychological Works of S. Freud". Hogarth Press, London.
Freud, S. (1922). "Introductory Lectures on Psychoanalyisis".
Gauguin, P. (1923). "The Intimate Journal of Paul Gauguin"
Glasgow Art Gallery and Museum (1985); Leaflet. "Salvador Dali: Christ of St John of the Cross".
Gombrich, E.H. (1972). "Symbolic Images". Phaidon, London.
Guilleminault, G.C., Billiard, M., Montplaisir, J. and Dement, W.C. (1975). Altered states of consciousness in disorders of daytime sleepiness. *Journal of Neurological Sciences*, **76**, 377-393.
Horowitz, M.J. (1964). The imagery of visual hallucinations. *Journal of Nervous and Mental Disease*, **138**, 513-523.
Huysmans, J.K. (1989). " A Rebords". Paris.
Jung, C.G. (1954). "The Interpretation of Dreams in Memories, Dreams and Reflections". (1963). Routledge and Kegan Paul, London.
Kadinsky, W. (19110. "Concerning the Spiritual in Art" . Trans. M. Sandleir. (1947). Wittenborn, New York
Klee, P. (1920). "Creative Credo". Reiss, Berlin.
Klein, R. (1917). *Zeitschrift für die gesamte Neurologie und Psychiatrie*, **36**, 323-340.
Koestler, A. (1959). "The Sleepwalkers: a History of Man's Changing View of the Universe". London.
Kokoschka, O. (1912). "On the Nature of Visions". Trans. H. Medlinger. Thwaites, London.
Krafft-Ebing, R. Von. (1899). "Psychopathia Sexualis". London.
Kroll, J. and Bachrach, V. (1982). Medieval visions and contemporary hallucinations. *Psychological Medicine*, **12**, 709-721.
Lucie-Smith, E. (1972). "Symbolic Art". Thames and Hudson, London.
Massie, S. (1978). "The Land of the Firebird". Hamish Hamilton, London.
Mills, L. (1936). Peripheral vision in arts. *Archives of Ophthalmology*, **16**, 208-209.
Penrose, R. (1958). "Picasso, his Life and Work". London.
Read, H. (1931). "The Meaning of Art". Faber and Faber, London.
Reitman, F. (1950). "Psychotic Art". Routledge and Kegan Paul, London.
Tolstoy, L.N. (1898). "What is Art". Trans. A. Maude. London.
Trevor-Roper, P. (1970). "The World through Blunted Sight". Thames and Hudson, London.
Vollard, A. (1924) "Paul Cezanne: his life and work".

# 13. The nature of music and musical hallucinations

J.D. Mitchell

---

### General Background

In common with other art-forms, music is difficult to define in precise terms. However, the closest that one can probably come to such a definition is that music is a definite and reproducible auditory stimulus which has the potential to induce a feeling of pleasure and satisfaction in those who hear it. One of the most remarkable aspects of music is that it has developed in virtually all known human societies. There is as much variation in musical form as there is in individual taste in differing cultures. A wide range of musical styles may exist even within comparatively well-defined social groups.

The idea that a sensory stimulus might evoke a feeling of pleasure is common in human experience. Aside from music, the parallel of visual art is obvious in this context. The concept that pleasurable sensory stimuli in defined modalities might be enhanced by concomitant experiences in others is also important. This phenomenon, known as synaesthesia, is a major component of culinary art where olfactory and gustatory modalities are so crucially interdependent. There is often an additional visual dimension. A dish of food can be made to look very much more attractive if it is neatly and artistically presented.

### Expression in Music

Music probably has a unique capacity to evoke feelings associated with a wide range of human experience. Some musical works are overtly descriptive of particular events, objects or stories. This is often implicit in the title. Other musical *oeuvres* employ various forms of "tone-painting" to draw the listener's attention to passages of particular descriptive significance. One way in which this can be achieved is by frank mimicry. The obvious example of this from the natural world is birdsong. The characteristic call of the cuckoo appears in the work of Delius and birdsong was also a central component of the inspiration of Olivier Messian.

Approximate imitation, such as the use of music to evoke natural sounds of indefinite pitch such as running water and thunderstorms, is also very common.

Such imitation permeates the whole of the Symphony No 6 in F (*Pastoral*) by Beethoven. There is also a recurring evocation of the sound of a babbling brook in the Song Cycle *Die Schöne Müllerin* by Schubert, and a representation of the incessant activity of the spinning wheel in the Spinnerlied from *Der Fliegende Holländer* by Wagner.

The third general category of tone-painting can be considered in terms of suggestion or symbolization. This is an attempt to produce a representation of a physical object, not itself associated with a specific sound, in purely auditory terms. Such "sound pictures" can be found in music from differing periods. The impressionist music of Debussy is especially relevant in this context. His set of Préludes for the piano contains short pieces with such evocative titles as *Des pas sur la neige*, *La fille aux cheveux de lin* and *La cathédrale engloutie*.

The distinction between these methods of producing sound pictures is necessarily artificial. All these devices sometimes occur within a single work. *Le Quattro Stagioni* by Antonio Vivaldi is one of the most popular *oeuvres* in the classical repertory. Not only is this work full of such imagery, but the musical manuscript is also annotated with descriptive sonnets relating to individual and specific passages in the music. *La Primavera* abounds in birdsong and also contains an attempt to reproduce the sound of thunder. *L'Inverno* emphasizes the sound of chattering teeth in the intense cold as well as the image of raindrops falling. Winds of various types also appear in *l'Inverno* with a vivid portrayal of ice skating leading up to the inevitable fall!

Most of these examples have depended mainly on pitch to achieve their effect although rhythm has also made a significant contribution in cases such as the chattering teeth and babbling brook. Rhythm can be of more central importance in the construction of tone pictures. The sounds of railway travel have traditionally been intrinsically rhythmic and may also have been a material factor in the rhythmic inspiration of some composers. The Czech composer, Dvorak, was well known as a railway enthusiast and, among his many works, the "Iron Horse" may have been a subconscious factor in his conception of the rhythmic figure which accompanies the melodic line of the trio section of the 3rd movement of his Symphony No 8 in G.

Even the most abstract musical work can conjure up an imagery of common experience. *Bolero*, a work by the French composer, Ravel was inspired by a Spanish Dance rhythm. It is characterized by a slowly progressive intensification of volume, energy and tension inexorably building up towards an inevitable final climax. Although this piece of music was entirely abstract in its inspiration, it has come to be strongly evocative of the human sexual act for many individuals, with the climax implicity signifying orgasm. In other musical works, eroticism may be more intentional. The energetic sexual exploits of the medieval galliards are graphically emphasized by the thrusting rhythms in *Carmina Burana* by Orff.

## The Elements of Music

Although Hindemith took the view that the impact of music was dependent on tensions which could be set up in terms of the three facets of pitch, rhythm and volume, the appeal of the music to the human psyche can essentially by considered to depend on the four main elements of pitch, rhythm, harmony and timbre.

In scientific terms, the first of these elements, pitch, is the frequency of the musical note. Certain specific sequences of notes are known as scales and form the basis of musical theory. Of the many types of scale the diatonic major is the best known. Many will remember this from school music lessons as the "tonic sol fa". This consists of a defined series of eight notes. The top and bottom notes are separated by one octave. The intervals between the notes of the diatonic major scale are not evenly spaced and comprise five whole tones and two half tones (semitones). While the diatonic major scale, along with its minor variant forms the essential basis of Western Classical Music, other scales exist.

The second element is rhythm, which is based on time. Rhythm and pitch are the two components of melody. The speed (or tempo) of the music is determined by the temporal frequency of the underlying rhythmic pulse or beat. Certain beats are accented, others are unaccented. The proportion of accented to unaccented beats is important in determining the mood and character of a piece of music. If every third beat is accented, the music often has the quality of a carefree dance with a general air of "easy grace". The waltz is a well known example of this. If every fourth beat is accented the character of the music is more march-like. Music written in quadruple rhythm often has a rock-like sense of inner strength. Modern composers have employed more novel rhythms to achieve other effects. One of the best known examples of this is "Mars" from the Suite *The Planets* by Holst. In this piece the accent falls on every fifth note producing a sensation of fierce and relentless energy. Quintuple rhythm is not necessarily associated with aggression. This rhythmic device was also employed by Tchaikovsky in a movement from his Symphony No 6 in B minor (*Pathetique*).

The third major element of music is harmony. This is the effect and sound which results from playing more than one note simultaneously. Such combinations of single notes are known as chords. An almost infinite number of possible combinations exists: some chords are pleasing in their sound (concordant), others unpleasant and astringent (discordant). Concords and discords are both widely used in musical expression. Harmonic effect is crucially dependent on the intervals between the constituent notes and harmonic style may enable the trained listener to recognize the era in which a work was composed and may even identify the composer.

The final element is timbre. This is the character of the musical sound and is predominantly related to the particular instrument on which the music is being played. The sound of the drum is clearly very different from that of the clarinet. Some instruments are even able to produce quite different timbres according to the style of playing. The violinist for example is able to produce a quite different sound according to whether he plays by plucking the string or drawing the bow across it. Certain timbres have some to be associated with certain moods and imagery. The sound of the organ often evokes images of religious devotion, the gong and cymbals are associated with things oriental and the xylophone with bones (as in "Fossils" from *Carnival des Animaux* by Saint-Saëns). In the 18th century world of Haydn and Mozart, the use of drums, cymbals and trumpets was particularly associated with "Turkish" or "Military" music (as in Haydn, Symphony No 100 in G).

## Hallucinations and Musical Inspiration

Much of the process of musical composition is inspirational. This covers a continuum extending from a deliberate and conscious attempt to reproduce a specific sound from some aspect of human experience to auditory hallucinations. Although it is unusual for a discrete hallucinatory experience to form the entire basis of the inspirational process, this probably has occurred rarely and as such is of obvious relevance to this essay.

Auditory hallucinations may consist of such varied sounds as the ringing of bells, a band playing, fragments of well-known songs or tunes or may take on the gigantic proportions of a symphonic or operatic work. Such synaesthetic relationships may be due to the emotional connotations of the percept or be part of multi-modality hallucinations involving auditory, olfactory or visual phenomena of varying degrees of complexity.

Perhaps the most accurate way of depicting such a wide range of auditory hallucinatory experiences is as a Venn diagram involving four overlapping circles: sounds, vocalizations, music and mixed hallucinations rather than as a spectrum of increasing complexity. Musical hallucinations have been encountered in clinical practice where they have mainly been associated with end-organ dysfunction, epilepsy, vascular, space-occupying and degenerative organic disorders, alcohol withdrawal states and psychoses.

An example of an auditory hallucination, probably associated with chronic end-organ dysfunction, as a material component of the inspirational process can be found in the work of the Czech, Smetana, who is widely believed to have suffered from neurosyphilis. Towards the end of his life he developed "partial paralysis" suggesting that he had the meningovascular type of the disease. During this period he experienced a persistent, high pitched, note in his ears which he identified as a particular musical note. This is immortalized in his late String Quartet *From my Life* for which he wrote an autobiographical programme (Greene, 1986). Specific themes in the work are associated with specific periods of his life. At the beginning of the finale he reminisces his younger days by recalling music which has been heard in previous movements. At this point, the 1st violin bursts in with a high, piercing E in the background of an A flat major chord which immediately and graphically illustrates the impact which this particular hallucination had on the composer. Its musical context also suggests that he retained some insight into the fact that the illness which eventually killed him had its roots in sexual indiscretions as a younger man.

Auditory illusions and hallucinations can also occur in relation to alcohol abuse. They can be encountered in a setting of alcoholic withdrawal or relative abstinence following chronic drinking (Mayer-Gross *et al.*, 1974). Patients may become aware of brief but intense rhythmic sounds – crankings, knockings, as subjective auditory disturbances in an otherwise clear sensorium. With time, the sounds may develop as vocalizations that become accusatory and an hallucinatory paranoid state may develop that bears close resemblance to some schizophrenic states. The importance of such hallucinations in the history of musical composition is impossible to gauge, but bearing in mind the propensity for composers to become dependent on alcohol they could well have been a major factor.

Little is known about the influence of drugs other than alcohol in the context of musical hallucinations and composition. The possible role of opium in the inspiration of one of the most familiar works of the symphonic repertoire, *Symphonie fantastique,* Op. 14, by the French composer Berlioz should however be considered. This work bears the subtitle "épisode de la vie d'un artiste", a phrase which betrays its autobiographical nature. The composer was well acquainted with de Musset's very free translation of de Quincey's "Confessions of an English Opium Eater". Berlioz describes experiencing hallucinations similar to those induced by opium in a letter to his father in 1830, a time at which he was involved in the composition of this work. It is possible that de Quincey's vision of a haunting figure of a girl whose reappearances bring an uneasy sense of doom may underlie the *idée fixe,* a rather discursive theme which is heard in different guises in each of the five movements of the work. Berlioz considered this as representing "a young musician of morbid disposition and powerful imagination who is plunged into a deep sleep accompanied by strange dreams in which sensations, feelings and memories are transformed in his sick brain into musical images and ideas" (Crabbe, 1980). The beloved is killed by her lover while under the influence of opium and is subsequently condemned to death and marched to the guillotine. The finale projects the dream into a nightmare of hellish spectres, an orgiastic dance of death and finally a parody of the ancient plainsong chant *Dies Irae* in which the beloved again appears horribly distorted and bedevilled beyond recognition (Macdonald, 1982).

The most quoted example of musical hallucinations in the course of a psychotic illness is that of the composer, Schumann. The subjective auditory phenomena which he experienced intermittently in his early years became progressively more persistent in his later life, particularly in the final years up to his tragic death. During one period his life was made a misery by a constant sound in his head which he recognized as the note A. He is said to have heard a particular trombone chord when his brother died. At times the sounds were sweet and fabulous but at others the inner voices and music "did not still the conflict of emotions but excited it" (Ostwald,

1985). There is talk of being "severely carried away" (*mitgenommen*) by these experiences and "strange afflictions of hearing" (*merkwürdige Gehöraffektionen*) are also described. In one instance the hallucinations were held at bay by the process of composition (Violoncello Concerto in A minor, Op. 129). In other cases they were a material factor in the genesis of new themes. One week in February 1854 his mind had no peace. From a solitary note grew strange music "more wonderful and played by more exquisite instruments than ever sounded on earth". During one night he leapt from his bed to commit this music to paper in a piano arrangement. This material is thought to be the basis for the main theme of the slow movement of Violin Concerto in D minor (Op. Posth.). The inspiration of many of his other works has also been thought to have been related to auditory hallucinations. *Kreisleriana,* Op. 16, has been described as a musical portrait of violence and madness. The *Spring Symphony* (Op. 38) and *Manfred* Overture (Op. 115) have also been mentioned in this context. On occasion the hallucinations consisted of sounds identifiable as the work of others. The "hearing" of *Eine Feste Burg,* a chorale from a cantata by J.S. Bach, was a particular example of this phenomenon.

There has been considerable debate as to the nature of Schumann's neuropsychiatric illness. Syphilis and schizophrenia have both had their proponents. The most credible diagnosis however seems to be manic depressive psychosis (Ostwald, 1985; Trethowan, 1977). The mood swings characteristic of this condition are immortalized in his music by his "two best friends", Florestan and Eusebius. The more audacious and self confident (hypomanic) side of his personality is found in Florestan: the shy and passive (depressive) aspect in Eusebius. These "friends" gave him ideas for various literary (*Neue Zeitschrift für Musik*) and musical projects and are an integral part of *Carnaval,* Op. 9, a work described by Schumann as being "a musical picture gallery of my many different mental states" (Ostwald, 1985). The extent to which alcohol was a factor in his hallucinosis is difficult to assess. This is not considered to have significantly influenced the content of the work of other composers such as the Finn, Sibelius, or the Russian, Moussorgsky, who are both thought to have consumed excessive quantities of alcohol. It seems clear that hallucinatory experiences were of critical importance in the artistic inspiration of Schumann.

In some ways, dreams might be considered as possessing features of both hallucinatory experience and rational, waking thought. Many composers claim to have heard music which came to them in dreams (Walker, 1979). Although most dreams are fragmentary, creative thought in a twilight or dream state is well recognized and does not necessarily imply anything pathological. During the composition of *l'Histoire du Soldat,* Stravinsky had such an experience in which he not only heard the music but saw the person performing it. A young gypsy was sitting by the edge of a road. She was playing the violin to amuse the small child sitting on her lap. The child showed appreciation by applause and Stravinsky was able to recall the music next morning, and included it in the *Petit Concert* (Craft, 1958). The Italian composer, Tartini, had a dream in Assisi (Tartini, 1765-6) in which he made a pact with the Devil for his soul and handed him his violin. The Devil took up the instrument which he played like sin (Greene 1986)! He played a sonata of such exquisite beauty as surpassed the boldest flight of Tartini's imagination. When Tartini awoke he seized his violin and tried in vain to reproduce the sound he had heard. He was nonetheless able to produce a sonata from this material. Although he considered this one of the best of his works, he thought it was still much inferior to what he had experienced in his dream! This sonata is known, for obvious reasons, as "The Devil's Trill" (Walker, 1979).

**The Psychology of Musical Expression: how does music convey its message to the listener?**

Music has the capacity to evoke an extremely wide spectrum of human sentiments.

One such sentiment is that of anguish. This has been expressed as a minor 6th falling to the 5th. Although the use of this figuration dates back to Josquin, it is also to be found in the setting of the *Crucifixus* in the B minor Mass of J.S. Bach and in the words "Mein Vater, mein Vater" in the song *Erlkönig* by Schubert. This figuration is also important in the powerful conclusion of *La Traviata* by Verdi.

Joy of a simple, innocent, blessed kind has been conveyed by a melodic sequence starting on the tonic followed by the 3rd, 5th, 6th, 5th degrees of the major scale.

This sequence appears in the *Pastoral Symphony* from the oratorio *Messiah* by Handel as well as the finale of *La Primavera* from *Le Quattro Stagioni* by Vivaldi. This has also been used in 20th century music in such passages as the settings for the words "So shalt thou enter in" and "Holy, Holy, Holy" from the morality *Pilgrim's Progress* by Vaughan Williams.

Major tonality is often thought generally to convey a mood of brightness as opposed to the minor which is considered to imply a mood of tragedy. There are however some striking inconsistencies in the context. The "Dead March" from the oratorio *Saul* by Handel is widely perceived as one of the most solemn pieces of music ever written. It is however cast in a major key. Despite this, the work conveys an intensely mournful impression which may well be related to the frequent use of minor 7th chords. The conclusion of Mahler's *Das Lied von der Erde* is also written in a major tonality. By contrast the "Fairy Music" from Mendelssohn's Overture to *Midsummer Night's Dream,* and the well-known *Badinerie* from J.S. Bach's Suite No 2, both very lively and extrovert works, are written in the minor. The key of C minor seems to be particularly associated with tragic music. Both the funeral march from the Symphony No 3 in E flat "Eroica" by Beethoven, initially conceived to mark the death of Napoleon, and the Masonic Funeral Music of Mozart are based around this tonality.

The musical expression of grief attains an added dimension of gravity in works such as the "Marcia Funébre Sulla Morte d'un Eroe" from the Piano Sonata in A flat, Op. 26 by Beethoven and the well-known funeral march which forms the slow movement of the Chopin B Flat minor piano sonata. The impact of both these works, as well as the slow movements of both the String Quartet in D minor "Death and the Maiden" by Schubert and the Beethoven 7th Symphony depend on the juxtaposition of a main section in the minor key with repetitive rhythmic figures and only a tentative movement of the melodic line away from the tonic against a more expansive trio section in the major.

There is an implicit sense of pleasure and security associated with the major triad. This comprises the tonic as well as the 3rd and 5th degrees of the diatonic major scale. In medieval times the major scale was merely one of so-called modes (Ionian) and became particularly associated with secular music, with only the more "severe" modes being used for liturgical purposes. Joy and pleasure is implicit in the sound of the major third, the crucial component of the major triad. The melodic setting of Schiller's "Ode to Joy" in the finale of the Symphony No 9 in D minor by Beethoven is critically dependent on the major third as is the Brindisi (drinking song) from *La Traviata* by Verdi and the popular song "Polly Wolly Doodle".

By contrast the sound of the minor third evokes a sense of sedate, stern and sober satisfaction, sometimes with an associated feeling of woe and melancholy. This interval forms the basis of the opening of Symphony No 5 in C minor by Beethoven, one of the most familiar, and yet most terse, musical ideas in the entire symphonic literature. It is also important in the thematic material of the Symphony No 5 in E minor by Tchaikovsky.

The impact of some works depends upon a conflict between the major and minor 3rd. This is exploited at the opening of the Symphony No 4 in F minor by Tchaikovsky – when A flat (minor of F minor) enharmonically becomes G sharp of the emotionally bright key of E major before becoming A flat once again and reverting to the gloom of minor.

A similar situation exist for major and minor 6th and their conflicts. The Hallelujah Chorus from Handel's *Messiah* is a familiar item in the choral repertory. The impact of this piece as an expression of confident joy is strongly dependent on the major 6th. The tension between the major and minor 6th is exploited by Beethoven in his opera *Fidelio*. This is illustrated by a duet in which Leonora sings of bitter tears (minor 6th) and Marcellina of sweet tears (major 6th).

The augmented 4th (identical to the diminished 5th) is not part of the major or minor triad, but has unique properties in terms of the sentiments which it can express. It has a devilish quality and has been referred to as the "Diabolus in Musica". Saint-Saëns achieved a considerable impact by making use of this device in his *Danse Macabre* as did Berlioz in the opening of the "Witches Sabbath" in the *Symphonie Fantastique*. Vaughan Williams used this figure to great effect in *Pilgrims Progress* not only to express the plaintive cry of *Christian in the City of Destruction* ("What shall I do to be saved?") but also to evoke the icy wastes of the Antarctic in *Sinfonia Antartica*. Holst, in contrast, used it to convey the image of war in his Suite *The Planets* (Mars).

If intervals between only two notes can give the impression of reflecting mood, series of more than two notes are much more complex in terms of emotional impact. The first three notes of the major triad (1, 3, 5,), with or without passing notes, is a particular example of a three note sequence which conveys a feeling of confident brightness. This is encountered in such works as "The Trumpet Shall Sound" (Handel, Messiah) and the Waltz *An Der Blauen Donau* by Johann Strauss. The notes of the major triad can also evoke pleasure in other combinations as in the *idée fixe* of the *Symphonie fantastique* by Berlioz (5, 1, 3). This musical theme permeates the whole work and is associated with the "beloved". The use of the notes of the primary triad of C major in this idea seems to convey an atmosphere in which the pleasurable feelings associated with the contemplation of romantic love are reinforced.

The sequential use of the notes of the minor triad (1,3,5) tends to convey a feeling of desperation as in the setting of the words "zu Hïlfe, zu Hïlfe, sonst bin ich verloren" with which a terrified Tamino cries for help in *Die Zauberflöte* by Mozart. When these notes are used in a different order however (5, 1, 3) the impression of utter tragedy can ensue as in the *St Matthew Passion* of Schutz ("My God, why hast thou forsaken me?"). This figure also appears in a slightly modified form at the opening of the finale of the Brahms D minor Piano Concerto (5, 1, 2, 3, 5, 1). While it is well know that the first movement of this work was conceived as an expression of the composer's grief for the psychotic illness of Schumann, the use of this sequence in this otherwise rumbustious movement does suggest that this grief permeates this concerto in a more general way than might at first be realized.

The sentiment of bitterness can sometimes be perceived in music containing a descending melodic sequence consisting of 5, (4), 3, (2), 1 in the minor key. This appears at the finale of the Symphony No 6 in B minor by Tchaikovsky as well as in the Arioso Dolent of the Piano Sonata in A flat, Op. 110 by Beethoven. Doleful desolation can also be portrayed by melodic figures which do not stray far from the tonic (1) particularly when they are cast in a minor tonality. This is exemplified by the Funeral March of Chopin's B flat minor Piano Sonata and the music evoking the "Doleful Creatures" in *Pilgrims Progress* (Vaughan Williams).

These examples attempt to illustrate how various melodic and harmonic devices can be associated with specific human sentiments and emotions. Many others could have been given and the figurations described here are by no means comprehensive; many more have been recognized. It is left to the reader, interest in this fascinating area whetted, to pursue these other aspects in more specialized texts.

**Musical Hallucinations in Clinical Neurology**

Coleman (1894) described hallucinations in the sane associated with local organic disease of the sense organs. He quoted a patient who, after some years of increasing tinnitus, heard not only noises but words, names of streets and songs. This patient subsequently developed hallucinations of smell and vision but throughout this period remained perfectly sane. The most common association in the literature is the development of musical hallucinations in a patient who has suffered from hearing loss and tinnitus for several years (Rozanski and Rosen, 1952; Ross *et al.*,

1975; Miller and Crosby, 1979; Hammeke *et al.*, 1983 and two personal cases). This may follow a prolonged antecedent history. Musical hallucinations can develop along with tinnitus after a head injury (Clovis, 1976), with retraction of the tympanic membranes in association with infection or persist until a plug of wax is removed from the external auditory meatus (Rhein, 1913).

A much rarer synaesthetic connection with ocular disturbances has also been described. Rhein (1913) reported the occurrence of musical phosphenes as a result of pressure on the eyeball and Ross *et al.* (1975) reported a deaf patient without tinnitus in whom the instillation of drops into the eye intensified musical hallucinations. These phenomena were unchanged following the surgical removal of a cataract. A most remarkable association between visual impairment and musical hallucinations was reported by Patel *et al.* (1981).

A lady of 86 with impaired vision developed vivid visual hallucinations with a clear sensorium. She would be pleasantly surprised by the presence of the visions which mainly occurred in the evening or dark or dim conditions. She would see children at play but when she tried to speak they never replied and if she tried to approach they disappeared. These visions were rightly regarded as being characteristic of the Charles Bonnet syndrome (Berrios and Brown, 1982). Soon she also started to see a circus with a tent, lights and acts which she could vividly describe and brought back memories of her childhood. Later, she began to hear the music which accompanied the acts and spent her evening enjoying the "circus". Although she remained a well adjusted person she was concerned with the "ring master", who she thought was the devil, following her around and because of this avoided bathing or using the toilet when she saw him watching her.

In a survey of 666 patients with temporal lobe epilepsy (TLE), 16% experienced auditory hallucinations as a part (or whole) of the ictus and crude auditory experiences were five times as common as more elaborate ones (Currie *et al.*, 1971). One of the contributors to this work later said that many of the more elaborate hallucinations possessed a musical quality (Henson, 1977). Such ictal sensations were often associated with emotional components or déjà vu phenomena (Currie *et al.*, 1971). Temporal lobe disorders may bring together several sensory modalities and the sounds themselves may have complex non-musical on non-linguistic linkages. Repetitive characteristics, movement to or away from the individual or a robot-like attraction may be encountered (Critchley and Rossall, 1981). The auditory hallucinations of TLE may be simulated by electrical stimulation of the right (more than left) temporal convolution at operation (Penfield and Rasmussen, 1953). Stimulation of the primary auditory areas could produce temporary deafness, buzzing or whistling sounds, and recollections of music were obtained in 17 of 40 experiential responses from the superior or lateral surface of the first temporal convolution (Penfield and Perot, 1963). Penfield in his Maudsley Lecture of 1955 quoted verbatim his patients' comments as they were recorded at the time of operation. Electrical stimulation appeared to evoke flashbacks or "strips of experience". Sometimes the event was recalled but more often it had faded from recollective memory but remained familiar and was acknowledged as a reminiscence of something past. One patient heard people coming in and the music – a funny little piece which had been the theme song of a children's programme. Others felt themselves present in a theatre, church or cafe and re-experienced the sense of the enjoyment of the original occasion. To another patient the experience was so vivid that she thought a gramophone had been turned on and that she was able to hum along with the orchestra. This is almost parallel to the patient described by Coleman in 1894.

> A man of 38 had right sided fits and heard bells ringing in his right ear. He complained of the presence of a musical box in the ward which was allowed to play in the night. He beat the rhythm of the music using his hand with a smile on his face.

Tumours, particularly meningiomas, of the temporal lobe (Tarachow, 1941), parietal lobe (Scott, 1979), and brainstem (Cascino and Adams, 1979) have been associated with musical hallucinations. They have also been reported following the removal of tumours.

> A right frontal meningioma (Keshaven *et al.*, 1988) was removed from a 43-year-old man. Postoperatively he made a slow recovery and was found to have infarcted part of the frontal lobe. He also had inappropriate ADH secretion. He became depressed and suspicious experiencing verbal auditory hallucinations of derogatory content as well as visual hallucinations. Six months later he was readmitted following drinking a bottle of Campho-Phenique to "anaesthetize" himself from the very distressing music that he had begun to hear. This consisted of hearing an orchestra in his head intermittently playing a monotonous march which was intolerable and caused sleep disturbance.

It is difficult to determine whether degenerative processes play a part in musical hallucinations associated with deafness but a vascular aetiology is suggested when the hallucinations start abruptly without obvious antecedent cause and then slowly regress spontaneously. Two illustrative cases are presented:

1   A 56-year-old woman woke in the early hours of the morning to the sounds of revelry, apparently from an adjoining house. The noise consisted predominantly of Country and Western music, with a hubbub of conversation in the background, and prevented her getting back to sleep. Over an hour, the music changed to traditional Scottish pipe music and then to hymn singing. She knew that her neighbours were not in the least religious and could not understand this development. She woke her husband and daughter who heard no noise. Only at that stage did she realize she was hallucinating. During this time her consciousness was clear and her judgement and affect unimpaired. There was no vertigo, deafness of other vestibular symptoms, no headache or other symptoms referable to the nervous system. She had no psychiatric symptoms and her daughter confirmed that there had been no change in her behaviour or personality apart from some anxiety engendered by her illness.

  Over a period of one week the hallucinations faded away, the music becoming less distinct, and she was left with tinnitus in the left ear. This consisted of a single musical note, which she characterized as a hum, and which persisted at the time of the neurological consultation. There were no physical signs in the nervous system or elsewhere. Rinne and Weber tests, pure tone audiometry and computerized tomography were all normal.

2   A lady sustained a subarachnoid haemorrhage at the age of 57 with a left temporal lobe haematoma, right hemiplegia and aphasia (Critchley *et al.*, 1989). She remained grossly aphasic but after 5 years showed considerable improvement with only occasional word finding difficulties. At the age of 63 she suffered a mild stroke with a right hemiparesis. CT scan showed a new area of infarction commensurate with the clinical picture. She began to complain of numbness in the left arm and leg at that time accompanied by auditory hallucinations which were described as "nattering inside her". The natterings consisted of a mixture of prayers, hymns and fragments of the Latin Mass she had learnt by heart as a girl when she used to sing in a church choir. At other times they would consist of words or sentences related to her current thoughts or to things she had just heard or read. These could sometimes be assimilated into the tunes and rhythms that were heard in her head at the time. The vocalizations and tunes would commence at a particular time of day (varying from week to week) and persist throughout the day except when talking, listening to others or reading aloud. Although annoying and highly embarrassing, there was no psychiatric illness, dementia, hearing loss or tinnitus. The noises stopped after five months for a period of four weeks but then returned.

Auditory illusions and hallucinations can occur in a setting of alcoholic withdrawal or relative abstinence following chronic drinking (Mayer-Gross *et al.*, 1974). When suffering from alcoholic hallucinosis, D.G. Rossetti was disturbed by the "chiming of cobwebs". With time such sounds may develop as vocalizations that become accusatory and an hallucinatory paranoid state may develop that closely resembles some schizophrenic states. An example of such a patient is:

Three days into a voyage in the North Sea, a 33-year-old fisherman noticed an irritating background noise which he could not characterize and did not immediately identify as an hallucination. This became more and more obtrusive, developing first into a buzz of conversation, then into a succession of pop tunes with chat from a disc jockey between them. He was able to recall some of the tunes, recognizing as being currently in the "charts", and identified the disc jockey as Tony Blackburn, a radio personality he particularly detested. Following this he developed the persistent and fixed idea that his wife was being unfaithful to him and became violent, demanding to be put ashore.

On admission to the local psychiatric hospital, the patient was alert, oriented and physically well. It transpired that he was a moderately heavy drinker and had been on a binge since his last trip, having necessarily abstained from alcohol after leaving port. He did not go on to develop frank delirium tremens and his auditory hallucinations and paranoia regarding his wife's fidelity resolved completely over several days.

Musical phenomena in this condition were regarded as rare (Victor and Hope, 1958) but Scott (1975) in a similar series of 70 patients, who gave a history of hallucinations during withdrawal from alcohol, reported that 44 described musical experiences in addition to other forms of auditory and visual hallucinations. These disturbances characteristically occurred early in the withdrawal phase, usually preceded other hallucinations, were more pleasant than frightening and tended to be chant-like and repetitive (Scott, 1975).

The common denominator for formed hallucinations in normal people seems to be a slowly progressive end organ failure. As in the Charles Bonnet syndrome of visual hallucinations, senility is usually a factor. Deafness is frequently followed by tinnitus which is only likely to be associated with a defined note in a trained musician. Musical hallucinations take longer to develop and may require more proximal degenerative changes in the brain. West (1975) has advocated a paradigm, based largely on the Hughlings Jackson concept of disinhibition, whereby sensory input suppresses myriads of quanta of nonessential information, including previously acquired memories (Miller and Crosby, 1978). The loss of this input permits "perceptual traces" to be released and re-experienced, either familiar or new – even bizarre combinations! Jingles from childhood and catchy tunes which stick in one's mind are particularly liable to be recalled. Most musical hallucinations are familiar and mundane except in those with highly trained and creative musical abilities. A parallel situation is described by Sacks and Kohl (1976).

> A 63-year-old woman had postencephalitic parkinsonism dating back to the age of 18. Levodopa therapy resulted in a dramatic release from the parkinsonism. She requested a tape recorder and over the next few days recalled the night clubs and music halls of her youth. When the increased excitement (erethism) necessitated a reduction of the dose of L-dopa she instantly "forgot" all these early memories.

When musical hallucinations arise suddenly in relation to epilepsy, electrical stimulation, head injury, vascular lesions or any other cause, the hallucinations first appear in external space and only when insight is gained do they retreat into internal space (i.e. head or ears).

> A woman of 78 who had been deaf for years without tinnitus developed musical hallucinations when she moved into a flat near where the Gas Board were using a pneumatic drill. She started to get headaches and a severe pain over the right eye. The hallucinations consisted of three tunes: "Happy Birthday", "Holding the Shoe" and something else. They were very troublesome to her. If she were mildly depressed the hallucinations would be particularly annoying, monotonous and repetitive. Such hallucinations seemed to be the most resistant to treatment with anticonvulsants, sedatives or antidepressants. She often played her radio loudly in an attempt to banish them but this was rarely helpful.

Other patients have been more fortunate and found ways of altering the experiences from those which have been annoying to more pleasurable sounds. Concentration on particular thoughts, talking or conversing, and ambient noises can produce such changes. Their enjoyment has been heightened in some cases by synchronizing with the music either by tapping, humming or singing along. The nature of the hallucination (i.e. rhythmic character, instrumental or vocal) does not seem to be a factor in determining the efficacy of such measures.

Musical hallucinations, whether arising as release phenomena or focal irritation, are basically similar. Focally triggered hallucinations are more liable to appear in external space in the first instance until the patient gains insight into their nature. In other circumstances they appear to be coming from the ears or the head (M.L. recognized them as her own vocalizations). Even with alcohol withdrawal hallucinosis, the music often appears pleasurable at first; irritation can be reduced by trick measures such as tapping or humming to the music but few patients have been able to suppress their hallucinations totally even for a brief period. Later the music can become insistent and all pervading until a psychotic or even a suicidal state is reached.

## References and Further Reading

Berrios, G.E. and Brook, P. (1982). The Charles Bonnet syndrome and the problem of visual perceptive disorders in the elderly. *Age and Ageing*, **11**, 17-23.

Cascino, G.D. and Adams, R.D. (1986). Brainstem auditory hallucinations. *Neurology*, **36**, 1042-7.

Clovis, W.L. (1976). They hear music. *American Journal of Psychiatry*, **133**, 1096.

Coleman, W.S. (1894). Hallucinations in the sane associated with local organic disease of the sensory organs. *British Medical Journal*, **1**, 1015-7.

Cooke, D. (1959). "The Language of Music". Oxford University Press, Oxford.

Crabbe, J. (1980). "Hector Berlioz. Rational Romantic". London

Critchley, E.M.R. and Rossall, C.J. (1981). Hallucinations. *In* "Practical Psychiatry". (Ed. S. Crown). pp. 21-5. Northwood Books, London.

Critchley, E.M.R., Young, A. and Ellis, A. (1989). Unusual vocal hallucinations following subarachnoid haemorrhage. *Journal of Neurology, Neurosurgery and Psychiatry*, **52**, 415.

Currie, S., Heathfield, K.W.G., Henson, R.A. *et al.* (1971). Clinical course and prognosis of temporal lobe epilepsy – a survey of 666 patients. *Brain*, **94**, 173-90.

Duncan, R. and Mitchell, J.D. and Critchley, E.M.R. (1989). Hallucinations and music. *Behavioural Neurology*, **2**, 115-24.

Greene, D.M. (1986). "Greene's Biographical Encyclopaedia of Composers". Collins, London.

Hammeke, T.A., McQuillen, M.P. and Cohen, B.A. (1983). Musical hallucinations associated with acquired deafness. *Journal of Neurology, Neurosurgery and Psychiatry*, **46**, 570-2.

Henson, R.A. (1977). Neurological aspects of musical experience. *In* "Music and the Brain". (Eds M. Critchley and R.A. Henson). pp. 3-21. Heinemann, London.

Keshavan, M.S., Kahn, E.M. and Brar, J.S. (1988). Musical hallucinations following removal of a right frontal meningioma. *Journal of Neurology, Neurosurgery and Psychiatry*, **51**, 1225.

Macdonald, H. (1982). "Berlioz". Dent, London.

Mayer-Gross, W., Slater, E. and Roth, M. (1974). "Clinical Psychiatry". 3rd Edn. (Eds E. Slater, and M. Roth). Bailliere, Tindall and Cassell.

Miller, T.C. and Crosby, T.W. (1979). Musical hallucinations in a deaf elderly patient. *Annals of Neurology*, **5**, 301-2.

Ostwald, P.F., (1985). "Schumann. Music and Madness". Gollancz, London.
Patel, H.C., Keshavan, M.S. and Martin, J. (1987). A case of Charles Bonnet syndrome with musical hallucinations. *Canadian Journal of Psychiatry,* **32**, 303-4.
Penfield, W. and Perot. (1963). The brain's record of auditory and visual experience. *Brain,* **86**, 598-696.
Penfield, W. and Rasmussen, T. (1952). "The Cerebral Cortex of Man". Macmillan, London.
Rhein, J.H.W. (1913). Hallucinations of hearing and diseases of the eye. *New York Medical Journal,* **97**, 123-8.
Ross, E.D., Jossman, P.D. and Bell, B. *et al.* (1975). Musical hallucinations in deafness. *Journal of the American Medical Association,* **231**, 620-2.
Rozanski, J. and Rosen, H. (1952). Musical hallucinations and otosclerosis. *Confin Neurology,* **12**, 49-54.
Sacks, O.W. and Kohl, M. (1970). Incontinent nostalgia induced by L-dopa. *Lancet,* **1**, 1394.
Scott, M. (1979). Musical hallucinations from meningioma. *Journal of the American Medical Association,* **241**, 1683.
Scott, R.T. (1975). Hallucinations of music in alcohol withdrawal. *Neurology,* **24**, 362.
Tarachow, S. (1941). The clinical value of hallucinations in localizing brain tumours. *American Journal of Psychiatry,* **97**, 1434-44.
Tartini, G. to Lalande, "Voyage d'un Francais en Italie". (1765-6), vol. 8, p.292. Paris.
Trethowan, W.H. (1977). Music and mental disorder. *In* "Music and the Brain". (Eds M. Critchley and R.A. Henson). pp. 398-432. Heinemann, London.
Victor, M. and Hope J.M. (1958). The phenomenon of auditory hallucinations in chronic alcoholism. *Journal of Mental and Nervous Disease,* **126**, 451-81.
Walker, A. (1979). Music and the unconscious. *British Medical Journal,* **2**, 1641-3.
West, L.J. (1975). A clinical and theoretical overview of hallucinatory phenomena. *In* "Hallucinations: Behaviour, Experience and Theory". (Eds R.K. Siegal and L.J. West). pp. 297-311. Wiley, New York.

# 14. Philosophy, knowledge and reality

Michael Ayers

---

As far as Europe is concerned, epistemology, i.e. serious and systematic thought about knowledge, belief and the general character of the processes involved in acquiring them, seems to have begun among the Greeks in the sixth century BC. From these beginnings, over centuries of continuous debate, were developed the various ancient approaches to the problems of knowledge and reality. Historically the most significant of such theories were those associated with five schools or tendencies: Platonism, Aristotelianism, Epicureanism, Stoicism and Scepticism both moderate (or Academic) and extreme (or Pyrrhonist). Medieval philosophers, Christian, Arab and Jewish, were chiefly impressed by Plato and Aristotle, whose theories they often interpreted as harmonious with one another, and which they cut to the shape of their preferred theological principles. Aquinas introduced a somewhat purer (if hardly pure) Aristotelianism in the 13th century, and this, in one form or another, was the dominant doctrine in European universities at the beginning of the modern period, despite the strong revival and development of other approaches, not least during the Renaissance.

The famous battle between "ancients" and "moderns" which continued through the 17th century, the battle which saw the birth of modern science as well as modern philosophy, was primarily between Aristotelianism and its critics. Yet for much of their explanatory theory the "moderns" were no less indebted to ancient philosophy than their entrenched opponents. Very roughly speaking, those early modern philosophers now called "rationalists" owed the basic structure of their epistemology to the tradition of Christian Platonism given authority by St. Augustine. "Empiricists", on the other hand, drew heavily on the epistemology of Epicurean atomism, splendidly set out by Lucretius in his great poem *De Rerum Natura,* and on the very imperfect record of the long debate between Stoics and Sceptics. As the modern argument proceeded, of course, such sources tended to be left behind, or modified virtually beyond recognition. Yet, just as modern atomic physics grew out of the revived Epicurean theory of atoms and the void, and may even be indebted for its existence to a Roman poet, so modern theories of knowledge, including models which psychologists as well as philosophers have commonly brought to the study of cognition, were first developed directly from ancient epistemology.

At the beginning of the 17th century a number of philosophers and scientists, such as Kepler, Galileo and Descartes' own early mentor, the Dutch scientist Isaac

Beeckman, saw the future of physics in the application of mathematics to nature. It is understandable that they were inclined to attribute the capacity for scientific knowledge to pure reason, i.e. to a grasp of rational or self-intelligible principles which are not drawn from the data of sense inductively, but may be perceived or understood independently of those data and employed in their interpretation. Such a view was developed and given a needed theological justification by another friend of Descartes, the monk Marin Mersenne, who called in aid what may be termed the "Augustinian triangle", St Augustine's conception of a relation between the human mind, the mind of the Creator and the nature of things. The basic thought is that God has created things in accordance with universal rational principles, "archetypes" or "essences" held in His mind (the theologically acceptable, God-dependent equivalent of Plato's transcendent universals or "ideas"), and that science is possible for us to the extent that he has created human minds in the image of His own. That we are capable of grasping the eternal truths of mathematics and other self-evident maxims independently of the deliverances of sense was, for Mersenne as for Augustine, indication that there is such a correspondence between divine and human reason, and therefore between human reason and the world. But Mersenne took the correspondence to be limited, ducking the crucial issue of the existence of "substantial forms".

For the Aristotelians, every natural substantial object or stuff consists in a specific "form" or nature embodied in "matter", neither of which could exist without the other. "Matter", in the last analysis, appears as an essentially characterless or undifferentiated substrate, the role of which is simply to make the instantiation of form possible. Knowledge is always of form, and scientific knowledge of any substance is achieved through an understanding and definition of that specific form which makes the substance the kind of thing it is, the "substantial form" which constitutes the thing. Mersenne did not reject this model outright, but argued that it leaves out of account God's employment of mathematics in creation. Mathematics admittedly does not give us the essences or natures of the multitudinous kinds of things in existence, but it does contain the principles of a general harmony which pervades the universe. About essences we may only speculate in the manner of Aristotelian science, but it is possible to explicate the divine harmony with comparative certainty in such "mixed" mathematical sciences as harmonics in the strict sense, geometrical optics and mechanics. This claim opposed the orthodox Aristotelian view that mathematics is a science which can tell us nothing about reality precisely because it abstracts from the nature of things, treating them as bare units or extensive quantities.

The radical and fundamental step taken by Descartes was his transformation of Mersenne's modest basis for a mathematizing research programme in physics by the claim that physics has just one object, the essence of which can indeed be captured mathematically, namely matter itself. Contrary to Aristotelianism, matter does have a nature, which is simply to be extended in three dimensions and so to be impenetrable and capable of motion. Bodies are not constituted by substantial forms as members of different species, gold or water, horses or oak trees. Every particular body consists of the same general substance as every other body, each appearing to us, and behaving, as one kind of thing or another according to its mechanical structure and the motion of its parts. In themselves bodies and their motions are fully describable in geometrical terms, and all motion is in accordance with certain simple and intelligible laws, the most fundamental of which is the law, unrecognized by the Aristotelians, that a body in motion or at rest continues in the same state until impeded or put in motion by some other body. The task of physics is to identify these general laws by analytical reasoning and then to employ them in the explanation of particular phenomena. It will be normal for any particular phenomenon to be explicable mechanically in several different ways, between which we may decide by experiment. To know the general principles of mechanics, however, experiment is unnecessary.

This austere, over-confident conception of physics supplies the main driving force behind Descartes' philosophy, but it is not expounded in his most famous work in epistemology and metaphysics, "Meditations on First Philosophy", published in 1641. Nevertheless Descartes was explicit that the purpose of that work was to provide philosophical foundations for his physics. The argument begins with his famous internal debate with the sceptic, a modified re-run of the Hellenistic debate as to whether there is a "criterion of truth." Unlike the ancient Epicurean and Stoic opponents of scepticism, Descartes takes it that the sceptic's reasoning successfully undermines our natural trust in the senses: I could be dreaming or, worse still, a deceiving God or demon could be creating the continuous illusion of a material world when there is nothing there. Even this supposition, however, leaves indubitable the basic fact of my own existence as a doubting, thinking thing, the point summed up in another work by the famous expression, "*Cogito, ergo sum*". This fact is something perceived or understood "clearly and distinctly", not by any kind of sense, but by the intellect or reason. Indeed, Descartes argues, even in our apprehension of material objects the intellect is as much involved as are the senses. Sensation gives us notice of changing sensible qualities, but the idea we have of one and the same extended, mutable thing or substance undergoing and surviving those changes is a purely intellectual idea underivable from the deliverances of sense and necessary for their interpretation.

Descartes then raises the question whether even intellectual understanding might not be illusory in any particular case. Could not a malign demon have made it appear to me that $2 + 3 = 5$, when in fact it does not? Such extravagant doubt is met with a proof "that God exists, ... that everything else depends on him, and that he is no deceiver; and that [therefore] everything which I clearly and distinctly perceive is of necessity true." The argument is notorious, not so much for the invalidity of the proof of God's existence, nor for the shaky premise that a perfect being will not deceive, as for its apparent circularity, since it is an employment of reason to validate reason. Yet Descartes' purpose seems to have been precisely to demonstrate that reason, when pressed, confirms rather than undermines itself, and that the confirmation rests on an Augustinian recognition that enlightenment by reason is enlightenment by God. Nevertheless the "Cartesian circle" left many of his successors persuaded that a validation of reason itself must be, since useless, then unnecessary; and some held not only that the deliverances of reason do not need validation, but that the same goes for the deliverances of the senses.

For Descartes himself our natural sensory beliefs are in themselves fatally vulnerable to doubt. Fortunately, however, we can distinguish within our complement of purely intellectual ideas the ideas of two distinct substances, extended substance or matter and thinking substance or mind, each capable of existing as such apart from the other. The possibility of scepticism with respect to the material world demonstrates this ontological independence of the thinking subject from matter. In human beings, however, mind and matter are conjoined, and sensation and imagination are to be understood as functions of their intimate union, occurring when the intellect "turns" or "attends" to images constituted by motions in the brain rather than to its own innate conceptions. Since there is a physical, mechanical process involved in sense-perception it is entirely intelligible that the senses, valuable as they are in our normal commerce with the world, should sometimes lead us astray. God does not thereby deceive us, however, since he has given us the faculty of intellect by which to discern, through our general understanding of their function and of physics, when the senses are to be trusted and when not.

Something should be said about Descartes' notion of an idea, which it is traditional to misrepresent as a pernicious novelty setting the problems of modern epistemology by driving a new kind of wedge, a *tertium quid,* between thought and its object. His extension of the term "idea" to the representative element in all thought whatsoever, i.e. beyond its usual reference to the "archetypes" or essences in the divine mind, and even beyond the human conceptions supposed to correspond to those essences, was mildly unorthodox but not unprecedented. The notion itself, however, was entirely orthodox, equivalent to the Scholastic notion of a concept. Echoing his predecessors, Descartes explained it through the notion of "objective" being, i.e. existence "in the mind" or, as it is still called in the late 20th century, "intentional" existence. Like others, he drew attention to the point that talk of an "idea" can be taken in two ways, either as a mental act or event or as the object or content of such an act. Hence the expression "my idea of the sun" may refer either to my act of conceiving of the sun or to the sun as I conceive of it, the sun as it is in my thought. All this simply reflects ordinary language and a feature of many terms where representation is involved. Thus a "belief" may be firm *qua* acceptance and improbable *qua* what is accepted. A "statement" may be the content stated, or the act of stating it. If it is said that Dürer's idea (or, for that matter, picture) of a rhinoceros was not much like a rhinoceros, the comparison is obviously not between a pachyderm and Dürer's act of thinking (or his drawing, taken as a physical object), but between a pachyderm as Dürer imagined (or depicted) it, and as it really is – between the rhinoceros in Dürer's mind (or in his picture) and a rhinoceros in nature.

Yet if Descartes' notion of an idea is just a version of ordinary ways of thinking about representation and reality, like them it raises certain questions about how it is to be interpreted. In giving the intentional object of a thought, e.g. a thought of green fields, it is plausible that we speak only of the thought, and not of what lies outside the thought. After all, it is possible to think about, even to "see", non-existent objects, such as ghosts or unicorns. We give, as it were, the inner direction of the thought or sense-experience, but are uncommitted as to whether anything lies in that direction. Descartes put this traditional point by defining an *idea* as "the form of any thought" – simply what makes it determinate. On the other hand, it seems right in general to *identify* the intentional object with the appropriate real object, even if they differ as the woman in Leonardo's picture may have differed from the woman who sat for him. There were not, after all, two different women, one ideal and one real, but a difference between the way a woman was painted and the way the same woman really was. It is this point which seems to be missed by Descartes' orthodox identification of idea *qua* act of thought with idea *qua* intentional object, since to accept that identification and *also* to identify intentional and real objects would seem to commit one to the absurdity of identifying real objects with acts of thinking.

This kind of problem, as to which aspects of our ordinary, slippery, seemingly incoherent model for thought should be taken seriously, was an old chestnut by Descartes' time, if exacerbated by his postulation of a great and systematic difference between the world as it appears to the senses and the bare, spare material world as (he supposed) it really is. Where Descartes differed sharply from the Scholastics was in what may be called his physics of intentionality. The Aristotelians thought of intentional existence as a special kind of physical existence of the form of the object in the appropriate organ or faculty. When we see something red, for example, the "sensible form" of red exists physically (if only intentionally, not "materially") in the organ of sight, later coming to exist as an object of memory – an "image" – in the organ of imagination. From this image the intellect (which was thought to have no need of a separate organ) may construct an "intelligible form" or universal notion for the purpose of abstract, scientific thought. This is taken to be an ultimate, irreducible account of what physically happens. For Descartes, however, all that ever happens in any material organ is motion, which only constitutes an "image", "object" or representation in so far as it gives rise to, or somehow enters into, a conscious idea in the mind. In other words, the material world is kept unpolluted by intentionality so as to be a suitable subject-matter for a purely geometrical, mechanistic physics. Intentionality is kicked upstairs as, with consciousness, an essential attribute of an immaterial substance whose very being is to think and *ipso facto* to represent.

Although Descartes simply took over the division of cognition between the faculties of sense (including "common sense"), imagination (including sensory memory) and intellect, he prided himself on maintaining a conception of the unity of the soul (and therefore its indivisibility and natural immortality) impossible in a system like the Aristotelians', which spreads the mind over a number of material organs or faculties. Sensation and imagination occur when the unitary, immaterial intellect responds to, or employs, brain-motions. A consequence is the paradox, immediately notorious among his critics, that animals are not conscious. They have only the material equivalent of sensation and imagination, which must be supposed to produce physical responses in a purely mechanical way. Yet this antecedent to behaviourism was not the only embarrassment to the theory, and the problem of the interaction between mind and brain remained a nagging difficulty for later Cartesians. One very general question, much canvassed by some critics, was how two separate substances, each subject to its own intelligible laws or principles, should constitute anything but two quite separate causal systems.

Yet there was also a more specific problem about the mind-brain relation in cognition. Sometimes Descartes wrote as if it consisted only in brute correlations set up by God between brain-events and mental events, a thought developed by such later writers as Arnold Geulinx and Nicolas Malebranche. More often, as has been suggested above, he saw the brain-event as itself a kind of immediate object of cognition. This may seem surprising, but it suited his analysis of sensory ideas: each involves a datum which is referred by the mind to an object. Thus (on an account proposed in a later work) a sensory idea of red is false if the given sensation is referred to an object supposed like the sensation, but true (although still obscure and confused) if it is referred to a supposed, but unknown cause, and both true and clear-and-distinct if it is referred to the actual mechanical cause. Yet his general view of thought – in particular his embracing the traditional principle that all thought involves ideas, i.e. is "of" something – leaves it mysterious how there could be, as an element of thought, a datum prior to representation or referral to an object. His solution seems to be that, on its own, the datum is not an element of thought but an image in the brain which can somehow be incorporated into thought in virtue of the intimate union of mind and body. Certainly the notion of a sensory datum interpreted by the intellect is a feature of Descartes' optical theory, and it is here that he expanded on the form supposed to be taken by the brain-image.

Despite his dualism, Descartes was sensitive to the fact that we experience ourselves as objects extended in space rather than as disembodied thinkers, whatever conception of ourselves can be achieved through metaphysical reflection on the sceptical predicament. Here he had a different kind of recourse to the notion of the intimate or, as he sometimes put it, "substantial" union of soul and body. The body is not just a tool of the mind but appears as the very subject of mental states such as pain, and in willing our bodies to move we appear to be directly moving our very selves. Nevertheless Descartes seems to have been committed to the view that this is no more than a practically useful illusion.

Yet another problem for Descartes was this. His theory was premised on the doctrine that we have innate interpretive ideas, not, of course, as actual conscious thoughts, but as dispositions or tendencies. As he himself said, they are innate as a predisposition to a disease may be innate. Yet, as the word "disposition" suggests, specific tendencies exist according to actual structures. What could the structure of the mind be, if not material? The thesis drawn from the *Cogito* that my essence is to think seems to entail that my present existence now consists in my present, actual thinking, yet how can that thinking be so structured as to sustain dispositional ideas and knowledge about what is not its current subject-matter? Descartes seems to have tried to pre-empt this point by suggesting that our innate ideas are all implicit in the very faculty of thought. For example, he assumed that all awareness involves awareness of the thinking subject; we are aware of the subject of our thought as limited or finite, but that negative concept presupposes the positive concept of an infinite being, i.e. an innate idea of God. Similarly, the innate idea of a substantial, enduring thing can be drawn from our ever-present idea of ourself as a substance. Perhaps understandably, this approach is never fully worked out, and no attempt is made to apply it to the innate idea of extension.

Issues raised by Descartes' theory set much of the agenda for philosophy for half a century or more. Perhaps the most spectacular and ingenious response was Spinoza's account of mind and knowledge, although Spinoza's main motivation was theological and moral rather than epistemological. In response to mind-body dualism, he argued in effect that all reality has (among an infinity of others unknown to us) both material and mental aspects. A "mind" is simply a part of nature under its mental, subjective aspect, and its "body" is the same part under its material aspect. A mind is constituted by its thoughts or ideas, so that it is, taken as a whole, itself an idea. Its body is not only identical with this idea, but is the object of the idea. So Spinoza identified the mind-body relation with the intentional relation between an idea and its object. It can help to understand this surprising mixture of panpsychism and materialism to relate it to Descartes' model of the mind attending to the image in the brain. For both philosophers an occurrence of sensing or imagining has a brain-process as its immediate object, which for Spinoza meant that it has its own material basis, i.e. itself under its material aspect, as its immediate object. We only perceive things outside the body mediately, through their effects on the body – i.e. through material images. Spinoza thought that sense-perception tells us more about our bodies – about how they are affected by external objects – than it does about external objects.

Nevertheless, all our experience gives us only "inadequate" ideas of our body. An "adequate" idea would incorporate knowledge of all its causes and effects, its whole place in nature. It would be an idea such as God has. Spinoza means this very seriously. For "Nature" is also "God" so that the mental aspect of the universe constitutes God's mind, the idea which embraces everything. Spinoza's panpsychism is pantheism. Human minds are parts of this universal mind, and of their very nature they do not comprehend the whole. Here Spinoza gives an ingenious explanation of the Cartesian innate, purely intellectual ideas. Certain features of reality pervade the whole, and can therefore be considered abstractly in any part of it. Thus, although I cannot form an adequate idea of my body or of my mind, I can form adequate ideas of matter and mind in general, i.e. of Nature in general under the attributes of extension and thought. These ideas exist in us just as they exist in the universal or divine mind, and truths involving them appear to us both necessary and universal, e.g. in doing geometry or mechanics.

Spinoza's system is perhaps the most astonishing and polished piece of virtuoso metaphysics in existence. Even the present resumé of a part of it may serve to show how, building largely on quasi-Cartesian principles, it neatly resolves some of the inherited problems. No longer are minds islands of a special substance in a peculiar, seemingly impossible causal relation to certain bits of the material universe, but, by means of a daring theology, mentality and intentionality are taken to be fundamental features pervading a seamless deterministic system – philosophical *explicantia* rather than *explicanda*. By the same token all processes, including human thought-processes, are brought under the laws of mechanistic physics. Animals are no longer denied conscious mentality, which becomes again a matter of degree, as it had been for the Aristotelians. Moreover, the traditional dilemma of intentionality is resolved: amazingly, a thought or experience becomes identical both with its intentional object, a brain-process as we conceive of it or experience it, and with the real object, the brain-process as it is in itself. The "Augustinian triangle" is collapsed along with the collapse of creator into creation, finite into universal mind. Innate, purely intellectual ideas, in us as they are in God, are indeed identical with God's ideas, and at the same time are themselves those very essences or universal principles in nature (even material nature) which are their subject-matter.

Leibniz, the other indisputably great "rationalist" metaphysician, was evidently impressed by Spinoza's resolution of the problems of dualism, but shocked both by the denial of a transcendent, personal God and by the vision of the human soul as (unless in its universal, purely intellectual and impersonal features) a somewhat edgeless correlate of an all too destructible body, both mere processes within "God or Nature". He was also dissatisfied with the Cartesian conception of matter as a substance definable purely geometrically, a conception which, he thought, generated not only the geometrical paradoxes of infinite divisibility, but also the metaphysical paradox of a fundamental substance which is not unitary, since always divisible. Moreover Descartes' geometrical matter is inert, since his intelligible laws of mechanics are presented as the simple, yet fertile principles according to which an immutable God may be supposed to keep matter in motion. A true substance, however, is for Leibniz something active, not something pushed about by God. Leibniz therefore postulated a world like Spinoza's in so far as mentality and intentionality are its fundamental, pervasive features, but unlike Spinoza's in consisting of a plurality of simple, active, independent substances.

In being active, substances are like Aristotelian forms rather than matter. As such, they are neither extended nor exist in space. Everything that happens within such a substance (which Leibniz called a "monad") flows from its own essence or nature, so that there is strictly no interaction between them. Indeed the notion of causal interaction is logically absurd, supposing that some attribute or "accident" (e.g. motion) should be transferred from one substance to another, i.e. should be detached from its possessor and come to belong to something else. Consequently both causal and spatial relations, which seem to be such important features of the world, are mere appearances. They are not, however, illusions, but grounded in reality, *phenomena bene fundata*. The truth of propositions expressed in terms of such relations depends ultimately on the possession of certain intrinsic, non-relative properties by simple substances.

It is in explanation of this last claim that Leibniz appealed to intentionality or representation as a fundamental feature of reality. He did so by exploiting certain truisms about perception. If a number of perceivers are all looking at one another, each will differ internally from the other according to its own point of view, i.e. according to its spatial relations to the others and the consequent effects of the others on its organs of perception. The perceptual state of each will therefore not only represent the other perceivers more or less well depending on its spatio-causal relations to them, but will also, *ipso facto,* reflect those relations themselves. Leibniz proposed that his form-like and atomic simple substances or "monads" are quasi-perceivers. A pre-established harmony holds between the perceptions of all monads, and a monad exists correspondent to every point in that *phenomenon,* infinitely divisible extension. His reductive claim is that monads and their internal representations are all that is truly real. The representative modifications of monads constitute the sole foundation of true propositions about causal and spatial relations between things rather as A's being off-white and B's being intensely white may constitute the sole foundation of the relational truth that B is whiter than A. The analogy between the intentional relation and a merely "extrinsic" relation such as *whiter than* holds only in part, however, just because A does not enter into the whiteness of B as the perceived object in some sense (i.e. intentionally, as its object) enters into the perceptual state. Yet the analogy does hold in part, in so far as it would be logically (although not, for Leibniz, metaphysically) possible for any of the mutual perceivers to exist as the sole occupant of a world, but with all the modifications it possesses in the actual world. Each monad internally represents, "contains" or constitutes both its "point of view" and its identity or individuality.

Leibniz, then, drew a firm distinction between the intentional object or *phenomenon* and the real or external object. He himself linked his model to his denial of the transmission of anything like "sensible forms" from one substance to another. Since there is no interaction in his system, change is explained as the progression within a substance from one perceptual modification to another in accordance with an internal law, force or tendency. Since what determines the state of a substance at any time can only be its own antecedent state, the whole of its future (and, Leibniz held, its past) lies in its present state. This tendency is analogous to desire or appetition in the soul, as "expression" is analogous to ordinary perception. (It also explains the possibility of innate ideas, as well as supplying the metaphysical basis for forces in nature.) Nevertheless there is a great difference between an ordinary monad and an animal soul. The latter is a monad in which representations achieve a degree of distinctness, coupled with a sort of retained echo, which constitutes sensation and memory. Human souls have not only such perceptions but also "apperception", a consciousness or reflexive knowledge of their perceptions. Unsurprisingly, Leibniz held that apperception, in ways we need not consider here, allows us to know the eternal truths, and so to be rational.

Although monads are the only absolute unities, in combination they constitute the relative unities which appear to us as material objects, most importantly animals and plants. They do so in virtue of the fact that some monads "dominate" other monads. Indeed, every monad is the principle of unity of an aggregate of other monads as the soul is the principle unifying the body. Reality is thus an infinite hierarchy of dominant and subordinate immaterial substances, quasi-souls and quasi-bodies. Although every monad "expresses" every other monad, a dominant monad expresses those subordinate monads which make up its own body "more particularly and more perfectly", or "more distinctly" than other bodies. The latter it expresses "according to the relation [they] have to its own body" and especially, in the case of animals, to those parts of its body that constitute its organs of sense. Rather like Spinoza, Leibniz thought that what we perceive most distinctly in sense-perception is what is happening in our own body.

The distinction drawn by Leibniz between bare "expression" on the one hand and animal sensation and human consciousness on the other makes it difficult to see what is left of the general analogy with perception. Faced with this problem, he appeals to his famous and influential notion of unconscious perception, which he takes to be familiar from our own case: e.g. we hear a multitude of sounds confusedly as one sound, or a sound that we do not consciously hear can nevertheless wake us up. The claim is that everything that affects us is really perceived, unconsciously if not consciously. It can be objected that not every change even in a conscious perceptual state counts as the perception of its cause: the drug that causes visions is not thereby perceived. Subliminal or unconscious perception of a sound in sleep counts as such just because of the causal role of the mechanism of conscious hearing ("blindsight" is analogous in this), not to speak of the sound's impinging on dreaming consciousness. Even less convincing is Leibniz's extension of the notion of "*petits perceptions*" below the level of consciousness to the infinity of monads which never consciously perceive anything at all.

Two features of Leibniz's systems deserve particular emphasis here. First, his conception of space as the form under which a non-spatial reality appears to us gave a radically new twist to the distinction between appearance and reality. The very framework under which things appear as real, external objects, subjects of mechanistic physics, is due to the structure of our minds rather than to things themselves. Second, his argument depends even more emphatically than Descartes' on the assumption that we can grasp our own nature and metaphysical status independently of our grasp of any other reality. It is from our own case that we understand, not only what "expression" is, the fundamental relation between substances, but also what a substance is, and the possibility that a unitary substance should be the subject of a variety of states. For he interprets the unity of consciousness, at one time and over time, as the self-awareness of a unitary substance undergoing variety and change. It supplies a paradigm of what a substance is.

Let us now turn back to consider the "empiricist" tradition. Descartes saw as his main obstacle the common-sense principle that all our knowledge has been acquired "either from the senses or through the senses". Among the invited critics of the "Meditations" were two prominent philosophers whose systems were built on just that principle, Pierre Gassendi and Thomas Hobbes. Gassendi, a monk like Mersenne, offered a learned and perceptive, if somewhat verbose modernization of Epicureanism, insisting that "the greatest evidence is the evidence of sense". If "reason" seems sometimes to be a superior faculty called in to correct and interpret the deliverances of sense, that is really the senses correcting themselves, since the principles or maxims reason employs are themselves derived inductively from experience. Even the principle that the whole is greater than its parts is believed because of our exceptionless experience that the sky is greater than one star, the body than one finger, and so forth. Gassendi also endorsed the Epicurean principle that, in an important sense, every sensation is true. The same thing's appearing different to different observers is no more a ground for scepticism than is the sun's melting one thing and hardening others. The different effects correspond to different mechanical relationships that the same thing has to the organs of sense in different conditions. Such effects may give rise to false beliefs in unwary observers, but every effect is a true sign of its actual cause, and it is the consequent judgement which is false. Gassendi's theory comes down to a causal analysis of the relation between sensation and object: a sensation's object is the total or, at least, sufficient cause of the sensations's having the character that it has. Since there always is such a cause, all sensations are true. Thus when water appears hot to one observer and cold to another, in each case the feeling is a true sign of the effect of the motion of the particles in the water on the motion of the particles in their hands.

Unlike Descartes, Gassendi took an interest in probability, which he also saw as the employment of "signs". Following ancient theory, he distinguished between "reminiscent" and "indicative" signs, the former arising from experience of constant conjunctions which enable us to infer the existence (actual or imminent) of something of a kind that has been perceived in the past. Indicative signs, however, allow us to infer the existence of what lies beyond perception, as analogy justifies the inference from the appearance of sweat on the skin to the existence of invisible pores. The theory of atoms and the void is not certain (as Descartes supposed his own physics to be), but is the most probable speculation based on such analogies. Gassendi denied knowledge of the nature of the mind – like the eye, it does not perceive itself – but in general he favoured materialism, partly because he saw no need to postulate a faculty of reason over and above sense and imagination, the faculties traditionally assigned material organs. In a late work, however, he allowed the thought that there is probably an immaterial element in the mind, if only because that supposition has the best chance of explaining the revealed fact of immortality.

Hobbes, on the other hand, was not only an unyielding materialist, but the proponent of an empiricism the terms of which allowed him to claim the same absolute certainty for his mechanistic physics as Cartesians claimed for theirs. Unlike Gassendi, Hobbes had a conception of mathematical or logical certainty to be set against the mere probability of judgements based on experience and induction. Such scientific certainty is possible, however, not because of some faculty of reason in addition to sense and imagination, but because the institution of language allows us to analyse experience into its most general or simple features, giving us the basic concepts of geometry and mechanics. At this level causal principles such as the laws of inertia become "manifest in themselves". Like Gassendi, Hobbes argued that when scientific theory corrects some immediate sensory judgement, the senses are really correcting themselves.

The role of language is explained in terms of a view of thought as a stream of images, "the discourse of the mind", which arise in accordance with certain principles of association: e.g. we think of St Peter when we hear of St Andrew "because their names are read together". Prior to language, the most important kind of association arises from experience of the constant conjunction of causes and effects, or "natural signs", which gives rise to a "presumption" about the past or the future. This happens more or less usefully and "prudently" in human beings and animals depending on their sensitivity to similarities and differences. "Names", however, introduce a new kind of "mark or sign" into the train of ideas, in so far as they are sensations or images not naturally, but arbitrarily or conventionally associated with other sensations and images. Through language, universality is possible, since a name is universal when it is a sign which is associated with, and stimulates, the images of many resembling things rather than just one thing. A proposition is "necessary" when nothing can be imagined which is named by the subject which is not also named by the predicate, and is "evident" (as it seems from Hobbes' somewhat unclear account) in so far as we can grasp the relationship which explains that impossibility, between the aspects or points of resemblance in virtue of which the two names are applicable. He explains necessity as a relation between meanings, a function of arbitrary definitions, but his account presupposes a prior relation between aspects or features. The task of the natural scientist is to define names which mark off the fundamental features of things, and so achieve necessary, analytic propositions which explicate things' naturally necessary operations. Some sciences, however, such as pure geometry and political theory, are *a priori*, possible as such because they are concerned with human constructs (political states or geometrical figures) rather than with natural objects.

The first modern empiricist to achieve anything like the authority of Descartes was John Locke, whose "Essay concerning Human Understanding" was published nearly fifty years after the "Meditations", in 1689. Like Gassendi, he held that the ideas and knowledge acquired through the senses are insufficient to give us a full understanding of nature, so that the physical theories of philosophers like Descartes and Hobbes, so far from being certain "science", are speculations which are not only unsubstantiated but for various reasons palpably inadequate for the purposes of explanation. The senses give us knowledge of the existence of things, but not of their essences. Like Hobbes, however, he made room in his theory for *a priori* universal knowledge, although such knowledge of the principles of physics (which, like his contemporaries, Locke conceived of mechanistically) lies beyond us. The *a priori* sciences to which we can attain, arithmetic, geometry and, as he thought, ethical and political theory, are possible, not because, as Hobbes suggested, the things they are about are constructed by us, but because they are about ideas constructed without any reference to reality, and so have no pretensions to be concerned with substantive things or their nature – an explanation which looks back to the Aristotelian view of mathematics. An important distinction is between "trifling" and "informative" truths. The former express mere definitions or part-definitions. The propositions of mathematics include informative truths, such as the proposition that the angles of a triangle equal the angle on a straight line, as well as definitions, but all those propositions about natural substances which have been proposed as principles of natural science, from the Aristotelians' "Man is a rational animal" to the Cartesians' "Body is extended", turn out to be merely trifling and arbitrary definitions. Locke was here rejecting both Hobbes' programme of language-aided analysis of experience and the whole conception (which Leibniz shared with Hobbes) of a science embodied in logically analytic propositions. In this, as we shall see, he had an important influence on Kant.

Locke's systematic analysis of the forms of knowledge and belief, of certainty and probability, was perhaps the most effective as well as the most complex of his century, but at its root lies a rather too neat causal model for both representation and sensory knowledge. The basic, quasi-Epicurean principle is that all simple ideas are "real", true and adequate. They are so precisely because they come from experience, being caused in us by objects operating on the senses in regular ways. As such effects, they serve in experience and thought as signs naturally signifying their causes, a kind of natural language of thought. Thus the sensory idea or image of yellow stands in thought as the sign of whatever it is in objects that regularly causes that sensation. Employing such a sign, we can adequately and dependably distinguish and think about a feature or "sensible quality" of objects without knowing just what that feature is in itself. In other words, we can have "sensitive knowledge" of the existence of such a feature, for in sensation we are directly aware, not only of a sensation or idea, but of something acting on us, causing that sensation, "though perhaps we neither know nor consider how it does it". This kind of knowledge of existence can be extended to attributes other than sensible qualities by means of the idea of power, together with experience of constant conjunctions. If we observe fire regularly melting wax, we can attribute to the fire the power to melt and to the wax the power to be melted, thus distinguishing certain attributes of fire and wax through their observable effects. We treat the wax's dependable melting in the proximity of the fire as a sign of something unobservable in each.

Locke also claimed that in sensation we can be aware of the "co-existence" of several sensible qualities, i.e., in one thing, and rejected Descartes' claim that we have to employ a purely intellectual idea of a substance in order even to be aware that we have some wax undergoing change in front of us. When we form such an idea explicitly, as we do in defining primitive noun-predicates such as "gold", "iron", "horse" or "spirit", it should be regarded, not as an innate idea of reason embodying some metaphysical knowledge of reality, but as a mere place-marker (in this like the idea of *power*) through which we conceive of the unknown cause of the union of certain sensible qualities and powers which we observe regularly to co-exist. There is some underlying nature in virtue of which what we call "gold" has the regularly conjoined properties included in our definition of gold, and when we define gold as "the thing or substance which is yellow, heavy, malleable, etc.", the term "thing or substance" does not reflect the mind's penetrating to some reality beyond the deliverances of the senses, but precisely to its not doing so: the term simply means "*whatever* is yellow, etc." Locke went on to suggest that we might distinguish the "substance" which is yellow, etc. from the "constitution" of that substance responsible for its specific attributes. He here had in mind the distinction between a common matter, the object of a universal physics, and the specific determinations of matter which might give rise to the observable differences between gold, water, iron and so forth. But his claim was that we are equally ignorant of both, despite the general plausibility of the atomic or "corpuscularian" speculation.

Perhaps the main fault of Locke's account of "sensitive knowledge" is that, although it recognizes that the apprehension of objects involves and interpenetrates the apprehension of causality (we do not first apprehend objects and then the causal relations between them, or *vice versa*), it seems to leave our perceptual knowledge as nothing but knowledge of collections of powers. Objects are known only through effects conceived of as blank sensory data. Locke, it is true, is famous for the claim that ideas of "primary qualities" (spatial attributes, including motion, together with solidity) *resemble* their causes as ideas of "secondary qualities" (colour, smell and the like) do not. Yet this distinction is presented as a reasonable hypothesis, and there is no theoretical recognition that the perception of secondary qualities (not to speak of their "co-existence") presupposes that their possessors are perceived as things in space. Perceived space provides the framework on which we can hang hypotheses (or confessions of ignorance) about the true physical nature of sensible qualities like colour. Space cannot itself be the subject of such an hypothesis, and sensory awareness is as much shot through with an awareness of spatial relations as it is with an awareness of causal relations. We simply could not be aware of things as mere "somethings" possessing powers to cause sensations in us.

An important area of Locke's philosophy concerns self-knowledge. First he accepted the traditional (and Cartesian) view of experience and thought as reflexive. The thinker is not only aware of the object of thought but, at least at some level, of the thought itself. Locke did not, however, follow the Cartesians in regarding reflection as a function of intellect, but treated it as a kind of internal sense which supplies ideas of our mental operations but which no more presents their fundamental nature, or the essence of mind, than the external senses present the true nature of colour, or the essence of matter. The subjective unity of consciousness, moreover, is far from being the consciousness of a simple enduring substance. It is simply a phenomenal or experienced unity, which is sufficient foundation for our "forensic" notion of a unitary self persisting through time and responsible for its actions (a "person"), but which may, for all we know, supervene on a flux of material or immaterial substance just as the unifying life of an animal supervenes on the perpetual replacement of the particles of its body. Faith projects the continuity of such a unitary moral agent beyond biological death, but personal immortality neither entails, nor is entailed by, the continuity of an immaterial, indivisible soul.

One of Locke's most significant critics, George Berkeley, often described as the founder of idealism (despite the rival claims of Leibniz), is also generally classified as a "British Empiricist". Yet the title is open to question, if only because he accepted a quasi-Cartesian conception of pure intellect, sharply distinguished from sense, as a faculty through which we achieve "notions" of ourselves and knowledge of our status as active, perceiving substances. Moreover, an important issue in his philosophy, as for the rationalists, concerns the relationship between divine and human ideas. On the other hand, he steered clear of any suggestion of innate concepts or knowledge, and restricted the term "idea" to sensory ideas conceived of on broadly Lockean lines (ideas are "things as they are perceived", but do not intrinsically point beyond themselves), cutting it away from the conception of an Augustinian universal archetype. Indeed he drew on the same empiricist tradition as Hobbes and Locke for his imagist theory of universal reasoning and knowledge. The truth is that Berkeley's epistemology is eclectic, subordinated to a metaphysical purpose. Rather like Leibniz and the earlier school of "Cambridge Platonists", Berkeley saw materialism as a dire threat to religion. But where Leibniz argued that body is really spiritual, and the Cambridge Platonists stressed the ontological inferiority of inert, senseless matter, Berkeley aimed to pull its sting by arguing that there is no such *substance* at all. Bodies exist, but as mind-dependent beings, and the only independent substance is spirit.

A part of his argument runs roughly as follows. Philosophers distinguish between things as we perceive or conceive of them ("ideas") and things as they are in themselves, assigning sense-relative qualities like colour to the former class, but supposing that other sensible qualities, such as extension, motion and solidity, exist not only as ideas in the mind, but outside the mind in an independent substance which they call "matter". This distinction, Berkeley claimed, is unknown to the vulgar, who do not postulate external qualities or material substance, but take it (with what truth will soon be considered) that the very things we perceive, i.e. ideas, have independent existence. Worse, it is impossible to make sense of the distinction between primary and secondary qualities. First, since it is impossible to conceive of (i.e. imagine) shape in abstraction from all sense-relative qualities, it is impossible to conceive of it as existing apart from them. Second, on examination spatial attributes turn out to be as relative to perception as secondary qualities.

Bodies are necessarily more or less large, motions are more or less swift, but that can only be true of bodies and motions as perceived, in relation to some observer. Indeed the notion of a finite extension is incompatible with the realist's view of space as infinitely divisible (a view which Berkeley made a special target in a famous critique of Newtonian infinitesimals).

Third, Berkeley argued at length, in an influential contribution to psychological optics, against an assumption which he took to be an important source of the distinction between primary and secondary qualities, i.e. that spatial properties are the common object of sight and touch, and are therefore relative to neither sense. Optics was of continuing importance in early modern philosophy, and Locke had argued, against Descartes' conception of "innate geometry", that the perception of distance and three-dimensional shape is "beholding to experience, improvement and acquired notions". He repeated, and made famous, a question asked by his correspondent William Molyneux, whether someone born blind and made to see would be able immediately to distinguish a cube from a globe by sight alone. Both answered negatively, arguing that three-dimensional vision involves a kind of habitual adjustment or interpretation of two-dimensional data as a result of our experience of a correlation between visual cues ("variety of light or colour") and felt distance and depth. Berkeley, however, pressed their shaky reason (the person "has not yet attained the experience that what affects his touch so or so, must affect his sight so or so") to yield the more general conclusion that *no* spatial judgements based on vision can be extended to touch, or *vice versa,* without such experiential inference. All that is given is a correlation between two distinct sorts of idea, tactual and visual, which have nothing whatever in common but a name. He applied similar principles to the explanation of a wide range of optical phenomena, and argued that the visual perception of the distance of objects is not truly the perception of them as external to, or distinct from the perceiver.

Berkeley insisted that his aim was not to undermine the senses, but rather to remove a temptation to scepticism by removing the conception of imperceptible "things in themselves", whether the geometrically defined matter of dogmatic Cartesians or the extended, solid "something" postulated by Locke as the object of physical speculation. "Real things" are not "matter" so understood, but the series of ideas of sense which arise in us independently of our wills and according to a dependable order. Since only spirits are active, the direct cause of these ideas is not "matter", but a wise, powerful and benevolent spirit. Since "real" ideas are independent of our wills, we are right to take them to exist distinct from human minds, but we are wrong to conclude that they exist independently of mind in general. They have been proved to be mind-dependent, and must therefore exist in a non-human mind, the mind of God. Real things and God's ideas are identical, revealed to us in sense-perception. The experienced regularities or laws that we ascribe to natural causality and the workings of material "essences" are nothing but correlations set up by God to allow us a kind of foresight and the possibility of adopting means to ends.

Berkeley was a dogmatic metaphysician, but his arguments made a great impression on a very different philosopher, the hero of 20th-century Positivism, David Hume. Hume wanted to demonstrate that all hopes of penetrating to the essences of things, to things as they are in themselves, are utterly futile. Dogmatic theology and metaphysics, including physics based on anything but the observation of regularities, should be "committed to the flames". The strategy he adopted, however, ensured a more general scepticism than that. His argument takes the form of an analysis and psychological explanation of human beliefs – the common-sense belief-system of the vulgar, the more sophisticated systems of metaphysicians, and the system of the most advanced natural philosophy or physics. The general framework of his explanations is much like Hobbes': there is a train of "impressions" and "ideas", i.e. sensations and images, the course of which is determined by principles of association between them, one of the most important kinds of association being set up by the experienced correlations we ascribe to cause and effect. Words enter the train, possessing meaning in virtue of their tendency to stimulate ideas and be stimulated by impressions and ideas. Belief consists in a certain force or vivacity possessed by some ideas with consequences for action.

There are, however, certain fundamental differences from Hobbes. First, Hobbes gave his account in the context of his materialism: sensations are motions produced in us by material objects. Hume, however, did not even allow himself Locke's principle that all our simple ideas are acquired through the senses, i.e. through physical sense-mechanisms. His version of the empiricist slogan was that every simple idea is a copy of an antecedent impression, impressions being identified simply by their greater vivacity. His point was, no doubt, that a scrupulous critique of beliefs through an analysis of their psychological natural history cannot start with the assumption that a certain set of beliefs is true, i.e. that there are material objects acting on the senses with particular effects. Consequently all Hume's explanations have to be internal to the train of impressions and ideas, in terms of principles of association capable of being discerned by the introspective observer, a programme which goes a long way towards determining its own astonishing results.

A second fundamental difference is that Hobbes's naturalistic programme was designed to demonstrate that all the functions commonly ascribed to the divine faculty of reason, including a grasp of the necessary principles of physical and moral science, can be explained in terms of sensation and imagination without supposing any more fundamental gulf between man and beast than is created by the human invention of language. Hume's programme, on the other hand, was designed to show that the belief-systems considered are due to, and imbued with, fundamentally irrational principles. Probably the most famous part of his system relates to causality. First, he claimed that all expectations ordinarily regarded as probable or certain, however sophisticated the "causal reasoning" on which they are based, derive ultimately from past experience as a matter of custom or habit. The mechanist view that we can see a "necessary connection" between the way a billiard ball strikes another and the consequent movement of the ball that has been struck is an illusion due to the projection of a subjective feeling of certainty onto the sequence observed. Unfortunately, however, this argument can mislead as to the depth of Hume's scepticism, since it can seem that his fundamental claim is simply that the justification of causal beliefs and predictions is always at bottom inductive (a view with which too many 20th century philosophers have been in agreement), and that he assigns such beliefs to custom rather than reason just because he has a narrowly deductive paradigm of reasoning. Yet it is only necessary to follow his crucial account of the belief of the vulgar in the continuous and, therefore, independent existence of their impressions (i.e. sensible objects), or the belief in the continuous existence of a unitary self, to find Hume evidently concerned to demonstrate that our ordinary apprehension of the world is the incoherent product of an imagination operating according to absurd and even contradictory principles. Moreover the account minimizes the role of inductive reasoning in the construction of our belief-system by stressing that, strictly considered, there are no constant conjunctions or correlations in experience. Our notion of reality cannot be explained, as Berkeley tried to explain it, in terms of lawlike correlations between impressions or ideas of sense, since there are no such correlations. How could there be when, for example, visual ideas, the objects of sight, cease to exist on the shutting of one's eyes? The very belief that we experience constant conjunctions derives from an irrational tendency to impose regularity on experience, the tendency which, together with others just as irrational (such as a tendency to confuse identity with similarity), gives us our supposedly "real things".

It has, indeed, been pointed out that the form of Hume's explanations owed something to the psychological and physiological explanations of madness given by medical writers, explanations consonant with earlier philosophers', especially rationalists', explanations of error. The imagination unconstrained by reason can make one man believe he is the second Messiah, another that he has attended a witches' sabbath, a third that he is made of glass. The Cambridge Platonist Henry More, the Cartesian Nicolas Malebranche and even Locke dilated, with many pathological examples, on the errors and absurdities, if not physiology of the imagination. Hume differs from these writers and resembles Hobbes in treating not just aberrations, but our entire belief-system, the world as we experience and conceive of it, as the product or construct of the associative imagination. The corpuscularian physics of a Boyle or Newton is as much an imaginative construct as the system of the vulgar. Yet in his evaluation of that product as error he effectively followed not Hobbes, but the rationalists. Science is just as incoherent as common sense, differing only in deriving from wider analogies in experience.

Nevertheless, Hume's scepticism is mitigated by a certain distinction between normal or healthy beliefs and abnormal or sick ones. Some principles of the imagination are "permanent, irresistable and universal", essential to human nature and to successful human life. Others are "changeable, weak and irregular", "neither unavoidable to mankind, nor... so much as useful in the conduct of life". Both the ordinary world-view and corpuscularian physics are built on the former kind of principle, but religious doctrines and metaphysical theories arise from tendencies which are "natural" only in the "sense, that a malady is said to be natural". As recent studies of Hume have demonstrated, his underlying model is this: our natural world-view is due to a hotch-potch of irrational principles, but it is practically sufficient because it has a certain functional correspondence with the unknowable way things really are. There is, for example, sufficient correlation for practical purposes between our imaginative beliefs in necessary connections and the unknown powers of things, the "secret connections" which must always remain unintelligible to us. The question is, however, how Hume can consistently allow himself, not just to hold this form of pragmatism, but even to think it. If the content of our concepts and beliefs is all to be explained in terms of the stream of impressions and copies of impressions, then it would seem impossible to step outside that stream even to postulate the existence of a real world bearing some real relation to it. If the very idea of causality, for example, involves an illicit imaginative projection, how can it be employed to think of that real relation? By adopting what might seem at first a methodology of unprecedented rigour, Hume leads us into a claustrophobic, incoherent vision of a brain capable only of contemplating or affirming its own irrational figments.

The last philosopher for present consideration, Immanuel Kant, was famously stirred from his dogmatic Leibnizian slumbers by reading Hume. The result, "Transcendental Idealism", is a profound and brilliant synthesis, not only of rationalism and empiricism, but also of scepticism and dogmatism, a synthesis which, in one updated version or another, still dominates the philosophy of the West. Kant agreed with the rationalists that there are certain rational principles which we bring to the interpretation of experience both automatically and after reflection. Broadly, we assume that experience will be of a system of substantial objects arrayed in three-dimensional space, interacting deterministically with one another and with us as observers. Kant did not accept that we can arrive at the laws of physics by intellectual analysis, but he saw physical speculation as constrained by *a priori* principles, e.g. we have to think of change as the modification, according to immutable laws, of a substance which is conserved through change. None of these principled presuppositions derives from experience. For how could experience ground our assumption of universal causality, when we rely on that assumption in sorting out which sensations to take seriously as experience, i.e. as veridical rather than illusory? Rather, these principles constitute our conception of reality, of what it is to experience a real world of independent objects. They are like Hume's laws of association in one respect: they are ordering principles according to which the imagination constructs our system of beliefs. Yet they are quite unlike Hume's principles in being inherently evident and necessary rather than merely natural and absurd.

For Kant, the mistake of empiricists like Hume and Berkeley was to deprive the ordering principles of their coherence and internal rationality, and to split up our apprehension of a world of objects into a train of sensations and images which owes such order as it possesses to chance or the arbitrary whim of God, and our natural interpretation of which is an error attributable to a contingent clutter of psychological tendencies. The mistake of the rationalists, on the other hand, was to employ these principles beyond their role in ordering and interpreting experience, as if they could enable us to penetrate beyond the observable to the unobservable and untestable nature of "things in themselves". The latter, Kant agreed with Hume, are utterly unknowable: we can conceive of them, and of the relations they bear to experience, only through such purely logical, empty concepts as that of a subject of predication, or the concept of the relation of ground to consequent. Such metaphysical doctrines as that the soul is naturally immortal, that reality is spiritual, or that our minds are related to the ideas of God, are illusions engendered, not merely by the imagination, but by reason employing principles beyond their proper function of defining reality for us as an object of perception and science.

Kant introduced his argument by means of a question employing a distinction drawn from Locke. Locke had claimed that we have no informative universal knowledge of natural substances, but nevertheless had assumed (and Kant agreed) that things consist of a universal extended substance the essence of which, if unknown to us, could in principle be unfolded in a deterministic physics. Kant also took the quasi-Cartesian view that in geometry we have systematic *a priori* knowledge of the nature of space. By what right can we presume to know such truths, regarded by Kant as both informative and necessary? Or, as he put it, how is synthetic *a priori* knowledge possible? His answer was that such knowledge corresponds to the structure of our apprehensive faculties, reflecting what the mind contributes to the product of its cognitive contact with reality. He divided responsibility for the synthetic *a priori* between sense and reason. First it is an absolute impossibility that the general object of external sense should be anything but a spatial array, or that consciousness should be anything but a temporal sequence of appearances or subjective representations. As Kant put it, space is the form of outer sense and time the form of inner sense. Indeed, since appearances of external objects will be among our inner states, time is the form of all appearance generally. This explains our synthetic *a priori* knowledge of space and time (e.g. that there is only one space or time) and also mathematical knowledge. Kant, following Locke, believed that the "evidence" of mathematics depends ultimately on the employment, at an abstract level, of the senses or sensory imagination, e.g. we can "see why" $2 + 1 = 3$ by visualizing one more dot being added to two existing dots. The need for such "intuition" does not make arithmetic an empirical matter since, although a child will commonly learn arithmetic from actual dots, blocks, oranges or whatever, the dots (or whatever) involved in *apprehending* an arithmetical relation can just as well be imaginary. Geometrical understanding Kant held, involves similar abstract intuitions of space.

Our understanding of what it is for something to possess empirically real existence in space and time, however, stems from more than intuition and the abstract forms of sensibility. It is also due to the system of abstract logical concepts involved in the very possibility of thought about a subject. Kant believed that the possible forms of propositional thought or judgement, when brought to bear on the subject-matter supplied by sensibility, generate what he called the "categories", i.e. the concepts or principles employed by the mind in constructing the empirically real (but "transcendentally" ideal) observable world. Thus the subject-predicate form of categorical judgement generates the duality of substance and accident, the conceptual constraint which ensures that we interpret the world as matter subject to determinate modifications. Similarly, the form of hypothetical judgement generates the concept of cause and effect, and so forth.

Perhaps Kant's most famous and pervasive line of argument, however, is based on the presupposition that experience and knowledge involve a consciousness which is unified both synchronically and diachronically. Like Locke, Kant rejected the Cartesian-Leibnizian view that the reflexivity of thought gives us knowledge of the nature of a unitary, enduring, immaterial self, a paradigmatic substance undergoing change. For Kant, the unity of consciousness is just that, involving the notion of a subject of experience but telling us nothing about that subject. The preconditions for the application of this abstract, almost empty, yet indispensable notion of a transcendental subject of self (conceptually distinct from the empirical self or human animal) do not comprise knowledge of the nature of the subject, but lie wholly within the *content* of its experience: i.e. it must have experience of an objective natural world. The argument is too complex for paraphrase here, but its tenor may be indicated by the famous "Refutation of Idealism" (i.e. of scepticism or "empirical idealism"). Descartes' doubter rejects the sensory presentation of a material world, but finds the existence of an enduring self or "thinking thing" unproblematical. Kant argued, in effect, as follows. The notion of such a subject involves conceiving of its states as ordered objectively in time. An objective time-order presupposes a natural order in which regular change occurs in a substance subject to law, such as, in the external world, the movement of the earth in relation to the sun (i.e. if there were no dependable laws of nature, there would be no dependable clocks or ways of measuring time). Yet the only laws available to us are the physical laws which govern matter, so that it is only through its relation to the material world that we can conceive of a perceiving self with states ordered in time. Therefore the Cartesian sceptic's position is incoherent – he rejects what he needs in order to conceive of himself as the pure subject of a unitary consciousness. What is wrong with this argument, however, is that it does not go far enough – it is still, in a sense, too "Cartesian". For it assumes that the unity of consciousness carries with it the notion of a self, even if a self of which we know nothing, conceptually distinct from the "empirical" or bodily self, the human being. Yet it is arguable that experience and thought are so much more integrated than even Kant claims, that it is the bodily self itself which is experienced as the subject of experience.

Nevertheless, like no other philosopher in the canon, Kant directs our attention to the interconnections and interdependencies between structural features of our experience and system of beliefs, and for this he can be thanked even by those who do not share his idealist view that the whole of that structure is due to us, and that none of it reflects the impingement on us of reality itself. Yet the comprehensiveness and *a priori* rigidity of his theory has made it as vulnerable as any dogmatic metaphysics. Non-Euclidean geometry, Relativity and Quantum Mechanics have seemed to disprove central Kantian contentions as to how we must think of an objective world. Consequently it is not surprising that neo-idealist theory has shaped itself round the idea of mutability: categories may be important, but they are open to amendment, gradual or revolutionary. The idea that even what seems fundamental in the structure of human thought is liable to change has in any case appealed to those philosophers after Kant who have been inclined to see at least a large part of the structure as socially and historically determined.

Both motives have tended to enhance the role ascribed to language. Within the analytic tradition neo-idealism commonly sees itself as concerned not with the transcendental structure of the mind, but with a mutable "conceptual scheme" realized in language. For current Pragmatism, generally speaking, the scheme is a quasi-scientific theory (even if a "folk" theory), and the pressure for change comes from the pressure to achieve successful predictions. For others, language owes its structure, not to quasi-scientific theorizing, but to the social practices or "language-games" in which it is employed. Idealism of either kind tends to give a blanketing, cover-all, if not dismissive response to a traditional inquiry of some interest: i.e. "How much of the world as we apprehend it, or of the structure of our experience and thought of it, is due to reality, how much to the mechanisms of perception and thought, how much to mutable theory or assumption, and how much to contingent human purposes, social structures or conventions?" Another view, more in the spirit of the realist naturalism of Hobbes or Locke than the constructivism of Hume, Kant, Wittgenstein or Quine (or, for that matter, Derrida or Rorty), is that that question deserves a more complex, sober and discriminating answer than idealism can give. Although a part of the correct answer may reveal itself in and through the structure of language, it is not simply a matter of the primacy of that structure. Here, indeed, it is appropriate for a philosopher to pause, and to pay attention to the observations and hypotheses of those who have engaged in the empirical study of cognition.

# 15. Hallucinations: selected historical and clinical aspects

G.E. Berrios

---

Hallucinations are here discussed as verbal reports of "sensory" experiences, with or without insight, not vouchsafed by a relevant stimulus (Berrios, 1985a). Hallucinations are a common occurrence in general psychiatric and neurological practice, and the issue of their clinical meaning remains an important one.

There are excellent accounts of the evolution of the concept of hallucination but few in the English language (Ey, 1973; Paulus, 1941; Quercy, 1930; Mourgue, 1932; James, 1986; Morsier, 1969). Experiences redolent of hallucinations are part of the common baggage of humanity (Quercy, 1930; Critchley, 1987). Reported under a variety of names, such experiences were, in earlier times, culturally integrated and semantically pregnant, i.e. their content was believed to carry a message for the individual or the world. That this feature of hallucinations has been mostly lost is a consequence of their "medicalization" during the 18th century. Classifications dating from this period started by regarding hallucinations as independent "diseases"; indeed, the view that they were "symptoms", i.e. fragments of behaviour which could be seen in different diseases is a 19th century invention.

The writings of two men, Nicolaï and Berbiguier, one German and the other French, set the stage for the 19th century debate on whether hallucinations necessarily were a sign of insanity (p. 77) (Ey, 1973). In 1791, Nicolai reported that he had been under much stress and "suddenly observed, at the distance of ten paces, the figure of a deceased person"; i.e. he seemed to be describing episodes of hallucinosis with preservation of insight. In 1821, Alexis Vincent Charles Bergiguier de Terre-Neuve du Thym[1] (for notes see end of chapter) reported complex hallucinatory and delusional experiences; his case became the paradigm for insane hallucinations during the 19th century.

Esquirol brought all hallucinatory phenomena under a common term. In doing so, he not only created an abstract concept but, by choosing a word whose etymology was linked to vision, imposed a restrictive "model" of perception to all sense modalities (Esquirol, 1817). Five of Esquirol's original cases had visual hallucinations. He stated: "If a man has the intimate conviction of actually perceiving a sensation for which there is no external object, he is in a hallucinated state:[2] he is a visionary (visionnaire)" (Esquirol, 1838). "Hallucinations of vision... have been called visions but this term is appropriate only for one perceptual mode. Who would want to talk about auditory visions, taste visions, olfactory visions?... A generic term is needed. I propose the word hallucination." (Esquirol, 1838).

Esquirol's view, borrowed from Condillac (1947) assumed that all sense modalities were symmetrical, i.e. that like vision and audition, they required a *public stimulus*.[3] Esquirol's insistence on the "central" origin of hallucinations was a major departure from the peripheralist views of Hartley and others.

Baillarger supported the view that there was an analogy between dreams and hallucinations. He felt, that two types of dream had to be distinguished: simple and "purely intellectual" and another "accompanied by sensory hallucinations". He also studied the mode of production of hallucinations and concluded that the initial element in all hallucinations had to be the intellect (Baillarger, 1846b).

In 1855, there was a famous debate at the Société Médico-Psychologique. Three issues were discussed: could hallucinations ever be considered as "normal" experiences? Did sensation, image and hallucination form a continuum? Were hallucinations, dreams, and ecstatic trance similar states? No firm conclusions were ever reached.

Tamburini (1881) published a classical paper suggesting that hallucinations were not a "psychiatric" problem. His paper: (1) brought under one explanation psychiatric and neurological hallucinations, (2) articulated a testable hypothesis (at least, in relation to hallucinations seen in neurological conditions), (3) legitimatized the use of the language and methods of neurophysiology in the field of insanity, and (4) simplified the old "insanity" view of hallucinations by developing a mechanistic account of their genesis, thereby doing away with preoccupations about meaning.

These four views have fared differently in the history of hallucinations. The first three have endured and govern research (mainly by neurologists) into hallucinations (Berrios, 1985b) for example, (Penfield and Porot, 1963; Gloor et al., 1982; Halgren et al., 1978; Hausser-Hauw and Bancaud, 1987). The great psychiatric question, however, has remained: are the findings of cortical physiology relevant to the hallucinations of schizophrenia, mania or psychotic depression? The fourth view has been much opposed; both psychoanalytic thinkers and conventional alienists have been loath to give up the semantic approach to hallucinations.

The unitary and reductionistic view suggested by Tamburini has since given way to the notion of "hallucinosis" (Berrios, 1985b). This category encompasses all hallucinatory experiences related to neurological disorder. Functional, psychiatric or psychotic hallucinations were, once again, set asunder on the psychological and semantic path.

But the neurologization of hallucinations also had negative consequences. It led to a reactive over-emphasis on semantics and psychodynamics and in the time elapsed between Freud and Ey, "insane hallucinations" (Faure, 1965) and "hallucinosis" (Ey, 1957) became different phenomena. This postponed the neurobiological analysis of psychiatric hallucinations. Neurologists, on their part, were given *carte blanche* to explore the symptom, apparently untrammelled by questions of meaning; thus, limiting the understanding of "psychotic" hallucinations (Morsier, 1938; Sutter, 1962). During the 1960s, interest in psychodelic drugs led to suggestions that an experimental model for all hallucinations might have been found (West, 1962; Keup, 1970; Siegel and West, 1975) but this came to nothing. Linguists (Castilla del Pino, 1984; Morenon and Morenon, 1991) and psychologists (Slade and Bentall, 1988) have done their best to offer new approaches, but the neurobiological dimension remains neglected. A positive result of Tamburini's work, however, was to reawaken interest in hallucinations in the sane. A typical example of this is the so-called Charles Bonnet syndrome.

## Charles Bonnet and his Syndrome

The report by the Swiss philosopher Bonnet [4] on the hallucinations affecting his grandfather has become as well known as the writings of Nicolaï and Berbiguier. Charles Lullin, an 89-year-old magistrate saw "without any external stimuli the image of men, women, birds, buildings that changed in shape, size and place but which he never accepted as real. The gentleman in question [having] had, at an advanced age, cataract operations on both eyes." (Bonnet, 1769). Although it is not clear from the text, it would seem that the operations had been performed *before* the hallucinatory episode. Bonnet concluded that these hallucinations "had their seat in the part of the brain which contains the organ of vision".

Morsier coined the eponym "Charles Bonnet syndrome" (Morsier, 1936) and endeavoured to show that there was "no correlation between onset of the visual hallucinations and eye pathology"; in five of his cases (out of 15), hallucinations had developed while the subject had normal vision (Morsier, 1967). He defined the syndrome as: "visual hallucinations in elderly patients, without evidence of cognitive impairment and unrelated aetiologically to peripheral problems of vision". He suggested that the cause was to be found in the brain itself.

The syndrome was introduced into Anglo-Saxon psychiatry in 1982 (Berrios and Brook, 1982; Damas Mora *et al.*, 1982). Since then, a much wider definition has been suggested consisting of any state of visual hallucinations in the elderly irrespective of accompanying symptomatology. For example, in spite of recent efforts to make it a meaningful phenomenon (Podoll *et al.*, 1989; Fuchs and Lauter, 1992) hallucinatory states related to dementia (Burgermeister *et al.*, 1964), ocular surgery (Ajurriaguerra and Garrone, 1965) and decreased visual acuity (Hécaen and Albert, 1978) are made to qualify for the title. It seems that there is little point in using such eponym to refer to all or any visual hallucinatory states in the elderly.

## Parapsychology, Statistics and Hallucinations

By the second half of the 19th century, it had become clear that single case studies were not sufficient. Help came from unlikely quarters in the shape of the Society for Psychical Research, founded in Cambridge 1882 by its three leading lights: Gurney, Myers and Sidgwick (Williams, 1985).

It started when Gurney[5] published in 1885 a review on hallucinations (Gurney, 1885; Gurney et al., 1886). Next came the Society's support for a survey into these experiences; the first "statistical inquiry" being carried out under the direction of Gurney, and its results reported in his book "Phantasms of the Living" (Parish, 1897). Parallel surveys had been carried out under the direction of W. James (1890) in the USA, L. Marillier (1890) in France, and Von Schrenck-Notzing in Germany. An important priming role was also played by James Sully's work who defined "illusions" in a wide sense,[6] and included information on perception, dreams, hallucinations, delusions and paramnesias. The Society for Psychical Research, however, was not interested in hallucinations *per se*, but in the fact that they might be a manifestation of the paranormal (Sidgwick, 1889-1894).

## Tactile Hallucinations

In current psychiatry, the psychopathology of touch has become subordinated to other symptoms and no longer commands diagnostic interest. This reflects both its relative infrequency and some uneasiness concerning the concepts involved in its definition. Since Greek times, touch has been a reluctant "fifth sense". Aristotle (1968) considered it as a primitive perceptual system and remarked upon the features setting it apart from the "distance" senses.[7] This view remained unchanged until the 17th century when British empiricism developed an interest in the epistemology of touch. Locke rejected the Cartesian view according to which extension constitutes the essence of material substance. He maintained also that all bodies possess the fundamental quality of "solidity" which he defined as: "the idea most intimately connected with and essential to body, so as nowhere else to be found or imagined but only in matter". This idea "we receive by our touch: and it arises from the resistance which we find in body to the entrance of any other body into the place it possess, till it has left it." (Locke, 1959).

The epistemological inquiry into what are the bodily components that suggest the idea of solidity led to the identification of "feelings of resistance" and "motor sensations" which conveyed superior information to "mere feelings". Armstrong (1962) has expressed it thus: "For all forms of sense perception beside seeing, hearing, tasting and smelling we employ the word feeling nevertheless it will be convenient to distinguish between at least two sorts of sense perception covered by the word 'feel': perception by touch and perception of our own bodily state". This distinction was introduced in psychology by Weber as *Tastsinn* (touch) and *Gemeingefuhl* (common sensibility) (Weber, 1846). These categories provided late 19th century psychiatrists with a framework to classify phenomena as widely apart as tactile hallucinations, neurasthenia, coenesthopathy, and depersonalization.

Descriptions of "imaginary itches" can be found in earlier literature. Darwin reported a case with diabetes who experienced "a hallucinated idea (an itch) so powerfully excited that it was not to be changed suddenly by ocular sensation or reason". (Darwin, 1796). In a Lockean vein, Esquirol (1838) wrote "touch, often appealed to by reason to correct the other senses may also deceive the insane. He may hallucinate rough surfaces or sharp ends hurting his skin, he may feel torn apart by cutting instruments." Sigmond observed that "hallucinations of touch vary exceedingly; it is singular enough to find an individual who believes that he has rats crawling over him, that spiders infest him." (Sigmond, 1848). Griesinger made the fundamental observation that in touch "hallucinations and illusions cannot be distinguished from each other; or rather the phenomena which constitute them, so far as they do not depend on anaesthesia, are in every case to be considered as illusions because the specific anomaly consists in the false interpretation of certain sensations." (Griesinger, 1861).

Brierre de Boismont stated "it is said that hallucinations of touch are difficult to investigate because they are apt to be confounded with neurological affections... there can be no question that there are some hallucinated persons quite capable of judging correctly of their sensations." (Brierre de Boismont, 1862; Azouvi, 1984). Brierre believed that on physical examination there was nothing neurologically wrong with patients experiencing tactile hallucinations. Tuke did not separate tactile from internal or corporal hallucinations and included under "tactile hallucinatory experiences" "electrical shock", "delusion of being changed or Lycantropy" and "sexual hallucinations" (Tuke, 1892). Storring (1907) included all these under "hallucinations of the cutaneous sense": "In delirium tremens patients often have hallucinatory sensations of spiders creeping over their skin, of ants running over them or of being covered by a fur." He also included more complex experiences "they frequently complained of electrical currents traversing their bodies. Others feel as if they were being kissed, or as if someone were lying by their side".

Classical writers already knew that cocaine could produce tactile hallucinations (Maier, 1928). For example, Magnan and Saury (1889) described how their patients tried to remove bugs from under their skin. De Clerambault (1942) described these as hypodermic, distal and punctiform hallucinations, and believed they were often accompanied by "sensations of movement" and involvement of consciousness. Tactile hallucinations following intoxication by *Atropa Belladona* were described by Moreau de Tours (1845) who reported a case who felt "that millions of insects were devouring his head." These states have been classically likened to feeling ants crawling under the skin. Terms coined to describe these sensations were *Psora Imaginaria* (Imaginary itch) (Darwin, 1796) and *formication*.[8]

## The Concept of Cénesthopathie

This very French notion (Dupré, 1913) reflects well the earlier German conceptual distinction between skin senses (*Tastsinn*) and common feeling (*Gemeingefuhl*). The latter refers to all the corporal sensations that remain once those associated with the skin (i.e. touch, temperature, pressure, and location) are separated off. Thus, it includes pain and "objectless" sensations such as well-being, pleasure, fatigue, shudder, hunger, nausea, organic muscular feeling, etc. This group of sensations was also called *coenesthesia* (Hamilton, 1859) and considered by some as the basis for a "sense of existence" (Gantheret, 1961). To explain such bodily feeling of "unity", two theories were put forward. Associationism stated that coenesthesia resulted from a *summation* of proprioceptive and interoceptive sensations (Taine, 1890); faculty psychology, on the other hand, postulated the existence of a hypothetic *brain centre* or function on which sensations converged; the resulting somatognostic pattern consisting in a Gestalt-type of account. This mechanism also provided the basis for the "body schema" (Schilder, 1923; Critchley, M. 1950; Gantheret, 1961; López Ibor and López Ibor, 1974). Soon after its inception, however, the functional territory of coenesthesia underwent erosion in that hunger, thirst, sexual pleasure, etc. began to be separated off and studied independently. In the end, all that was left were sensations common to various organs such as deep pressure, pain, and unanalyzable sensations such as "tickling" or "stuffiness" (Titchener, 1901).

It is at this stage that the term *cénesthopathie* entered into French psychiatry as a "local alteration of the common sensibility in the sphere of general sensation, corresponding to hallucinosis in the sphere of sensorium." (Dupré, 1913). Two large groups of coenesthopathies – "painful" and "paraesthesic" – were recognized and each divided into cephalic, thoracic and abdominal. Patients in the painful group felt their organs "stretched, torn, twisted"; and in the paraesthesic group experienced itching, hyperaesthesiae, paraesthesiae, etc. The syndrome was never accepted in Anglo-Saxon psychiatry where such symptoms were recatalogued as hypochondriasis, neurasthenia or dysmorphophobia (Reilly and Beard, 1976; Thomas, 1984). In France itself some *coenesthopathies,* for example *topalgie* (or cephalic coenestopathy), were later reclassified as "neurovegetative dystonias" (Bernard and Trouve, 1977) or psychosomatic syndromes (Ey, 1950). Others studied the same phenomena as "disorders of the corporal scheme", "subjective disorders of sensibility" and "psychoneuroses" (Ladee, 1966). Other states, such as chronic tactile hallucinosis or delusional parasitosis became quasi-independent entities.

## Delusional Parasitosis

This complex clinical phenomenon, alternatively considered as a hallucinosis or a delusional state, consists of complaints, in clear consciousness, of body infestation by insects or parasites; visual hallucinations may complicate the picture. Early descriptions of "itchy dermatoses" (Brocq, 1892), "acarophobia" (Thiébierge, 1894) and "parasitophobia" (Perrin, 1896) have given the impression that the syndrome was a phobia or a neurosis. This is not so (Berrios, 1994). Initially phobia, obsession and delusion were closely linked (as fixed ideas). Thus, Perrin considered "parasitophobia" as a hallucinatory state unaccompanied by anxiety or other affective disturbance! (Perrin, 1896). Perrin remained undecided as to whether the primary disorder was an "alteration of intellectual faculties" (i.e. a delusion) or a hallucination thereby starting an ambiguity which has remained to the present day. (For the subsequent history of these concepts see Berrios, 1982, 1985a; Leon et al., 1992).

## The "Hallucination of the Double"

One of the better known subtypes of hallucination is the so-called "phenomenon of the double" (also called autoscopy, heautoscopy, Doppelganger, etc.). It is defined by most as a report of a perception (usually visual but occasionally "affective" or "emotional") or an image of the self present in public space, "as if reflected in a mirror". The vision may be fleeting or durable, of the whole person or parts thereof, fully-bodied or transparent and veil-like, and is accompanied by an emotional response: the subject may interpret it as a portent, as a provider of comfort, or (often enough) feel it to be an extension of his own body.

Three conclusions impress themselves on anyone perusing the literature (both medical and non-medical) on heautoscopy: one is its repetitiveness; another its vagueness and lack of definition (i.e. several phenomena seem to be talked about); yet another that its size far exceeds any hard clinical knowledge.

This is not surprising. Medical writings on heautoscopy would be thin indeed if they did not borrow cases from fiction writers who either experienced it themselves (McCulloch, 1992) or used the phenomenon as a trick to create an emotional atmosphere (Tymms, 1949; Miller, 1985). Indeed, no proper clinical series [9] seems to have been published so far, the medical literature being based on anecdotal reports repeated again and again.[10] Little is known on the natural history, clinical presentation, meaning and aetiology of this phenomenon; indeed, it is not even clear whether it should always be classified as a hallucination. At this stage, therefore, the medical importance of heautoscopy cannot be said to match its putative socio-anthropological, psychodynamic, or even para-psychological significance (Rank, 1971; Abse, 1976).

Whether medical or not, the concept itself is embedded in a wider nest of beliefs. The widest concerns "bilocation", i.e. the reported capacity of some people to be in two places at the same time. This para-normal rather than medical phenomenon, is based on the assumption that human beings may dissociate into two material bodies or into a material and an "aetherial" moiety. Bilocation is related to another paranormal notion, namely, the "astral body": this refers to a hypothetical "body" of fine matter constituting a link between the terrestrial body and a high astral representation. Since the times of Paracelsus and Du Prel (if not before) it has been believed that such astral body is the carrier of psychical energy (indeed, most religions and cultures seem to include in their belief-system analogical forms of such "meta organism") (Bonin, 1976).

Heautoscopy is also related to another belief, the "out-of-body" experience, which [11] is defined as "an experience where the mind or awareness is separated from the physical body" (Twemlow et al., 1982) and which may occur in near-death situations. Once again, this notion assumes that some sort of temporary dissociation has taken place: indeed, some writers have included the criterion that the spiritual component of the experience must "see" the somatic body from its position in space (Green, 1968).

In addition to para-normal states, heautoscopy has been reported as associated with "clinical" concepts such as depersonalization, derealization, déjà vu, hypnagogic and dissociation states, misidentification syndromes, hysteria (McConnell, 1965) grief (Maack and Mullen, 1983) mental handicap (Collacott and Deb, 1988), puerperium (Craske and Sacks, 1969), and neurological disease (Hécaen and Green, 1957; Nouet, 1923; Conrad, 1953).

There is no *a priori* reason to believe that the experience of seeing the image of one's self is historically recent or culturally dependent upon Western ideas. Most writings on heautoscopy refer to the fact that Aristotle had already reported the case of a man who persistently saw his image.[12] It matters little when the experience was first described. By the time descriptive psychopathology was being constituted during the 19th century, the symptom was well known: Wigan reported one case (Todd and Dewhurst, 1955), Griesinger (1861) two,[13] and following the German, Brierre de Boismont called it *deuteroscopie*.[14] The term *Doppelganger,* used (incorrectly) to refer to heautoscopy was coined by Jean Paul Richter[15] early in the 19th century to refer to the phenomenon of "bilocation" (called *Varödgr* by the Norwegians).[16] *Austocopie* (Féré, 1891; Lemaitre, 1902; Sollier, 1903) was used up to the early 20th century, but it was felt that it did not actually refer to the perception of the self by self, and was replaced by *héautoscopie* (Menninger-Lerchenthal, 1935; L'Hermitte, 1951*b*; Hécaen and Ajuriaguerra, 1952). The terms *hallucination spéculaire* (Féré, 1891) and *Spiegelphantom* (Conrad, 1953) did not catch on.

Between 1890 and the first World War, the main features of the phenomenon were described (Féré, 1891; Lemaitre, 1902; Comar, 1901; Sollier, 1903, 1908*a,b*; Naudascher, 1910) and most publications since have simply footnoted earlier discoveries. This impasse will only be overcome when adequate case-series are reported and both clinical and neurobiological markers duly collected.

## Clinical aspects

There is little evidence (other than its surface description) that the experience of the double reported by creative writers is necessarily related to that seen in patients with functional or organic psychiatric disease. Economy of thought and the need to offer a common explanatory hypothesis have encouraged writers to bring these experiences together.

The experience itself seems to include the following features: a subject (no gender effect has been reported) will suddenly "see" (occasionally "feel") in front of him (usually few yards away, although doubles walking or standing on the side of the individual have also been reported) a figure which is recognized (either immediately or after some observation) as being that of the self. Recognition is not necessarily based on its being an exact copy; indeed, the image may be with its back to the observer or not well formed – nonetheless it is "felt" to be the self. Occasionally, only parts of the body (usually head or bust) are seen, a curious feature being that the surroundings may occasionally be "seen" through the "eyes" of the double.[17]

The experience may occur when the subject is alert or when tired and dreamy or when in fact he is asleep (it is probably unwise to lump this latter experience with the others). The vision may occur once in a life time or repeat itself; it is mostly involuntary, although on a few occasions individuals might elicit it at will; it tends to last only few seconds, although it may be persistent to the point that the observer has time to approach the image, shake hands, or talk to it. The image is mostly silent although the observer, somehow, feels that he knows what it is in "its mind"; indeed, often it is the double that holds all thoughts, is active and full of energy whilst the observer feels passive and empty (this has given rise to the belief that heautoscopy occurs during depersonalization). The double may be stationary, recede from the observer, or come to him. Commonly, the double is perceived as an image reflected in a mirror (although it may not look identical, not be a "mirror-image" nor be dressed as the observer; this is the origin of the French notion of *image spéculaire*.

The emotional reaction of the observer tends to consist of a feeling of bewilderment and/or warmth (rather than fear). Somehow, he feels "linked" or joined to the double in a particular way: sometimes as a projection of the self, or as its complementary part. Again, since the time of Sollier (1903) this feeling of belonging has been considered as specific. On occasions, particularly when the observer is in an anxious or depressed state of mind, the vision of the double may offer comfort.

## Associations and mechanisms

No statistical information is available as to the incidence or prevalence of this phenomenon, nor on its co-morbidity. To judge by the number of cases reported in the medical literature (and their repetitive nature) it can be concluded that the phenomenon is rare. So, there might be little point in trying to identify a particular disease or mechanism with which heautoscopy is particularly associated. As far as this writer knows, no neurobiological markers have been reported: this partially results from the fact that some cases date from the time when neuro-imaging and other techniques had not yet developed; furthermore, few of these ever reached the post-mortem slab. The fact that some of the 19th century writers who reported the experience were known to suffer from epilepsy, neurosyphilis, or acute infectious diseases, led to the speculation that these conditions may increase the likelihood of heautoscopy. However, the phenomenon is nowadays rarely if ever reported in relation to epilepsy; whether or not general paralysis of the insane is important is unlikely to be known as not enough cases can be mustered for an adequate study.

However, there is little reason to believe that these diseases provided special pathological conditions for the symptom to develop. As to other mental and neurological disorders, all that can be said is that although they remain common, heautoscopy is rarely counted amongst their symptoms. This has drawn attention to personality characteristics or psychodynamic mechanisms (or both), and interestingly enough, the literature on the latter is more extensive than on the former. Indeed, little can be said on "type" of personality unless some empirical research (and this is hampered by both the small number of patients and the bluntness of the measuring instruments) is carried out. Of course, it is not difficult to propound that subjects with a tendency to anxiety, depersonalization, dissociation, suggestibility, and eidetic imagery are prone to experiencing heautoscopy; there is, however, little evidence to support any of these speculations. What is worse, whilst this type of personality is common, heautoscopy is very rare.

**Other Types of Hallucination**

Although early in the 19th century Baillarger offered a clear description of *unilateral hallucinations,* these interesting phenomena became a popular field of investigation only after 1880 (Hammond, 1885; Higier, 1994; Lamy, 1895; Wormser, 1895; Féré, 1896; Joffroy, 1896; Lugaro, 1904). This is likely to have been due to Tamburini's return to a peripheralist explanation (Robertson, 1881, 1901; Regis, 1881; Toulouse, 1892). Recent work seems to suggest that musical hallucinations are more common in elderly females suffering from deafness; acute and short lived *musical hallucinations* are seen in stroke and depression and rarely need treatment; persistent states, such as those seen accompanied by deafness and minor cognitive impairment may lead to much unhappiness and reactive depression and must be treated; some cases, particularly those related to epileptic foci, respond well to carbamazepine (Berrios, 1990*a*).

*Peduncular hallucinations* were first described by L'Hermitte (1922) and because of this is was said that "he had opened the new chapter of mesencephalic psychiatry." (Van Bogaert, 1927). In two papers, L'Hermitte described florid visual hallucinations, without insight, which he put down to a disorder of dreaming caused by a lesion in the red nucleus and/or neighbouring areas: "The hallucinated patient is therefore someone who is dreaming whilst awake, someone in whom the function of sleep is severely disordered." (p. 434) (L'Hermitte, 1932). The hallucinations tended to get worse in the evening and it is likely that some of these subjects were in a delirious state.

*Lilliputian hallucinations* consist in the "vision of small people, men or women of minute or slightly variable height. They are mobile, coloured, generally multiple. Sometimes it is a theatre of small marionettes, scenes in miniature... the subject sometimes hears the small people talk, when the voice assumes a lilliputian tone." (Leroy, 1922). The hallucinations have no diagnostic value and can be seen in both organic and functional disorders.

*Hallucinations of smell and taste* were described by Baillarger and considered to be rare. This may be one explanation why little attention was and is paid to these disorders; yet another explanation may have to do with the general point that there seems to have been in France a cultural and scientific ambivalence towards the phenomenon of olfaction itself (Corbin, 1986). In 1905, Leroy reported the case of a woman who smelt around her a terrible smell and also heard voices (Leroy, 1905) and Wedensky (1912) reported that olfactory hallucinations might herald bouts of drinking in alcoholics. Durand (1955) has offered a full historical review of these important phenomena (Bullen, 1899; Ey, 1973).

Although the *phantom limb phenomenon* was well described earlier in the 19th century (and indeed before), it only became of interest during its second half.[18] In 1861, Gueniot called the experience "subjective heretotopia of the limbs" and a "hallucination" (p. 423) (Gueniot, 1861). Mitchell (1871) is credited with having coined the term "phantom limb" ten years later. Major monographs have been published on the topic (Arondel, 1902; Culbetian, 1902; Katz, 1992).

## Hallucinations in the Elderly

Based on the fact that no firm experimental evidence has yet become available that subjects reporting having a hallucination are necessarily experiencing or reading-off a percept, the existence of the symptom has occasionally been called into question, and the suggestion made that it may often be a form of "sensory delusion" (Ey, 1973). This view is particularly applicable to "true" or "psychiatric" hallucinations, where the reported features of the "percept" seem to violate the rules of perception (as, for example, in unilateral, extracampine or composite hallucinations). "Organic" hallucinations or hallucinosis such as those accompanying delirium tremens or drug intoxication, i.e. (Berrios, 1985b; Morsier, 1938) seem, a different phenomenon. Such hallucinations can be experimentally induced (Siegel and Jarvik, 1975) and have, since the last century, been related to dreaming breaking into consciousness (Lasègue, 1971). Although separate types of hallucination have been singled out for special study such as Lilliputian, peduncular, functional, extracampine, heautoscopic, negative, verbal and unilateral hallucinations (Berrios, 1985b) this has rarely led to the identification of a firm clinical predictor.

In the elderly the distinction between psychiatric and organic hallucinosis becomes less clear-cut. The type of hallucinations often seen in this age group also leads to another clinical problem, namely, that of separating hallucinations occurring in sense modalities related to public (vision and audition) and private stimuli (touch and proprioception): i.e. that of differentiating between a real and a hallucinated itch. This is particularly problematic when cognitive impairment is present.

Hallucinations in the elderly (Berrios, 1992) involve all sense modalities, and remain a cause of concern amongst care-givers (Haley, 1987). Prevalence figures, once again based on hospital samples, range between 15% (Eastwood and Corbin, 1983) and 30% (Berrios and Brook, 1984). The differential strength of risk factors such as age, pre-morbid personality, sensory deficits, and sex remains unclear. However, a recent study suggests that visual hallucinations increase with age (Anonymous, 1990). In regard to pre-morbid personality, Eastwood and Corbin (1983) reported that hallucinators tended to be single, to have been living alone prior to admission, and have an "independent" or "reclusive" personality. Other reports suggest that sensory deficits (Slade, 1976) and being female (Berrios, 1990a) increase the risk of hallucinations.

Conventional classifications of hallucinations by sense modality, disease, presence of insight, and/or accompanying symptoms may be less adequate in the elderly for, as mentioned above, a shift has taken place in this age group towards the organic end of the causal continuum. In order to construct a proper database in this area, it would seem advisable simply to describe the hallucination and its context. The latter may range from states of apparent cerebral normality (so-called Charles Bonnet syndrome), to those where there is clear brain pathology. As mentioned above, confusion reigns in regard to the Charles Bonnet syndrome (Berrios and Brook, 1982; Podoll et al., 1989); for example, some seem to believe that sensory deprivation is the essence of this phenomenon, so that an apparently "normal" elderly subject who hallucinates but has no eye-sight troubles is denied the appellative (Schneck, 1990). The issue remains, however, whether visual impairment alone is a sufficient and necessary cause for hallucinations in subjects otherwise showing no evidence of neurological or psychiatric disease: one problem with this view is the obvious discrepancy between the high frequency of peripheral visual defect in the elderly and the rarity of the Charles Bonnet phenomenon. It is likely, therefore, that a second, central factor is in operation; what this factor may be is conjectural, and may range from some unknown genetic tendency to hallucinate – coded, say, by what one could speculate to be a hallucinator's gene – to the more likely presence of (undetected) cerebral pathology.

"Provoked" or drug-induced hallucinations are common in the elderly as attested by papers reporting toxic hallucinations – both simple or formed – and in all sense modalities (Brown et al., 1980; Chinisci, 1985; Sonnenblick et al., 1982; Gardner and Hall, 1982). It is in the nature of anecdotal clinical reporting that these studies are uncontrolled and hence suggest little by way of risk factors. For example, is the triggering of hallucinations dose-related? What are the relevant host variables? etc.

Hallucinations in the elderly can be seen as a unitary symptom such as delusional parasitosis (Berrios, 1982, 1985a; Bourgeois et al., 1986) and the hallucinations of widowhood (Olson et al., 1985) or as part of another condition such as Alzheimer's disease. In regard to the latter, it is not widely known that the first "case" ever reported exhibited auditory hallucinations (Berrios and Freeman, 1991). Recent interest in the "psychiatric aspects" of Alzheimer's disease (Wragg and Jeste, 1989) has led to a series of papers some suggesting that senile dementia of the Lewy body type (SDLT) is more often accompanied by visual hallucinations than Alzheimer's disease (Perry et al., 1990a) and that a reduction in cortical choline acetyl-transferase is more marked amongst hallucinators (Perry et al., 1990b). This finding ties in well with what is known of the role of acetylcholine in the control of REM (rapid eye movement) sleep activity.

Hallucinations in the elderly are likely to be multidetermined. Explanations originating in experimental psychology (Bentall, 1990) and neurobiology, albeit attractive, are articulated at a high level of generality, and hence are not readily applicable to individual cases. Explanations originating in clinical psychiatry tend to be anecdotal and mostly based on casual correlations. There are reasons for this divorce between the theoretical and clinical approach: first, since the 19th century, no real improvement has taken place in the quality of the concepts marshalled to examine hallucinatory phenomena (Mourgue, 1932; Berrios, 1982; Paulus, 1941); second, advances made on the experimental psychology (Slade and Bentall, 1988) and neurobiology of perception have been only partially tried in the field of hallucinations; indeed, a great specialist in the physiology of perception once told this writer that hallucinations had little to do with his field of inquiry; third, the type of statistical analysis used in most psychiatric studies does not allow any causal connections to be drawn. Finally, even the putative relevance to diagnosis of sensory modality and/or theme has been called into question (Lowe, 1973).

In the case of the elderly, all explanatory models seem to apply. This is, for example, the case with the views put forward by Jackson (Marazzi, 1962; West, 1962) according to which the release of "lower" centres and consequent "experiencing" of hallucinations might be due to a loss of inhibition; and also with the deafferentation model suggested by Fischer (Fischer, 1969; Fischer *et al.*, 1970), based on the view that hallucinations result from a loss of balance between sensory/sensory or sensory/motor inputs. In this regard, the elderly present the best examples of cases where there is both a decline in sensory input (caused by deficits in the windows of perception) and motor activity (caused by physical disabilities). Equally applicable to the elderly is the model according to which hallucinations result from mechanical and/or electrical irritation of relevant brain sites (Miller *et al.*, 1987; Tamburini, 1881; Berrios, 1990*b*). Indeed, there is evidence that strokes, tumours, and epilepsy might play a role (Berrios, 1990*a*).

In summary, there seems to be an increased incidence and prevalence of hallucinations in the elderly, and this regardless of whether cognitive impairment is present, the effect being more marked in women. Two hypotheses are available to explain this high frequency: one says that hallucinations are disease-related, the other that they are ageing-related. No concepts specially tailored to account for hallucinations in the elderly are available but models developed for the young seem to apply; these include the mechanisms of release, de-afferentation, loss of balance between sensory and motor inputs, and irritation.

## Notes

1   See excellent account by Lechner (1983).

2   Esquirol brought into circulation a term with an ambiguous etymology for which three origins have been suggested. Firstly, *hallucinatio* or *hallucinari* which means to err or to abuse; secondly the Greek "alo" meaning "uncertainty" or "licentiousness of spirit"; and finally, *ad lucem, adlucinor, hallucinator* i.e. terms relating to light or illumination (see p. 77, Christian, 1886, *op. cit.*)

3   Thus, Esquirol built into his definition of hallucination as a "perception without object" the logical requirement of an absence of external and public object. This has created problems for the rest of sensory modalities such as taste, touch and internal sensations where the public criterion cannot be implemented and hence the distinction between a real itch and a halucinated one becomes impossible unless external criteria (not belonging in the definition) are used.

4   Charles Bonnet (1720-1793) was a Swiss naturalist and philosopher, and a follower of David Hartley's theory of association of ideas.

5   Edmund Gurney (1847-1888) was a fellow of Trinity College, Cambridge. A restless scholar, he studied classics, music, medicine, and the law, but stayed at none. One of the founders of the Society for Psychical Research, he participated in the survey on apparitions and extraordinary forms of human communication. He suffered from a cyclothymic personality, and died in Brighton after having taken an overdose of sleeping pills.

6   James Sully (1842-1923) was an English psychologist who became Grote professor of mind and logic at the University of London. He wrote: "The phenomena of illusion have ordinarily been investigated by alienists, that is to say, physicians who are brought face to face with their most striking forms in the mentally deranged. While there are very good reasons for this treatment of illusion as a branch of mental pathology, it is by no means certain that it can be a complete and exhaustive one"...[however] "there is the view that all men habitually err, or that illusion is to be regarded as the natural condition of mortals", p.2, Sully, 1895, *op. cit.*

7   "But there is a difference between the object of touch and those of sight and hearing, since we perceive them because the medium acts upon us while we perceive objects of touch not through the agency of the medium but simultaneously with the medium, like a man who is struck through the shield" (Aristotle, 1968).

8   Formication has been used in medicine since the time of Ambrosio Paré who described *pouls formicant* (formicant pulse) as "a weak, frequent pulse that gives the sensation of crawling like an ant" (Littré, 1878). The earliest usage in dermatology dates back to 1707 (Oxford English Dictionary).

9   The great original works in this field are: Sollier (1903), Féré (1891), Lemaitre (1902), Menninger-Lerchenthal (1935), Hécaen and Ajuriaguerra (1952), and Lunn (1970). Later papers, are heavily dependent upon these works: e.g. Lukianowicz (1958), Damas Mora *et al.* (1980), Faguet (1979), and Grotstein (1982).

10   For example: L'Hermitte (1951a,b), Dewhurst (1954), Todd and Dewhurst (1955), Dewhurst and Pearson (1955), Pearson and Dewhurst (1954).

11   The literature on this is also large; for history and lists of references see: Green (1968) and Twemlow et al. (1982).

12   It seems as if there has been some confusion as to where this report occurs. Some have related it to Antiphron, a madman whose delusions Aristotle reports in "Memory and Recollection". The report, in fact, occurs in *Meteorologica,* iii, 4 (McCulloch, 1992).

13   The cases of Tasso "who carried on a long conversation with his protecting spirit" (*Schutzgeist*) and "Van Helmont who saw his own soul with a human face (*mit menschlichem Gesicht*)" (p. 92) (Griesinger, 1861).

14   "Goethe reports having one day perceived the image of his own person coming to meet him. German psychiatrists have given the name of deuteroscopie to this variety of illusion" (p. 55) (Brierre de Boismont, 1862). Boismont does not give a reference to the German alienists in question. Interestingly enough, as late as 1877, deuteroscopie still appears in Littre's Grand Dictionary (Vol 2) with his earlier meaning of "nervous condition in which the patient purports to see objects which are in the future."

15   Better known as *Jean Paul*; see Doppelgänger in Bonin (1976).

16   So-called when the double is perceived only by hearing (see Smith, 1974).

17   This is clearly seen in the case of Zutt's (1953) epileptic young man who would see his own body from a point in the ceiling where he once was fixed before getting into a trance.

18   Charles Bell wrote: "The man whose arm has been amputated, has not merely the perception of pain being seated in the arm, but he has likewise a sense of its position. I have seen a young gentleman whose leg I amputated, making the motion of his hands to catch the leg and place it over the knee" (Bell, 1830; Furukawa, 1990).

**References**

Abse, D.W. (1976). Delusional identity and the double. *Psychiatry,* **39,** 163-175.
Ajurriaguerra, J. and Garrone, G. (1965). Désafferentation partialle et psychopathologie. *In* "Desafferentation Expérimentale et Clinique". (Symposium Bel Air II), pp. 91-157. Georg, Geneva.
Anonymous (1990). Psychiatrische symptomatologie en leeftijdsafhankelijkheid. Een preliminaire A.M.D.P. IV Studie bij 140 psychogeriatrische patienten. *Acta Neuropsychiatrica,* **3,** 55-60.
Aristotle, (1968). "De Anima," Books II and III (translated by D.W. Hamlyn). Clarendon Press, Oxford.
Armstrong, D.M. (1962). "Bodily Sensations". Routledge and Kegan Paul, London.
Arondel, A. (1898). "Sur les Hallucinations des Moignons". pp. 1-44. Paris.
Azouvi, F. (1984). Des sensations internes aux hallucinations corporelles: de Cabanis a Lélut. *Revue Internationale d'Histoire de la Psychiatrie,* **2,** 5-19.
Baillarger, J. (1846). Des hallucinations. *Mémoires de la Académie Royale de Médicine,* **12,**

273-475.
Bell, C. (1830). "The Nervous System of the Human Body". Longman, London.
Bentall, R.P. (1990). The illusion of reality: a review and integration of psychological research on hallucinations. *Psychological Bulletin*, **107**, 82-95.
Bernard, P. and Trouve, S. (1977). "Sémiologie Psychiatrique". Masson, Paris.
Berrios, G.E. (1982). Tactile hallucinations: conceptual and historical aspects. *Journal of Neurology, Neurosurgery, and Psychiatry*, **45**, 285-239.
Berrios, G.E. (1985a). Delusional parasitosis and physical disease. *Comprehensive Psychiatry*, **26**, 395-403.
Berrios, G.E. (1985b). Hallucinosis. *In* "Handbook of Clinical Neurology". Vol. 2. (46). (Ed. J.A.M. Frederiks). pp. 561-572. Elsevier, Amsterdam.
Berrios, G.E. (1990a). Musical hallucination. A historical and clinical study. *British Journal of Psychiatry*, **156**, 188-194.
Berrios, G.E. (1990b). A theory of hallucinations. *History of Psychiatry*, **1**, 145-150.
Berrios, G.E. (1992). Psychotic symptoms in the elderly: concepts and models. *In* "Delusions and Hallucinations in Old Age". (Eds C. Katona and R. Levy). pp. 3-14. Gaskell, London.
Berrios, G.E. (ed.) (1994). Anxiety and phobias. *In* "History of Mental Symptoms". (G.E. Berrios). Cambridge University Press, Cambridge (in the press).
Berrios, G.E. and Brook, P. (1982). The Charles Bonnet syndrome and the problem of visual perceptual disorders in the elderly. *Age and Ageing*, **11**, 17-23.
Berrios, G.E. and Brook, P. (1984). Visual hallucinations and sensory delusions in the elderly. *British Journal of Psychiatry*, **144**, 662-664.
Berrios, G.E. and Freeman, H.L. (Eds). (1991). "Alzheimer and the Dementias". Royal Society of Medicine, London.
Bonin, W.E. (1976). "Lexikon der Parapsychologie und ihrer Grenzgebiete". 2 Vols. Scherz, Bern.
Bonnet, Ch. (1769). "Essai Analytique sur les Facultés de l'Ame". 2nd Edn. Vol. 14, Fauche, Neuchatel.
Bourgeois, M., Rager, P., Peyre, F., Nguyen, L.A. *et al.* (1986). Fréquence et aspects du syndrome d'Ekbom enquête auprès des dermatologues francais. *Annales Médico-Psychologiques*, **144**, 659-668.
Brierre de Boismont, A. (1862). "Des Hallucinations". Baillière, Paris.
Brocq, L. (1892). Quelques apercus sur les dermatoses prurigineuses. *Annales de Dermatologie et Syphiligraphie*, **3**, 1100.
Brown, M.J., Salmon, D. and Rendell, M. (1980). Clonidine hallucinations. *Annals of Internal Medicine*, **93**, 456-457.
Bullen, F.S. (1899). Olfactory hallucinations of the insane. *Journal of Mental Science*, **45**, 513-533.
Burgermeister, J.J., Tissot, R. and Ajuriaguerra, J. de. (1964). Les hallucinations visuelles des ophthalmopathies. *Neuropsychologie*, **3**, 9-38.
Chinisci, R.A. (1985). Auditory and visual hallucinations as a medication side effect: recognition and management. *Clinical Gerontologist*, **3**, 71-73.
Christian, J. (1886). Hallucination. *In* "Dictionnaire Encyclopédique des sciences médicales". Vol. 48. (Eds S. Dechambre and L. Lereboullet), pp. 77-120. Masson, Paris.
Castilla de Pino, C. (1984). "Teoría de la Alucinación". Alianza, Madrid.
Clérambault, G. de (1942). "Oeuvre". Vol. 1. Presses Universitaires de France, pp.145-210. Paris.
Collacott, R.A. and Deb, S. (1988). Autoscopy, mental handicap and epilepsy. *British*

*Journal of Psychiatry*, **153**, 925-827.
Comar, G. (1901). l'Auto-représentation de l'organisme chez quelques hystériques. *Revue Neurologique*, **9**, 490-495.
Condillac, E.D. (1947). Traité des Sensations. *In* "Oeuvres Philosophiques de Condillac". Vol. 1. 1st Edn. (1784). Presses Universitaires de France, Paris.
Conrad, K. (1953). Uber ein eigenartiges Spiegelphantom. Heautoskopisches Phénomenen als Dauerzustand by Hypophysentumor. *Nervenarzt*, **24**, 265-270.
Corbin, A. (1986). "The Foul and the Fragrant: odor and the French Imagination". Harvard University Press, Cambridge MA.
Craske, S. and Sacks B.I. (1969). A case of "Double Autoscopy". *British Journal of Psychiatry*, **115**, 343-345.
Critchley, E.M.R. (1987). "Hallucinations and their Impact on Art". Carnegie Press, Preston.
Critchley, M. (1950). The body-image in neurology. *The Lancet*, **i**, 335-340.
Culbetian, C. (1902)."Hallucinations de Moignon". Paris.
Damas Mora, J., Skelton-Robinson, M. and Jenner, F.A. (1982). The Charles Bonnet Syndrome in perspective. *Psychological Medicine*, **12**, 251-261.
Damas Mora, J.M., Jenner, F.A. and Eacott, S.E. (1980). On heautoscopy or the phenomenon of the double: case presentation and review of the literature. *British Journal of Medical Psychology*, **53**, 75-83.
Darwin, E. (1796). "Zoonomia". Vol. 2. U. Johnson, London.
Dewhurst, K. (1954). Autoscopic hallucinations. *Irish Journal of Medical Science*, **1**, 263-267.
Dewhurst, K. and Pearson, J. (1955). Visual hallucinations of the self in organic disease. *Journal of Neurology, Neurosurgery and Psychiatry*, **18**, 53-57.
Dupre, E. (1913). Les Cénestopathies. *Mouvement Médical*, **23**, 3-22.
Durand, V.J. (1955). Hallucinations olfactives et gustatives. *Annales Médico-Psychologiques*, **113**, 777-813; and 249-264.
Eastwood, M.R. and Corbin, S. (1983). Hallucinations in patients admitted to a geriatric psychiatry service: review of 42 cases. *Journal of American Geriatrics Society*, **31**, 593-597.
Esquirol, E. (1817). "Hallucinations". (Panckouke Dictionary), Paris.
Esquirol, E. (1838). "Des Maladies Mentales". Baillière, Paris.
Ey, H. (1950). Hypochondrie. Etude No17. *In* "Etudes Psychiatriques". Vol. 2. Desclée de Brouwer, Paris.
Ey, H. (1957). Les hallucinoses. *l'Encéphale*, **46**, 564-573.
Ey, H. (1973). "Traité des Hallucinations". Vol.2. Masson, Paris.
Faguet, A. (1979). With the eyes of the mind: autoscopic phenomena in the hospital setting. *General Hospital Psychiatry*, **1**, 311-314.
Faure, K. (1965). "Hallucinations et Réalité Perceptive". Presses Universitaires de France, Paris.
Féré, Ch. (1891). Note sur les hallucinations autoscopiques ou spéculaires et sur les hallucinations altruistes. *Comptes Rendus de la Société de Biologie*, 451-453.
Féré, C. (1896). Un spasme de cou coïncidant avec des hallucinations visuelles unilatérales. *Comptes Rendus de la Société de Biologie*, **3**, 269-271.
Fischer, R. (1969). The perception-hallucination continuum. *Diseases of the Nervous System*, **30**, 161-171.
Fischer, R., Kappeler, T., Wisecup, P. and Thatcher, K. (1970). Personality trait-dependent performance under psilocybin. *Diseases of the Nervous System*, **31**, 91-101.

Fuchs, T. and Lauter, H. (1992). Charles Bonnet Syndrome and musical hallucinations in the elderly. *In* "Delusions and Hallucinations in Old Age". (Eds C. Katona and R. Levy). pp. 187-200. Gaskell, London.
Furukawa, T. (1990). Charles Bell's description of the phantom limb phenomenon in 1830. *Neurology,* **40**, 1830.
Gantheret, F. (1961). Historique et position actuelle de la notion de schéma corporel. *Bulletin de Psychologie,* **15**, 41-44.
Gardner, E.R. and Hall, R.C.W. (1982). Psychiatric symptoms produced by over the counter drugs. *Psychosomatics,* **23**, 186-190.
Gloor, P., Olivier, A. and Quesney, L.F. (1982). The role of the limbic system in experiential phenomena of temporal lobe epilepsy. *Annals of Neurology,* **12**, 129-144.
Green, C. (1968). "Out-of-the-Body Experiences". Hamish Hamilton, London.
Griesinger, W. (1861). "Die Pathologie und Therapie der psychischen Krankheiten". Krabbe, Stuttgart.
Grotstein, J.S. (1982). Autoscopic phenomena. *In* "Extraordinary Disorders of Human Behaviour". pp. 65-77. Plenum Press, New York.
Gueniot, M. (1861). D'une Hallucination du Toucher (ou hétérotopie subjective des extrémitée) particulière à certains amputés. *Journal de Physiologie de l'Homme et des Animaux (Brown-Sequard),* **4**, 416-430.
Gurney, E. (1885). Hallucinations. *Mind,* **10**, 162-199; 316-317.
Gurney, E., Myers, F.W.H. and Podmore, E. (1886). "Phantasms of the Living". Vol. 2. Trubner, London.
Haley, W.E., Brown, S.L. and Levine, E.G. 91987). Family caregiver appraisals of patient behavioural disturbance in senile dementia. *Clinical Gerontologist,* **6**, 25-34.
Halgren, E., Walter, R.D., Cherlow, D.G. and Crandall, P.H. (1978). Mental phenomena evoked by electrical stimulation of the human hippocampal formation and amygdala. *Brain,* **101**, 83-117.
Hamilton, W. (1859). "Lectures on Logic and Metaphysics". Vol.4. William Blackwood and Sons, Edinburgh.
Hammond, W.A. (1995). Unilateral hallucinations. *Medical News (New York),* **47**, 681-689.
Hausser-Hauw, C. and Bancaud, J. (1987). Gustatory hallucinations in epileptic seizures. *Brain,* **110**, 339-359.
Hécaen, H. and Ajuriaguerra, J. (1952). "Méconnaisances et Hallucinations corporelles" (Intégration et desintégration de la somatognosie), Masson, Paris.
Hécaen, H. and Albert, M.L. (1978). "Human Neuropsychology". John Wiley, New York.
Hécaen, H. and Green, A. (1957). Sur l'Héautoscopie. *l'Encéphale,* **46**, 581-594.
Higier, H. (1894). Uber unilaterale Hallucinationen. *Wiener Klinik,* **20**, 139-170.
James, A.R.W. (1986). l'Hallucination simple? *Revue d'Histoire littéraire de la France,* **6**, 1024-1037.
James, W. (1890). "Principles of Psychology". Vol. 2. Macmillan, London.
Joffroy, A. (1896). Las hallucinations unilatérales. *Archives de Neurologie,* **4**, 97-112.
Katz, J. (1992). Psychophysiological contributions to phantom limbs. *Canadian Journal of Psychiatry,* **37**, 282-298.
Keup, W. (Ed). (1970). "Origin and Mechanisms of Hallucinations". Plenum Press, New York.
Ladee, G.A. (1966). "Hypochondriacal Syndromes". Elsevier, Amsterdam.
Lamy, H. (1895). Hémianopsie avec hallucinations dans la partie abolie du champ de la vision. *Revue de Neurologie,* **3**, 129-135.

Lasegue, C. (1971). "Ecrits Psychiatriques". (First published 1881), Privat, Toulouse.
Lechner, J. (1983). A.V.C. Berbiguier de Terre-Neuve du Thym, "l'Homme aux Farfadets", Thèse de Médecine, Louis Pasteur, Strasbourg.
Lemaitre, A. (1902). Hallucinations autoscopiques et automatismes divers chez des écoliers. *Archives de Psychologie*, **1**, 357-379.
Leon, J., Anthelo, E. and Simpson, G. (1992). Delusion of parasitosis or chronic tactile hallucinosis: hypothesis about their brain physiopathology. *Comprehensive Psychiatry*, **33**, 25-33.
Leroy, E.B. (1905). Préoccupations hypocondriaques avec hallucinations obsédantes de l'Ouïe et de l'Odorat. *Comptes Rendus du Congrès de Médicines Aliénistes*, Masson, Paris.
Leroy, R. (1922). The syndrome of lilliputian hallucinations. *Journal of Nervous and Mental Disease*, **56**, 325-333.
L'Hermitte, J. (1922). Syndrome de la calotte du pédoncule cérébral. Les troubles psychosensoriels dans les lésions du mésocéphale. *Revue Neurologique*, **29**, 1363-1364.
L'Hermitte, J. (1932). l'Hallucinose pédonculaire. *l'Encéphale*, **27**, 422-435.
L'Hermitte, J. (1951*a*). "Les Hallucinations". Doin, Paris.
L'Hermitte, J. (1951*b*). Visual hallucinations of the self. *British Medical Journal*, **1**, 431-434.
Littré, E. (1878). "Dictionnaire de la Langue Francaise". Vol. 2. Hachette, Paris.
Locke, J. (1959). "An Essay Concerning Human Understanding". (Ed. A.C. Fraser). Dover Publication, New York.
López Ibor, J.J. and López-Ibor Alino, J.J. (1974). "El Cuerpo y la Corporalidad". Gredos, Madrid.
Lowe, G.R. (1973). The phenomenology of hallucinations as an aid to differential diagnosis. *British Journal of Psychiatry*, **123**, 621-633.
Lugaro, E. (1904). Sulle allucinazioni unilaterali dell'udito. *Rivista di Patologia Nervosa e Mentale*, **9**, 228-237.
Lukianowicz, N. (1958). Autoscopic phenomena. *Archives of Neurology and Psychiatry*, **80**, 199-220.
Lunn, V. (1970). Autoscopic phenomena. *Acta Psychiatrica Scandinavica*, **46**, 118-125.
Maack, L.H. and Mullen, P.E. (1983). The Doppelganger, disintegration and death: a case report. *Psychological Medicine*, **13**, 651-654.
Magnan, V. and Saury, M. (1889). Trois cas de cocainisme chronique. *Comptes Rendus, Séances et Mémoire de la Société de Biologie*, 60-63.
Maier, H.W. (1928). "La Cocaine", Payot, Paris.
Marillier, L. (1890). "Statistique des Hallucinations, Congrès Internationale de Psychologie". Paris.
Marazzi, A.S. (1962). Pharmacodynamics of hallucination. *In* "Hallucinations". pp. 36-49. Grune and Stratton, New York.
McConnell, W.B. (1965). The phantom double in pregnancy. *British Journal of Psychiatry*, **111**, 67-89.
McCulloch, W.H. (1992). A certain archway: autoscopy and its companions seen in Western writings (edited and introduced by T. Dening). *History of Psychiatry*, **3**, 59-78.
Menninger-Lerchenthal, E. (1935). Das Truggebilde der eigene Gestalt (Héautoscopie, Doppelgänger) Abhandlungen aus der Neurologie, Psychiatrie, Psychologie und ihren Grenzgebieten. *Monatschrift für Psychiatrie und Neurologie*, **74**, 1-196, Karger, Berlin.
Miller, K (1985). "Doubles". Oxford University Press, Oxford.

Miller, F., Magee, J. and Jacobs, R. (1987). Formed visual hallucinations in an elderly patient. *Hospital and Community Psychiatry*, **38**, 527-529.
Mitchell, S.W. (1871). Phantom Limb. *The Lippincott Magazine*, **8**, 563-569.
Moreau de Tours. (1845). "Du Haschisch et de la Aliénation Mentale", Poiters, Paris.
Morenon, M. and Morenon, J. (1991). l'Hallucination appartient au système de la langue. *l'information Psychiatrique*, **67**, 633-642.
Morsier, G. (1967). Le Syndrome de Charles Bonnet. Hallucinations visuelles des vieillards sans déficience mentale. *Annales Médico-Psychologiques*, **125**, 677-702.
Morsier, G. de (1936). Les Automatismes visuels. *Schweizer Medizinische Wochenschrift*, **66**, 700-708.
Morsier, G. de (1938). Les hallucinations. *Revue d'Oto-Neuro-Ophtalmologie*, **16**, 241-352.
Morsier, G. de (1969). Etudes sur les hallucinations, histoire, doctrines, problèmes. *Journal de Psychologie Normale et Pathologique*, **66**, 281-317.
Mourgue, R. (1932). "Neurobiologie de l'Hallucination". Lamertin, Bruxelles.
Naudascher, G. (1910). Trois cas d'hallucinations spéculaires. *Annales Médico-Psychologiques*, **11**, 284-294.
Nouët, H. (1923). Hallucinations spéculaires et traumatisme cranien. *l'Encéphale*, **18**, 327-329.
Olson, P.R., Suddeth, J.A., Peterson, P.J. and Egelhodd, T. (1985). Hallucinations of widowhood. *Journal of the American Geriatrics Society*, **33**, 543-547.
Parish, E. (1897). "Hallucinations and Illusions". London, Walter Scott (improved translation of Parish E. (1984) Uber die Trugwahrnehmung. *Schriften der Gessellschaft für Psychologischen Forschung*, 1-246).
Perry, R.H., Irving, D., Blessed, G., Fairbairn, A. and Perry, E.K. (1990a). Senile dementia of Lewy body type. A clinically and neuropathologically distinct form of Lewy body dementia in the elderly. *Journal of Neurological Sciences*, **95**, 119-139.
Perry, E.K., Marshall, E., Perry, R.H., Irving, D., Smith, C.J., Blessed, G. and Fairbairn, A.F. (1990b). Cholinergic and dopaminergic activities in senile dementia of Lewy body type. *Alzheimer Disease Association Disorders Journal*, **4**, 87-95.
Paulus, J. (1941). "Le Problème de l'Hallucination et l' Evolution de la Psychologie l'Esquirol à Pierre Janet". Les Belles Lettres, Paris.
Pearson, J. and Dewhurst, K. (1954). Sur deux cas de phénomènes autoscopiques. *l'Encéphale*, **43**, 166-169.
Penfield, W. and Porot, P. (1963). The brain's record of auditory and visual experiences. *Brain*, **86**, 595-696.
Perrin, L. (1896). Des névrodermies parasitophobiques. *Annales de Dermatologie et Syphiligraphie*, **7**, 129-138.
Podoll, K., Osterheider, M. and Noth, J. (1989). Das Charles Bonnet-Syndrom. *Fortschritte der Neurologie und Psychiatrie*, **57**, 43-60.
Quercy, P. (1930). "Etudes sur l'Hallucination". Alcan, Paris.
Rank, O. (1971). "The Double". North Carolina Press, North Hill.
Regis, E. (1881). Des hallucinations unilatérales. *l'Encéphale*, **1**, 43-74.
Reilly, T.M. and Beard, A.W. (1976). Monosymptomatic hypochondriasis (letter). *British Journal of Psychiatry*, **129**, 191.
Robertson, A. (1881). On unilateral hallucinations and their relation to cerebral localization. *In* "Transactions of the International Medical Congress". Vol III, (Ed. W. McCormac). pp. 632-633. Kolckman, London.
Robertson, A. (1901). Unilateral hallucinations: their relative frequency, associations, and

pathology. *Journal of Mental Science,* **47**, 277-293.
Schilder, P. (1923). "Das Körperschema". Springer, Berlin.
Schneck, J.M. (1990). Visual hallucinations as grief reaction without the Charles Bonnet syndrome. *New York State Journal of Medicine,* **90**, 216-217.
Sidgwick, H. (1889-1894). The census of hallucinations. *Proceedings of the Society for Psychical Research,* 1889-1890, **4**, 7-25; 429-435; 1891-1892, **7**, 429-435; and a final report on the census of hallucinations. *Proceedings of the Society for Psychical Research,* 1984, **10**, 25-252.
Siegel, R.K. and West, L.J. (Eds). (1975). "Hallucinations". John Wiley, New York.
Sigmond, G. (1848). On hallucinations. *Journal of Psychological Medicine and Mental Pathology,* **1**, 585-608.
Slade, P.D. and Bentall, R.P. (1988). Sensory deception. *In* "A Scientific Analysis of Hallucinations". Croom Helm, London.
Slade, P. (1976). Hallucinations. *Psychological Medicine,* **6**, 7-13.
Sonnenblick, M., Weissberg, N. and Rosin, A.J. (1982). Neurological and psychiatric side effects of cimetidine. Report of 3 cases with review of the literature. *Postgraduate Medical Journal,* **58**, 415-418.
Siegel, R.K. and Jarvik, M.E. (1975). Drug-induced hallucinations in animals and man. *In* "Hallucinations". (Eds R.K. Siegel and L.J. West). pp. 81-162. Wiley and Sons, New York.
Smith, S. (1974). "Die Astrale Doppelexistenz". Bern.
Société Médico-Psychologique (1855-56). Reports of Sessions between 26th February 1855 and 28th April 1856. *Annales Médico-Psychologiques* 1855, **i**, 526-550; **ii**, 126-140; 1856, **i**, 281-305; **ii**, 385-446.
Sollier, P. (1903). "Les Phénomènes d'Autoscopie". Alcan, Paris.
Sollier, P. (1908a). Quelques cas d'autoscopie. *Journal de Psychologie Normale et Pathologique,* **5**, 160-165.
Sollier, P. (1908b). Autoscopie interne vérifiée expérimentalement. *Journal de Psychologie Normale et Pathologique,* **5**, 354-358.
Störring, G. (1907). "Mental Pathology in its Relation to Normal Psychology". Swan Sonnenschein and Co., London.
Sully, J. (1895). "Illusions". Kegan Paul, London; Trübner, Trenck.
Sutter, J.M. (1962). l'Apport de la neurologie a la psychopathologie des hallucinations. *l'Evolutions Psychiatrique,* **27**, 501-535.
Taine, H. (1890). "De l'Intelligence". Vol. 2. Hachette, Paris.
Tamburini, A. (1881). La theorie des hallucinations. *La revue scientifique de la France et de l'Etranger,* Third Series, **1**, 138-142, (Tamburini A. (1990). A theory of hallucinations. *History of Psychiatry,* **1**, 145-156).
Thièbierge, G. (1894). Les Acárophobes. *Revue Générale de Clinique et de Thérapeutique,* **32**, 373.
Thomas, C.S. (1984). Dysmorphophobia: a question of definition. *British Journal of Psychiatry,* **144**, 513-516.
Titchener, E.B. (1901). Common sensation. *In* "Dictionary of Philosophy and Psychology". Vol. 1. (Ed. J.W. Baldwin). Macmillan, London.
Todd, J. and Dewhurst, K. (1955). The double: its psychopathology and psychophysiology. *Journal of Nervous and Mental Disease,* **122**, 47-55.
Toulouse, E. (1892). Les hallucinations unilatérales. *Gazette des Hopitaux,* **65**, 609-618.
Tuke, D.H. (Ed). (1982). "Dictionary of Psychological Medicine". Churchill, London.

Twemlow, S.W., Gabbard, G.O. and Jones, F.C. (1982). The out-of-body experience: a phenomenological typology based on questionnaire responses. *American Journal of Psychiatry*, **139**, 450-455.

Tymms, R. (1949). "Doubles in Literary Psychology". Bowes and Bowes, Cambridge.

Van Bogaert, L. (1927). l'Hallucinose pedonculaire. *Revue Neurologique*, **1**, 608-617.

Weber, E.H. (1846) Der Tastsinn und das Gemeingefuhl. *In* "Handwörterbuch der Physiologie". Vol. III. (Ed. R. Wagner).

Wedenski, J.N. (1912). Des hallucinations olfactives comme signes précurseurs de l'accès dipsomaniaque. *Revue Neurologique*, **24**, 416-617.

West, L.J. (ed). (1962). "Hallucinations". Grune and Stratton, New York.

Williams, J.P. (1985). Psychical research and psychiatry in late Victorian Britain: trance as ecstasy or trance as insanity. *In* "The Anatomy of Madness". Vol. 1. (Eds W.F. Bynum, R. Porter and M. Shepherd). pp. 233-254. Tavistock, London.

Wormser, A.A. (1895). "Des Hallucinations Unilatérales". Paris.

Wragg, R.R. and Jeste, P.V. (1989). Overview of depression and psychosis in Alzheimer's disease. *American Journal of Psychiatry,* **146**: 577-587.

Zutt, J. (1953). "Aussersichsein" und "auf sich selbst zurückblicken" als Ausnahmezustand. *Nervenarzt*, **24**, 24-30.

# 16. Delusions: selected historical and clinical aspects

G.E. Berrios

---

Delusions are here defined as speech acts, unwarranted in logic and/or in reality, purporting to carry information about the world or the self (Berrios, 1991). Delusions are often met with in general psychiatric and neurological practice, and the issue of whether they are always pathological remains a recurrent clinical nightmare. Literature on their nature and meaning continues growing apace; much selectivity has been, therefore, exercised to write this chapter; not surprisingly, this has been governed by the author's ideas, and results of his own clinical research.

Much of the confusion concerning the concept of delusion stems from its chequered history and from the national differences which still beset its understanding.

**Matters Historical: British views**

The symptom "delusion" has for centuries been the keystone of the concept of insanity. Before the 19th century, to have delusions was to be mad (and vice versa). Indeed, ambiguity can be found up to the 1850s in languages like French and German where Délire and Wahn, respectively, could refer both to madness and to delusion, and in the case of French, also to delirium (in the sense of organic confusion).

The English philosopher Hobbes' views on madness are important as they influenced the work of Locke (Blakey, 1850). In "Leviathan" he suggested that delusions were a hallmark of madness: "If some man in Bedlam should entertain you with sober discourse; and you desire in taking leave, to know what he were, that you might another time requite his civility; and he should tell you, he were God the father; I think you need expect no extravagant action for argument of his Madnesse." (p. 141) (Hobbes, 1968).

Locke's "Essay", however, is the classical place for the most influential definition of delusions and madness before the 1820s: "whereas madmen, on the other side, seem to suffer by the other extreme. For they do not appear to me to have lost the faculty of reasoning, but having joined together some ideas very wrongly, they mistake them for truths; and they err as men do that argue right from wrong principles. For, by the violence of their imaginations, having taken their fancies for realities, they make right deductions from them." (Book II, Chapter XI, 13) (Locke, 1959)

David Hartley, (Hoeldtke, 1967; Oberg, 1976), proposed a neurophysiological mechanism for Locke's view on delusion. He also defined madness as an "imperfection of the rational faculty". (p.253) (Hartley, 1834).

The Scottish clinician William Cullen[1] (for notes see end of chapter) (Bouman, 1975) wrote: "delirium, then, may be more shortly defined, – in a person awake, a false judgement arising from perceptions of imagination, or from false recollection, and commonly producing disproportionate emotions." (p. 167) (Cullen, 1827). Cullen distinguished two kinds of delirium: "as it is combined with pyrexia and comatous affections, or as it is entirely without such a combination. It is the latter case that we name insanity."

Haslam (1809) on insanity and delusion, represents a view from the shop-floor: "If a cobbler should suppose himself an emperor, this supposition, may be termed an elevated flight, or an extensive stretch of imagination, but it is likewise a great defect in his judgement, to deem himself that which he is not, and is certainly an equal lapse of his recollection, to forget what he really is." This analysis assumes the novel point that there is an interaction between mental faculties and that delusions result only when all three mental functions are affected.

In their textbook, Bucknill and Tuke (1858) wrote: "The word delusion is generally used by English writers, to include all the various errors to which reference has been made, whenever those errors are not corrected by the understanding." (p. 127). They believed that it would be advantageous to distinguish between hallucinations, illusions and delusions and defined the latter as:

a person may (independently of false inductions) have certain false notions and ideas, which have no immediate reference to the senses... as for example, when he believes himself or other person to be a king or a prophet; or that there is a conspiracy against his life; or that he has lost his soul. Or as another example, he may believe himself to be a tea-pot, without seeing or otherwise perceiving any change in his form. In all examples under this last head, a man is necessarily insane. He cannot have a false belief, (not simply a false induction, but) the result of disease, and unconnected with the senses, without the mind itself being unsound. When there is no pre-morbid perception, but only a false conception, the French employ the expressions, *conceptions fausses, conceptions délirantes*, and *convictions délirantes*.

In view of the Continental influence operating at the time on British psychiatry, it is not surprising that their analysis is carried out in the light of the ongoing French debate on delusions. Little has been left of the old Lockean ideas. Blount (1856) writing on the definition of delusion, illusion, and hallucination states that "we have been as much pleased with the general clearness in the use of these terms in all the French works we have studied, as we have been disappointed in our own authors."

The only original view on delusion to appear in Britain for the rest of the century was put forward by a neurologist, Hughlings Jackson, as an offshoot of his model for symptom-generation. This model was built on four conceptual pillars: (1) evolutionism (and its counterpart, dissolution), (2) the belief that in the human higher mental functions were sited on the cortex, (3) the doctrine of "concomitance", a crude form of dualism, and (4) the assumption that mental and brain functions were organized in a hierarchical manner. The diseases on which he successfully tried this mechanism had been stroke and epilepsy in which both negative symptoms (caused by the abolition of a function) and positive symptoms (caused by the adaptative release of inhibited functions) could be easily demonstrated.

But, then, Jackson applied his model to "mental disorder" (a concept which, incidentally, he considered "nonsense"). Surprisingly, his views only found fertile ground in France, in the work of Ribot (Delay, 1957) and Janet (Rouart, 1950), and have survived in the work of H.Ey (1975) (Evans, 1972). During the late 19th century Jackson had almost no followers in English-speaking psychiatry (except, perhaps, MacPherson, 1889) and none during the 20th (Stengel, 1963; Berrios, 1977). He tried to account for obsessions, dementia and delusions (Savage, 1917): "illusions, delusions and extravagant conduct, and abnormal emotional states in an insane person signify *evolution* not *dissolution;* they signify evolution going on in what remains intact of the mutilated highest centres – in what disease, affecting so much dissolution, has spared." (Taylor, 1931) or "disease only causes the (physical condition for the negative element of the mental condition; the positive mental element, say a *delusion,* obviously an elaborate delusion, however absurd it might be, *signifies activities of healthy nervous arrangements,* signifies evolution going on in what remains intact of the highest cerebral centres." (my italics) (Taylor, 1931). The crucial questions, remain: which function had to be abolished and which "released" for the delusion to appear? In regard to the latter he suggested that: "certain very absurd and persistent delusions are owing to fixation of grotesque fancies of dreams in cases where a morbid change in the brain happens suddenly, or when one increases suddenly, during sleep." (p. 482) (Taylor, 1931). This explanation was perhaps plausible for organic delirium in cerebral vascular accidents or epilepsy, but was it valid for ordinary delusions? Jackson never said. In regard to the issue of function abolished he wrote:

> Suppose a patient imagines, to take one delusion as a sample of his mental condition, that his nurse is his wife. It is not enough to dwell only on the positive element, that he supposes the person attending on him is his wife, for this delusion of necessity implies the coexisting negative element that he does not know her to be his nurse (or some woman not his wife). His "not-knowing" is a sample of the result of disease (dissolution of A); his "wrong- knowing" is a sample of the outcome of what is left intact of his highest cerebral centres." (Taylor, 1931).

Jackson's model was interesting for he proposed that delusions were not themselves a manifestation of diseased brain tissue but the expression of healthy tissue released by the abolition of function in some higher centre. This view differed markedly from any which was (and is) being currently entertained.

## Matters Historical: Continental views

At the end of the 18th century, the word delirium referred to three notions: insanity, organic delirium (Phrensy) and delusion proper. Their common basis was a disorder of reasoning and judgement considered to result from organic disease of the brain. Organic delirium was different only in that it was accompanied by fever and was transitory; insanity was chronic and without fever; delusion *was not yet recognized as a separate symptom.*

Pinel's views on delusions reflect well the French reaction against the ideas of Locke and Condillac (Riese, 1969). "I used to think likewise but I have been surprised to find patients without any impairment of the understanding who are victims of attacks of excitement as if only the affective faculties were involved (*comme si les facultés affectives avoient été seulement lésées*)." (pp 155-156) (Pinel, 1809).

To Landre-Beauvais (1813)[2] – *délire* was a form of perverted understanding: "the perversion of the functions of human understanding leads to: 1. the patient joining together ideas which are incompatible, and taking these combinations as truths; these constitute diverse forms of *délire;* and 2. the patient developing false ideas in regard to one or to a series of objects." (p. 281) .

Esquirol's earliest conception of *délire* was wide and included hallucinations: "A man has a *délire* when his sensations are not in keeping with external objects, when his ideas are not in keeping with his sensations, when his judgements and decisions (*déterminations*) are not in keeping with his ideas, when his ideas, judgements and decisions are independent from his will." (Esquirol, 1814). *Délire* may be found: (1) affecting the self and personality of the individual, (2) relating to sensations and ideas, (3) leading to false judgements, (4) leading to bizarre action, and (5) resulting (apparently) from a specific impairment of the will. (p. 254) (Esquirol, 1814). This view of *délire,* which was to influence French psychiatry for the rest of the century, involved all mental functions, i.e. intellect, emotions and will, and is alien to conventional and narrower (delusional) British views.

Georget[3] was, perhaps, the one writer of this period who captured more clearly than anyone else the difficulties involved in defining *délire*:

> the available definitions of *délire* are either vague, unintelligible or incomplete and nonspecific. This is because it is difficult, not to say impossible, fully to distinguish between groups or separate the normal from the pathological, or indeed place boundary stones between reason and *délire*, without feeling that some phenomena do not fit into the groups, that reasonable actions can be seen as *délire*, or *délire* as a reasonable action. (Georget, 1835).

Falret's[4] contribution is important: he criticized Esquirol's definition and insisted on the need to consider lack of insight as a central criterion. *Délire* was shaped by four factors: (1) the state of the brain, (2) the intellectual and moral character of the patient, (3) circumstances surrounding the onset of *délire*, and (4) ongoing sensations (both internal and external) (p. 361) (Falret, 1864).

Feuchtersleben (1847) discussed delusion and delirium from two perspectives.

The first was the conventional one: "delirium is the erroneous combination of manifold ideas often united with the patient's own inclinations, without his being aware of the error or being able to overcome it". He proposed that various forms of delirium be formed according to four polar behaviours: fixed vs wandering, quiet vs excited, cheerful vs wild, and acute vs chronic.

Griesinger (1861), reminded his readers that insanity was not necessarily accompanied by delusions. Delusions were always secondary: "the false ideas and conclusions, which are attempts at explanation and vindications of the actual disposition in its effects are spontaneously developed in the diseased mind according to the law of causality." He believed that

> the insane ideas of patients are distinguished from the erroneous views of the normal not only by the circumstances of their relation to the diseased subject himself, but also by numerous other characteristics: they are always part of a general disturbance of mental processes (e.g. emotions), they are opposed to views formerly held by the patient, he cannot get rid of them, they resist correction by the testimony of the senses and the understanding, they depend upon a disturbance of the brain which is also expressed in other symptoms (sleep disorders, hallucinations).

Baillarger offered, many years before Jaspers (1948) a clear account of *primary delusions*. He differentiated false judgements on normal sensations from illusions, believing that in the former there was no "illusion" for the perception was normal, i.e. patients interpret "in a particular manner" a sensation which is real, they make a false judgement or rather develop a "delusional idea on the occasion of a [normal] sensation" (Sérieux and Capgras, 1909).

Lasègue[5] in 1852, suggested that paranoid delusions (*délire de persécutions*) might constitute a separate disorder. He accepted the classification of delusions into general and partial but believed that further subdivisions were unwarranted: "delusions do not have either the homogeneity suggested by textbooks nor the variety hinted at by dramatists." He then described typical persecutory delusions which he believed constituted a new form of insanity.

Until the 1840s, it was believed that delusion always was a "pathological" phenomenon, i.e. never seen in the sane. However, Moreau de Tours (1845) suggested that there was a continuity between normality and alienation. To make his view plausible, Moreau identified a third group of subjects suffering from "intermediate" mental aberrations. Observation of subjects intoxicated with hashish suggested that *délire* and hallucinations had in common a *fait primordial*. Moreau's contribution is important in four respects. In spite of his biological phenomenon, i.e. as a symptom which could be found in a number of conditions. Delusions were identical to dreams and could result from excited imagination itself caused by intoxication with hashish and other factors. Because this could happen to any one, there was no discontinuity between the sane and the madman, indeed, such intermediate states were found in clinical practice.[6]

To Ball and Ritti (1881) the crucial issue was to "delimit *délire* from the normal state." We see a new language appearing during this period and the notion of unconscious cerebration, expounded by Laycock and Carpenter, was used to explain delusions (Davies, 1873; Hall, 1979; Leff, 1991; Young, 1970):

> All observers are now in agreement that there exist a number of manifestations of cerebral activity – frequently very complex – that constitute what has been called unconscious cerebration (*cérébration inconscient*) which differ from conscious and voluntary cerebral functions in that they occur automatically. This automatism of some cognitive acts is kept going by habit and transmitted by heredity. Cerebral automatism is of great help to conscious work; but it must not be allowed to get the upper hand as its preponderance would cause anarchy that is *délire*.

Then, rather incongruously, (for Carpenter's "unconscious cerebration" was subcortical) (see Walshe, 1957), these authors localized delusions on the cortex: "the cells of the cortical mantle, we are told, are the organ of intelligence; it is, therefore, right that to their disorder, whether anatomical or physiological, that the production of delusions should be attributed." (Ball and Ritti, 1881). They still iterated the French view, so difficult to translate into Anglo-Saxon concepts: "Which are the psychological functions affected in delusion? We know that psychological life includes four orders of function: sensation, thinking, emotion, and action. Each of these can be impaired, so that there can be a sensory delusion (*délire sensoriel*), an intellectual delusion (*délire de la pensée*), an emotional delusion (*délire de sentiments*) and a delusion of acts (*délire des actes ou délire inpulsif*)." In the first group, Ball and Ritti included hallucinations; in the second, typical delusions (the *primordial Deliren* of the *Germans*) and obsessions; in the third, anhedonia-like experiences, and also made-emotions; and in the fourth, impulsions. Four criteria for *délire* were listed: spontaneity, bizarreness, conviction, and personalized meaning of the idea (p. 349).

Ball and Ritti classified *délire* into non-vesanic (delirium) and vesanic; the later corresponding to insanity: "we considered as vesanic those patients with delusions who on post-mortem are found to have no lesions in the brain." Vesanic delusions can be general or partial, the former referring to generalized episodes of madness, the latter to hallucinations and delusions proper.

Jules Cotard (1891) wrote two original papers on delusion. In the earlier paper (1891), he argued that the mechanical classification of delusions according to theme or whether or not they were systematized was not sufficient, and that delusions should be studied in relation to the individual who suffered from them. This did not mean searching for meaning but associating the delusion to other symptoms. He suggested that delusions may simply be the cognitive expression of motor function. Increases in motor behaviour, such as in mania, may influence the colour and content of delusions and make them grandiose; nihilistic delusions would be generated by the motor retardation of depressed patients.

Cotard later resorted to ongoing models of aphasia according to which the loss of motor and sensory "images" of words gave rise to motor and sensory aphasia, respectively. He believed that images were present in all motor and sensory activities, and hence the loss of "mental vision" characteristic of psychotic melancholia could also result from a loss of images: "it can be concluded that the impossibility of invoking images, the loss of mental vision, both frequent symptoms in melancholia, might be explained by a psychical paralysis as well as by an anaesthesia of the sentiments." (p. 421) (Cotard, 1891). The important point in Cotard's speculation is his emphasis on the relationship between motor activity, thinking, and mental content.

By the early 20th century, French psychiatry had recognized four sources of delusions: hallucinations (*délire hallucinatoire*), intuition (*intuition délirante*), interpretation (*interpretation délirante* or *délire d'intérpretation*), and fabulation or imagination (*délire d'imagination*) (p. 178) (Porot, 1975).

Magnan and Sérieux (1892) put forward their view on "chronic delusional states with a systematic evolution". Four stages to this condition were recognized: incubation (delusional mood), crystallization of the persecutory delusions, appearance of grandiose delusions and dementia (mental defect). A subgroup of these patients, representing the more bizarre and hebephrenic end of behaviour, was masterly described by Auguste Marie the same year (Marie, 1892). However, clinical vignettes included in the book by Magnan and Sérieux show that the new diagnostic category *cut across* what currently would be called schizophrenia, psychotic depression and delusional disorders.

Parallel to these nosologic developments, other French alienists continued analysing delusions in isolation from other symptoms. Vaschide and Vurpas (1903) dealt with the history and definitions of *délire* and its relationship to dreaming, and mapped its ever narrowing evolution from wide category to specific *trouble du raisonnement*. They also studied its nosological role in regard to *délire chronique,* paranoia, and mental confusion.

In 1909 Paul Sérieux published, with Joseph Capgras, an important volume on the "delusion of interpretation" moving away from the over-arching category proposed by Magnan: "we shall try to detach from it a condition we want to call *délire d'intepretation* because it is easily separable. Whilst the psychoses leading to dementia include chronic hallucinations, our cases have exclusively delusions." They were, therefore, characterized by: "(1) multiple and organized delusions, (2) absence or poverty of hallucinations, (3) normal intellect, (4) chronic course, and (5) incurability without terminal defect." In other words, the authors were describing paranoid or delusional disorders.

In the best study on *intuitions délirantes,* Targowla and Dublineau (1931) published a review that included 60 case reports. They concluded that intuition was a form of automatism and that delusions, originated by this mechanism, were totally unrelated to perceptions. The new symptom was: "a judgement that suddenly and spontaneously appears in consciousness, beyond the control of the will, which has no intellectual or sensory origin and which is completely formed, self-evident and requiring no proof."

In 1905 Dupré coined the term *mythomanie* to refer to severe confabulatory delusions, which he subdivided into mythomania of vanity, and malignant and perverse mythomania; he later also described a "wandering mythomania" shown by young subjects who in addition to their confabulations exhibited *Wanderleben* (Dupré, 1925).

Philippe Chaslin (1890) wrote papers on *délire* exploring the question of why persecutory delusions are more often accompanied by auditory hallucinations, whilst visual hallucinations are more commonly seen with religious delusions. To account for these associations, Chaslin suggested a neurophysiological hypothesis based on Tamburini's theory of hallucinations (Tamburini, 1890) "Delusion, like hallucination, is a physiological phenomenon of pathological origin; this genesis prevents the idea from corresponding to the reality of things... I shall try to show that at the beginning of the disease the auditory hallucination and the delusion are the same phenomenon only of different intensity... the content of the predominant hallucinations is determined by the mental content of the delusion... however abstract an idea might be it always contains an obscure image which in certain conditions may become distinct." Chaslin, influenced by Cotard's ideas on the genesis of delusions, believed that delusions and hallucinations were two sides of the same psychological and neurophysiological coin.

Chaslin (1912) went on describe delusions (*idées délirantes*). Concepts were illustrated by a clinical vignette. He wrote that "delusions may present isolated or combined with hallucinations. Clusters of delusions may appear in the same patient, and these I call delusional states (*délire*). Delusions may be unconnected or form a system, these clinical states I call incoherent and systematized delusional states, respectively." The former, he thought, were typically seen in subjects with low intelligence or dementia although a form of incoherence (*discordance générale, désharmonie entre les différents signes de l'affection*) (Lantéri-Laura and Gros, 1992) was seen in conditions such as dementia praecox. Primary and secondary paranoia were the best examples of systematized delusional states, in which, according to Chaslin, there was a relative preservation of intellectual functions. Secondary paranoia was the remnant of a severe psychotic state, and could signify a transition to dementia.

Chaslin also took a different view of the genesis of delusions:
delusional ideas seem to have their source in the emotions of the patient, of which they are a symbolic representation. The difference between primary and secondary delusions may simply be one of intensity and presentation rather than of emotional origin. One could illustrate the origin of delusions by recollecting the mechanisms of dreaming. Propensities, desires, and feelings from the waking state reappear in dreams in symbolic scenes... Freud has shown this to be the case. (p. 178) (Chaslin, 1912).

Finally, Chaslin explored the question of delusional contagion and concluded that it was rare, and that it occurred in people living closely together, particularly when one member was weaker than the other (p. 179) (Chaslin, 1912).

## The 20th Century

All aspects of delusion had been fully discussed during the 19th century. Why is it, then, that in Anglo-Saxon psychiatry (it is otherwise in the Continent) there is still the belief that we owe everything to Karl Jaspers?[7] It would be tempting to ascribe this to historical ignorance, but the explanation is likely to be less simple, and has probably to do with the influence of the great group of German emigrés who arrived in Britain during the 1930s.

Jaspers' first writing on delusion appeared in 1910. It dealt with delusions of jealousy and is an attempt to deal with the question of whether they result from a development of personality or a disease. The article included eight clinical reports, a presentation of the descriptive psychopathology of delusions of jealousy, and some nosological considerations. In a paper on disorders of perception (1912) and another on pseudohallucinations (1911), Jaspers dealt tangentially with the issue of delusional belief and insight. Finally, in a superb short paper on the "feelings of presence", which he called "vivid cognitions" (*Leibhaftige Bewusstheiten*), Jaspers studied the issue of differentiating intuitive from cognitive claims and their pathological changes (1913). It was, however, in "General Psychopathology" (pp. 78-90) (1948) where he offered the longest account of delusions. The only point to be repeated here is that – as shown above – all his types and definitions had already been discussed.

## The 1950 World Congress

Since the time of the First World War, little new was said on delusions in German (Schmidt, 1940) or reasons that led to the decision to make delusions the central theme of the 1950 First World Congress of Psychiatry (Morel, 1950). At this meeting, held in Paris, great men attended: Mayer-Gross, Guiraud, Morselli, Rumke, Delgado, Ey, Gruhle, Minkowski, Skransky, and Baruk. Gruhle, then a grand old man, re-asserted the very definition that, since Hagen, had been a commanding view in German psychiatry (Schmidt, 1940): "delusion is an interpretation without reason, an intuition without cause, a mental attitude without basis. It represents neither sublimated desires nor repressed wishes but is a sign of cerebral dysfunction. It is not secondary to any other phenomenon and has no relationship to the patient's constitution." (Morel, 1950).

Based on the work of Monakow and Mourgue, Guiraud offered a "biological model" according to which delusions resulted from a failure of "primordial psychological activity (*atteinte de l'activité psychique primordial*) distorted and masked by human cognitive and affective superstructures". (Morel, 1950). The primordial activity itself was a composite of psychological functions which included the feeling of existence, of nutrition, of reproduction, of vigilance and of growth. These "pulsions" were organized by the self that adapted their satisfaction to reality according to logical rules. Focal or diffuse pathological changes in the central nervous system might then cause selective or global failures (*une anomalie partielle ou globale du dynamisme psychique primordial*). This, in turn, might cause a collapse in the logical organization of the self (Morel, 1950).

Mayer-Gross stated that the choice of delusions as theme for the Congress was "appropriate" for at the time there was a "relatively low ebb of interest in the psychopathology of delusions." He noted that the conventional criteria were not useful in practice and identified the two ways in which this difficulty could be solved: "one can call a delusion pathological or, as Bumke put it, an error of morbid origin; or one can insist that delusions do not differ from other human beliefs in principle, that no line of demarcation exists. As Bleuler, whose views have so widely influenced psychopathological thinking all over the world, has pointed out, delusional ideas correspond to and are directed by the patient's affects and emotions." (Bleuler, 1906).

E. Morselli attempted a review of the neurobiological bases of delusional states but did not go beyond listing toxic and metabolic states. H.C. Rumke undertook an analysis of the symptom delusion which he defined as an "artificial abstraction." His contribution was, perhaps, the most important in that Rumke showed the uselessness of defining delusions as "beliefs" and also the weakness of the conventional criteria.

**The Pre-delusional State**

The fact is that, so far, analysis of the form and content of crystallized delusions has given no clues as to their brain localization (Cummings, 1985). Since the 19th century, alienists have pondered over the clinical relevance of experiences (not often reported by patients) occurring before they finally are taken over by the "wrong belief". These experiences, which have been variously called "delusional mood" (Schmidt, 1940) "perplexity" (Störring, 1939) "trema" (Conrad, 1858) and "*delusion viva*" (Llopis, 1969), last from seconds to weeks, and are often ineffable, i.e. patients do not have the words or experiential notions to describe them in any detail. Indeed, psychiatrists themselves do not seem to have the right clinical categories to classify and understand them either. On account of their "raw" quality, these experiences may be better indicators of the brain sites involved in their pathological origin than the delusions themselves (which are likely to be much distorted by psychosocial noise).

Unfortunately, empirical analysis of these experiences has proved difficult. Because they are often fleeting and strange, and are likely to occur during states of subtle cognitive disorganization (Llopis, 1946; Ey, 1954), pre-delusional experiences are not analyzable in the here and now. For the same reason they may not be memorable enough and hence escape retrospective study. This explains why current information on the nature of these states comes from single case studies or anecdotal reports. It is likely that experiences superficially so different as delusional mood, perplexity or trema are, in fact, the same phenomenon; differences resulting from the perspective from which they have been analyzed (e.g. emotional, behavioural or intellectual, respectively). As Bleuler suggested, it might be that these experiences are all "affective" in nature. They may, indeed be related, (Oepen *et al.* 1989), to limbic dysfunction on the non-dominant hemisphere. Should this be the case, the old distinction between primary and secondary delusions may, after all, be unwarranted as all delusions may arise "secondary" to affective changes (whether the latter be fleeting or longer lasting).

**Current Clinical Views**

The view that delusions are "abnormal belief systems" (for a criticism of this view see Berrios, 1991) has led to the suggestion that probabilistic models (Iversen, 1984) may explain the manner of their origin or persistence. Fischhoff and Beyth-Marom (1983) suggest that inferential failures may originate at each stage of the Bayesian procedure. Two difficulties beset this approach: one relates to the assessment of *a priori* probabilities, and the other to the determination of what counts as *a posteriori* evidence. In fact, Hemsley and Garety (1986) show that failures at each stage of the inferential procedure lead to "phenomenological" situations resembling delusional "beliefs".

Delusions have been variously explained in organic, (Arthur, 1964; Cummings, 1985; Mourgue, 1932) psychodynamic, (Faure, 1971) and cognitive terms (Winters, 1983; Oltmanns and Maher, 1988). Currently, the clinical event in which identifiable brain changes seem to be causally related to delusions is dubbed "organic delusional syndrome" (ODS) in DSM III-R (APA, 1987). The usefulness of this category is yet to be demonstrated, particularly in the elderly where functional and organic psychoses often coincide. Some authors have gone as far as diagnosing ODS in the presence of cognitive impairment and confusion or impaired sensorium (Cornelius *et al.*, 1991), others have suggested that late paraphrenia may be a form of ODS (Miller *et al.*, 1986).

**Delusions and Brain Sites**

Current views are less speculative than earlier ones. The temporal and the frontal lobes have been particularly investigated with the occasional finding that subjective experiences, held with some conviction, may be evoked by cortical and subcortical stimulation to either side of the brain during neurosurgery for epilepsy (Gloor *et al.*, 1982; Halgren *et al.*, 1978). In general, however, evidence linking delusions to the temporal lobe is based on few significant correlations, for example, that short-lived delusional ideal may episodically occur in temporal lobe dysfunction (Tucker *et al.*, 1986)

Changing views on the lateralization of brain functions have also played a role: thus, attempts were made to link schizophrenia-like states to the dominant-hemisphere (Berrios, 1989; Trimble, 1984). Contradictory claims have also been marshalled, for example, by Peroutka *et al.* (1982) that strokes affecting the non-dominant temporal lobe may lead to delusional experiences. More recently,

Cutting (1990) has endeavoured to make a case for linking delusions (and the misidentification syndromes) to the non-dominant hemisphere. But the recent interest in the "executive" functions of the frontal lobes has led some to suggest that delusions, after all, might be sited in that region of the brain (Benson and Stuss, 1990).

Delusions seem common in the elderly, a view recently summarized in Katona and Levy (1992), and based on epidemiological and hospital reports but not confirmed in community studies. Studies do not provide separate figures for delusions and hallucinations, let alone specify subtypes for the former (Cunha *et al.*, 1985). The problem arises as to whether the traditional primary-secondary dichotomy holds in the case of the deluded elderly. Delusions seen in the context of what is believed to be a schizophrenic (or paraphrenic) illness are assured to be "primary", whilst those seen in mania, involutional melancholia (Sims, 1988) or "organic" states, "secondary" (Cummings, 1985). In the elderly with cognitive impairment, typing of delusions is difficult as most subjects are likely to be suffering from some form of brain disease, and hence it should conventionally be concluded that his/her delusions are secondary. It has been claimed that an adequate level of cognition may be relevant to both the appearance and maintenance of delusions (Berrios and Brook, 1985). However, there are few reports of an increase in delusions as the illness worsens (Drevets and Rubin, 1989)

In the elderly without cognitive impairment, delusions are found alone or combined with other mental symptoms; in either case, sensory deficits and a particular type of pre-morbid personality are said to play a role. Cases without affective or thought disorder, and where sensory deficits do not seem to play an important role, have a prevalence of about 8% and have been variously classed as late paraphrenia, paranoia, persecutory states, late onset schizophrenia, etc. (Post, 1966). No consistent causal factor seems to have been found for this group (Moore, 1981). It has been believed since Kraepelin (Cooper *et al.*, 1974; Soni, 1988) that deafness leads to delusions; as may "hypersensitive" (Kretschmer, 1918; Rasmussen, 1978) and "paranoid" personalities (Schweighofer, 1982; Koehler, 1981).

## Notes

1   This was at the time the accepted view. For example, Pargeter states: "The definition of madness, by the consent of all writers, is delirium [i.e. delusion] without fever" p.vi, Pargeter (1792).

2   Landre-Beauvais (1772-1840), disciple of Pinel and professor of Medicine at La Salpêtrière, was the author of a famous and influential book in which the symptoms of mental disorder were integrated with those of general medicine. This work, which went through numerous editions, can be considered as the first written from the point of view of a "semiology" of disease.

3   E.J. Georget (1795-1828), described as one of the great promises of early 19th

century French psychiatry, died young. He qualified from Tours and Paris, and received his psychiatric training at the Salpêtrière under Esquirol, in whose arms he died.

4   Jean Pierre Falret (1794-1870) trained under Esquirol and wrote on hypochondria and suicide, on administrative psychiatry, and against the concept of monomania. He was the father of Jules Falret (1824-1902), another important alienist.

5   Ernest Charles Lasègue (1816-1883) trained first as a philosopher but influenced by Claude Bernard and Morel (with whom he had shared digs as a student), he switched to Medicine and trained as a psychiatrist under Jean Pierre Falret. He is better known for his work on delirium tremens and anorexia nervosa.

6   Jacques Joseph Moreau de Tours (1804-1884) trained under Esquirol; he became interested on the effects of drugs (hashish) on mental state after accompanying a patient to the Near East.

7   Karl Jaspers (1883-1969) was a German philosopher who worked as a psychiatrist up to the First World War. In his early thirties, he abandoned psychiatry to dedicate himself to writing books on philosophy, and also political issues and intellectual biography. His psychiatric ouput includes 10 articles all written before 1913, when the first edition of General Psychopathology "Allgemeine Psychopathologie" was published. This book went through seven editions, the last in 1959. After the third edition, Jaspers had little to do with the book, delegating its upgrading to Kurt Schneider. This is important to those attempting a conceptual analysis of the 1963 English translation (in fact, the seventh German edition).

## References

APA. (1987). "American Psychiatric Association Diagnostic and Statistical Manual of Mental Disorders". 3rd Edn Revised. American Psychiatric Association, Washington D.C.

Arthur, A.Z. (1964). Theories and explanations of delusions: a review. *American Journal of Psychiatry,* **121**, 105-115.

Ball, B. and Ritti, E. (1881). Délire. In "Dictionnaire Encyclopédique des Sciences Médicales". Vol. 26, (Eds A. Dechambre and L. Lereboullet). pp. 315-434. Masson, Paris.

Benson, D.F. and Stuss, D.T. (1990). Frontal lobe influences on delusions: a clinical perspective. *Schizophrenia Bulletin,* **16**, 403-411.

Berrios, G.E. (1977). Henri Ey, Jackson et les Idées Obsédantes. *l'Evolution Psychiatrique,* **42**, 685-699.

Berrios, G.E. (1989). Epilepsia y Psiquiatria: aspectos generales y su relación con la depresión. *Revista de Psiquiatria Facultad de Medicina de Barcelona,* **16**, 35-43.

Berrios, G.E. (1991). Delusions as " Wrong Beliefs": A conceptual history. *British Journal of Psychiatry,* **159**, (suppl. 14), 6-13.

Berrios, G.E. (1991*b*). Negative and Positive Signals: a conceptual history. In "Negative vs Positive Schizophrenia Symptoms". (Eds A. Marneros, N.C. Andreasen and M.T. Tsuang). pp. 8-27. Springer, Berlin.

Berrios, G.E. and Brook, P. (1985). Delusions and psychopathology of the elderly with dementia. *Acta Psychiatrica Scandinavica*, **72**, 296-301.

Blakey, R. (1850). "History of the Philosophy of Mind". Vol. 2. pp. 206-215. Longman, Brown, Green, and Longmans, London.

Bleuler, E. (1906). "Affectivität, Suggestibilität, Paranoia". Carl Marhold, Halle.

Blount, J.H. (1856). On the terms delusion, illusion, and hallucination. *Asylum Journal of Mental Science*, **2**, 494-505; **3**, 508-516.

Bouman, I.E. (1975). "William Cullen and the Primacy of the Nervous System". PhD Dissertation, Indiana University.

Brazier, M.A.B. (1984). "A History of Neurophysiology in the 17th and 18th Centuries. From Concept to Experiment". Raven Press, New York.

Bucknill, J.C. and Tuke, D.H. (1858). "A Manual of Psychological Medicine". John Churchill, London.

Chaslin, Ph. (1890). Contribution à l'Etude des Rapports du délire avec les hallucinations. *Annales Médico-Psychologiques*, **12**, 45-70.

Chaslin, Ph. (1912). "Eléments de Sémiologie et Clinique Mentales". Asselin and Houzeau, Paris.

Conrad, K. (1958). "Die beginnende Schizophrenie". Thieme, Stuttgart.

Cooper, A.F., Curry, A.R., Kay, D.W.K. *et al*. (1974). Hearing loss in paranoid and affective psychoses in the elderly. *Lancet*, **ii**, 852-854.

Cornelius, J.K., Day, N., Fabrega, H. Jr., Mezzich, J., Cornelius, M.D. and Ulrich, R.F. (1991). Characterizing organic delusional syndrome. *Archives of General Psychiatry*, **48**, 749-753.

Cotard S. (1891). De l'origine psycho-sensorielle ou psycho-motrice du délire. *In* "Etudes sur les Maladies Cérébrales et Mentales". Baillière, Paris.

Cullen, W. (1827). "The Works of Thomas Cullen". William Blackwood, London.

Cummings, J.L. (1985). Organic delusions. *British Journal of Psychiatry*, **146**, 184-197.

Cunha, V.G., Barros, O. and Siqueira, A.L. (1985). Levantamento epidemiologico psicogeriatrico em Asilos. *Jornal Brasileiro de Psiquiatria*, **34**, 389-394.

Cutting, J. (1990). "The Right Cerebral Hemisphere and Psychiatric Disorders". University Press, Oxford.

Davies, W.G. (1873). Consciousness and unconscious cerebration. *Journal of Mental Science*, **19**, 202-217.

Delay, J. (1957). Jacksonism and the work of Ribot. *Archives of Neurology and Psychiatry*, **78**, 505-515.

Drevets, W.C. and Rubin, E.H. (1989). Psychotic symptoms and the longitudinal course of senile dementia. *Biological Psychiatry*, **25**, 39-48.

Dupré, E. (1925) "Pathologie de l'Imagination et de l'Emotivité". Payot, Paris.

Esquirol, J.E. (1814). Délire. *In* "Dictionnaire des Sciences Médicales, par une Société de Médicins et de Chirurgiens". pp. 251-259. Panckoucke, Paris.

Evans, P. (1972). Heri Ey's concepts of the organization of consciousness and its disorganization: an extension of Jacksonian Theory. *Brain*, **95**, 413-440.

Ey, H. (1954). Structure et destructuration de la conscience. *In* "Etudes Psychiatriques". pp. 653-760. Desclée de Bouwer, Paris.

Ey, H. (1975). "Des Idées de Jackson a un Modèle Organo-Dynamique en Psychiatrie". Privat, Paris.

Falret, J.P. (1864). "Des Maladies Mentales et des Asiles d'Aliénés". pp. 321-424. Bailliière, Paris.

Faure, H. (1971). "Les Appartenances du Délirant". Presses Universitaires de France, Paris.

Feuchtersleben, E. (1847). "The Principles of Medical Psychology". (First German edition, 1945). Sydenham Society, London.
Fischhoff, B. and Beyth-Marom, R. (1983). Hypothesis evaluation from a Bayesian perspective. *Psychological Review*, **90**, 239-260.
Georget, E.J. (1835). Délire. *In* "Dictionnaire de Médicine ou Répertoire Général des Sciences Médicales Considérées sous les Rapports Théoriques et Pratiques". Vol. 10, 2nd Edn. Bechet, Paris.
Gloor, P., Olivier, A., Quesney, L.F., Andermann, F. and Horowitz, S. (1982). The role of the limbic system in experiential phenomena of temporal lobe epilepsy. *Annals of Neurology*, **12**, 129-144.
Griesinger, W. (1861). "Die Pathologie und Therapie der Psychischen Krankheiten für Aerzte und Studirende". Adolph Krabbe, Stuttgart.
Halgren, E., Walter, R.D., Cherlow, D.G. and Crandall, P.H. (1978). Mental phenomena evoked by electrical stimulation of the human hippocampal formation and amygdala. *Brain*, **101**, 83-117.
Hall, V.M.D. (1979). The contribution of the physiologist William Benjamin Carpenter (1813-1885) to the development of the principles of the correlation of forces and the conservation of energy. *Medical History*, **23**, 129-155.
Hartley, D. (1834). "Observations on Man, His Frame, His Duty, and his Expectations". (First edition 1749). Thomas Tegg and Son. London.
Haslam, J. (1809). "Observations on Madness and Melancholy". Callow, London.
Hemsley, D.R. and Garety, P.A. (1986). The formation and maintenance of delusions: A Bayesian analysis. *British Journal of Psychiatry*, **149**, 51-56.
Hobbes, T. (1968). "Leviathan". Penguin Book, London.
Hoeldtke, R. (1967). The history of associationisms and British medical psychology. *Medical History*, **11**, 46-64.
Iversen, G.R. (1984). "Bayesian Statistical Inference". Sage, London.
Jaspers, K. (1910). Einfersuchtswahn. Ein Beitrag zur Frage: "Entwicklung einer Persnlichkeit oder Prozess". *Zeitschrift für die Gesamte Neurologie und Psychiatrie*, **1**, 567-637.
Jaspers, K. (1911). Zur Analyse der Trugwahrnemungen (Leibhaftigkeit und Realitätsurteil). *Zeitschrift für die gesamte Neurologie und Psychiatrie*, **6**, 460-534.
Jaspers, K. (1912). Die Trugwahrnemungen. *Zeitschrift für die gesamte Neurologie und Psychiatrie, (Referate und Ergebnisse)*, 4, 289-534.
Jaspers, K. (1913). Uber Leibhaftige Bewusstheiten (Bewusstheitsstäuschungen). Ein psychopathologischen Elementarsymptom. *Zeitschrift für Patho-Psychologie*, **2**, 151-161.
Jaspers, K. (1948). "Allgemeine Psychopathologie". 5th Edn. Springer, Berlin.
Katona, C. and Levy, R. (eds). (1992). "Delusions and Hallucinations in Old Age". Gaskell, London.
Koehler, K.G. (1981). The Schreber case and affective illness: a research diagnostic re-assessment. *Psychological Medicine*, **11**, 689-696.
Kretschmer, E. (1918). "Der sensitiver Beziehungswahn". Springer, Berlin.
Landre-Beauvais, A.J. (1813). "Séméiotique ou Traité des Signes des Maladies". 2nd Edn. Brosson, Paris.
Lantéri-Laura, G. and Gros, M. (1992). "Essai sur la discordance dans la psychiatrie contemporaine". Epel, Paris.
Lasègue, Ch. (1852). Du délire des Pérsecutions. *Archives Générales de Médicine*, **28**,

129-150.
Leff, A. (1991). Thomas Laycock and the cerebral reflex: a function arising from and pointing to the unity of nature. *History of Psychiatry*, 2, 385-408.
Locke, J. (1959). "An Essay Concerning Human Understanding". (First Edition 1690). Dover Publications, New York.
Llopis, B. (1969). Sobre la delusión y la paranoia. *In* "Afectividad, Sugestibilidad, Paranoia". (Ed. E. Bleuler). (Translated by B. Llopis) Morata, Madrid.
Llopis, B. (1946). "La Psicosis Pelagrosa". Editorial Científico-Médica, Barcelona.
MacPherson, J. (1889). On the dissolution of the functions of the nervous system in insanity, with a suggestion for a new basis of classification. *American Journal of Insanity*, 45, 387-394.
Magnan, V. and Sérieux, P. (1892). "Le Délire Chronique Evolution Systématique". Masson, Paris.
Marie, A. (1892). "Etude sur Quelques Symptoms des Délires Systématisés, et sur leur Valeur". Doin, Paris.
Miller, B.L., Benson, D.F., Cummings, J.L. and Neshkes, R. (1986). Late life paraphrenia: an organic delusional syndrome. *Journal of Clinical Psychiatry*, 47, 204-207.
Moreau de Tours, J.J. (1845). "Du Hachisch et de l'Aliénation Mentale". Fortin, Masson et Cie, Paris.
Morel, F. (ed). (1950). "Psychopathologie des Délires". Paris, Hermann; Ey, H., Marty, P. and Dublineau, J. (1952). Psychopathologie Générale. *Comptes Rendus Des Séances. Premier Congrès Mondial de Psychiatrie*, 1, Hermann, Paris.
Moore, N.C. (1981). Is paranoid illness associated with sensory defects in the elderly? *Journal of Psychosomatic Research*, 25, 69-74.
Mourgue, R. (1932). "Neurobiologie de l'Hallucination". Maurice Lamertin, Bruxelles.
Oberg, B.B. (1976). David Hartley and the association of ideas. *Journal of the History of Ideas*, 37, 441-454.
Oepen, G., Harrington, A., Spitzer, M. and Funfgeld, M. (1989). "Feelings" of conviction: on the relation of affect and thought disorder;. *In* "Psychopathology and Philosophy". (Eds M. Spitzer, F.A. Uehlein, G. Oepen). pp. 43-55. Springer, Berlin.
Oltmanns, T.F. and Maher, B.A. (eds). (1988). "Delusional Beliefs". Wiley, New York.
Pargeter, W. (1792). "Observations on Maniacal Disorders". Murray, London.
Peroutka, S.J., Sohmer, B.H., Kumer, A.J., Folstein, M. and Robinson, R.G. (1982). Hallucinations and delusions following a right temporoparieto-occipital infarction. *Johns Hopkins Medical Journal*, 151, 181-185.
Pinel, Ph. (1809). "Traité Médico-Philosophique sur l'Aliénation Mentale," 2nd Edn., Brosson, Paris.
Porot, A. (1975). "Manuel Alphabétique de Psychiatrie". Presses Universitaires de France, Paris.
Post, F. (1966). "Persistent Persecutory States of the Elderly". Pergamon Press, Oxford.
Rasmussen, S. (1978). Sensitive delusion of reference, "sensitiver Beziehungswahn". *Acta Psychiatrica Scandinavica*, 58, 442-448.
Riese, W. (1969). "The Legacy of Philippe Pinel". Springer, New York.
Rouart, J. (1950). Janet et Jackson. *l'Evolution Psychiatrique*, 25, 485-501.
Savage, G. (1917). Dr Hughlings Jackson on mental disorder. *Journal of Mental Science*, 53, 315-328.
Schmidt, G. (1940). Der Wahn in deutschsprachigen Scrifttum der letzten 25 Jahre. *Zentralblatt für die gesamte Neurologie und Psychiatrie*, 97, 113-193.

Schweighofer, F. (1982). Der Fall Schreber. *Psychotherapie Psychosomatische Medizine Psychologie*, **32**, 4-8.

Sérieux, P. and Capgras, J. (1909). "Les Folies Raissonnantes. Le Délire d'Interprétation". Alcan, Paris.

Soni, S.D. (1988). Relationship between peripheral sensory disturbance and onset of symptoms in elderly paraphrenics. *International Journal of Geriatric Psychiatry*, **3**, 275-279.

Smith, C.U.M. (1967). David Hartley's Newtonian neuropsychology. *Journal of the History of the Behavioural Sciences*, **23**, 123-136.

Stengel, E. (1963). Hughlings Jackson's influence in psychiatry. *British Journal of Psychiatry*, **109**, 348-355.

Störring, G. (1939). "Wessen und Bedeutung des Symptoms der Ratlosigkeit by psychiaschen Erkrankungen". Leipzig, Barth.

Tamburini, A.A. (1990). Theory of hallucinations. Introduced and translated by G.E. Berrios *History of Psychiatry*, **1**, 145-156. (First Published, 1881).

Targowla, R. and Dublineau, J. (1931). "l'Intuition Délirante". Maloine, Paris.

Taylor, J. (ed.) (1931). "Selected Writings of John Hughlings Jackson". Vol. 2. Hodder and Stoughton, London.

Trimble, M. (1984). Interictal psychoses of epilepsy. *Acta Psychiatrica Scandinavica*, **69**, (Suppl. 313) 9-20.

Tucker, G.J., Price, T.R.P., Johnson, V.B. and McAllister, T. (1986). Phenomenology of temporal lobe dysfunction: a link to atypical psychosis. A series of cases. *Journal of Nervous and Mental Disease*, **174**, 348-356.

Vaschide, N. and Vurpas, Cl. (1903). "Psychologie du Délire dans les Troubles Psychopathiques". Masson, Paris.

Walshe, F.M.R. (1957). The brain stem conceived as the "Highest Level" of function in the nervous system; with particular reference to the "Automatic Apparatus" of Carpenter (1850) and to the "Centrencephalic Integrating System" of Penfield. *Brain*, **80**, 510-539.

Winters, K.C. and Neale, J.M. (1983). Delusions and delusional thinking in psychotics: a review of the literature. *Clinical Psychology Review*, **3**, 227-253.

Young, R.M. (1970). "Mind, Brain and Adaptation in the Nineteenth Century". Clarendon Press, Oxford.

# 17. Delusions, schizophrenia (as illustrating a breakdown in the boundaries of reality), psychosis and neurosis

Alice M. Parshall

---

This chapter addresses several facets of the interrelationship between psychiatry, the discipline of the deranged human mind, and reality. Other contributors have discussed paradigms of reality. Psychiatry rarely dares look closely at the normality used as the yardstick against which to identify abnormal states of mind, let alone at the relationship of that normality to reality.

The areas covered here, delusions, schizophrenia, psychosis and neurosis are conceptually contrasting. Delusions fall into the category of psychiatric symptoms and are broadly false or unreal beliefs; schizophrenia is a psychiatric syndrome whose nosology remains unclear, but in the phenomenology of which delusions sometimes occur; psychosis is a word of multiple application, which can be nicely defined as a state of mind ensuing from faulty reality testing; neurosis in this application can be seen as a corollary of psychosis in that it is a state of mind in which the individual may experience tension and anxiety about events and their implications but can still test and recognize reality. In other words, the reality of thoughts and thinking is of central importance when considering delusions, and delusions may be seen in schizophrenia, while the capacity to recognize an external or internal reality and to test it against one's own beliefs and perceptions differentiates the non-psychotic or neurotic from the psychotic condition. Reality is thus a central issue in the delineation of key psychiatric states. But what that reality is vis-à-vis the external world, let alone the internal is a perplex to all those who thoughtfully consider the human predicament.

> In likening those trees that I had seen in the garden to strange deities, had I not been mistaken like Magdalen when, in another garden, on a day whose anniversary was soon to come, she saw a human form and "supposed it was the gardener." Treasurers of our memories of the golden age, keepers of the promise that reality is not what we suppose.... (Proust, 1954)

Psychiatry may not always be able to offer a definition of the reality with which it negotiates, but it continues to fight its corner as a didactic discipline. And since a large portion of its work concerns the identification and treatment of those individuals whose personal relationship with reality is sufficiently at variance with others to have caused a communication or behaviour which has come to attention and aroused concern, there is a supposed model of reality in the head of most psychiatrists. Moreover, most psychiatrists have enough confidence in that model of reality to assume it will be shared by most other people and to take issue with the opposing view of patients. Thus two central features of this notion of reality emerge. It should be demonstrable by scientific methods and it should be agreed upon by most.

On the one hand then the reality of psychiatry strives to be that which is scientific and of the external, objective world. There is something unsatisfying about that opinion however, and those in many areas of art and those of psychodynamic persuasion would contend that it was actually antithetical:

> So often, in the course of my life, reality had disappointed me because at the instant when my senses perceived it my imagination, which was the only organ that I possessed for the enjoyment of beauty, could not apply itself to it, in virtue of that ineluctable law which ordains that we can only imagine what is absent. And now, suddenly, the effect of this harsh law had been neutralized, temporarily annulled, by a marvellous expedient of nature which had caused a sensation – the noise made by both the spoon and the hammer. (Proust, 1954).

Conventional psychiatry has more loyalty to physiology, and prefers that that which is seen should be something which reflects light, which is then incident upon the retina, that that which is heard should be that which is transmitted in waves and stimulates the inner ear and that that which is felt should be that which is capable of stimulating the sensory nerve endings in the skin. A perception occurring in the absence of a stimulus is a hallucination, and as such "unreal". The psychotic symptom, "hallucination" is not however, dealt with in detail in this chapter. Its partner "delusion", which is dealt with in detail below, has a deceptively reliable definition stating broadly that it is an unreal belief if it can be proposed that a delusion occurs because of unreal logic, it follows that there is an objectively testable and real logical or cognitive process which the normal do follow and the abnormal do not. But this has not seemed compelling to some either.

> This book (of life), more laborious to decipher than any other, is also the only one which has been dictated to us by reality, the only one of which the "impression" has been printed in us by reality itself. When an idea – an idea of any kind – is left in us by life, its material pattern, the outline of the impression that it made upon us, remains behind as the token of its necessary truth. The ideas formed by the pure intelligence have no more than a logical, a possible truth, they are arbitrarily chosen. The book whose hieroglyphs are patterns not traced by us is the only book that really belongs to us. Not that the ideas which we form for ourselves cannot be correct in logic; that they may well be, but we cannot know whether they are true. (Proust, 1954).

Both hallucinations and delusions occur in schizophrenia, and it is a hypothesis available for development that there is a single fault underlying these two which results in inability to appraise reality outside the mind or inside it. There are of course, other symptoms of schizophrenia and faulty reality testing is more definitive of psychosis than of schizophrenia, an important distinction which has been mentioned and which will be expanded below.

On the other hand the notion that the real, *ergo* sane, state of affairs can be authorized by consensus is strong in conventional psychiatry. So much so that traditionally it is regarded as good practice to enquire of informants whether a state of affairs reported by a patient really is so. For example, were there *really* problems with talkative and grumbling neighbours, or would any other family member *really* have shared a belief that a deceased relation was available as a source of advice. The reality of the many being seen as more convincing than the reality of the individual. So the reality of psychiatry takes a fair bit and probably most of its credibility from being that declared, seen or perceived by the majority – the men on the Clapham omnibus. It is a sort of average but not clearly modal, mean or median. Whether that is safe or satisfactory is a separate debate. Whether because an opinion or percept is held by many it becomes real regardless of any other factors, or whether there is a quintessentially real logic or perception which most people are likely to share has preoccupied philosophical thinkers.

In any event this socially defined or consensus reality has dangers. There are profound social dangers because those deemed to be psychiatrically "ill" attract penalties of opportunity and freedom. There is always in a free society, anxiety, intermittently reinforced, that psychiatry has got it wrong and X was not mad after all. In an oppressed society there is fear likewise, sometimes justified, that psychiatry is allied with authority and that which is deemed not the right view is being perverted into not the real view, and so "mad". And moreover, since usually only one or a few psychiatrists see a given patient there exists the possibility that the psychiatrist's view is deviant, unreal or mad. And there is an ever present risk of misidentifying individual intellectualism as madness. And so on.

No doubt emerging partly in response to this, there are other schools of psychological thought which are less committed to social reality as the norm, and which do not regard testable external reality as the appropriate yardstick by which the human condition should be measured. The phenomenological, empathetic school ascribes weight to the meaning of the individual patient's mental set and indeed takes the view that the relevant reality is that of the individual (Jaspers, 1959). The psychodynamic schools likewise respect greatly the meaning of an individual's beliefs and deductions to them. The "antipsychiatry" schools attempt a different approach to the same issues, along the line that there is no pathological problem if an individual's world view is at variance with others or with that commonly upheld and any resulting dissonance is the responsibility of the matrix of society. Whether any of these views can function as a categorical alternative to that of conventional psychiatry should provoke thought.

Let us now look at how the notion of reality has impinged upon the development of topics in psychiatry introduced above.

## Delusions

Delusions are a special sort of unreal belief. Jaspers described then as the basic characteristic of madness and psychiatrists are considerably attached to them as important symptoms or signs. The identification of a delusion is accepted as evidence that an individual is psychotic, although whether this is of much real significance is argued below. In that respect delusions may be more phenomenologically basic than hallucinations, since true hallucinations are distinguished from pseudohallucinations (in one sense of that term) by the presence of a delusional belief in the reality of the hallucinatory perception.

Delusions are also respected as stigmata of mental abnormality in wider fields. They are the *sine qua non* of insanity in many of its forensic applications and depending on their content may result in the compulsory detention of the holder.

It might therefore be expected that there is a clear conception of what a delusion is. There is at least an agreed definition. Students in psychiatry learn the catechism response that a delusion is a false, unshakeable idea or belief which is out of keeping with the patient's educational, cultural and social background and is held with extraordinary conviction and subjective certainty (Sims, 1988). In other words the deluded person has a belief which he holds to be true while others think it false. The three separate components of the definition do however, need to be borne in mind. Jaspers (1959) summarized them in his description of a delusion as a perverted view of reality, incorrigibly held.

Delusions are traditionally divided into primary and secondary. These categories are not clear, but as discussed by Sims (1988), a primary delusion is probably best understood as one which cannot be ascribed to a response to another psychopathology, and does not reflect a disturbance of perception or intelligence. Primary delusions are regarded as autochthonous, and in phenomenological notation are un-understandable, that is to say not meaningful in any interpretation of the individual's biography or personality. Secondary delusions are those which do not fulfil the criteria above, in other words they may have strong affective colouring or accompany organic brain disease or be understandable products of the holder's development or environment. The difference between primary and secondary delusions is imprecise, not least because it may be established on the strength of how much is known about the patient. It is not surprising that some authors claim that all delusions are understandable and therefore secondary if one knows enough about the patient. Because of such difficulties, not all primary delusions are first rank symptoms of schizophrenia, although they are at the same time deemed to be pathognomonic of that condition! Jaspers regarded primary delusions as true delusions and called secondary delusions "delusion-like ideas."

While Jaspers' vocabulary is not in common use, most psychiatrists would suggest that primary delusions, whatever they may be, suggest something particularly odd occurring in the mental apparatus at the time of their inception and deserving of special attention. It is worth reiterating the triad of constituents of a delusion: there is an abnormal sequence of thought, which leads to notions which have no foundation in reality and which are adhered to despite the presentation of reality based alternative evidence. Thus a breakdown in proper utilization of reality-data occurs in more than one way in the production of a delusion, and although it is possible to hurry on by saying that a delusion results from faulty reality testing of a cognition, this does not advance things much. The components of the delusional process deserve more attention.

Four types of primary delusion are identified. First is the *autochthonous delusion* or delusional intuition. Such ideas arise in a single stage, out of the blue, are usually self referent and of huge import to the patient. Second is the *delusional percept* (which is a first rank symptom of schizophrenia) and is a two-stage development. A normal perception is invested with delusional meaning so that in the first stage the object becomes meaningful in the field of sensations and in the second it becomes invested with delusional significance. Third is *delusional mood* (atmosphere) when the individual experiences a global sense that something portentous is going on. Fourth is *delusional memory* (retrospective delusion), which may have characteristics of the above but which is attributed to the past.

But dissecting the category "delusion" does not reveal a unique, shared and definitive characteristic of the group and indeed this proves extremely difficult to state in terms of reality or anything else. "Delusion" may ultimately prove to be a polythetic category. For the time being however, contributors keep trying to characterize the category in their own vocabularies. The cognitive schools suggest that true delusions are underpinned by a rearrangement of meanings in the face of desymbolization and emerge as an attempt to explain a new, otherwise incomprehensible status quo. Others, following Schneider (1949) have suggested that delusions only occur because there is brain abnormality, for others following Bleuler the foundation is an alteration in the mood state. Yet others following Kretschmer (1927) suggest delusions develop from a preexisting personality configuration. Followers of Freud have emphasized the comprehensibility of so-called delusions and would therefore not suggest that they needed a status separate from that of "psychotic" and the antipsychiatrists would suggest that a delusion was an adaptive response to intolerable psychosocial stress.

On the one hand one can only be impressed although not surprised that the same avenues have been explored in attempts to gain some understanding of psychosis (*q.v.*), but on the other one is really no further forward in identifying the essence of delusion. As Roberts (1992) points out "attempts to understand its pathogenesis have been dominated by unsubstantiated speculation." Winters and Neale (1983) consider existing theories of delusion formation fall into two camps: the motivational and the defective. In the former the delusion arrives to explain or relieve an aberrant state of mind, presumably when contact with reality has already been lost, in the latter it reflects a cognitive-attentional deficit, presumably when reality cannot be appraised.

Roberts (1992) provides a useful review of the various theories about the origin of delusions and points out that it is essential that researchers in this field do not fall into the trap of thinking that reliable operational descriptions, which may refine diagnostic opportunity, are actually theories (see also Persons, 1986). Roberts suggests that some of the difficulties in achieving a useful overview of the topic arise because separate contributors are unable or unwilling to synthesize their hypotheses, but also points out that there has in the past never been an adequate model to facilitate experimental research into delusions, a state of affairs which the cognitive school is able to go some way to redress. Roberts presents a general, parsimonious model of the formation of delusional belief based on the assumption that this follows a temporal sequence and may progress through a number of stages. That model is divided into pre-psychotic, acute, and chronic phases, representing the vulnerability, inception and increasing complexity of delusional development.

Re the pre-psychotic phase: attention is drawn to pre-disposing factors which, although expressed in multifarious vocabulary, can be summarized as a blurring of the ability to keep apart the internal and the external world together with a blurring of the ability to keep apart fantasy and reality. The individual has some awareness of this which causes hypervigilance and the paranoid conclusion that outside agencies are threatening an already tenuous control. Frith and Done (1989) propose that delusions (and hallucinations) arise from a disorder of internal monitoring, resulting in the failure to recognize internally generated acts as such. These same authors demonstrate experimentally that patients with delusions of alien control had impaired monitoring of internal selection of motor action. They proposed that the deficit arose because of impaired neurological connections between the mesial temporal lobe and the frontal cortex.

More traditional sources suggest that the prepsychotic state is the result of regressed pre-symbolic thought process – either infantile or phylogenetically primitive. This line was developed by Arieti (1964) who proposed that delusions emerged as a defence against overwhelming anxiety generated by regression from Aristotelian logic to Paleologic. The cardinal feature of the latter is that things are thought to be identical because they have in common a single feature. This paralyses symbolization and results in gross classification errors by the individual to whom the notion of reality is then redundant.

Satisfying though this may be it does not gain much support from experimental studies – the logical processes of the deluded are not demonstrably different from those of the non-deluded, unless one integrates into this the very particular "illogicality" of formal thought disorder, which would be a sleight of hand. It can however, perhaps be observed that this pre-psychotic stage is an awareness by the individual that he is on the verge of losing his grip on the appraisal of reality – his own and that of the world about him. Why some patients suffer delusions whereas others do not remains an enigma.

Suggestions as to what may precipitate a delusion in the predisposed individual are if anything even wider! Roberts suggests that the host of factors can be said to share an ability to disrupt previous patterns of meaning, to create experimental novelty or to produce arousal. It has also been the observation that delusional states may emerge in relationship with demonstrable coarse organic brain disease. Tantalising though this is, it has not been possible to use the findings to generate any very substantial hypotheses about neuropathological associations of delusions because they are seen in so many disorders of the central nervous system. The phenomenological division of delusions into "organic" and "functional" does not hold up well, which may suggest there is no such natural division. There is now focused interest on abnormalities of the limbic and subcortical structures in "functional" illness which will be discussed further in the section on schizophrenia. One can meanwhile, share the conclusion of Roberts that the contribution of organic factors to delusional development may be represented in a specific vulnerability and a non-specific precipitant and to recognize that the most cohesive explanation for the inauguration of a delusion is a profound affective stressor which provokes disintegration of previous structures and a drive to reduce anxiety.

Even having set this stage of pre-psychotic panic it is difficult to formulate what occurs to make a delusion. Bleuler discusses the breakdown of associative threads between thinking and feeling with a reduction in the capacity for logic coinciding with increased emotionality. The result of this is that logical thinking with its purchase on reality is put at the service of affective needs and delusions emerge as the new meaning attributed to the changed view of the world. In other words, for Bleuler the primary problem is the unreal logic of thought disorder.

Beyond this stage of delusion formation it is not essential to suggest there is an abnormal process, merely that the individual casts around for explanation for the utterly bizarre experience above, which of the static types of primary delusion outlined is closest to delusional mood. Explanations are assembled from fragments of the individual's acquired knowledge, from his biography, from fiction and media (and presumably, sometimes by chance from the reality in which case others do not note any abnormality).

Roberts reports some work that suggests that there may in addition be abnormalities in the attributional style of the deluded, characterized by a readiness to jump to conclusions, to invest coincidence with meaning, to make external attributions for aversive experience and to exhibit high level of certainty in decision making tasks. These may of course be *post-hoc* developments.

Considered too are the factors which influence whether a delusional system is elaborated or becomes chronic. It is clear that the less intellectually dilapidated a patient is, the more elaborate his delusional system is likely to be and indeed a chronic and coherently expressed delusional system is associated with a relatively good psychosocial prognosis. In juxtaposition to this are the conditions proposed by Berner (1986) under which an acute certitude becomes chronic, viz. that the environment reacts with suspicion, depriving the patient of corrective experiences, there is post-psychotic dynamic depletion such that the individual loses the intellectual ability to test reality or there is coexisting organic impairment which has the same effect. These conditions should be considered in the light of those patients whose delusions remain transient, discussed in the section on psychosis in this chapter. They should also be considered in the light of the proposal of many authors who note that a perpetrated delusional system has many benefits (see Roberts 1991 for review) and that loss of delusion may force an individual into a painful re-entry into reality based appraisal of life which is much the theme of the quotations cited from "Remembrance of Things Past".

The relationship of delusion formation to contact with reality remains obscure. One can propose from the above that the severance from reality in the delusional process seems to occur with affect dominating logic rather than the "normal" obverse, and that the "new" reality established is extremely convincing to the subject. One can suggest, feebly, that this probably has neurobiological correlates and is then psychologically elaborated.

Fulford (1989) takes a considerably more robust view of the uncertainty around the meaning of delusion above. He appraises the conventional triadic definition of delusions, viz. that they are false beliefs, incorrigibly held and culturally atypical and challenges whether any of these is valid (*a priori* to substantiate the intuitive moral grounds of compulsory treatment for the deluded). In short he concludes they are not. He gives several examples of beliefs which while true are nevertheless delusional, a conundrum well recognized in clinical practice. He reminds the reader than many delusions are not beliefs at all but value judgements, and emphasizes that to judge as false another individual's value judgement is treacherous. Fulford considers the criterion of incorrigibility weak because mere conviction is not a mark of pathology and that to consider as pathological a view that is "culturally atypical" is paternalistic and totalitarian. Noting that even with unequivocable delusions there is usually no defect of logical thinking as such, he points out that those who would retain delusions as the hall-mark of psychosis or of mental illness are on thin ice. He posits an alternative hypothesis – that delusions are (or derived from) a species not of defective reasoning but of defective reasons for action, which puts a very different complexion upon the matter.

Attention will now be turned to psychosis, of which so called condition delusions may be an indicator. After an introduction there will be a divergence into first a discussion of psychosis as it relates to the state disorder schizophrenia, and then to a discussion of psychosis as it is variously used in psychiatry and as it relates to the trait neurosis.

**Psychosis**

Psychosis is a phenomenological finding and is thus neither a putative illness nor a symptom. Nevertheless, there is a feeling in psychiatry that, while little is certain, it should at least be clear whether a patient is or is not psychotic. In conventional psychiatric classification the presence of psychosis separates "major" from "minor" disorder. The former includes the organic brain syndromes in which, in a hierarchial system (Foulds, 1976; Parshall and Priest, 1993), psychotic symptoms are expected and allowed, and the so-called functional psychoses, schizophrenia and manic depressive disorder, in which of course psychotic symptoms are a key feature. The latter, which clinically may be by no means minor, includes neurotic and personality disorder.

Maverick conditions which challenge this divide haunt nosologists, for example the so-called atypical psychoses, borderline personality disorder of which transient psychosis is the most reliable feature, and severe psychosomatic disturbance, for example anorexia nervosa. In these there are apparently psychotic symptoms which are not only completely atypical in terms of duration and diffuseness, but also occurring in "minor" illnesses. In other conditions, e.g. so-called negative-symptom schizophrenia, there is an alternative embarrassment. The condition seems clearly to be more closely related to major than minor disorders and evidence supporting this can be recruited from reputable disciplines such as genetics and neuroimaging, but yet the psychotic phenomena are absent. One is forced to conclude that either the current conception of "psychosis" is wrong or at least too weak to be of use in the face of information taken from other sources or that the framework of psychiatry is wrong despite other data.

This demands a brief review of what is understood by psychotic. It is odd but true that so widely though the word is used in psychological medicine, it has no well established definition. Broadly it implies "very" disturbed, for example the Oxford dictionary offers that psychosis means severe mental derangement involving the whole personality. A quantitative definition can however, offer little to psychiatric classifications, particularly those such as the ICD which strive to be aetiologically guided.

"Psychosis" in the setting of contemporary psychiatry is embedded in an essentially "medical" tradition. There is a tendency, with historical antecedent, to acknowledge that the presence of psychosis suggests brain disease. This view is usually first ascribed to Griessinger who in fact had a more encompassing view, asserting that "psychological diseases are diseases of the brain" (1861).

For the next half century views diversified as observers became more occupied by the psychological components of psychosis. The Swiss school including Bleuler and Jung maintained that organic brain disorder underlay psychosis. Bleuler emphasized that brain disease was responsible for the primary symptoms of the disorder – the disorder in this case being a very broad view of schizophrenia which was seen as effectively synonymous with psychosis. But Bleuler's primary symptoms of schizophrenia psychosis were those of the personality, viz. "Autism, Ambivalence, loosening of associations and affective-ideational splitting". Bleuler regarded reality distortion symptoms like delusions and hallucinations as secondary, the individual's psychological response to the primary features, which should recall the discourse on delusion formation above. Since it is these symptoms which conspicuously demonstrate a rent in the individual's appreciation of (other people's) reality, this position also relegates the central importance of this.

## Psychosis and its relationship to schizophrenia

Schneider (1959) took an opposing position in his reclassification of overt symptoms, the presence of which, in the absence of overt brain disease, help circumscribe schizophrenia. These familiar "first rank" symptoms include delusional perception, hallucinatory voices in the form of a running commentary and passivity experience. These all lean heavily on the concept of a patient's relationship with reality for definition. Adoption of first rank symptoms has not however, resulted in a strict definition of a syndrome of schizophrenia with a uniform prognosis, nor is it entirely successful in differentiating schizophrenia from other conditions.

If psychotic symptoms are understood to be plesiomorphic, i.e. generally distributed, and only more specific to schizophrenia than to other functional psychosis, it is not surprising that they occur commonly in manic depressive psychosis. They occur also however, in 9% of people with so called neurotic and character disorders (Carpenter et al., 1973). This emphasizes that psychotic symptoms really do not conveniently define the functional psychoses as they are currently understood, and does suggest that it is methodologically more prudent not to see them as of relevance in illuminating the coherence or aetiology of schizophrenia or any other nosological entity, but rather as an indicator of a thought or perceptual aberration which may or may not be of unitary genesis. A useful corollary of this would be to separate the word psychosis from its association with the currently recognized major psychiatric disorder, or as several more radical authors suggested, ban the noun altogether and use the adjective, "psychotic" a great deal more specifically.

Despite the convenience and common usage of schneiderian first rank symptoms in practical psychiatry it is recognized by most that appraisal of information garnered from techniques more modern than phenomenology (although not necessarily superseding it as a methodological tool) has invited new hypotheses of the category schizophrenia and its subdivisions to be explored. The current mainstream would probably cautiously concur that schizophrenia is a neurodevelopmental disorder for which there can be a considerable genetic vulnerability and which is often associated with disarray in the mesial temporal, limbic and frontal cytoarchitecture and widespread accompanying disturbance of neural and psychosocial function. The cause of course remains obscure.

Recommended subdivisions of schizophrenia are legion and are covered by standard reference texts. In the past two decades however, classifications of schizophrenia have often resulted in a division between those forms in which psychotic symptoms, i.e. hallucinations and delusions are prominent and those in which these symptoms, and indeed aspects of the personality, are conspicuous by their underrepresentation. The paradigm for this being "positive" versus "negative" symptom schizophrenia, but the same theme emerges in the "Type I versus Type II" division and is implied when "active" schizophrenia or a defect state is discussed. This does little more than emphasize that severance from reality is *not* a very effective tool in the investigation of schizophrenia. However, because there has been a wave of research into the neuropathology of schizophrenia and its subtypes, there has been a parallel interest in the neuropathological relationship of hallucination and delusion.

Liddle *et al.* (1992) summarize and contribute to this work. Previously Liddle had segregated, on neuropsychological findings, three putative syndromes of schizophrenia. He proposes that a psychomotor poverty syndrome is associated with dysfunction of the left dorsal pre-frontal cortex, that a disorganization syndrome is associated with dysfunction of the right ventral pre-frontal cortex and a reality distortion syndrome comprising hallucinations and delusions is associated with an abnormality of the medial temporal lobe. Regional Cortical Blood Flow (rCBF) data, as made available from PET scanning, are presented and support these syndromes. In the case of reality distortion there is a correlation between syndrome score and rCBF in the left parahippocampal area which is in line with a progressive body of evidence implicating this part of the brain as of central importance in schizophrenia. There are reports of SPECT imaging on schizophrenic patients with auditory hallucinations, showing increased tracer uptake in the left temporal lobe while the patients are hallucinating.

Suffice it to say that contemporary psychiatry is able to suggest focal brain damage associated with, if not necessarily causing, the experiences during which an individual is said to be cut off from reality.

## Psychosis and its relationship to neurosis

If the concept of a psychosis is separated from the concept of "major" psychiatric diagnosis, and thereby the concept of specific organic aetiology, widespread emergence of psychotic symptoms becomes less disquieting. The atypical psychoses do not, as some authors have suggested (Vaillant, 1964), have to be regarded as variants of schizophrenia, and can be considered independently.

Some traditions have used this freedom to interpret the severance from reality which seems to underlay the formation of psychotic symptoms as the result of overwhelming psychological stress, allowing that psychosis can be purely psychogenic, even if the major psychiatric disorders are organic. Boenhoffer (1911), for example, suggests that mental processes of an emotional kind can call into being and maintain psychotic process in personalities already vulnerable on account of their constitution or disposition. Binder (1955) posits that some delusions and hallucinations, not just their contents, are but the exaggeration of a normal psychic development. In this school, a progression can be traced from normal conviction to overvalued idea to delusion, in a comprehensible, empathically understandable way. In other words, in contrast with the conclusions drawn here on the likely origins of delusions, there is no need to consider an organic contribution to all psychotic symptoms. Following this path schizophrenia is different because in this the delusions are absurd, a view naturally contested by both the phenomenological and psychoanalytic factions.

The atypical psychoses to which to some borderline personality disorder is close, have represented such a perplex to those who encounter them that it is probably not surprising that they should have attracted somewhat perorative names and reputations, for example, "hysterical", "factitious" or "malingering". If the concept of psychosis is set against a concept of neurosis, let alone attached to a concept of organicity, then the nosological status of these conditions, becomes an issue close to the psychiatrist's dignity. Various authors have examined representatives of the group in detail to see whether "true" psychotic symptoms can be shown to disappear under scrutiny. True in this respect implies delusions or hallucinations, the hard, narrow, symptoms of psychosis, as opposed to depersonalization and derealization which are seen as softer, wider symptoms. Phenomenological studies of Pope *et al.* (1985) and Chopra and Bateson (1986) concluded that it is possible to demonstrate psychotic symptoms in clusters of patients who do not have schizophrenia and do not categorize into any of the diagnoses above, and even more striking are the findings of Chapman and Chapman (1986) on socially integrated college students in whom they identified a significant proportion with hard as well as soft psychotic symptoms.

From the above it is to be concluded that psychotic symptoms are apparently widespread in expression and distribution in clinical syndromes and in non-clinical controls. What is less clear is whether there is a continuum between the psychotic and non-psychotic experience, and in order to examine this it is relevant to focus more closely upon the characteristics of the psychotic state which have been promoted as definitive of it, viz. insight, voluntary control and, most germane here, reality testing.

Insight is roughly a patient's recognition that he is suffering from a mental illness, and is assumed to be faulty in psychosis. Identifying insight is not easy. David (1990) looked at components of insight as they are operationalized in clinical practice and was led to the conclusion that it was not an all or nothing phenomenon. Earlier authors have also been impressed by "intermediate level of disbelief in the reality of abnormal perceptions and convictions" (Strauss, 1969).

Fulford (1989) provides a discourse on why insight is unlikely to stand up as a hard character, because our formulation of it is wrong. That author points out that the presence of severe (often read as psychotic) mental illness is taken as grounds for application to the Mental Health Act, compulsory detention and treatment. He comments, fairly, that there is underlying this an assumption that mental illness is different from physical illness, since there is no Physical Illness Act. However, the conventional psychiatric school is usually more concerned with promoting the similarities between severe mental illness, and in particular psychosis and organic illness, than the differences between them. Fulford has suggested that if an Illness Model is interpreted as a Dysfunction Model, mental illness is a better illness paradigm than physical illness, and moreover psychotic mental illnesses are paradigm mental illnesses.

Despite this however, as Fulford points out there is something about psychotic mental illness which is significantly at variance with other illnesses to allow special medico-legal consequences. He points out that intuitively it would be argued that it was lack of insight, or reality testing, that constituted this difference, in other words, non-psychotic patients (characteristically) recognize that they are mentally ill, while psychotic patients (characteristically) do not. But therefore, it would seem as if the psychotic's particular irrationality is that he gets his diagnosis wrong. He is as it were wrong on various points of fact to do with data, knowledge and the correct perception of signs and symptoms. On these grounds, the insight which the psychotic lacks is no different from that lacked by patients who do not correctly notice or appraise physical illness. Both groups can be said to have failed to test reality, and reality testing then seems meaningless as a key characteristic at the psychotic/non-psychotic interface. Indeed, Fulford concludes, in line with Aubrey Lewis, that this is a distinction without a difference which has lost whatever usefulness it may once have had, and should be abandoned. He promotes an alternative hypothesis that the concept of psychosis is better understood not in terms of the conventional view of disease = dysfunction, but rather in terms of disease = action failure. So much for the meaningfulness of insight!

However compelling the arguments against the reality of psychosis, it remains the case that there is extreme reluctance to drop the notion of a psychotic/non-psychotic divide. While DSM III and ICD IO give it little nosological respect it is still implicated and there is a general feeling that it would be difficult to do without it. One solution is to try to drop the concept of psychosis, since this, as any sort of category, let alone illness, seems too vague to be of use, and to continue to try to grasp what may be coherent about the psychotic state.

Other authors have given more credence than Fulford to reality testing in this regard. Frosch (1964) asserts that the existence of psychosis "hinges mainly on the loss or retention of the ability to test reality". Frosch separates for examination, three aspects of the association of the self with reality. These are relationship with reality, feelings of reality and reality testing. The differences between these can best be appreciated by their impairment. Disturbances in the relationship with reality include perceptual distortions such as illusions and hallucinations. The feeling of reality breaks down in depersonalization and derealization. Testing of reality which is crucial for the psychotic/non-psychotic divide, refers to a patient's evaluation of these experiences.

As discussed in the section on delusions, psychoanalysis also accepts the phenomenological view that psychosis is a break from reality, formulated in the language of that discipline as a withdrawal of the cathexis of the ego from the external world. The rent in reality is then occupied by a symptom such as a delusion or a hallucination. Psychoanalysis postulates however, that while there is rupture with external reality, there is continuity of the inner or psychological reality of the subject, and following this therefore the content of psychotic experiences is meaningful in the symbolic or biographical sphere of the patient. Thus a psychological continuity is established between the normal and psychotic states of mind, and psychoanalysts would argue that there is a measure of continuity between psychosis, neurosis and normality. Analysts would argue that dreams and hallucinations are very similar. And thus, the hall-mark of psychosis, the dismissal of reality, is psychotic only in its extreme form because everybody, neurotics and normals included, distorts to some degree and fails to correct completely their distortions. Psychotics radically replace reality with an internal psychological production, then confusing internal with external, while neurotics modify it to a lesser degree through affect charged fantasies et cetera.

In psychoanalysis, the concept of psychosis extends beyond the symptom criteria. For the schools of thought following Klein (1946) or Bion (1957) and Kernberg (1981), psychotic refers to a type of mental functioning, potentially present in every body and clinically evident in different individuals under different circumstances. Psychotic and non-psychotic parts of the personality coexist, and a psychoanalyst may demonstrate psychotic enclaves in apparently normal individuals. Moreover, in psychoanalysis, the word psychotic is also used, informally, to describe extremely intense psychic disturbance of any type. It is used to warn of those patients who, it is predicted, may break down in analysis – classically those with the borderline configuration – and it is also used to describe infantile psychological states.

## Conclusion

Having introduced this chapter by suggesting that the concept of reality is of central importance in the definition of key psychiatric states, I would not conclude differently. The reality in question for conventional psychiatry is that of consensus and physiological perception, reflecting neatly psychiatry's dual affiliations to medicine and sociology. Loss of reality testing is the only phenomenon which should retain the adjective psychotic, the neurotic-psychotic divide is not graded but psychosis is a graded condition.

It seems that an individual's proper relationship with and capacity to test reality is maintained through integrity of mesial temporal structures. These can dysfunction temporarily, chronically or permanently, and the breakdown occurs with a flood of pure limbic affect. Indeed this may be close to the affective-ideational splitting of Bleuler. At our current state of knowledge it seems that this dysfunction can occur in many states of mind and does not enlighten psychiatric nosology.

Beyond this it seems appropriate to assume that all consequences of an individual losing touch with his reality testing should be interpreted as secondary. Hallucinations and illusions can be understood as psychological elaborations constructed to make sense of the new reality as it is perceived vis-à-vis the external world. These co-exist with retained normal perceptive ability. Thought disorder can be seen to be a cognitive rearrangement assembled to explain a new appearance of the internal world and this co-exists with retained normal logical capacity.

How an observer describes and discusses these phenomena will depend upon his perspective, be it sociological, legal, philosophical, psychodynamic or cognitive. Some of these discussions have been observed in this chapter. Such discussions may be extremely interesting and enlightening and seem to have contributed as much to "human" thought as any topic one can think of. Perhaps that is their adaptive function and that that is what keeps us all going.

What is also clear is that the loss of ability to test reality is often more apparent to and of more concern to those who witness it than those who undergo it, despite the heavy direct and indirect social penalty which it can attract. One suspects that an intact ability to test reality, tedious though it often is, is fundamental to the maintenance of a secure, cohesive and evolving society. This would be a further adaptive function.

Nevertheless there is an impression that most if not all people can switch if only partially into a psychotic mode of functioning and that this is often an agreable and cosmic experience quested after, for example, by those enjoying hallucinogenic drugs. The experience of new internal and external reality seems, at best, to have the joy of novelty and to be bathed in feeling. Possibly some artistic productions can elicit an echo of that feeling in others allowing some respite from their own human reality.

But this discovery which art obliges us to make, is it not, I thought, really the discovery of what, though it ought to be more precious to us than anything in the world, yet remains ordinarily for ever unknown to us, the discovery of our true life, of reality as we have felt it to be, which differs so greatly from what we think it is that when a chance happening brings us an authentic memory of it we are filled with an immense happiness? In this conclusion I was confirmed by the thought of the falseness of the so-called realist art, which would not be untruthful if we had not in life acquired the habit of giving to what we feel a form of expression which differs so much from, and which we nevertheless, after a little time take to be, reality itself. (Proust, 1954).

## References

Arieti, S. (1964). "Interpretation of Schizophrenia". Crosby Lockwood Staples, London.
Arthur, A.Z. (1964). Theories and explanations of delusions: a review. *American Journal of Psychiatry,* **121**, 105-115.
Berner, P., Gabriel, E., Kieffer, W. et al. (1986). Paranoid psychosis: new aspects of classification and prognosis coming from the Vienna Research Group. *Psychopathology,* **19**, 16-29.
Bion, W.R. (1957). Differentiation of the psychotic from the non-psychotic personalities. *International Journal of Psychoanalysis,* **38**, 266-275.
Bleuler, E. (1911). "Dementia Praecox or the Group of Schizophrenias" (transl. Zinkin, J.) International Universities Press, New York.
Boenhoffer, K. (1911). How far should all psychogenic illnesses be regarded as hysterical? (transl. Candy, J) *In* "Themes and Variations in European Psychiatry". (Eds S.R. Hirsch and M. Shepard, 1974). University of Virginia, Charlottesville.
Carpenter, W.T., Strauss, J.S. and Mulich, S. (1973). Are there pathognomic symptoms of

schizophrenia? *Archives of General Psychiatry,* **28**, 847-52.

Chapman, L.J. and Chapman J.P. (1986). Scales for rating psychotic and psychotic-like experiences as continua. *Schizophrenia Bulletin,* **6**, 476-88.

Chopra, H. and Bateson, J. (1986). Psychotic symptoms in Borderline Personality Disorder. *American Journal of Psychiatry,* **143**, 1605-7.

David, A. (1990). Insight and psychosis. *British Journal of Psychiatry,* **156**, 798-808.

Frith, C.R. and Done, D.J. (1989). Experiences of alien control in schizophrenia reflect a disorder in the central monitoring of action. *Psychological Medicine,* **19**, 359-63.

Foulds, G.A. (1976). "The Hierarchical Nature of Personal Illness". Academic, London and New York.

Frosch, J. (1964). The psychotic character. Clinical psychiatric considerations. *Psychiatric Quarterly,* **38**, 1-16.

Fulford, K.W.N. (1989). "Moral Theory and Medical Practice". Cambridge University Press.

Jaspers, K. (1959). "General Psychopathology". (transl. J. Hoenig and M.W. Hamilton, 1963). Manchester University Press, Manchester.

Kernberg, O.F. (1981). Structural interviewing. *In* "Borderline Disorders". *Psychiatric Clinics of North America,* **4**, 1, 169-195.

Kretschmer, E. (1927). The sensitive delusion of reference (transl. J. Candy). *In* "Themes and Variations in European Psychiatry". (Eds S.R. Hirsch and M. Shepherd, 1974). John Wright, Bristol.

Liddle, P.F., Friston, K.J., Frith, C.D. et al. (1992). Patterns of cerebral blood flow in schizophrenia. *British Journal of Psychiatry,* **160**, 179-87.

Parshall, A.M. and Priest, R.G. (1993) Nosology, Taxonomy and the Classification Conundrum of the functional psychoses. *British Journal of Psychiatry,* **162**, 227-236.

Persons, J.B. (1986). The advantages of studying psychological phenomena rather than psychiatric diagnoses. *American Psychologist,* **41**, 1252-1260.

Pope, H., Jonas, J., Hudson, J.I., Cohen, B. and M. Tohen, (1985). An empirical study of psychosis in Borderline Personality Disorder. *American Journal of Psychiatry,* **142**, 1285-90.

Proust, M. (1913-27). "Remembrance of Things Past". (Transl. C.K. Scott Moncrieff, 1954). Chatto and Windus, London.

Roberts, G.A. (1991). Delusional belief and meaning in life: a preferred reality? *British Journal of Psychiatry,* **159** (suppl. 14), 20-29.

Schilder, P. (1951). On the development of thoughts. *In* "Organization and Pathology of Thought". (Ed. D. Rappaport). Columbia University Press, New York.

Schneider, K. (1949). "The concept of delusion". (transl. J. Candy). *In* "Themes and Variations in European Psychiatry". (1974). John Wright, Bristol.

Schneider, K. (1959). "Clinical Psychopathology". 5th edn. (transl. Hamilton, M.W.). Grune and Stratton, New York and London.

Sims, A. (1988). Delusions and other erroneous ideas. *In* "Symptoms in the Mind. An introduction to descriptive psychopathology". pp. 82-104. Balliere Tindall.

Strauss, J.S. (1969). Hallucinations and delusions as points on continua function. *Archives of General Psychiatry,* **21**, 581-586.

Tarnapolsky, A. and Berelowitz, M. (1987). Borderline personality: a review of recent research. *British Journal of Psychiatry,* **151**, 724-34.

Tarnapolsky, A., Chesterman, L.P. and Parshall, A.M. What is psychosis? Manuscript.

Vaillant, G.E. (1964). An historical view of the remitting schizophrenias. *Journal of Nervous and Mental Disorders,* **138**, 48-56.

Winters, K.C. and Neale, J.M. (1983). Delusions and delusional thinking in psychotics: a review of the literature. *Clinical Psychology Review*, **3**, 227-253.

# 18. Hysteria and conversion

Christopher J. Mace

## Introduction

"Hysteria" remains one of the most puzzling concepts within medicine. Ilza Veith has pointed out that its story runs the full length of medical history (Veith, 1965). However, hysteria continues to attract criticisms of its usefulness and validity, even though Lewis' (1965) remark that it tends to outlive its obituarists remains as true as ever.

In modern medicine, hysteria has become subdivided into syndromes, but in practice the distinctions between these have not always been drawn as clearly as they might. This chapter will present the often confusing subject of hysteria in terms of a series of ways in which what is "hysterical" seems opposed to what is "real". It is hoped that, in understanding some of the varied challenges hysteria poses to accepted ideas of reality, some light can be shed on hysteria's extraordinary longevity, its contentiousness, and its apparent indispensability. At the same time, a new logic within the rather arbitrary divisions to which it has been subject may become apparent.

## Reality and the Attribution of Illness

In medicine, as elsewhere, the nature of "reality" has to be arbitrated through agreements and disagreements between people. This is particularly evident with the concept of mental illness, where a deviant sense of reality can be an indication of illness. It has been remarked that at least three people are needed before it is possible for anyone to be called "mad". At least two people have to agree about what should pass for reality, and to agree also that whatever this reality is, the remaining person's grasp of it is deficient. Agreements of this sort do inform the idea of mental disorder, and the different sorts of disorder have been distinguished. It is notoriously difficult to identify these agreements accurately, even when they are apparently explicit. For instance, medical students are commonly taught that the anxious or "neurotic" patient possesses a grasp of reality that the mad or "psychotic" patient lacks. But a distinction on these grounds may seem shaky in the harsher light of clinical practice: many "neurotic" patients, although they may have a greater awareness that they are ill or in need of help, have thoughts and expectations that are no less bizarre or handicapping than those of the patient who is "psychotic". If this neat distinction is more problematic than it first appears, the way questions of reality bear upon diagnosis is likely to be complex. Yet the fraught diagnosis of "hysteria" seems to provide a particularly good vehicle for any attempt to unravel some of these complexities.

One way in which real circumstances differ from those of a trio setting out to label one of their number as "mad" *ab initio* (apart from cultural norms in which judgments about others are inevitably embedded) is that at least one professional group will have a special responsibility for diagnosing illness of all kinds. Its members, usually doctors, make sanctioned judgements about who is ill according to differences between normative standards applying to the population at large, and anyone from that population having a particular illness. For ordinary purposes, the judgements about ill health that result are quite independent of whether the doctor belongs to the group of the ill, rather than the rest of the population, and the judgements are taken for those that the reasonable person would make if they had the professional's education and his knowledge of the particular case.

However, when possession of an aberrant sense of reality becomes a qualification for a diagnosis, disagreements between the people involved are inevitable. Nevertheless, the general assumption holds that when people are deemed to be ill on these grounds, they are ill by virtue of differences between their experience and that of the rest of the population. But an important fact intrudes here. The professional arbiters of illness make up a distinct group whose members will also structure reality in ways peculiar to themselves. This introduces sources of possible disagreement other than conflicts between the "ill" and the "healthy", which may have important consequences for diagnostic practice. Among these, two are particularly relevant to a discussion of hysteria.

First is the possibility that groups of doctors, whose own handling of reality may differ in some respects from most other people, will experience conflict with some other groups of people whose handling of reality is no more aberrant, but happens to clash in key particulars with the medical standpoint. If so, there is a danger that specific conflicts of this sort might nevertheless be used by doctors as evidence of ill health among the people identified with the incompatible standpoint, even though their outlook may seem much less odd to most people.

A second possibility is that, as doctors develop demarcation criteria within their field of expertise, illness, their view of what counts as illness, may become refined until it clashes with the reactions of a layman. The internal logic of medical thinking could prompt doctors not only to see people as ill who do not appear so to most people, but to deny that some groups of people are "really" ill, even though most people might find little to distinguish them from people who doctors did accept had "real" illnesses.

## What is Hysteria?

Currently, it is fair to say that "hysteria" is a medical label that is both suspect and fragmented. While adjustments continue to be made in the formal classification of hysterical disorders, three broad kinds of hysteria have been commonly recognized. These differ not only in the sort of features they are associated with, but also in terms of whether the hysteria is seen as an illness, or as something that refers to a type of person.

### Hysteria as an illness

To say hysteria can be an illness is to see it as an undesirable affliction that has relatively specific effects on a person's state of mind or body. After a clear point of onset, an illness can be expected to follow a definable course in which there may be remissions, relapses, cure or exacerbation. Two main types of hysterical illness have been distinguished, according to whether symptoms are predominantly psychological or neurological.

In dissociation hysteria, psychological changes are attributed to a reversible division of awareness. This frequently results in an amnesia which is then referred to as "psychogenic" (Mace and Trimble, 1991). The dissociation may also be associated with evident alterations in conscious awareness, apparently undirected wandering, and changes in the sense of personal identity giving rise to the varieties of dissociation hysteria known as somnabulism and fugue states.

The other type of hysterical illness, conversion hysteria, is what doctors usually mean when they refer to "hysteria", and is associated with physical symptoms. These most commonly take the form of seizures, paralyses, losses of bodily sensation, aphonia, and blindness, and mimic neurological illnesses although they have no apparent physical cause. (Some forms of pain are often, but not universally, also regarded as common symptoms of conversion hysteria).

The symptoms of both dissociation hysteria and conversion hysteria are ones which are associated with other conditions also. However, whether these are amnesias or paralyses, their form is regarded as untypical of those associated with a known underlying pathology. Instead, the symptoms of either have been accounted for as having a psychological origin through unconscious mechanisms.

### Hysteria as a disorder of personality

An alternative way of construing hysteria has been as an inherent and relatively unchangeable aspect of a person, as in the epithet "hysteric". The medical concept of "personality disorder" designates instances where aspects of somebody's behaviour, while distressing to themselves or others, appear inherent to their personal make-up rather than a consequence of some external affliction. A personality disorder is manifest through certain traits that might be modified, but not removed, and for which, unlike the effects of an illness, the affected person is felt to remain responsible. Because a personality disorder lacks the clarity of an illness which may come and go, the concept is open to abuse, and care has to be taken to ensure that there has been a history of abnormal development, in which the distressing traits were emerging before adulthood.

The traits that have been specifically associated with a hysterical (or "histrionic") personality disorder have included changeable, dramatising and attention-craving behaviour as well as indiscriminate flirtatiousness. In practice, these have not always been clearly separated from the symptoms of hysterical illness, being mistakenly taken as evidence of conversion hysteria. In fact, only about 20% of patients with conversion hysteria seem to have a hysterical personality type (Kretschmer, 1926; Merskey, 1979).

## The grid of hysteria

While the diagnoses of dissociation hysteria, conversion hysteria and hysterical personality disorder usefully stake out the range of findings that may be subsumed under "hysteria", they are not absolutely exclusive. There are cases for which neither the ideas of illness nor personality disorder seem appropriate by themselves. For instance, some people appear to be persistently subject to dissociative mechanisms from an early age, and the development of their personality may be affected as a result. In cases where this appears to leave them relating to others through two or more personalities, each having its own associated behaviours and memories and displacing the other(s) in turn, some practitioners would make a diagnosis of "multiple personality disorder". However, this is an entity that moves uncertainly from the illness of dissociation hysteria towards the status of a personality disorder.

Similarly, some people are subject from an early age to multiple somatic complaints which have no evident physical cause. Attempts have been made to replace the diagnosis of conversion hysteria by redefining hysteria in terms of a chronic disposition to suffer from a wide range of unexplained physical symptoms. The rubrics of "hysteria" (Perley and Guze, 1962) "Briquet's hysteria" (Guze, 1970) and, currently, "somatoform disorder" (APA, 1980) have denoted disorders of this sort. However, their candidate symptoms are very broad in range and quite unspecific to the diagnosis. The designation marks a trait that might therefore be better expressed in terms of a particular pattern of behaviour (a compulsive form of doctor-shopping) rather than the physical complaints. It makes sense to see "somatoform disorder" as a further variety of personality disorder rather than a type of illness.

Given these continuities, the ambit of hysteria might best be summarized on a two-dimensional grid. One separates syndromes according to whether they resemble a discrete illness rather than a pervasive personality disorder; the other distinguishes the extent to which the presenting features are predominantly somatic or psychological in nature:

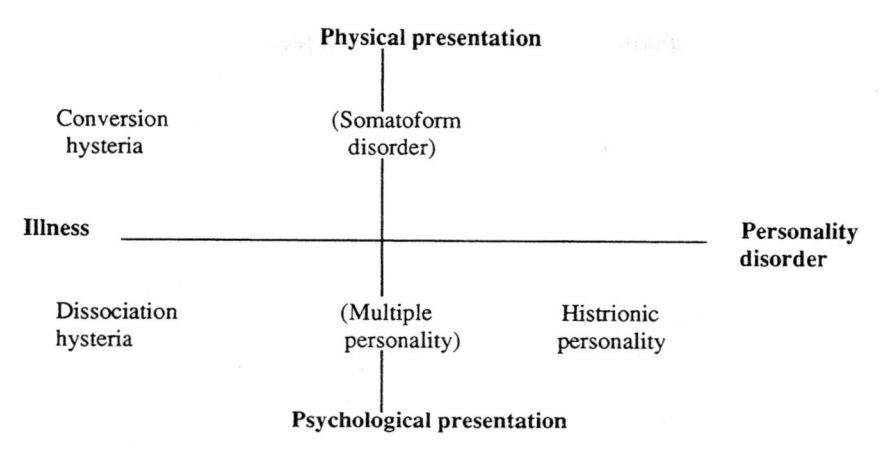

```
                    Physical presentation
                            |
  Conversion          (Somatoform
   hysteria            disorder)
                            |
                            |
  Illness  _____  Personality
                            |                     disorder
                            |
  Dissociation        (Multiple        Histrionic
   hysteria           personality)     personality
                            |
                  Psychological presentation
```

FIG. 1. The grid of hysteria.

## Hysteria and Reality

One of the reasons hysteria seems to be very closely bound up with questions of reality is that each of the major subtypes raises different issues about the nature of reality and who defines it. In brief, dissociation hysteria designates a set of states in which the patient attaches a changed sense of reality to his own experience; in hysterical personality disorder a patient is experienced by his doctor as being unreal in comparison to other people; in conversion hysteria, the doctor's training leads him to see these patients' illnesses as unreal compared to cases of "true" neurological illness.

## Hysterical dissociation and the experience of being unreal

The range of dissociation hysteria has been referred to already, while more detailed discussions of special forms such as psychogenic amnesia and fugue states will be found in other chapters within this section. Whether or not psychological dissociation has a specific impact on a patient's memory or his sense of identity, subjective feelings of detachment from his stream of experience are likely to be present. A distinction is often made here between detachment from one's own mental processes and/or body, termed depersonalization, and derealization, in which there is detachment from one's immediate environment (or distortion in the way it is experienced as a whole, e.g. as reduced in size). Both depersonalization and derealization refer to loss of a prior sense of reality, a change that marks the sufferer out from people who are not in a dissociative state.

It is important to remember here that not all dissociative states, whose range encompasses religious or hypnotic trances among other examples, fall within the illness of dissociation hysteria. Those that do do so on the presumption that the state is debilitating to the person experiencing it, and that the person's changed apprehension of reality is a less objective one (whether or not he experiences it as such himself). Although these judgements may be contentious, they are not different in kind to those involved in identifying other forms of psychological disorder. The comparisons that are crucial to dissociation hysteria lie between the prospective patient's sense of reality and that of people deemed "normal" within the culture at large. The fascination of its phenomena notwithstanding, hysterical dissociation provides a relatively uncomplicated instance of diagnosticians making clinical judgements consistent with widely shared convictions about reality, rather than prejudices that may be special to them as a group.

## Hysterical personality and the unreal persona

Many different, and often pejorative, traits have been attributed to the hysterical personality in addition to those cited above. They have included suggestibility, dissembling, frigidity, shallowness, and a preoccupation with appearances. These may seem ill-assorted, and research has questioned whether they do occur as a genuine cluster (Walton and Presley, 1973). Conversely, attempts to reinforce the concept have, following Shapiro (1965), added the idea that hysterical personality can be linked to a specific cognitive style as well as distinctly "soft" behavioural characteristics. (It is claimed that the hysterical person has a style of thought and speech that is characteristically impressionistic and lacking in detail, and this has received some empirical support (Miller and Magaro, 1977)).

However, it may be easy to overlook a vein running through the various qualities attributed to the hysterical personality type. This was summarized eloquently by a master psychopathologist, Karl Jaspers in 1923:

> To characterize the type more precisely we have to fall back on *one basic trait:* Far from accepting their given dispositions and life opportunities, hysterical personalities crave to appear, both to themselves and others, as more than they are and to experience more than they are ever capable of. The place of genuine experience and natural expression is usurped by a contrived stage-act, a forced kind of experience. This is not contrived "consciously" but reflects the ability of the true hysteric to live wholly in his drama, be caught up entirely for the moment and succeed in seeming genuine. All the other traits can be understandably deducted from this. In the end the hysterical personality loses its central "core" as it were, and consists simply of a number of different exteriors.

The abiding character of hysterical personalities is therefore a lack of authenticity: as people, they are unreal. Of course this is a savage judgement, and hard to validate. Like criticisms of the pejorative nature of descriptions of the hysteric ("a male psychiatrist's caricature of femininity" (Chodoff and Lyons, 1958)), it smacks of partiality. But it can also be a judgment that reveals as much about the doctors' values as their patients'.

In a little-known piece, Eliot Slater, already infamous for denouncing the concept of hysteria as an illness (Slater, 1965) speculated, at the end of his career, on the reasons why hysterical character was outlined in opprobrious terms in principle, and why the young and attractive females who attracted the label received such a frosty reception from their doctors in practice (Slater, 1982). Although their evident sexual forwardness, emotional receptivity and manipulative skill were, in his view, socially adaptive and "biopositive", they made the physician feel personally uncomfortable when these qualities intruded into a consultation. The doctor's response was not only to deny these were positive qualities, but to rationalize his unease by pathologizing them. Slater hints that this kind of attitude is rather a hypocritical one for psychiatrists in particular to adopt, since, in a "quiet kind of way", he felt a manipulative use of charm was very helpful to them. Nevertheless, because the typical doctor was vulnerable to having his "defences against unpermitted feelings" shaken, he became less able to carry through the routines of careful, unflustered judgment in which he had been trained and on which he prided himself.

The sort of clash between the hysteric and her doctor that Slater was referring to does not seem one that can be explained in terms of sexist stereotyping, especially as female clinicians can be equally susceptible to such rejecting reactions. Rather, it is as if the traditional hysterical personality comprised a potent blend of traits which represent an inversion of the ideal of detached, responsible and rational action that informs the medical persona. Confrontations with others who embody the underdeveloped, shadowy aspects of the persona should be expected to involve a mixture of fascination and fear, which may be fended off through a brusque dismissal of the provocateur. It is small wonder that, when seen by clinicians reacting from an excessively rational standpoint, people with "hysterical" traits have been dismissed as essentially "unreal".

On this account, the label of hysterical personality may conceal a drama based on a specific clash between people whose ways of viewing the world and whose personal priorities within it are directly opposed. The reality and values of one are not necessarily any more remote from those of the general population than those of the other. As a variant of hysteria, it seems distinct from the illness of dissociation hysteria not only on account of its chronicity, but in the partiality of the comparisons on which it is based.

## Conversion hysteria versus real neurological illness

Most doctors feel they have a good sense of what conversion hysteria ought to look like. The patient does not just have one or more neurological signs and symptoms in the apparent absence of underlying disease. These findings and complaints are expected to express symbolically conflicts to which the patient is subject; their occurrence is likely to represent an attempt by the patient to manipulate their immediate situation ("secondary gain"); and the patient may well be curiously indifferent to the apparent severity of his or her plight ("la belle indifference"). So far so good. But compare these widely prevalent ideas with the diagnostic criteria of conversion disorder being currently recommended by the American Psychiatric Association (APA, 1987):

TABLE 1. *Diagnostic criteria for Conversion Disorder*

| | |
|---|---|
| A | A loss of, or alteration in, physical functioning suggesting a physical disorder. |
| B | Psychological factors are judged to be etiologically related to the symptom because of a temporal relationship between a psychosocial stressor that is apparently related to a psychological conflict or need and initiation or exacerbation of the symptom. |
| C | The person is not conscious of intentionally producing the symptom. |
| D | The symptom is not a culturally sanctioned response pattern and cannot, after appropriate investigation be explained by a known physical disorder. |
| E | The symptom is not limited to pain or to a disturbance in sexual functioning. |

(American Psychiatric Association, 1987)

The traditional features of the conversion symptom that have just been cited are no longer to be found. Their exclusion has been consistent with clinical research that has shown them to be of little diagnostic validity (Lewis *et al.*, 1965; Lazare, 1981), and has been the outcome of gradual attrition over successive revisions of the diagnostic criteria. Furthermore, the only one of these modified criteria that still justifies the idea that conversion hysteria is a psychogenic condition – criterion B, that a stressor is temporally related to a symptom's appearance – has been shown to be such an unreliable discriminator (Ford, 1985) that its inclusion could be criticized just as strongly. It seems to be have been retained to provide a relatively simple means of judging a symptom to be psychologically induced, with no presumption of how this would occur.

This is very different from the way that introduction of the diagnosis of conversion hysteria had originally relied heavily upon psychoanalytic theory, with evidence of the defensive and communicative functions of conversion symptoms being demanded for diagnosis (cf. Mace, 1992*b*). With the removal of these requirements, no useful rule remains, when arguing for the diagnosis of a physical symptom as hysteria, by which a psychological contribution can be confirmed.

This development is not wholly negative, however. It is tempting to infer that, because the psychological theory of conversion has been abandoned as a basis for diagnosis, the diagnostic category itself should be dispensed with. But an important historical fact should not be ignored, namely that the theory of conversion pioneered by Freud was introduced only in order to explain *post hoc* how a group of symptoms might have arisen that were already puzzling (Mace, 1992*a*). Before attempting to explain hysteria in terms of depth psychology, Freud had clarified the relationship between hysteria and other disorders to a greater degree than his own mentor in the field, Charcot. Whereas Charcot had viewed the signs of hysteria as the sequelae of neuropathology, albeit of a more subtle sort than obtained ordinarily, Freud emphasized how hysterical symptoms actively contradicted all known processes of pathogenesis, the essence of the condition being that, in the forms adopted by its symptoms and bodily signs: "hysteria behaves as if anatomy did not exist" (Freud, 1888).

The real launching point for conversion hysteria had been this recognition that candidate symptoms defied the templates on which diagnostic practice was based (Mace, 1992a). The crucial insight was barely mentioned by Freud once he moved on to elaborate a psychological model of hysteria's etiology. But that theory was independent of it, and indeed does not provide the only model compatible with the idea that a hysterical symptom is not simply unusual, but makes no sense in terms of the general rules of pathology (cf. Merskey, 1979). Once any psychological theorizing is put to one side, this underlying characteristic remains. It amounts to a recognition that the features of an hysterical illness, although they often have a visible and disabling impact, fail to be "real" to a medical mind that requires them to be interpretable within the framework provided by anatomy, physiology and pathology.

The apprehension of hysterical complaints as less than real is enshrined in medical terminology, particularly in references to "pseudo-" symptoms. Hysterical seizures are frequently referred to as pseudoseizures. The implication is that, while a pseudoseizure is a form of seizure, a "true" seizure can only be one that has a clear organic basis, usually some form of epilepsy. Fenton (1986) has suggested that for clinical purposes it would be preferable to talk here of "pseudo-epileptic seizures", but this ignores the way in which the term "pseudoseizure" implies a general opposition between hysterical complaints and real ones. This is more explicit when, in the American literature especially, the entire class of conversion symptoms is increasingly referred to as "pseudo-neurological" symptoms. The neurological symptom has an organic basis, the pseudo-neurological symptom does not. The neurological symptom is real, the hysterical symptom is not.

This incompatibility between the symptoms of hysteria and the symptoms of neurological disease has an important corollary. This is that any symptom that can be satisfactorily explained in terms of neuropathology can no longer be viewed as hysterical. Clinical practice bears this out. Marsden (1986) described how several complaints, including dystonia musculorum deformans, blepharospasm, spasmodic dysphonia, stiff-man syndrome and paroxysmal kinesigenic dyskinesia became viewed as "organic" rather than hysterical over one decade. One might turn now to revisions in epileptology for additional instances, where such "hysterical" features as bizarre thrashing movements, pelvic thrusting or ophisthotonus during seizures, have all recently been associated with complex partial seizures of frontal lobe origin (e.g. Kanner *et al.*, 1990; Fusco *et al.*, 1990) instead of pseudoseizures. As soon as there is some basis for supposing that a symptom might be "organic", it must cease to be hysterical.

Despite this, intermittent attempts continue to try to find a general neurophysiological explanation of the symptoms collectively attributed to conversion hysteria. It is not only the superficial resemblance of hysterical signs and symptoms to those of neurological disease that provoke this. Up to two-thirds of patients with hysterical symptoms can have evidence of independent neuropathology (Whitlock, 1967; Merskey and Buhrich, 1975), while the curious tendency of conversion symptoms to prefer the left side of the body when they are unilateral (Stern, 1977) has invited speculation about a central neurological mechanism for over a hundred years (Briquet, 1989; Flor Henry, 1973). However, while modern techniques such as evoked potentials are pressed into pursuit of a neurological mechanism (e.g. Levy and Mushin, 1972), the results remain contradictory and inconclusive (Howard and Dorfman, 1985). It is interesting that none of these accounts recognizes that the goal of explaining the physical pathogenesis of hysterical symptoms is inevitably a mirage. Any substantial success would entail a drastic erosion, if not abandonment, of the concept of hysteria as a pseudoneurological illness.

Instead of simply taking the resemblance of the symptoms of conversion hysteria to those of true neurological illness to mean this form of hysteria must intrinsically have something to do with the nervous system, it may be important to recognize that it has a special affinity for neurology as opposed to other branches of medical practice and ask why this is. Certainly, one outstanding feature of neurology during the era of conversion hysteria has been its precision: the correlations between structural or physiological changes and neurological signs and symptoms have simply been far more specific, reliable and consistently explicable than those in other specialties. Cases that contradict these expectations are going to pose more of an anomaly, and call to be dealt with in exceptional ways, such as attributing them to illnesses that seem to exist but cannot be accepted as real. The diagnosis of conversion hysteria arose as a necessary artefact of medical thinking (Mace, 1992*b*). As such, it differs from other variants of hysteria not only because it refers to somatic symptoms, but because it highlights the extent to which medical judgments about the reality of illness differ from an uninformed view.

## Summary

Hysteria is presented as a medical condition that illustrates how medical practice can impose its own constraints upon reality, as well as studying differences between people who have a given condition differ and those who do not. In particular situations, medical perceptions, and the portraits of syndromes they give rise to, may be tainted either by differences between the outlook characteristic of the diagnostician and that of a given group of would-be patients, or by idiosyncracies that distinguish the diagnostician's outlook from the common man's ways of construing reality. Historically, the portrayal of "hysteria" as a disease within medicine has been problematic, and led to separation of three components, viz. dissociation hysteria, conversion hysteria and hysterical personality. These are described, and it is argued that whereas dissociation hysteria reflects psychological differences between a group of patients and most other people, the concept of hysterical personality begs an additional difference between the described group and their doctors. Similarly, the diagnosis of conversion hysteria, a condition that doctors see uniquely as both real yet less than real, owes as much to differences between their perception and that of most other people, as to differences in kind between this group of patients and any other.

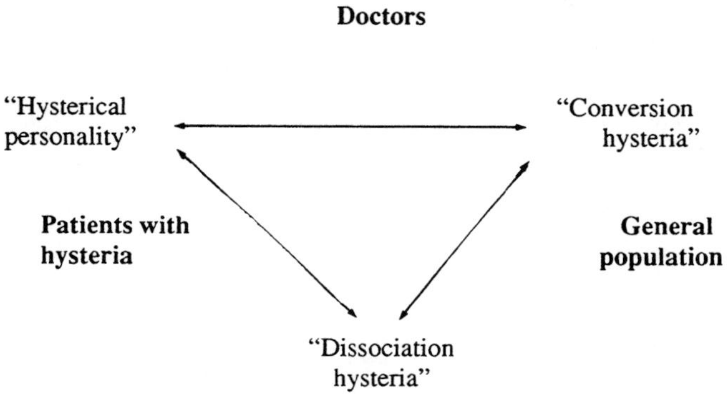

**Doctors**

"Hysterical personality" ←———————→ "Conversion hysteria"

Patients with hysteria          General population

"Dissociation hysteria"

FIG. 2. The triangle of reality, illustrating how the three major concepts of hysteria each highlights a different contrast between two sets of people concerning what is real.

## References

American Psychiatric Association (1980). "Diagnostic and Statistical Manual of Mental Disorders" 3rd Edn. APA, New York.
American Psychiatric Association (1987). "Diagnostic and Statistical Manual of Mental Disorders" 3rd Edn, revised. APA, New York.
Briquet, P. (1859). "Traité de l'Hystérie" Bailliere, Paris.
Chodoff, P. and Lyons, H. (1958). Hysteria, the hysterical personality, and "hysterical" conversion. *American Journal of Psychiatry*, **114**, 734-40.
Fenton, G. (1986). Epilepsy and hysteria. *British Journal of Psychiatry*, **149**, 28-37.
Flor Henry, P. (1983). Hysteria. *In* "The Cerebral Basis of Psychopathology". pp. 263-299. Wright, Bristol.
Ford, C.V. (1985). Conversion disorders: an overview. *Psychosomatics*, **26**, 371-383.
Freud, S. (1888). Hysteria. *In* "The Complete Psychological Works". Vol 1. Standard Edn. (Ed. J. Strachey). pp. 39-59. (1966). Hogarth Press, London.
Fusco, L., Iani, C., Faedda, M., Manfredi, M., Vigevano, F., Ambrosetto, G., Ciarmatori, C. and Tassinari, C. (1990). Mesial frontal lobe epilepsy: a clinical entity not sufficiently described. *Journal of Epilepsy*, **3**, 123-135.
Guze, S.B. (1970). The role of follow-up studies: their contribution to diagnostic classification as applied to hysteria. *Seminars in Psychiatry*, **2**, 392-402.
Howard, J.E. and Dorfman, L.J. (1986). Evoked potentials in hysteria and malingering. *Journal of Clinical Neurophysiology*, **3**, 39-49.
Jaspers, K. (1923). "General Psychopathology". (Transl. J. Hoening and M.W. Hamilton),

Manchester University Press (1963), Manchester.

Kanner, A.M., Morris, H.H., Luders, H., Dinner, D.S., Wyllie, E., Medendorp, S.V. and Rowan, A.J. (1990). Supplementary motor seizures mimicking pseudoseizures. *Neurology*, **40**, 1404-1407.

Kretschmer, E. (1926). "Hysteria Reflex and Instinct" (Transl. V. Baskin and W. Baskin). (1960). Philosophical Library, New York.

Lazare, A. (1981). Conversion symptoms. *New England Journal of Medicine*, **305**, 745-748.

Levy, R. and Mushin, J. (1972). The somatosensory evoked response in patients with hysterical anesthesia. *Journal of Psychosomatic Research*, **17**, 81-84.

Lewis, A. (1975). The survival of hysteria. *Psychological Medicine*, **5**, 9-12.

Lewis, W.C., Berman, M. and Madison, W.I.S. (1965). Studies of conversion hysteria: I. Operational study of diagnosis. *Archives of General Psychiatry*, **13**, 275-282.

Mace, C.J. (1992a). Hysterical conversion I: a history. *British Journal of Psychiatry*, **161**, 369-377.

Mace, C.J. (1992b). Hysterical conversion II: a critique. *British Journal of Psychiatry*, **161**, 378-389.

Mace, C.J. and Trimble, M.R. (1991). Psychogenic amnesias. *In* "Memory Disorders: Research and Clinical Practice". (Eds T. Yanagihara and R.C. Petersen). pp. 429-453. Dekker, New York.

Marsden, C.D. (1986). Hysteria – a neurologist's view. *Psychological Medicine*, **16**, 277-288.

Merskey, H. (1979). "The Analysis of Hysteria". Bailliere Tindall, London.

Merskey, H. and Buhrich, N.A. (1975). Hysteria and organic brain disease. *British Journal of Medical Psychology*, **48**, 359-366.

Miller, I.W. and Magaro, P.A. (1977). Toward a multivariate theory of personality styles: measurement and reliability. *Journal of Clinical Psychology*, **33**, 460-66.

Perley, M. and Guze, S.B. (1962). Hysteria – the stability and usefulness of clinical criteria. *New England Journal of Medicine*, **266**, 421-426.

Shapiro, D. (1965). "Neurotic Styles". Basic Books, New York.

Slater, E. (1965). The diagnosis of "hysteria". *British Medical Journal*, i, 1395-9.

Slater, E. (1982). What is hysteria? *In* "Hysteria". (Ed. A. Roy). pp. 37-40. Wiley, Chichester.

Slavney, P.R. (1990). "Perspective on 'Hysteria'". Johns Hopkins University Press, Baltimore.

Veith, I. (1965). "Hysteria: the History of a Disease". University of Chicago Press, Chicago.

Walton, H.J. and Presley, A.S. (1973). Use of a category system in the diagnosis of abnormal personality. *British Journal of Psychiatry*, **122**, 259-267.

Whitlock, F.A. (1967). The aetiology of hysteria. *Acta Psychiatrica Scandinavica*, **43**, 144-162.

# 19. The psychology and interrelationship of twins

Alison M. Macdonald

---

People have always been fascinated by twins. Multiple births are not the usual way for humans to produce offspring. However, while nowadays the delivery of twins or higher multiples is regarded as a normal variation in conception and pregnancy, most societies have at some stage viewed such births with a mixture of awe and fear (Corney, 1975). In some cases this has led to development of customs and rituals, presumably to help adjust to the threat aroused by such an abnormal event. In our present-day individualistic Western society the relationship of pairs of twins may be idealized; they are often seen as having a special bond, and people may have strong views about the differential treatment or separation of twins, and about paranormal concepts such as telepathy, which are reinforced by media images of twins.

This chapter describes how various aspects of the twin relationship, with each other and the outside world, have been documented. It examines some of the different historical representations of twinship and how these may affect our present ideas about twins, related, wherever possible, to scientific investigations. However, in spite of a vast literature accumulated over the last century on the biological aspects of twinning, and the medical complications of twin pregnancy and delivery (MacGillivray *et al.*, 1988), and also on the study of twins as a research tool in genetics (Neale and Cardon, 1992) there has been very little scientific examination of twinship *per se*. This fact led Zazzo (1976) to write that "there is no gemellology".

Since most of the information available is qualitative in nature, and many small studies have not been replicated, this chapter gives, inevitably, a highly personal view. The reasons for this paucity of research stem from current paradigms of scientific investigation; most scientific interest in twin similarities and differences has arisen from genetics, in which twins are useful as a tool for disentangling the effects of genes and environment on diseases and other characteristics. The only interest that most geneticists have had in twins themselves, until recently, has been in establishing that, as a group, twins are comparable with singletons for the measures of interest, thereby allowing results obtained from twin studies to be generalized to the wider single-born population. The other empirical field which should claim interest, psychology, has focused on individual differences.

Zazzo (1976) is one of few psychologists who have shown interest in the relationship of twins, naming it the couple effect. He points to twinship as the extreme example of a couple situation because of the lack of effect of age, sex or genetic differences in monozygotic (MZ) twins which would even be found in studies of closely spaced siblings. He suggests that twins should be studied for themselves, so that we might learn about the psychology of couples in an extreme situation. We could then use such results to feed back into genetic studies, increasing the knowledge to be gained from them.

**Twin Conception and Birth**

Monozygotic (MZ) twins arise through the division of a single fertilized egg (the zygote), and, although there are different types of MZ twin placentation according to the timing of division of the zygote, the basic biological similarity arises through the fact that these twins are effectively "clones", that is they share the same genes; any differences between them thus arise from genetic changes after division and differing environmental influences, including those which occur during the prenatal period. The cause of MZ twinning remains a mystery, and some would classify it as a congenital abnormality. Dizygotic (DZ) twins, on the other hand, are genetically equivalent to siblings, being, the result of fertilization of two separate eggs by two different sperms, but unlike other siblings they also share a womb and are the same age. Although we know the reason for DZ twins, the factors which lead to release of two eggs rather than one, and the apparently variable incidence of this at different times and across different cultures, are not understood. The existence of a third intermediate type of twins produced by the division of an egg and subsequent fertilization of the two identical halves by different sperm remains a theoretical possibility without any scientific data, and I shall thus disregard it. Twinning therefore remains one of nature's unsolved mysteries though human beings have long tried to find explanations for these siblings who shared a womb, and who, in some cases, share identical features and biological makeup.

There are many hazards attached to twin birth (MacGillivray et al., 1988). Pre-and perinatal mortality is historically higher in twin conceptions, and it is only in relatively recent times that it has become expected that both twins in a pair will survive. This applies particularly to MZ twins who are at higher risk of a variety of problems, including the fetofetal transfusion syndrome. In past times, the occurrence of a pair of twins, particularly MZ, both of whom survived to adulthood, must have been a far less common event than it is today. Thus the birth of twins would have been a time of mixed emotions and surviving twins (and their parents) were the objects of considerable attention.

## Epidemiology of Twinning

The twinning rate in England and Wales was just over 10 per 1000 maternities in the 1980s (Botting *et al.*, 1990), and ranges between 8 and 20 per 1000 maternities in most countries, of which between 3 and 4 per 1000 and are identical twins (Bryan, 1992). There is secular variation in twinning rates, most of the reasons for which are still unknown apart from a recent increase in multiple births resulting largely from infertility treatments. There are also wide ethnic differences, from as low as 4.3 per 1000 maternities in Japan to as high as 46 per 1000 maternities among the Yoruba of Ibadan, Nigeria (Nylander, 1975). However, where the variation has been investigated, it seems to be in non-identical (fraternal, binovular or dizygotic, DZ) twinning rates, identical (uniovular or monozygotic, MZ) rates remaining apparently stable across cultures.

## Types of Differences between Twins and Singletons

It is a truism that growing up as a twin is psychologically different from growing up as a singleton (Rutter and Redshaw, 1991). The ways in which it is different include growing up with a same age sibling as a unique form of sibling relationship. Twins have to share parental attention from the beginning and relate in a triadic rather than the usual dyadic system with mother, as well as experiencing a different sort of family interaction. Twins share a womb, and in some cases a placenta; this may have unique biological and psychological consequences. Twins receive special attention, both positive and negative, from other people, particularly if they are identical, and they are exposed to comparisons from the start, both overt and covert; everything they do will be contrasted with their same age sibling. Differences and similarities will inevitably be noted, whether they are encouraged or dismissed.

## Myths and Customs Associated with Twinning

Before the advent of modern obstetric and perinatal medicine, twin birth would frequently be followed by the death of both infants, or the survival of a single sickly child. The arrival of twins must have signalled some problems for the family – two mouths to feed instead of the expected one (a fact which may still cause hardship today). This explanation has often been used to account for some of the customs associated with twin birth which included killing one or both of them and their mother, adopting one, and purification rituals of the land and parents (Frazer, 1925; Gedda, 1961; Scheinfeld, 1973; Corney, 1975). However, other writers (Devereux, 1960) have noted that such customs did not seem to be associated with areas of either particularly high or low twinning rates, suggesting that the event was universally a threatening one to the whole community. The combination of emotions evoked and the responses were thus at a more primitive than pragmatic level. In particular, because animals were known to have plural births, the event was degrading for the mother, family or the whole group, and also led to suspicion that the mother had been unfaithful, either with another man or with an evil spirit. Many societies had structures with strict seniority and the birth of two people the same age caused problems. Primogeniture is a concept as old as humankind and remains important in the organization of our family structures. Twin births, upsetting the "normal" expectations, met differing responses, which might be widely variant even in relatively small geographical areas.

The myths and rituals which have surrounded twin birth form a background to the beliefs and attitudes to twinning and are likely to shape our preconceptions about twins and their relationships affecting the environment which twins encounter even today. Frazer (1925) describes magic, taboos and myths all over the world. From his descriptions, the magic associated with twins seems to emanate from the fact that their plural birth was an abnormal event, similar customs often arising around infants born breech, in a caul or with some congenital abnormality. I can find little reference to magical telepathy in twins in ethnological reports, even though the belief in the sympathetic influence of one individual on another at a distance is the essence of magic; however, such beliefs may underlie the attribution of one soul to twins by certain peoples, and even the killing of one to preserve the life of the other by preventing susceptibility to simultaneous illnesses which has been reported. Twins have been widely credited with other special powers, perhaps more significant to the societies in which they lived.

Many North and South American Indian and African tribes believed that twins had special power over the weather, particularly rain, and in some cases twins were thought to be children of lightning or of the sky. In Japan, where twinning is rare due to a low rate of DZ twinning, some tribes believed that one twin was fathered by a spirit and there was uncertainty about which member had spiritual paternity. Other Japanese peoples detested twins and would not allow anything to be bought or borrowed from their mother. Information about a twin birth was suppressed and one twin given away (Corney, 1975).

In modern Japan, twin births are now more widely accepted especially since their increased occurrence due to infertility treatment. The Japanese word for a twin pregnancy which is still used in rural areas, is "chikusho-bara" and means "animal belly" (Yoshida, personal communication) harking back to the degrading comparison with animal plural births. In earlier centuries this expression was one of the most obscene insults (Veith, 1960), which has parallels in some African peoples (Corney, 1975). Veith also notes that, historically, the medical literature on multiple birth in Japan refers to the aversion to it as natural, thereby offering no speculation, and no allusions to any special powers or portents of twinship.

In medieval Europe twins were thought to be due to two fathers, thus the mother must have unfaithful to her husband. In Scotland and England infertility was believed to follow a twin birth and the twins themselves might be childless. They were thought to die within a short time of each other, but if one did survive he might have healing powers. In Wales, until early this century, twins were associated with good luck and fertility, and in demand to attend weddings to ensure luck to the couple.

Some peoples rationalized the dual birth by a belief that twins had one soul or personality. In the Yoruba of Nigeria, who probably have the highest twinning rate in the world (Nylander, 1975) the combination of a high rate of birth and death led to development of a set of customs (the Ibeji cult) which presumably served to transform the fear and sadness surrounding twin birth into joy (Corney, 1975). Customs included the carving of effigies of a dead twin, or sometimes of both when they lived, to be carried by the mother or the surviving twin. There is an implicit recognition of the supernatural power of the twin bond in these customs.

Two other sources of twin mythology, the Old Testament biblical stories and Greek mythology, provide strikingly different views of twinship (Beit-Hallahmi and Paluszny, 1974). The Old Testament emphasizes differentiation and competition between the twins while from Greek myths comes the view of fusion and closeness in twin personalities. The Old Testament provides examples of themes using the good twin- bad twin. Such themes are elaborations of the simple hero myth common to all cultures, and using twins may be seen as a tool for combining tales of hostile brothers with tales of good's triumph over evil. Jacob and Esau in the book of Genesis were born as a result of divine intervention as Rebekah, their mother, was previously barren. They began competition in the womb, and later competed for their mother's love, the younger twin, Jacob, triumphing. Pharez and Zarah, sons of Tamar and Judah (Jacob's son and her father-in-law), also began to compete in the womb, and the twin who was born second again won primacy. A variety of explanations has been offered for the biblical victories of the younger twin, from casting the hero in the weaker role as one who must overcome ordeals to ensure survival, to archaic customs in which the first born was sacrificed because of beliefs that he was the offspring of a deity, or simply the denial of the reality of the weaker younger twin.

In Greek mythology the best known pair of twins is Castor and Pollux, the Gemini constellation and also known as the Dioscuri. The tale expresses well the ambivalence and confusion aroused by a twin birth (and there are different variations of the story). Castor and Pollux were sons of Leda, one said to have been fathered by Zeus, and the other by Leda's husband, Tyndareus. In spite of their divided paternity these half-brothers were regarded as Dioscuri, as twins and as close friends. Many legends describe their devotion to each other, and their fates were inseparable in life and death. There are similar stories of twins in the Vedic mythology of India, and some authors have speculated on the significance of these widespread myths (Harris, 1913).

Zeus fathered other twins, Apollo and Artemis, Amphion and Zethus, and one other pair with a divine and mortal impregnation, Hercules and Iphicles. The stories about these twins all emphasize their unique bond, their harmony and love, and twins are an exception to traditions of sibling rivalry in Greek myths.

## Twins in Literature

I have a strong impression, not backed by my empirical investigations, that twins are over-represented in literature. Perhaps it is simply that I notice them, but on the other hand, as in mythology, they do offer a special type of intimate relationship which may be used to highlight characteristics such as sibling rivalry or fraternal loyalty, and to demonstrate the contrast of good and evil. Mistaken identity was a common early theme, used by the Greek dramatists, but also notably by Shakespeare in the *Comedy of Errors* and in *Twelfth Night, or What You Will*. Gedda (1961) reviews the use of twins in classical and early 20th century literature, and Abbe and Gill (1980) also explore the use of twins in art photography.

Some writers are motivated to write about twinship through their own experience. Thornton Wilder's life and work are thought to have been influenced by the fact that he was the survivor of a pair of twins, supposedly identical. His brother, Theophilus, died a few hours after birth, and clearly his family was rather unusual in that the dead child not only was named but also had a nickname, Pax, and thus it seems likely that they talked about him to a remarkable degree. Glenn (1986) is one of a number of writers who have explored the themes in Wilder's writing, concluding that not only does some of his work relate directly to his fantasies about his dead twin brother, like "The Bridge of San Luis Rey", but that the themes in "Theophilus North" (an overt use of his twin's name and a partial anagram of his own) are probably deeply autobiographical, the hero seen as Wilder's *alter ego*, or perhaps as his lost twin.

In France there is a legend that "the Man in the Iron Mask" was actually the twin brother of Louis XIV, and Alexandre Dumas made use of this in his novel. Mark Twain was intrigued by the idea of exchanging twins at birth, and of pseudo-twins – unrelated individuals who look so alike they could pass for identical twins. Twain is said to have enjoyed pretending he was a twin and to have confused a newpaper reporter by telling him "My twin and I got mixed up in the bathtub when we were only two weeks old, and one of us drowned but we didn't know which. Some think it was Bill, and some think it was me". When asked what he himself thought, he replied "I would give worlds to know... But I'll tell you a secret... One of us had a peculiar mark – a large mole on the back of his left hand; that was me. That child was the one that drowned".

There are many examples of twins used in recent literature. Bruce Chatwin focuses on the relationship of a pair of male MZs in "On the Black Hill" (1982), describing their interdependent rivalry and loyalty in intricate detail, together with the intense anxiety caused by the possibility that one of them might marry. Angela Carter invokes no fewer than five sets of twins in her bawdy novel of the theatre, "Wise Children" (1991), primarily about a wonderfully individual pair of MZ twin ex-chorus line actresses who both enjoy the narcissistic pleasures of looking alike and dressing alike, but are as different as chalk and cheese in character, and quite able to function as individuals. The novel is cleverly narrated from both points of view, and the use of twins allows development of the touching, but unsentimental, intimacy of their relationship in combination with their differing perspectives.

Scheinfeld (1973) observed that twins have been given numerous comedy roles in books, plays and films but that they have been principals in relatively few tragedies, which he felt was as if should be, twinship being more productive of mirthful situations than of sad ones. Perhaps it is part of a changing culture that some more recent popular works (e.g. the film *"Dead Ringers)"* have used twins in more sinister roles to emphasize conflict.

## Psychological Studies of Twin Relationships

Most studies of temperamental development in twins are primarily concerned with the similarities and differences in MZ and DZ pairs, and the extent to which these reflect genetic and environmental contributions to temperament. Few studies have examined the intra-twin pair relationship for itself. Those that have done so tend to be small and difficult to interpret because of methodological insufficiencies such as poor zygosity determination, unspecified or biased ascertainment, and especially, small numbers of pairs. Also, almost all such studies focus on infants and children in families, with little or no work addressing the continuing adult relationship of twins.

A major difference for twins and their parents from other families of single-born children is that, from the first, parents have to learn to relate to two infants, to distinguish them as individuals, and to communicate with them both, often as part of a larger family of young children. We might speculate on a range of possible reactions arising from prior expectations and in reaction to the characteristics of the twins themselves – from a rigid system of trying to treat the twins absolutely equally and identically, to respond to them simultaneously and ignore any differences between them, to a conscious effort to treat as individuals and maximize differences through attending to their needs separately. The mechanisms of such responses are little researched, and may vary from one family to another according to the particular structure and attitudes to parenting, etc., as well as to the characteristics of the twins themselves. However it seems likely that some patterns will be observable; interaction with parents, parental preferences, and the effects of and on other siblings of twins have been studied.

One of the most reliable, and well-replicated, findings in this area is from observation of parent (usually mother)- child interaction. Some authors have reported that mothers of twins engage in both quantitatively and qualitatively different styles of interaction and, in particular, speech from that of mothers with single-born children. Lytton *et al.* (1977) observed that the most important differences between twins and single-born infants were that mothers and fathers of singletons simply spoke more to their children than twin parents did to theirs. This was not a result of more behaviour overall, since the total number of actions was greater for twins. Parents of twins also engaged in more control behaviour – they used more commands and prohibitions, more reasoning, more suggestions, perhaps because they had to. They were more consistent in enforcing rules laid down, showed less affection and less "positive action". There were more interventions from twin mothers, but they were non-verbal rather than verbal. The twins themselves showed less speech, less mature speech, and lower internalization of standards than age matched singletons. The MZ twins were significantly inferior to DZ twins in vocabulary IQ, rate of child speech, and rate of speech by parents to a child. This was not related to a simple class effect, nor to pre- and perinatal complications, but to the mother's education level.

Breland (1974) found that close spacing of siblings means more adverse effects on intellectual development of the younger one. Schaffer and Liddell (1984) examined the behaviour of adults and unrelated children in a dyadic (adult-single child) and a polyadic (adult-four children) interaction. They found that while in the larger group there was an overall increase in the children's demand for adult attention, the necessarily fragmented attention led to a reduced response of the adult in the polyadic situation. The style of response also changed – adults were more controlling, and participation in a child's activities reduced in frequency and duration. The change was not just quantitative but qualitative too. This parallels the observations of a parent and twins, a triadic situation. These factors, therefore, are not unique to twins, but as Zazzo suggested we are seeing the twin situation as an extreme form of couple effect. It seems that twins, especially MZ twins, experience a different type of communication with their parents from single-born children, and especially with their mother, which may tend to make them rely on each other more. This can have detrimental effects on language development (Hay and O'Brien 1984), but will presumably also affect their sibling relationship.

The demands of the twin situation also affect mothers of twins. Thorpe et al. (1991) examined rates of emotional distress in a large cohort of mothers of children aged 5 years. They found that mothers of twins had significantly higher scores indicative of depression than mothers of singletons of the same age, and that this was even the case if compared with mothers of closely spaced singletons. Interestingly, the highest rates of distress were in those mothers who had lost one twin, confirming that the stresses of coping with both the demands of a newborn infant and the grief of losing another have a long term impact on the mother's wellbeing.

Minde et al. (1982) examined maternal preferences for same-sexed premature twins. In an observational study of 18 intact pairs, each twin having a birthweight below 1500g, they found that mothers developed a preference for one twin within 3 weeks of birth and it was almost invariably the healthier twin (there were no significant differences in birthweights of the first and second born twins in this group). The preferred twin (measured by maternal preoccupation, favourable comparison with the co-twin, and higher emotional tone) at 3 and 6 months showed significantly more social behaviours than the nonpreferred twin. In the two opposite sex pairs examined, maternal preference corresponded to the sex of the mother's wish during pregnancy. Observation indicated that mothers behaved differently towards the preferred twin, and in most cases in favour of the preferred twin. In pairs where there was no preference, actual behaviour was more democratic.

Minde *et al.*'s findings are in contrast to an earlier small study by Allen *et al.* (1971) which found that fathers preferred the first born twin and the one with a higher apgar score, while mothers preferred the second born and neurologically inferior twin. However, this was expressed preference, not assessed through observation. Another study of maternal preferences by Spillman (1984) found that mothers tended to prefer the heavier twin. Hay and O'Brien (1987) found that in cases where newborn twins came home from hospital separately, parents' perceptions of the twin who came home first were more favourable than the one who came home second (apparently independently of medical problems which might relate to the different length of hospitalization).

Goldbert *et al.* (1986) conducted an observational study of maternal behaviour and attachment in low birth-weight twins and singletons, including a sample of single surviving twins. They found that even in this vulnerable group the majority of mothers and infants formed secure attachments, and that twinship *per se* did not affect attachment status. Some subtler variations among the subjects led the authors to suggest that the presence of a same aged peer may compensate for possible less optimal maternal care, but these aspects need further research.

Goshen-Gottstein (1981) conducted an observational study of maternal behaviour with opposite-sexed twins, triplets and quadruplets. She found that from early infancy male and female infant twins and supertwins were treated differently in some areas, often unconsciously. There was differential reinforcement of proximity seeking, independent of the children's behaviour. The boys' needs were positively reinforced, the girls' less often so. There are problems generalizing the results of this study, as the families were largely from a traditional Jewish environment where the male child is favoured for cultural and socioeconomic reasons.

The relationship between a pair of twins may begin to develop before birth, while they are sharing their mother's womb. Intrauterine experiences are likely not only to be different for twins from single-born infants because of the many additional biological risks incurred by two fetuses sharing one womb (see for example, Price, 1950; Bryan, 1992) but also because, from an earlier stage of life, they are in close proximity to a separate human being other than their mother. Piontelli (1989) has observed both singleton and twin pregnancies using a series of ultrasound scans followed by weekly observations of the infants for one year after birth. Piontelli was interested in whether individuality of temperament was already evident in the fetuses, and whether the fact of there being two *in utero* might entail a more precocious awareness of another person than found in single-born infants. She concluded, presenting detailed observations of two pairs of opposite sex DZ twins, that each twin seemed to have his/her own temperament from an early stage and that the pattern of their interaction was also established early, patterns which seemed to continue in the same direction after birth. For example, in one pair the boy was withdrawn and rebuffed his sister's attempts at contact while she was active and lively, patterns which continued after birth. Piontelli did not consider, however, that being a twin *per se* precipitated a more precocious awareness, rather that, for example, if the twin displays a lively interest in exploring the womb then she would also take pleasure in contact with her twin.

The La Trobe Twin Study in Australia (Hay and O'Brien, 1983) has as its specified aim the study of twins for themselves, to help twins and their families. From this group come observations which require replication in other centres. They suggest that not only are twins different from single-born children in a variety of ways, but some types of twins, particularly MZ males, have different patterns of development from others. Hay and O'Brien (1984) found that not only were MZ males different on a range of cognitive tests but that temperamentally they were less interested, less eager, less fluent, and less articulate than female twins. Bryan (1992) has also commented on the behavioural problems of MZ male infants, though overall risk for socio-emotional behavioural disturbance in twins seems to be very similar to that in singletons (Rutter and Redshaw, 1991). There is, however, considerable evidence that twins experience a disproportionate level of language and reading difficulties in childhood (Hay and O'Brien 1984).

Hay and O'Brien (1984) also noted that the single-born brothers of twins were less likely to have a close relationship with one of the twins than were sisters. Similarly Sandbank (1988) found sex differences in the response of the older sibling; older sisters were preferred by twins and older brothers disliked their younger twins more than older sisters. Older siblings of MZ twins resented the twins more than siblings of DZ pairs. Parental ratings of young twins indicated that they perceived the first born twin as easier to manage, less fussy and healthier and the parents felt closer to him/her. This was not the case in mixed sex pairs, and was more marked in girl pairs and MZ pairs. Hay and O'Brien (1984) suggest that this may be because parents use birth order to distinguish twins when nothing else is available. Individuals may be separated in mixed sex pairs on the basis of sex, while in same sex DZ pairs there are often sufficient physical or behavioural differences to categorize the infants. These studies suggest that, as with other pairs of siblings, we cannot regard all twin pairs as alike; differences among them are due not only to individual differences but also to differences in the family structure in which they grow up. Dibble and Cohen (1980) hypothesize that "subtle differences" between the twins may have lasting effects on the parents' perceptions. In turn, these perceptions may have lasting effects on the twins.

**Behaviour Genetics and Twins**

Many twin studies of temperament, cognitive abilities, personality, and psychopathology have been conducted over the last 50 years or so. Such studies focus on comparison of the within and between pair differences in MZ versus DZ twins, and have shown that genetic factors contribute in varying degrees to the development of psychological characteristics from sociability to introversion and intelligence to creativity (Plomin, 1986). One common finding of behaviour genetic studies of personality is that although both genes and environment influence most characteristics, there is little evidence that the environmental factors shared by pairs of twins or siblings act to make them more alike.

Hoffman (1991) concludes that objective and subjective family experiences vary for siblings as a function of factors such as birth order, gender and others (*vide infra*) and hence that what may appear to be "family environment" may in fact be experienced differently by siblings or twins and thus actually form part of their idiosyncratic experience. It may be that the extent of differences and similarities in siblings (and hence twins) is tied to whether outcomes are influenced by a general "family style" or by an individually experienced specific environment.

Little scientific attention has been paid to twin interaction effects until recently. With the development of model-fitting techniques it has become possible to begin to tease apart some of the effects which being raised in the same family and with a same age sibling might have on personality structure (Eaves, 1976; Hopper and Culross, 1983; Carey, 1986) but on the whole these efforts have been applied to examining the difference between MZ twins and DZ twins, which is crucial to use of the twin method in genetics. One recent analysis of criminality which allowed for "reciprocal twin influence" (Carey, 1992) showed that twins do seem to influence each other in this area, with MZ twins having a more powerful influence than DZ same sex, and both more than DZ opposite sex twin pairs. When such a factor was taken into account in a genetic analysis the influence of genetic factors on criminality was considerably less than found in previous traditional twin studies which did not allow for sibling interaction effects.

One could hypothesize that any characteristic which was partly heritable and in which peer group effects were important would show similar results, with a marked "twin" effect, graduated by zygosity and sex. The dual effects of closeness and rivalry, or cooperation and competition as they tend to be called in behaviour genetics, may be difficult to detect because both may be acting to balance one another out.

It is also possible that genotypic effects on joint behaviour, or other social behaviour, may be different from genotypic effects on individual behaviour (Fuller and Hahn, 1976). One early study by Von Bracken (1934) gave twins tasks to complete and assessed both the output and efficiency of MZ and DZ twins. He concluded that MZ twins worked to preserve or restore harmony or equality; when the twins worked together the "stronger" one would allow the "weaker" one to catch up. For DZs, there was a striving towards superiority or excellence in a joint situation, in competition with the partner, if the actual difference in individual ability was minimal. Segal (1984) tested the competition, cooperation and altruism of MZ and DZ pairs in experimental situations. She found that, on the whole, there was evidence of greater cooperation and altruism in MZ pairs (the pairs were selected for concordance of IQ scores, and the average age of the two groups was similar). Required jointly to complete a difficult puzzle, 94% of MZ pairs did so, but only 46% of DZ pairs, suggesting that the MZs were more able to combine their efforts effectively, the DZs less able to do so. In those DZ pairs who did succeed, the activity was dominated by one child, essentially solving the puzzle individually.

It seems that, as Lytton *et al.* (1977) observed "Twinship, as an enduring ecological factor, has a considerable impact – possibly a greater one than social class – on children's socialization experiences and development".

## Psychodynamic Studies of Twin Individuation

In psychodynamic theory, one of the fundamental processes in the personality development of an infant is individuation and this requires a separation of the infant from the mother (Bowlby, 1960). General psychodynamic theory assumes this applies to development of an individual resulting from a single birth. For twins, individuation not only involves maternal separation but also separation from the twin.

In analytic terms, the first object for a twin is not the mother, as it would be for a single-born infant, but the other twin, so that from the first twins are in a triadic rather than a dyadic relationship with their mother. Twins have a symbiotic relationship with each other from which they must emerge as individuals in order to complete the process of psychological maturation. In early infancy twins confuse their identities (Burlingham, 1952; Leonard, 1961; Zazzo, 1960) for example by recognizing mirror reflections of themselves as belonging to their twin, or sucking each other's thumbs. Athanassiou (1985) considers that while this symbiotic aspect may be more pronounced in MZ twins, the intensity is largely due to whether the parents, especially mother, encourage it by treating the two children as a single individual. She seems to view the separation from the twin as inherently fraught with problems because, while a mother is usually able to help her child to emerge from the symbiotic stage, each twin experiences a similar symbiosis with his own twin, with the additional complication of mother as both another symbiotic object and, conversely, someone who disturbs the symbiosis between the twins.

Adelman and Siemon (1986) examine the emotional separation of adult twins, recognizing that the understanding of issues surrounding such "intense attachment" may throw light on other sibling ties. They comment that much of the psychodynamic literature on individuation is anecdotal and emphasizes the more extreme and pathological aspects of the twin bond, as well as ignoring the social milieu of the twins. The paradox of the intimacy of twins is described – to be together or to separate. Twins are envied by others for their closeness and companionship, but if twins find this so satisfying and necessary that it excludes others and interferes with individual development, then it may limit rather than enhance their lives. These authors accept that preconceptions about twins idealize their closeness which may make it difficult for them to achieve a redefinition of their relationship to allow them intimacy without dependency, and separateness without estrangement. Their influence on each other may not always appear positive – twins may be locked into a rivalry involving bickering and fighting which appears to confirm their separateness but in fact maintains them in an enmeshed pattern of interlocked behaviour. While other types of separation in families, of children from their parents, have celebrations and social rituals attached to them (confirmation, graduation, marriage) there are no such rituals attached to the loosening of sibling bonds.

Like other close couples, twins use a restricted code to signal intimacy and the exclusiveness of their relationship. Like such codes in married couples, use affirms the strength of "we" above "I". Although a "secret" language (idioglossia or cryptophasia) may occur in extreme cases, mostly "twin language" is some form of subtle and implicit restricted code, giving them a private shorthand way of communicating complex ideas. This may be seen in adult life as an ability to complete each other's sentences, which can make other people feel excluded, intentionally and unintentionally, and serve to amplify the bond between the twins.

The use of an elaborated code in communication (that is, explicit verbal description of feelings and perceptions rather than the assumption of tacit understanding) may facilitate separation, but retain affection by allowing the twins to talk about themselves. As such a use of language actually implies separateness, it may be very difficult for twins to begin to use. It may also be difficult for twins to form intimate relationships with other non-twins – there may be an expectation that there will be a tacit understanding of what the other person is feeling, and so no need to explore the alternative experiences and realities, so again use of an elaborated code for communication is necessary, at least in the early stages of new relationships. Twins themselves report problems sometimes in other love relationships, because they assume that a partner will understand them as well as their twin, who has a lifetime of practice (Rosambeau, 1987). I have on occasion found that the spouses of close identical twins can be extremely angry and resentful of the intimacy shared by the twins from which they feel excluded. Some studies (Galton, 1874; Zazzo; 1960) have found that twins are slightly less likely to marry, and this used to be thought to be associated with decreased fertility, a now discredited notion, a psychological explanation seeming more plausible.

## Twins as Siblings: can studies of non-twin siblings tell us more about twinship?

Some psychologists have investigated the relationships between siblings empirically. Initially this was through observations that birth order seemed to affect the outcome for children in a family differentially. Galton (1874) triggered interest in primogeniture, noting in his studies of "eminent men" that they were more frequently first born children. Over the last century, examination of sibling relationships has changed from simple correlations of achievement with primogeniture to natural observational studies of parent-child interaction, and more recently to sibling-sibling-parent interaction. Such studies have considerable relevance for twin interaction if twins are viewed as an extreme form of sibship. One of the most striking findings of sibling studies is that far more information is obtained about the siblings when the whole family structure is examined.

Schacter (1982) found that adjacent siblings usually judge themselves as different from each other, but that this occurs more often if they are the first two in a family than in later closely spaced pairs. It also happens more often in same rather than opposite sex pairs. Schacter suggests this is a defence against sibling rivalry, which is more extreme among earlier than later born sibs and those of same sex role.

Bank and Kahn (1982) examine a concept they call intense sibling loyalty which may characterize the popular view of an "ideal" twin relationship − that is a Hansel and Gretel type relationship of loyalty, attachment and devotion to each other. They conclude that sibling loyalty is promoted by the example of at least one nurturing parent, relatively harmonious and equitable interactions between the siblings from infancy, being reared together, and closeness in age. Also important are the "fit" of personalities, roles, styles, and interests, in a lock and key fashion. Thus some reciprocal needs are important. Unavailability of parents also promotes such a close relationship. If one extrapolates these findings to the normal twin situation, then clearly many twins start with a high level of the factors which promote such closeness − they are identical in age, grow up together and, particularly for MZ twins given their genetic identity, are likely to "fit" more often then many siblings. Unavailability is defined by Bank and Kahn as abandonment, an extreme version, but we might hypothesize that parents of twins are more emotionally "unavailable" than other parents through necessity: in a traditional nuclear family mother may be kept busier by the physical demands of two infants, and father may have to work longer hours to support his larger family, whilst in one parent families these stresses may be even more marked. Such factors might promote the closeness of the twins, and their mutual interdependence.

Ross and Milgram (1982) looked at the concept of closeness in lifespan terms. They found that closeness as a family was more frequently reported than closeness to specific siblings, and was more stable than specific sibling relationships which changed over the lifespan. Family framework was the factor most powerful in the origin of sibling closeness. Factors which prevented closeness were when siblings were far apart in age, separated in childhood, and some family relationships. "Surrogate parenting" by siblings led to close relationships between the pair, and critical incidents like death or divorce lead to a variety of outcomes. Common or complementary interests and enhanced physical proximity − sharing bedrooms, attending the same school, or geographical isolation − all increase childhood closeness. When children shared significant time in groups, forming childhood cliques either within a large family or with other children, the nature of the groups was affected by age spacing, gender, personality characteristics, interests and the number in the family. Again we see that twinship provides a ready made maximization of these factors promoting closeness.

Sibling rivalry on the other hand, seemed to have two dynamics. Overt comparison by adults, whether positive or negative, and covert comparison. The latter occurs when a child observes an adult's preferential treatment of another child, and perceives that greater value is placed on the comparison child by the adult. Such comparisons may be adult initiated or sibling generated. The latter are especially important in adolescence or childhood, and in vying for attention, recognition and love of parents. The comparison of siblings on their accomplishments is also important in development of sibling rivalry. Once again, extrapolation to the twin situation indicates that there may be ample opportunity for rivalry to develop. By the nature of a couple, comparisons, overt and covert, will occur. The effort to distinguish individual twins will often lead to comparisons, even if these are apparently non-judgemental, simply drawing attention to difference rather than "better" or "worse". Research on preferences for twins (*vide supra*) suggests that covert comparison could easily arise.

To conclude, while such studies of siblings do not directly examine twins, they do take account of many factors directly relevant to the twin situation. From such empirically based work we may conclude that twinship *per se* maximizes many factors likely to lead to a close sibling relationship, and, on the other hand, to sibling rivalry. These conditions are not mutually exclusive, and twin relationships may be a delicate balance of cooperation and competition, which is certainly evident from anecdotal accounts (e.g. Rosambeau, 1987).

**Twin Relationships that go Wrong**

The popular media are fascinated by the idea that twins are bound by an invisible bond, which is seen to lock them inevitably into a life of closeness and identity, dependence and intimacy. Alternatively twins must be rivals, bound by a mutual dislike which must explode in violence and criminal acts. These extremes, which seem to be not unlike the opposing Biblical and Greek myths, are perpetuated in stories about twins in newspapers, and magazines. The voyeuristic aspects of these articles reflect a primitive interest in things we do not understand. Twins seem most often to arouse comment in the press if both get the same marks in an exam, or have the same dream, if they die within a short time of each other or provide some other example of their indissoluble bond. Most often of interest are pairs of twins for whom their close relationship has had extreme results.

The Kray twins, Reggie and Ronnie, whose activities dominated the East End of London gangland scene in the 1950s and 60s, have provided seemingly endless copy for the media. The Kray twins grew up in a poor area of London, in a matriarchal family with an often absent father. They had an older brother Charlie, who is also part of their criminal story. The twins' rise to power was in part due to their coupledom; their closeness and loyalty to the "Firm" was the essence of all gang culture but magnified in this pair of blood brothers, and they also had a very strong sense of rivalry and competition with each other. In one of many books about their lives by Pearson (1972), after Ronnie murdered George Cornell, a member of an opposing gang, he is said to have had the idea of using murder as a test of loyalty, a rite of initiation and a bond, like a group called the Leopard Men he had heard about in Nigeria. From Pearson's account, it seems highly likely that Jack "the Hat" McVitie was murdered by Reggie in response to Ronnie's taunts – he had to kill to show that he was as hard as Ronnie, but also to unite them, because they shared everything. The combination of Ronnie's episodes of paranoid psychosis, their physical strength (both boxed), heavy drinking and a culture of violence and fear, coupled with the relationship of the twins to each other has resulted in a real life crime story which has already passed into myth.

As told by Pearson (1972) they were always dressed alike, always together, and showed a degree of interdependent self sufficiency from an early age. No-one but their mother could tell them apart as children, they were addressed as "twins" and later known as the "Terrible Twins". Both had diphtheria at age 3, resulting in their first separation as Ronnie, the second born twin, stayed in hospital longer until his mother took him out against medical advice to reunite him with his family. From then on a slight difference seems to have entered their relationship; their mother is said to have felt she must compensate for Ronnie's illness. Reggie was brighter and talked more, Ronnie shyer, moodier and clumsier but nevertheless always had to outdo his brother. They competed, initially for their mother's attention, and watched each other like hawks. As the tale of their adult lives is told, Reggie emerges as the more controlled and rational twin, but lacked the power to oppose his brother's ideas. Under the influence of drink he indulged his hatred and violence and the twins become like one person; sober, Reggie found it harder to be like Ronnie.

For these twins, while twinship alone probably was not responsible for their behaviour, it seems to have influenced it, and in turn they were influenced by others' reactions to them as twins. Their story contains elements of what all good gangster tales should: confused identity, family bonds and rivalry, money, glamour and violence on an epic scale. That it is true, though much of it seems to have passed into East End mythology, makes it all the more fascinating.

Another pair of twins, June and Jennifer Gibbons, who developed a restricted code of communication to a degree which completely excluded the outside world have been described by Wallace (1986). These twins seem to have become caught in a spiral of behaviour, culminating in violence and destructiveness of themselves and property from which they could not escape. Wallace writes "June and Jennifer emerge... as two human beings who love and hate each other with such intensity that they can neither live together nor apart. ...If they come too close or drift apart, both are destroyed. So the girls devised games and strategies and rules to maintain this equilibrium". The so-called "Silent Twins" communicated little with anyone but each other. Under adult scrutiny, they would sometimes be frozen immobile, unable to move other than in synchrony, each waiting for the other to move first. Their "secret language" to each other was a rapid patois of distorted English, but they also used a highly developed code of tiny facial movements to control each other and preserve their identicalness. These twins believed they were identical in mind and communicated telepathically but Wallace had access to their detailed and intricate diaries, recording the same events from each of their perceptions. In their distorted world, their thoughts and feelings about each other showed that they did not fit exactly, their interpretations were different. Their struggles, to control the differences, to dominate, to remain one and at other times to break away, were expressed in a violence towards each other, themselves, and their surroundings. And they had a powerful effect on those around them, splitting staff responsible for their welfare over whether or not the response to their behaviour should be separation, and arousing strong feelings that they had one mind.

At a less extreme level, in the course of corresponding with and interviewing hundreds of twins I have been impressed by the variety of reactions to their twinship. I have met (rarely) pairs for whom their dependence on each other has become a handicap. One pair of male MZ twins lost their jobs when altered working conditions dictated that they should separate; after a lifetime of reinforcement of their togetherness and identity at all times they were unable to do this and the resulting distress and problems caused led to their dismissal. A pair of female MZ twins, both with anorexia nervosa, compete with each other to lose weight, and hospitalization of one tends to leave the other well and coping, but the positions are reversed as the hospitalized twin recovers. Similar patterns may sometimes be observed in pairs of alcoholic twins, though often one of the pair will become teetotal to avoid becoming like his twin.

Such cases are unusual. There are plenty of examples of bizarre and criminal behaviour in single-born people to match these, but it does seem that twinship can sometimes have lasting and destructive effects. Perhaps surprisingly in the light of some of the literature discussed here, that is rarely the case. Space precludes a thorough examination of the family structures, events, peer groups and interactions that occurred in the lives of the sets of twins described, but the books cited both provide plentiful material, which accords with many of the dimensions encouraging closeness and rivalry discussed above; such strong and distorted twin bonds could arise and be developed, and like any closed relationships, cut off from the real world and involving secret games and rituals, the outcome might be sinister.

In the few studies which examine the question, it does not appear that twins are more or less frequently affected by emotional problems than single-born people (Paluzsny *et al.*, 1977; Chitkara *et al.*, 1988). This may be an over simplification arising from group comparisons, as it is possible that in some cases twinship does precipitate or maintain major psychiatric problems and that in others it actually provides a close supportive relationship which prevents problems in otherwise vulnerable individuals. Certainly, if the twin relationships are viewed as an extreme form of couple, subject to intense forms of rivalry and/or closeness and dependency then it would be expected that there will be some people for whom their twinship is a significant source of distress.

## Telepathy: coincidence or sixth sense

Even nowadays, the idea of separating twins can arouse unease, or sometimes frank dismay; this probably stems from a feeling that there is a possibility that their relationship goes beyond the conscious level, and sharing of a birth, age, features, etc. Many fictional stories of twins use telepathy and extrasensory perception, and the media welcome apparently authentic stories. Rosambeau (1987) in her investigation of a sample of volunteer twins found that 183 out of 600 participants claimed to have some sort of telepathic experience. Others had similar experiences but attributed them to coincidence. Rosambeau divided up the experiences, finding that most of them fell into three categories. Twins seemed to report the simultaneous expression of identical thoughts (including answering questions the other has not yet asked, finishing sentences, getting the same marks in exams, buying the same clothes in different towns), sympathetic pain (sickness, pain and even swelling during the other's pregnancy, having the same operation at different places) and an ability to anticipate imminent contact (telephoning simultaneously so the line is engaged, sensing when a twin will visit).

The most robust test of a "twin bond", and the possibility that it extends into the paranormal, must be the remarkable coincidences reported by twins who have grown up apart. The most well known current series of such twins is examined by Professor T.J. Bouchard and his team at the Minnesota Twin and Adoption Centre (see e.g. Tellegen *et al.*, 1988). Members of the team have often been present at the emotional reunions of adult twins, separated soon after birth, and endeavour to investigate the twins before their contact with each other "contaminates" their behaviour and perceptions. Some of the similarities in the twins are remarkable and have attracted a lot of media attention. Often, despite their separation at birth and upbringing in different areas and by quite different families, their lives may show remarkably similar patterns, perhaps marrying at similar ages, even to spouses with the same name, and having the same number of children in the same gender order. Their likes and dislikes may be similar, and mannerisms and speech patterns are sometimes disconcertingly indistinguishable.

Some of the similarities may be due to the biological similarity of the twins; food preferences for example may be partly genetically determined, although most studies have shown that the amount of contact the twins have is more important (Fabsitz *et al.*, 1978). Many such experiences which appear to be extrasensory perception may be entirely coincidental. Watson (1981) explores the nature of coincidence and the odd, apparently inexplicable happenings that twins sometimes report, focusing on some of Bouchard's pairs of reared apart twins. He shows that statistically many such events could occur and that patterns which may appear to have meaning often arise in numerology. He cites Zimbardo's "small world" phenomenon, whereby two strangers meeting anywhere in the world would, after some discussion, eventually find a common acquaintance or experience, leading them to say "it's a small world". This almost universal experience is explicable simply through numbers and coincidence, combined with a search for common ground which rapidly narrows the field. Some coincidences, however, are easier to understand from the perspective of psychodynamic theory, which allows for the unconscious mind as well as the conscious, in affecting our communication, recall, denial and attributions.

Both Watson (1981) and Rosambeau (1987) cite the work of J.B. Rhine in North Carolina, testing possible thought transmission between twins. The tests used are said to involve one person looking at successive cards printed with symbols and the other at a distance attempting to state which symbol is involved. Twins were not found to differ according to zygosity, nor were they better or worse than pairs of friends or other family members. Rhine himself did not believe that the apparently exceptional cases of telepathic communication sometimes reported in MZ twins were any more outstanding than others involving a mother and daughter, a young couple in love or another close relationship of affection and friendship. I have not been able to find accounts which contradict this view.

Eaves and Last (1980) attempted to assess empathy in twins, by studying their reciprocal perceptions of each other's social attitudes. Both twins in 34 pairs, and in separate rooms, completed a social attitude scale as they thought their twin would answer, and then for themselves. Twins were not particularly good at predicting each other's responses, and how good they were seemed to depend neither on sex nor on being MZ. What emerged from analyses was that twins tended to rate their co-twins more like themselves than they actually were, especially if they were MZ. There was a small contribution of a real ability of twins to predict their co-twin's responses, but this study does not allow any examination of whether this is greater than would be found in any kinship pair. Another small study (Paluszny *et al.*, 1977) also examined the projections of one twin onto the other, using a measure of depression, and found that MZ twins were more likely to rate their co-twin like themselves than were DZ twins.

There have been reports of cases of simultaneous Sudden Infant Death Syndrome (SIDS) in twins, which if unexplained could add to the feeling that twins' fates are linked. No excess has been noted among MZ twins as compared with DZ (Spiers, 1974). An examination of a series of 13 pairs of healthy twins who died together of no apparent cause (Bass, 1989), searching for noxious environmental agents in the homes of the twins, concluded that all 13 sets died from injuries (hyperthermia, asphyxia, suffocation, or smothering) unintentional or otherwise, and that most of the deaths were preventable. It is also possible that simultaneous death of infant twins could be caused by infections, which are presumably likely to affect both twins when they are in close physical proximity, and which would accord with the lack of any difference between MZ and DZ twins.

**Conclusions**

Twins grow up surrounded by the same multifarious influences as single-born children, but with some additional factors. The fact of their multiple birth, as an abnormal event in itself for humans, the presence of a same age sibling, the divided attention of parents, comparison by family, peers and others and the later need to separate, all make the twin situation different. For identical twins, the additional fact of sharing similar, sometimes indistinguishable, physical features, must be perhaps the most unusual aspect. For all twins, but especially MZs, the reactions of other people (stemming from their own preconceptions and/or ignorance about twins) must vary from enjoyable and amusing to tiresome and sometimes distressing. One might conclude that it is surprising that so many twins develop quite normally. To do so would be to underestimate the influence of twinship, and to negate the positive aspects of it.

Twins are only twins to the outside world when seen together, preferably MZ and identically dressed. One researcher with considerable experience of treating twins psychodynamically said at a conference that he had never been able to diagnose a person as a twin just from speaking to the individual. So, twinship is inherently about the couple, the relationship of the couple, and how that is viewed and how it affects behaviour and individual psychology and other interactions. For individual twins however, they are always twins, with or without their partner, after the death of one of them, and not being a twin is a condition they have no experience of. It is normal for them, part of who they are.

The more uncanny aspects of twinship, the telepathy, coincidence, ESP or whatever one might choose to call it, arise, I believe, from a primitive need to explain the incomprehensible, and to mystify historically valued concepts of sibling loyalty and primogeniture. For some, they are easily dismissed or explained away. Genetic similarity and common environment probably account for the bulk of such experience; unconscious levels of communication for yet more. It would be interesting to know if those twins who believe in telepathic communication were also those with a more vested interest in their identity as twins, the "we-self", and whether those who did not were more individuated. Science knows little about the way such constructs are generated and maintained.

Further information on the making and breaking of twin bonds has come from studies of siblings, especially within their wider family structures. From these we learn that the closeness and rivalry of pairs of siblings are not simply different according to birth order and sex but also because of their position in the larger family group, and according to the way they are treated. The factors which seem to promote both the closeness and rivalry of sibling pairs are maximized in twins and their relationship may be a delicate balance or interplay of the two dimensions, which in some cases will cause problems, but in many others will lead to an enriching close relationship. Studies of the interactions of twins with their mothers further show how the couple both affect and are affected by the triadic interaction.

From art and mythology we obtain pictures of idealized twin relationships, by which twins and their families will be influenced to a greater or lesser degree. Individualizing the twins can be taken to an extreme, denying their twinship, just as well as attempts, perhaps caused by a sense of fairness, to maintain identity and ignore differences. It is important not to forget that twins can have something denied to the single-born population, a readymade friend and companion to support and help them through life, if the conditions exist for such a relationship to prove mutually beneficial. Perhaps this is why twins seem not to have more psychological problems than single-born people, as seems to be the case from the small amount of evidence available. There may be protective effects to counterbalance the less positive aspects of twinship. Twin survivors of the holocaust (Segal, 1985) subjected to horrific experiments in Auschwitz at the hands of Dr Josef Mengele, told of a dual urge to survive, in the knowledge that death of one of them meant almost certain killing of the other for anatomical comparison; such distortion of symbiotic twin bonds is almost unthinkable.

I have tried to show, drawing on many widely different sources, how the nature of coupledom, inherent in twin relationships, the attitudes of parents and the wider society, with the biological relationship of twins may shape their interactions and give rise to the so-called twin bond, to a greater or lesser degree. I hope that what this disparate information shows is that there is no one way of viewing twins; one pair is likely to be as different from another as any two individuals, and their relationship with each other is influenced by a multitude of factors. At times this leads to a special and close tie, for life, a bond which some will envy and others fear, probably depending on their own preconceptions about twinship and experience of family relationships. In other cases rivalry will result, and the twins will not be affectionately close but may be caught in an equally interlocked system. For most twins, successful individuation will allow enjoyment of a special intimate bond hand in hand with the experience of their own lives as separate individuals.

I hope that twins who read this will not consider themselves or their relationship diminished in any way by attempts to describe and explain some of the more "uncanny" aspects of twinship. The amount of attention that idealized and "magical" aspects of the twin bond are afforded in the popular media has long called for a closer examination of what makes twins such objects of speculation and curiosity. From my own perspective, that of behaviour and psychiatric genetics, I wholeheartedly agree with the sentiments of Carey (1992) that although discussion of the interaction of twins may be interpreted as challenging the utility of the twin method, "paradoxically, ... large scale studies of twins are exceptionally important for the study of sibling interactions. The twin method is not at fault; the problem is the inappropriate use of the twin method".

## Acknowledgements

My thanks to Elizabeth Bryan, Bina Coid, Ian Harvey, Robin Murray and Lyn Pilowsky for their helpful comments on earlier drafts of this chapter, and to all the twins who have contributed to our research projects, stimulating my interest in twin relationships.

# References

Abbe, K.M. and Gill., F.M. (1980). "Twins on Twins". Clarkson N. Potter, New York.
Adelman, M.A. and Siemon, M. (1986). Communicating the relational shift: separation among adult twins. *American Journal of Psychotherapy*, **40**, 96-109.
Allen, M.G., Pollin, W. and Hoffer, A. (1971). Parental, birth and infancy factors in infant twin development. *American Journal of Psychiatry*, **127**, 1567-1604.
Athanassiou, C. (1985). A study of the vicissitudes of identification in twins, 329-335.
Bank, S. and Kahn, M.D. (1982). Intense sibling loyalties. *In* "Sibling Relationships: their Nature and Influence across the Lifespan". (Eds M. Lamb and B. Sutton-Smith), Lawrence Erlbaum Assoc Inc, Hillsdale, New Jersey.
Bass, M. (1989). The fallacy of the simultaneous sudden infant death syndrome in twins. *American Journal of Forensic Medicine and Pathology*, **10**, 200-205.
Beit-Hallahmi, B. and Paluszny, M. (1974). Twinship in mythology and science: ambivalence, differentiation, and the magical bond. *Comprehensive Psychiatry*, **15**, 345-352.
Bloch, A-M. A. (1969). Remembrance of feelings past: a study of phenomenological genetics. *Journal of Abnormal Psychology*, **74**, 340-347.
Botting, B.J., MacFarlane, A.J. and Price, F.V. (1990). "Three Four and More: a Study of Triplets and Higher Order Births". HMSO, London.
Bowlby, J. (1960). Separation anxiety. *International Journal of Psychoanalysis*, **41**, 89-112.
Breland, H.M. (1974). Birth order, family configuration and mental achievement. *Child Development*, **45**, 1011-1019.
Bryan, E.M. (1992). "Twins and Higher Multiple Births: A Guide to their Nature and Nurture". Edward Arnold, Sevenoaks.
Burlingham, D.T. (1949). The relationship of twins to each other. *Psychoanalytic Study of the Child*, **3**, 57-72.
Burlingham, D.T. (1952). "Twins". International University Press, New York.
Carey, G. (1986). Sibling imitation and contrast effects. *Behavior Genetics*, **16**, 319-341.
Carey, G. (1992). Twin imitation for antisocial behaviour and implications for genetic and family environment research. *Journal of Abnormal Psychology*, **101**, 18-75.
Chitkara, B., Macdonald, A.M. and Reveley, A.M. (1988). Twin birth and adult psychiatric disorder: an examination of the case records of the Maudsley Hospital. *British Journal of Psychiatry*, **152**, 391-398.
Corney, G. (1975). Mythology and customs associated with twins. *In* "Human Multiple Reproduction". (Eds I. MacGillivray, P.P.S. Nylander and G. Corney). Saunders, London.
Dibble, E.O. and Cohen, D.J. (1980). The interplay of biological endowment, early experience, and psychosocial influence during the first year of life: An epidemiological twins study. *In* "The Child and his Family". (Eds E.J. Anthony and C. Chiland). Wiley, New York.
Eaves, L.J. (1976). A model for sibling effects in man. *Heredity*, **34**, 132-136.
Eaves, L.J. and Last, K.A. (1980). Assessing empathy in twins from their mutual perception of social attitudes. *Personality and Individual Differences*, **1**, 174-176.
Fabsitz, R.R., Garrison, R.J., Feinleib, M. and Hjortland, M.A. (1978). Twin analysis of dietary intake; evidence for a need to control for possible environmental differences in MZ and DZ twins. *Behavior Genetics*, **8**, 15-25.
Frazer, J.G. (1925). "The Golden Bough. A study of Magic and Religion". 3rd Edition. Macmillan, London.

Fuller, J. and Hahn, M.E. (1976). Issues in the genetics of social behaviour. *Behavior Genetics*, 6, 391-406.
Galton (1874). "Hereditary Genius".
Gedda, L. (1961). "Twins in History and Science". Charles C. Thomas, Springfield, Illinois.
Glenn, J. (1986). Twinship themes and fantasies in the work of Thornton Wilder. *Psychoanalysis and Studies of Children*, 41, 627-651.
Goshen-Gottstein, E.R. (1981). Differential maternal socialization of opposite-sexed twins, triplets and quadruplets. *Child Development*, 52, 1255-1264.
Harris, J. R. (1913). "Boanerges". The University Press, Cambridge.
Hay, D.A. and O'Brien, P.J. (1983). The La Trobe Twin Study: a genetic approach to the structure and development of cognition in twin children. *Child Development*, 54, 317-330.
Hay, D.A. and O'Brien, P.J. (1984). The role of parental attitudes in the development of temperament in twins at home, school and in test situations. *Acta Geneticae Medicae et Gemellologiae*, 33, 191-204.
Hoffman, L.W. (1991). The influence of the family environment on personality: accounting for sibling differences. *Psychological Bulletin*, 110, 187-203.
Leonard, M.R. (1961). Problems in identification and ego development in twins. *Psychoanalytic Study of the Child*, 16, 300-320.
Lytton, H., Conway, D. and Sauve, R. (1977). The impact of twinship on parent-child interaction. *Journal of Personality and Social Psychology*, 35, 97-107.
MacGillivray, I., Campbell, D.M. and Thompson, B. (Eds). (1988). "Twinning and Twins". Wiley, Chichester.
Minde, K.K., Perotta, M. and Corter, C. (1982). The effect of neonatal complications in same-sexed premature twins on their mother's preference. *Journal of the American Academy of Child Psychiatry*, 21, 446-452.
Neale, M.C. and Cardon, L.R. (1992). "Methodology for Genetic Studies of Twins and Families". NATO ASI series D: Behavioural and Social Sciences. Vol 67. Kluwer Academic Publishers, Dordrecht, Netherlands.
Nylander, P.P.S. (1975). Frequency of multiple births. *In* "Human Multiple Reproduction". (Eds I. MacGillivray, P.P.S. Nylander and G. Corney). Saunders, London.
Paluszny, M., Selzer, M.L., Vinokur, A. and Lewandowski, L. (1977). Twin relationships and depression. *American Journal of Psychiatry*, 134, 988-990.
Pearson, J. (1972). "The Profession of Violence: the rise and fall of the Kray twins". Weidenfeld and Nicolson, London.
Piontelli, A. (1989). A study on twins before and after birth. *International Review of Psychoanalysis*, 16, 413-426.
Plomin, R. (1986). "Development, Genetics and Psychology". Lawrence Erlbaum Assoc, Hillsdale, New Jersey.
Price, B. (1950). Primary biases in twins studies. A review of prenatal and natal difference-producing factors in monozygotic pairs. *American Journal of Human Genetics*, 2, 293-352.
Rosambeau, M. (1987). "How Twins Grow Up". The Bodley Head, London.
Rosenberg, B.G. (1982). Life span personality stability in sibling status. *In* "Sibling Relationships: their Nature and Influence across the Lifespan". (Eds M. Lamb and B. Sutton-Smith), Lawrence Erlbaum Assoc Inc, Hillsdale, New Jersey.
Ross, H.G. and Milgram, J.I. (1982). Important variables in adult sibling relationships: a qualitative study. *In* "Sibling Relationships: their Nature and Influence across the

Lifespan". (Eds M. Lamb and B. Sutton-Smith), Lawrence Erlbaum Assoc Inc, Hillsdale, New Jersey.

Rutter, M. and Redshaw, J. (1991). Annotation: growing up as a twin: twin-singleton differences in psychological development. *Journal of Child Psychology and Psychiatry*, **32**, 885-895.

Sandbank, A.C. (1988). The effect of twins on family relationships. *Acta Geneticae Medicae et Gemellologiae*, **37**, 161-171.

Schacter, S. (1982). *In* "Sibling Relationships: their nature and influence across the lifespan". (Eds M. Lamb and B. Sutton-Smith), Lawrence Erlbaum Associates Inc., Hillsdale, New Jersey.

Schaffer, H.R. and Liddell, C. (1984). Adult-child interaction under dyadic and polyadic conditions. *British Journal of Developmental Psychology*, **2**, 33-42.

Scheinfeld, A. (1973). "Twins and Supertwins". Pelican Books.

Segal, N.L. (1984). Cooperation, competition, and altruism within twin sets: a reappraisal. *Ethology and Sociobiology*, **5**, 163-177.

Segal, N.I. (1985). Twin survivors of the holocaust. *Twins*. Nov/Dec. 28-31.

Siemon, M. (1980). The separation-individuation process in adult twins. *American Journal of Psychotherapy*, **34**, 387-400.

Spiers, P.S. (1974). Estimated rates of concordancy for the sudden infant death syndrome in twins. American *Journal of Epidemiology*, **100**, 1-7.

Spillman, J.R. (1984). "The Role of Birthweight in Maternal-Twin Relationships". MSc thesis. Cranfield Institute of Technology.

Sutton-Smith, B. (1982). Birth order and sibling status effects. *In* "Sibling Relationships: their Nature and Influence across the Lifespan". (Eds M. Lamb and B. Sutton-Smith), Lawrence Erlbaum Assoc Inc, Hillsdale, New Jersey.

Tellegen, A., Lykken, D.T., Bouchard, T.J., Wilcox, K.J., Segal, N.L. and Rich, S. (1988). Personality similarity in twins reared apart and together. *Journal of Personality and Social Psychology*, **54**, 1031-1039.

Thorpe, K., Golding, J., MacGillivray, I. and Greenwood, R. (1991). Comparison of prevalence of depression in mothers of twins and mothers of singletons. *British Medical Journal*, **302**, 875-878.

Veith, I. (1960). "Twin Birth: Blessing or Disaster. A Japanese View", 230-236.

Von Bracken, H. (1934). Mutual intimacy in twins. Types of social structure in pairs of identical and fraternal twins. *Character and Personality*, **2**, 293-309.

Wallace, M. (1986). "The Silent Twins". Chatto and Windus, London.

Watson, P. (1981). "Twins: an uncanny relationship?" The Viking Press, New York.

Zazzo, R. (1960). "Les Jumeaux: le couple et la personne". Tome II. l'Individuation psychologique. Presses Universitaires de France, Paris.

Zazzo, R. (1976). The twin condition and the couple effects on personality development. *Acta Geneticae Medicae et Gemellologiae*, **25**, 343-352.

# 20. Perception of sexuality

John M. Kellett, Margaret R. Hilton and W. Falkowski

## Sexuality

*Love is merely a madness*
*Shakespeare*

Literature abounds with memorials to the compulsive, and at times irrational nature of erotic love. Shakespeare tells of love pursued relentlessly despite risk (*Romeo and Juliet*), love based on mistaken identity (*Twelfth Night*), and love aroused by magical potions (*A Midsummer Night's Dream*), with more than a hint of perversion in Titania's adoration of Bottom transformed into an ass. The adage "love is blind" warns those destined to taste its nectar.

So what is the nature of this "madness"? Is it programmed prenatally, lovemaps causing us to be attracted to particular types of people, or activities, as suggested by Money (1986)? Does our erotic arousal depend on our ability to surmount the oedipus complex and castration anxiety as suggested by the Freudians? Do we search for a partner who satisfies the female need for power, and the male for fecundity?

When two people meet and are attracted, is this based on pheronomes, a template of our opposite sexed parent, or is it the effect of our orgasm-releasing endorphins, to which we become addicted and the lack of which causes the despair of losing our lover?

Probably our most fundamental task is to decide our own sex.

## Gender identity

The first words of the midwife after delivery usually announce our sex for life. Today this knowledge is often already available through amniocentesis or ultrasound. There are, of course, many ways of defining gender which are laid out in the following table:

*Categories of gender*

Physical: Genetic
          Gonadal
          Genital morphology
          Hormonal

Secondary sexual characteristics
  Internal morphology (presence of uterus, prostate, etc.)
Psychological: Gender identity (feeling male or female)
  Social sex role (masculine or feminine)
  Public sex role (dress)
  Sexual orientation

## Mechanisms of sexual differentiation

The central nervous system controls and sustains the viscera, musculature and organs of the body (a) directly through the peripheral and autonomic nervous systems, and (b) indirectly via the endocrine system. The master gland of the endocrine system is the pituitary, situated beneath the brain to which it is joined by the pituitary stalk conveying neural and hormonal messages from the hypothalamus. Circadian rhythms, responsible for stimulating pituitary activity, are innate but are also influenced by external factors: by feedback mechanisms from the endocrine system, by the eye's perception of the hours of daylight (particularly for those living in northern latitudes as on the island of Spitzbergen) affecting the frequency of conception, and by psychological factors – thus the ratio of boys to girls born in times of war differs from that in peacetime.

How psychological factors can cause changes in human sexual differentiation remains unexplained; but psychological factors undoubtedly pervade sexual recognition. Phenotypic sex can be different from perceived or emotional gender identity, and herein lies the interest in our pursuit of the boundaries of reality. Psychological factors connected with sex which can also influence the interaction of the individual with the reality of his milieu include the stability of his sexual role, whether orthodox or deviant; the uncertainty of his self esteem in that role; and any guilt feelings which may have a sexual basis, e.g. due to nocturnal emissions in a chaste religious setting, remorse caused by masturbation, or the psychological turmoil of a victim of rape or sexual abuse.

Clear evidence of the role of the brain in sexual differentiation comes from the rat. At birth the hormonal activity of the hypothalamus is feminizing (MacLusky and Naftolin, 1981). Would-be-male rats then produce a burst of testosterone secretion, some of which is metabolized within the hypothalamus to dihydrotestosterone and aromatized to oestrogen. It is the production of oestrogen locally which blocks the release of luteinizing hormone (LH) (the female response).

Though a similar mechanism has been found to operate in the hamster, in rhesus monkeys masculinization is produced by testosterone directly. It has been suggested that there is a difference between defeminization produced by the effect of oestrogens, and masculinization produced by androgens. Defeminization stops bisexual behaviour in the male but masculinization allows it, thus leaving remnants of female behaviour (McEwen, 1981). Clearly the defeminization or masculinization of the female brain does more than block the LH response to oestrogens. Areas of the rodent brain affected include preoptic nuclei, amygdala, ventromedial hypothalamus, hippocampus, and suprachiasmatic nucleus with a potential change in their sensitivity to sex hormones in adult life. These areas of the brain have been specifically examined in the attempt to find a physiological foundation for homosexuality.

If brain organization is determined *in utero* by androgen production why should females born with adrenogenital syndrome, who are treated from birth with cortisone, thus reducing the production of androgenic hormones, develop quite normally? At least this is true as far as menstruation and gender identity are concerned but perhaps not so true of their behaviour. Ehrhardt and Meyer-Bahlburg (1981) claim that there is an excess of boisterous, hoydenish behaviour, i.e. of tomboys.

Hormones also play a major role in the development of sexual organs. Children deficient in 5 alpha reductase, cannot produce dihydrotestosterone which is necessary for the development of the penis and the descent of the testes. Gonadal differentiation depends particularly on the SRY gene carried on the Y chromosone, though other genes may be involved (Lancet, 1990).

Proceptive and receptive sexual behaviour characterize the sexual stereotypes of the human male and female respectively. The proceptive actively seeks sexual contact, has a relatively constant sexual appetite and is easily aroused by visual stimuli. The receptive may welcome a sexual encounter and is easily aroused by such attention, but can tolerate sexual abstinence with relative ease. Most of us regard this concept as a trans-Atlantic caricature but to others it is a matter to be treated with gravity. Nyborg (1984) found that very masculine men also had poor spatial ability, and this ability was highest in people whose phenotype was more androgynous (intermediate). Other characteristics of the male such as aggression, energy expenditure, and preference for play with objects rather than people is dependent on prenatal priming and less affected by the post-natal hormone profile. In stark contrast, Greer (1972) takes the view that recognizable differences between males and females, apart from their genitalia, are politically rather than scientifically determined. Anthropologists would disagree (Reynolds, 1991): if females were to be better at verbal skills, to take more pleasure playing with other children, and to be quicker to react to extraneous stimuli like the cry of a child, these would seem to be excellent adaptations to motherhood.

## The transsexual

The transsexual, despite normal physique, is convinced that he is of a different sex from his body. In this he differs from most effeminate boys who accept their sex with reluctance. As he enters adolescence he may still harbour the belief that his true sex will out and express disappointment about the absence of the desired secondary sexual characteristics. From infancy he has preferred the toys and company of girls and sooner or later their clothes. Cross dressing may have been done at the behest of mother or with her consent, but by adolescence it becomes a secret activity. Erotic fantasies are of being a woman penetrated by a male and there is little attraction to girls. Before a final decision is made to abandon the morphological sex some subjects seek refuge in hypermasculine activities like motor racing, or mountaineering, which they may combine with marriage. By the late twenties this defence mechanism fails, the marriage breaks up, and the patient turns to genital reassignment surgery.

The female to male follows much the same course, with less pressure from peers to conform than is applied to the male. The onset of menstruation is a major stress, but the adoption of male dress and patterns of behaviour is more easily tolerated. A steady sexual relationship with another woman is frequent.

As with most sexual minorities there is strong pressure to accept a biological origin, which can be used to justify surgical intervention, and deny the value of psychological attempts to change gender to that of the body. However, if it were biological, one would expect that its prevalence would be similar in different countries with different cultures. Furthermore one would also expect the sex ratio to remain constant. Ross *et al.* (1981) tested this hypothesis by comparing the known prevalence in Sweden and Australia. Australia seems to put more emphasis on sexual stereotypes, thus making it more difficult for effeminate men to fit into the culture. Bearing in mind the difficulty of estimating actual incidence they found it nearly three times higher in Australia, with a sex ratio of males: females of 5:1 compared to a more equal ratio in Sweden. They conclude that the transsexual is someone with low levels of appropriate masculinity or femininity who is forced totally to reject his own sex by social pressures. Societies which place greatest value on a clear cut distinction between males and females end up, paradoxically, with larger numbers of identified transsexuals.

Freund *et al.* (1974) found a similar dynamic, in both transsexuals and homosexuals, which differed significantly from heterosexuals. However, there may be significant differences in the feminine behaviour demonstrated by the transsexual and a proportion of homosexuals (Rosen *et al.*, 1977). The latter are not so much feminine as effeminate, exaggerating the feminine mannerisms of adult women, a behaviour increased by stress and difficult to suppress. Feminine behaviour, such as a preference for playing with dolls, is more easily suppressed, thus enabling the transsexual to adopt the male role more easily than the effeminate homosexual.

The suggestion that transsexuals are homosexuals seeking social acceptance for their changed role is an oversimplification. If that were the case one would expect those with a strong libido to be more determined to seek reassignment than those who can lead an asexual life. This is not born out. My first encounter with a transsexual was with a 60-year-old American who had retired from her male business career and adopted the female role without obtaining surgery. As far as she was concerned "what mattered was between my ears, and not what was between my legs." Probably the most articulate transsexual is Jan Morris (1974) who describes her change of sex in "Conundrum". Though marrying, and fathering five children, sexual intercourse never assumed the preoccupation of many males. Rather he obtained his "sensual satisfaction from buildings, landscapes, pictures, wines and certain sorts of confectionery". Though his conviction that he was a woman took form under a piano at the age of three or four, and remained an increasing preoccupation throughout his childhood and adult life, he adopted the surprisingly male life style of foreign correspondent, at one time being the only newspaper correspondent on the first expedition to climb Everest (and was responsible for that news reaching the British public on the day of the coronation). Such travelling also provided an alibi against the husband role in his marriage. Hormonal treatment and genital surgery freed him from this unhappiness and allowed her to express herself in the way she had always intended. With oestrogens she describes the first subtle changes thus: "The first result was not exactly a feminization of my body, but a strippide [stripping away of the rough hide] in which the male person is clad. I do not mean merely the body hair, nor even the leatheriness of the skin, nor all the hard protrusion of muscle: all these indeed vanished over the few years, but there went with them something less tangible too, which I know now to be specifically masculine – a kind of unseen layer of accumulated resilience, which provides a shield for the male of the species... This suggestion, for it is hardly more, was stripped from me, and I felt at the same time physically freer and more vulnerable. I had no armour. I seemed to feel not only the heat and the cold more, but also the stimulants of the world about me. I relished the goodness of the sun in a more directly physical way, and for the first time in my life saw the point of lazing about on beaches. The keenness of the wind cut me more spitefully."

Elizabeth Wells (1986) writes more briefly of her experience of becoming a woman making many of the same points as Morris. She also opted for male occupations from the army to deep-sea fishing, mining, sawmilling and truck-driving. The decision to change sex and have surgery transformed her life and "the real tragedy of the problem was that it had stifled so much of my potential. I was almost totally self-centred because of it, impatient with other people's problems (they looked so trivial compared with mine), bitter about my own, and cynical and negative. So much time and effort had been wasted." As with Morris, sexual expression had been muted until surgery; neither identifying themselves as homosexual, though tolerant of that persuasion.

Stoller (1985) has studied such patients from a psychoanalytical viewpoint and came to the conclusion that the development of masculinity depends on the ability of the child to separate from its mother and hers to allow this. "The longer, the more intimately, the more mutually pleasurable is a mother-infant son symbiosis, the greater the likelihood the boy will become feminine." He sees many so-called masculine traits as a defence against this symbiosis. These include a fear of intimacy, and a rejection of feminine attributes, such as tenderness and emotional expression. He cites the notorious culture of Sambia, in New Guinea, in which the male children are finally separated from their mothers between the ages of 7-10 and made to fellate the adolescents and swallow semen which is thought to provide the power of masculinization. Thus prepared, the young males enter a society where there is extreme separation of roles: the male a warrior, the female the nurturer. Though fellatio may be going too far, the childhood of the upper class English male, snatched from his nanny at seven and sent away to a boarding preparatory school, is not so dissimilar! In the female transsexuals Stoller studied he found in every one that the mother infant bond had been broken by illness in the mother. The child had been forced to care for mother and the father had assumed the role of buddy in some ways setting up a similar symbiosis to the mother with her effeminate son.

Despite the opportunities for biological sex to go awry there is little evidence for this occurring in the transsexual (Rekers et al., 1979). Many believe that the conviction of the body being incorrectly matched to the brain is induced by well meaning parental pressure.

**Homosexuality**

Having established our own sex, we normally seek to combine with the other to create a unit which has the attributes of both. A significant minority seeks solace with its own sex. Four per cent of men and 1% of women are exclusively homosexual though 37% of men and 6% of women have experienced homosexual orgasm, usually during adolescence (Kinsey, 1948, 1953).

The word "homosexual" is both a noun and an adjective, the root coming from the Greek "homo", the same. Homosexuality can be defined as erotic attraction for the same sex. Whilst in the animal kingdom there is reckoned to be no exclusive homosexuality, in the human there is a continuum between the two extremes of exclusive homosexuality and heterosexuality.

## Historical perpective

Two thousand years ago homosexuality was accepted as the norm in Greece and Rome. Plato praised the virtues of male homosexuality, and suggested that pairs of homosexuals would make the best soldiers (in contrast to current service policy in the UK). In the early days of the Roman empire marriages between men or women were legal. Several emperors, including Nero, were married to men.

The Catholic church based its position on the writings of Augustine and Aquinas, who suggested that sexual acts which did not lead to conception were unnatural, and hence sinful. Subsequently in the Middle Ages the accusation of homosexuality lead to the Inquisition, and the convicted were subject to severe punishment.

The medicalization of deviance is usually the prelude to acceptance. Krafft-Ebing's "Psychopathia Sexualis" (1886) linked homosexuality to genetic flaws and a predisposing abnormality of the central nervous system, a view which was accepted until Hitler's Germany turned such a view into a justification for extermination.

In more recent times tolerance has again gained impetus, with the Wolfenden report in 1957 recommending that laws against any form of sexual behaviour between consenting adults in private should be repealed. However the epidemic of AIDS has undoubtedly increased hostility to this group (Masters and Johnson, 1988).

## Aetiology

Psychoanalytic theories make interesting reading; Freud's "Three Essays on Sexuality" (1905) considered that man was universally bisexual, as evidenced by the homosexual behaviour in prisons and on ships where men are denied the company of women. Male homosexuality is dependent on the castration complex, identification with mother, and anal fixation.

Some authors have emphasized the effect of upbringing, the absent or weak father and the dominant mother (e.g. Bieber *et al.*, 1962). Bell *et al.* (1981) interviewed 293 homosexual and 140 heterosexual women, and 686 homosexual and 337 heterosexual men. They found that sexual preference was strongly established by adolescence, and rarely changed during adult life. Homosexual boys avoided physically demanding sports, preferred female playmates and feminine games. They found no support for the weak father, dominant mother concept, seduction by another homosexual, or by lesbians choosing their father as a role model. Van Wyk and Gerist (1984), using Kinsey's sample, consider that sexual orientation becomes fixed at 18 for men and 21 for women. Noting the preference for opposite sexed playmates they suggest that such familiarity may cause an incest taboo. The first love object is a relative stranger. Adolescent masturbation by another male is slightly more likely in the latent homosexual male, but in girls early exposure to heterosexual intercourse is more likely to cause homosexuality, possibly as such early experience is not necessarily pleasurable, especially if the partner was an adult male.

Behavioural theories are supported by the evidence from prepubertal sexual behaviour but do not explain the initial choice. Genetic theories were supported by the finding of Kallmann (1952) of 100% concordance in 37 pairs of male monozygotic twins, compared to 12% in 26 pairs of dizygotes. Subsequent studies have failed to replicate these results (Zuger, 1976; Heston and Shields, 1968) though a recent one still suggests a genetic component (Bailey and Pillard, 1991). Here 52% (26/56 pairs) of monozygotes were concordant for homosexuality, 22% (12/54) dizygotes, 11% (6/57) of adopted siblings, and 9.2% (13/142) of biological, male siblings. The higher figures for adopted compared with biological siblings suggest an environmental influence. There is no evidence for chromosomal abnormality.

Dorner's (1976) finding that male homosexuals responded to oestrogen with a rise in luteinizing hormone (LH) unlike other males, was partially supported by Gladue *et al.* (1984). Gooren (1986) found no significant difference in LH surge after oestrogen between 23 male homosexuals and 15 heterosexuals. However 11 homosexuals and 5 heterosexuals showed a female type response which was attributed to lower response of the testosterone production to LH; and there was still an excess of female type response in the homosexuals. Dorner et al. (1991) now suggest that lower levels of pre–natal testosterone predispose to male homosexuality whilst high levels in females to female homosexuality or bisexuality.

## Comparisons of personality and physique

Early studies on the personality of homosexuals were conducted on prison populations, or psychiatric patients, and the results generalized to all homosexuals.

Later, more scientific, studies tend to show that homosexuality *per se* is not associated with mental illness, nor are there major differences in personality (Reiss, 1980). Thus Hooker (1957) excluded prisoners and psychiatric patients in her sample of 30 male homosexuals matched for age, intelligence and education with heterosexual men and found no significant differences between the groups.

Saghir and Robins (1973) extended investigations further by not only excluding psychiatric patients but using single heterosexuals as their control group, as they have higher rates of psychiatric illness than their married counterparts. They concluded that the majority of homosexuals was well adjusted, but there was an increase in the rate of alcoholism in the female homosexuals.

Bell and Weinberg (1978) studied 979 homosexual men and women, describing 36% of males and 16% of females as "dysfunctional" or "asexual". These were unhappier than heterosexual subjects, being lonely, and needing professional help in their lives.

Whilst appearance and behaviour can suggest, in a small proportion of homosexuals, their orientation (e.g. "butch" short-haired trouser wearing females, and effeminate males) such characteristics can also be found in heterosexuals and their orientation cannot be so identified unless they specifically wish to "advertise" it.

## Self-discovery of homosexuality

Though some date this from early childhood, most become aware of their orientation in adolescence. This discovery often causes confusion and distress for the individual brought up in a heterosexual environment. The discovery may be gradual, based on the degree of sexual arousal induced by heterosexual or homosexual stimuli. Others make the discovery following a physical homosexual experience. A few only make this discovery after a heterosexual marriage, thus causing great pain to both partners. It is reckoned that a fifth of homosexual men and a third of lesbians have been married at least once (Bell and Weinberg, 1978; Masters and Johnson, 1979).

Though some are proud to "come out" many homosexuals are upset by the discovery, see it as illness, and seek treatment. Many keep the discovery secret for fear of losing their job and friends, or upsetting their families. Some mothers confronted by the homosexuality of a son undergo a grief reaction similar to that experienced at death.

**Paraphilias and Unlawful Sex**

Because of the tremendous range of idiosyncratic practices, only the most common are described below. Many such as bestiality, necrophilia, and coprophilia cause revulsion in the majority; others, such as sexual asphyxia, a sense of incredulity that people should indulge, given the risk of accident or death. The oddities of the human species are perhaps no more clearly exposed than in the area of sexual behaviour. The practices described are not peculiar to the male sex, though they are often represented as being so.

## Solitary activities

### 1. Fetishism

This is the deviation which raises most mirth, in response to descriptions of men sexually fixated on stiletto heels, rubber suits, underwear, and so on. The term refers to the use of objects as the repeatedly preferred, or exclusive method of achieving orgasm and often involves textures with strong sexual associations such as shininess, wetness, and furriness. An example was a young man unable to masturbate to ejaculation without using the lining of a stolen jacket. He had been sexually abused at the age of five by a family friend, which he continued to resent. His father left home when he was about 10 leaving the family poor, so that he was kept warm at night by being covered by his father's jacket. It is not difficult to imagine how, as he began to develop sexually, he became fixated on this source of comfort during his early experience of sexual arousal and masturbation. The fact that the jackets had to be stolen from men he found attractive might be linked with the anger he still harboured from his abuse, and the sense of revenge and triumph that the theft of the jacket presented. Such fetishes usually start very early in life and are very resistant to change.

### 2. Transvestism

This can be seen as another fetish, in which sexual arousal is heightened by wearing women's clothes. Again there is an early age of onset, often before the age of 10, and it is usually well established by mid-adolescence. As with most paraphilias there is a continuum from people who occasionally use objects of clothing as part of normal sexual activity or masturbation, to those who dress up regularly in the privacy of their own homes, to those who spend much of their lives cross dressing and obtain a particular excitement from being accepted as women. There is no desire to be a woman, and treatment is usually sought because of objections from their partner.

## Activities involving non-consenting victims

### 1. Exhibitionism

Exposure of the penis in order to elicit some reaction from the observer is perhaps the most common deviation. If one follows Freud one might imagine that the male proudly displays his penis to excite envy and humiliation in his victim. However such men are usually described as timid and make no attempt to enter into any kind of relationship with the victim though a small minority proceeds to rape. A study by Bluglass (1980) found that 79% of those convicted of indecent exposure had no previous sexual offence, and over a four year follow-up only 20% were re-convicted of a similar offence. Those who do re-offend do so repeatedly from adolescence onwards. Though exhibitionists are often socially unskilled, some are married. Mooning, which is exposure of the buttocks, is usually confined to adolescence.

Another disorder of courtship is frottage, where the male rubs his genitals against women in a crowd, and touching breasts or buttocks of strangers.

### 2. Voyeurism

The voyeur achieves sexual pleasure by peeping at unsuspecting women in a state of undress, or watching coital couples. There is no attempt to attract attention; voyeurs are considered to be socially and sexually inhibited, their only motivation is to obtain sexual arousal. A few attract attention to themselves as a prelude to sexual assault. Female voyeurism at wrestling matches, male striptease, or in the female equivalent of "girlie" magazines has become a recognized social fact.

### 3. Obscene phone calls

A paraphilia in which the victim is kept at a greater distance involves making obscene and threatening phones calls. A variation encountered in clinical work was of a man who pretended that he had the daughter of the victim captive and that unless she engaged in masturbation the daughter would be injured. Clearly such calls can be extremely alarming and even with milder forms, such as heavy breathing, women can feel invaded. Most calls go unreported so their incidence is unknown. However surveys suggest that most women have experienced such calls, several repeatedly. Recently telephone helplines such as the Samaritans have become objects of such calls. The motivation would seem to be the gaining of a sense of power to compensate for a feeling of inadequacy. In the case mentioned above for instance, the man involved was of low intelligence, epileptic, over-weight, and with poor social skills, so that his ability to attract a partner was compromised. Harassment is not exclusively related to the female sex.

### 4. Erotomania (Clerambault's Syndrome)

This is the only paraphilia which is more common in the female. It is, fortunately, a relatively rare syndrome in which an individual develops a delusional belief that a particular person is in love with them. As with all delusions, this belief is resistant to rational argument, and characteristically the woman becomes increasingly preoccupied with the relationship, interpreting even letters of rejection as a coded message of love designed to put his wife off the scent. Though occasionally due to paranoid schizophrenia, it occurs in those with no mental illness. A related delusion is morbid jealousy, where a person believes that their partner is being unfaithful, in the absence of any evidence. Again the individual does not respond to rational argument, and may become dangerous to their partner or attempt to keep them a prisoner to ensure that they remain faithful.

### 5. *Sado-masochism (S/M)*

Dominance and submission are the major themes of this perversion, which involves inflicting pain or suffering on another individual, or being the recipient of abuse and humiliation, including chastisement and bondage, in order to achieve sexual arousal. Gosselin (1987) provided a detailed and fascinating account of sado-masochistic relationships and the precautions to be taken to ensure the safety of the participants. He emphasizes the care and trust involved in the teasing and tantalising of consenting couples who engage in S/M practices, and contrasts this with the behaviour of psychopaths who aim to inflict real pain and humiliation. Storr (1990) likens the dominant submissive pattern involved to that experienced in the parent-child relationship, and considers it to be an immature expression of sexuality, which replays earlier dynamics. He also considers such practices to be encouraged by the inhibitions, guilt and uncertainty about sex common in Western societies, and argues that they are not to be found in preliterate groups.

The wealth of S/M pornography and the existence of specialist S/M clubs implies a widespread practice. At the extreme is a group which relishes and exploits its power over another to the point of rape or murder.

### 6. *Paedophilia*

Those who sexually abuse children divide into two main types: those whose primary sexual orientation is to children, and see nothing wrong in their behaviour, and those who are deeply ashamed and only offend under stress. Again dominance/submission is a major theme, children being selected for their innocence and vulnerability. Howells (1979) used the repertory grid technique with a sample of heterosexual paedophiles and controls, to examine their attitudes to children. Paedophiles saw adults as threatening, and were much more comfortable with children, who, they felt, were likely to be uncritical and show love unconditionally. They expected the children to have a similar attitude to sex as adults, with an equal ability to consent, and even initiate sexual play. It is common, in clinical practice, to find paedophiles who resent the legal restraints, and also the children for "seducing" them. Until recent years an organization called "Paedophile Information Exchange" existed to try to change the law on sexual activity with children, as the Wolfenden report achieved for homosexuals. The group was made illegal following a widely reported child abduction.

The growth of concern about the prevalence of child sexual abuse has heightened tension in this whole area, making it difficult to avoid over-zealousness, at times, in professionals charged with protecting children from risk.

## 7. Rape

The fear of rape is a preoccupation of many women today. Debate continues about whether rape is the result of abnormality, or as Brownmiller (1975) would argue "a conscious process of intimidation by which all men keep all women in a state of fear". Certainly research has failed to identify particular characteristics of rapists. A study by Malamuth (1981) raised concern when a third of students said they might commit rape if they were certain they would not be caught. Further studies have underlined how often men use a level of coercion on some occasions to achieve coitus. Quinsey et al. (1981) set up an experiment in which half the subjects were told it was normal to be aroused by rape. When shown rape scenes, this group showed as much arousal as rapists and much more than controls. This result emphasizes the danger of the recurrent depiction of sexual violence in the media, which also "give permission".

Cross cultural studies (Rattray, 1923) have shown that societies where the emphasis is on sexual equality, cooperation and sharing have very low levels of rape. In contrast societies characterized by male dominance, and negative attitudes towards women have high levels (Sanday, 1981) Men are seen as committing rape when their masculinity is threatened and as a way of gaining symbolic control over childhood trauma (Holmstrom and Burgess, 1980).

## Aetiology of the Paraphilias

### Biological theories

Flor-Henry (1987) and Langevin (1990) have reviewed theories of the importance of brain function in determining sexual expression. It has been argued that the preponderance of sexual deviation in the male results from differences in the process of cerebral lateralization in males and females. As, ultimately, lateralization is more complete in the male, there is a reduced capacity for one hemisphere to take over the functions of the other if damaged. A link between temporal lobe disturbance and many types of deviation has been found in several studies (Kolarsky et al., 1967; Flor-Henry, 1980). Furthermore some paraphilias appear for the first time after brain damage (Cummings, 1985).

Other hypotheses link the superior visuospatial abilities of men, and their proceptive sexuality, to the greater use of fantasy to initiate and maintain arousal. Over time eccentric fantasies can be embellished to become more arousing, with a need to act out these fantasies in reality. The importance of fantasy rehearsal has been illustrated by MacCulloch et al. (1983) among a group of sadistic psychopaths. Fantasy rehearsal has been associated with a variety of deviations and is commonly a focus of treatment.

In most perverse activity there is at least some element of aggression; and in some forms of abnormal expression, particularly sexual assault, rape, and sadistic murder, aggression is the key. The similarity of physiological responses during aggression and sexual expression as well as the common focus in the hypothalamus and limbic system activity, underline the importance of pursuing research into constitutional causes of the paraphilias.

## Social learning theories

Learning theory argues that sexual deviations can be conditioned by the juxtaposition of sexual arousal and/or orgasm with a certain stimulus, which may be a particular object or person. It further argues that early experiences associated with pleasure are more likely to be repeated. For instance a young boy may in later life adopt a pattern of abusing younger boys, in order to maximize his own arousal and because he expects them to respond as he did himself. Such a theory fails to explain the difficulty of eradicating paraphilias when more powerful stimuli are available.

Social learning theory incorporates the view that influences throughout early development determine attitudes and behaviours which are later re-enacted. This mostly occurs by modelling ourselves on others, especially parents, but also on models in books, magazines and films. To this extent the portrayal of sexual aggression in all forms of media must be of concern. Experts differ as to whether deviant pornography satisfies the needs of the paraphiliac, preventing their fantasies from being acted out, or whether it feeds the fantasies until circumstances allow their enaction. The fact that rapists usually have large quantities of violent pornography can be interpreted either way, but just as banning the publication of racist literature has made a more tolerant society, so one may regard the distribution of violent pornography with concern (see Murrin and Laws (1990) and Check and Malamuth (1986)).

Clinical experience suggests that many sexual deviants have been subject to sexual or physical abuse in childhood (see Rada (1978) and Groth and Burgess (1979)). Much sexual aggression appears to be motivated by a need to triumph over a childhood trauma. A man who had been repeatedly persecuted and humiliated by an alcoholic mother, later felt excited and triumphant when rehearsing rape fantasies. Sometimes patients have flash backs to their own sexual abuse when attempting intercourse, with the result that they feel an urge to attack the partner whose identity at that time cannot be separated from that of the abuser. Women are more likely to react in self-destructive ways, such as in eating disorders, drug abuse/overdose or by self mutilation.

As well as being humiliated by others, some sexual deviants are prevented from socializing by physical deformity. Poor self esteem, fuelled by socially stigmatizing conditions, has been particularly reported in fetishists, and those making obscene phone calls, enabling them to avoid face to face contact with others in the practice of their deviation.

Inadequate social training can lead to a lack of understanding of sexual mores. This especially applies to those with learning disabilities brought up in institutions where their behaviour was tolerated as relatively harmless. When such people are re-housed in the community, they can be suddenly confronted by the full force of the law without realizing their offence.

Marshall and Barbaree (1990) have presented an integrated theory of the aetiology of sexual offences, combining biological and hormonal factors, quality of parenting, sociocultural attitudes, and situational factors. They echo a common, but by no means universally accepted view that men are born with a propensity for sexual aggression which must be overcome by appropriate experiences of socialization. Laws and Marshall (1990) further explore the role of social learning theory to explain the conditioning of the paraphilias.

## Sociobiological theories

Sociobiology provides two mechanisms whereby deviance can become resistant to relearning. The first is imprinting where there is a critical period during which the brain is especially sensitive to learning. Imprinting is a form of sudden learning not unlike the conversion experiences achieved by evangelists. They create increased suggestibility by causing their audience to hyperventilate, and the hyperventilation of orgasm may have the same effect of reinforcing the stimuli present at the time. Wilson (1987) suggests that male children need to imprint on female genitalia, learning which is prevented by our taboo of nudity. Second there are innate releasers which allow the male to be aroused by the female physiognomy without imprinting. Unfortunately these releasers are of necessity abbreviated so that a smooth hemisphere may be a female breast or buttock, but could also be a wetsuit.

## Conclusion

The theory of evolution makes the ability to reproduce our first priority. The advantage of sexual reproduction in increasing diversity and reducing the selection of an unfit mate nevertheless leaves the process of sexual union open to the maverick. Some paraphilias may be seen as a means by which the unfit are satisfied, and prevented from disrupting society. Whatever the reason, or cause, we experience our sexuality as a fundamental part of our personality, with the result that, whatever the deviation, its practitioners will usually insist that its origin is biological, and its practice, though a problem for society, must be accommodated. It is fashionable to decry the possibility of altering sexual orientation, even though there are effective remedies. Problems of gender identity are more fundamental, and here, as with the more socially acceptable deviations it may be wiser to help the individual to fulfil his aspirations, than deny them. As Anatole France has written "Of all sexual aberrations, chastity is the strangest".

## References

Bailey, J.M. and Pillard, R.C. (1991). A genetic-study of male sexual orientation. *Archives of General Psychiatry*, **48**, 1089-1096.
Bell, A.P. and Weinberg, M.S. (1978). "Homosexualities". Simon and Schuster, New York.
Bell, A.P., Weinberg, M.S. and Hammersmith, S.K. (1981). "Sexual Preference: Its Development in Men and Women". Bloomington, Indiana University Press, Indiana.
Bieber, I., Dain, H., Dince, P., Drellich, M., Grand, H., Gundlach, R., Kremer, M., Rifkin, A., Wilbur, C. and Bieber, T. (1962). "Homosexuality: A Psychoanalytic Study". Basic Books, New York.
Bluglass, R. (1980). Indecent exposure in the West Midlands. *In* "Sex Offenders in the Criminal Justice System". (Ed. D.J. West). Institute of Criminology, Cambridge.
Brownmiller, S. (1975). "Against Our Will: Men, Women, and Rape". Simon and Schuster, New York.
Check, J.V.P. and Malamuth, N.M. (1986). "Pornography and Sexual Aggression: A social learning theory analysis. *In* "Communication Yearbook 9". (Ed. L. McLaughlin), pp. 181-213. Sage, Beverly Hills, CA.
Cummings, J.L. (1985). "Clinical Neuropsychiatry". Grune and Stratton, New York.
Dorner, G., Rhode, W., Stahl, F., Krell, L. and Masius, W. (1976). A neuroendocrine predisposition for homosexuality in men. *Archives of Sexual Behavior*, **4**, 1-8.
Dorner, G., Poppe, I., Stahl, F., Kolzsch, J. and Uebelhack, R. (1991). Gene- and environment-dependent neuroendocrine etiogenesis of homosexuality and transsexualism. *Journal of Experimental and Clinical Endocrinology*, **98**, 141-150.
Ehrhardt, A.A. and Meyer-Bahlburg, H.F.L. (1981). Effects of prenatal sex hormones on gender-related behavior. *Science*, **211**, 1312-1318.
Flor-Henry, P. (1980). Cerebral aspects of the orgasmic response: normal and deviational. *In* "Medical Sexology". (Eds R. Forleo and W. Pasini). Elsevier, Amsterdam.
Flor-Henry, P. (1987). Cerebral aspects of sexual deviation. *In* "Variant Sexuality; Research and Theory". (Ed. E. Wilson). Croom Helm, London.
Freud, S. (1905). Three essays on sexuality. *In* "Freud S." 1991. Vol. 7, pp.33-155. Penguin Books, London.
Freund, K., Langevin, R., Zajac, Y., Steiner, B. and Zajac, A. (1974). Parent child relations in transsexual and non-transsexual homosexual males. *British Journal of Psychiatry*, **124**, 22-3.
Gladue, B.A., Green, R. and Hellman, R.E. (1984). Neuroendocrine response to estrogen and sexual orientation. *Science*, **225**, 1496-9.
Gooren, L. (1986). The neuroendocrine response of L.H. to estrogen administration in heterosexual, homosexual and transsexual subjects. *Journal of Clinical Endocrinology and Metabolism*, **63**, 583-588.
Gosselin, C.C. (1987). The sadomasochistic contract. *In* "Variant Sexuality: Research and Theory". (Ed. G.D. Wilson). Croom Helm, London.
Green, R. (1976). One hundred and ten feminine and masculine boys: behavioural contrasts and demographic similarities. *Archives of Sexual Behaviour*, **5**, 425-46.
Greer, G. (1972). "The Female Eunuch". Paladin, London.
Groth, A.N. and Burgess, A.W. (1979). Sexual trauma in the life histories of rapists and child molesters. *Victimology*, **4**, 10-16.
Heston, L. and Shields, J. (1968). Homosexuality in twins. *Archives of General Psychiatry*,

**18**, 149-160.

Holmstrom, L.L. and Burgess, A.W. (1980). Sexual behaviour of assailants during reported rapes. *Archives of Sexual Behaviour*, **9**, 427-440.

Hooker, E. (1957). The adjustment of the male overt homosexual. *Journal of Projective Techniques*, **21**, 18-31.

Howells, K. (1979). Some meanings of children for paedophiles. *In* "Love and Attraction". (Eds M. Cook and G. Wilson). Pergamon, London.

Kallman, F.J. (1952). Comparative twin study on the genetic aspects of male homosexuality. *Journal of Nervous and Mental Diseases*, **115**, 283-298.

Kinsey, A.C., Pomeroy, W.B. and Martin, C.E. (1948). "Sexual Behaviour in the Human Male". Saunders, Philadelphia.

Kinsey, A.C., Pomeroy, W.B., Martin, C.E. and Gebhard, P.H. (1953). "Sexual Behaviour in the Human Female". Saunders, Philadelphia.

Kolarsky, A., Freund,K., Machelk, J. and Polak, O. (1967). Male sexual deviation: association with early temporal lobe damage. *Archives of General Psychiatry*, **17**, 735-43.

Krafft-Ebing, R. von, (1886). "Psychopathia Sexualis". Translation 1965. Stein and Day, New York.

*Lancet* (leader) (1990). The secret of sex. **2**, 348.

Langevin, R. (1990). Sexual anomalies and the brain. *In* "Handbook of Sexual Assault". (Eds D.R. Laws and H.E. Barbaree), Plenum Press, New York.

Laws, D.R. and Marshall, W.L. (1990). A conditioning of the etiology and maintenance of deviant sexual preference and behaviour. *In* "Handbook of Sexual Assault". (Eds W.L. Marshall , D.R. Laws and H.E. Barbaree). Plenum Press, New York.

MacCulloch, M.J., Snowden, P.R., Wood, P.J.W. and Mills, H.E. (1983). Sadistic fantasy, sadistic behaviour and offending. *British Journal of Psychiatry*, **143**, 20-29.

MacLusky, N.J. and Naftonlin, F. (1981). Sexual differentiation of the central nervous system. *Science*, **211**, 1294-1303.

McEwen, B.S. (1981). Neural gonadal steroid interactions. *Science*, **211**, 1303-1311.

Malamuth, N.M. (1981). Rape proclivity among males. *Journal of Social Issues*, **37**, 138-157.

Marshall, W.L. and Barbaree, H.E. (1990). An integrated theory of the etiology of sexual offending. *In* "Handbook of Sexual Assault". (Eds W.L. Marshall, D.R. Laws and H.E. Barbaree). Plenum Press, New York.

Masters, W.H. and Johnson, V.E. (1979). "Homosexuality in Perspective". Little Brown, Boston.

Masters, W.H. and Johnson, V.E. (1988). "Crisis: Homosexual Behaviour in the Age of AIDS". Grove Press, New York.

Money, J. (1986). "Lovemaps: clinical concepts of sexual/erotic health and pathology paraphilia and gender transposition in childhood, adolescence and maturity". Irvington, New York.

Morris, J. (1974). "Conundrum". Penguin, London.

Murrin, M.R. and Laws, D.R. (1990). "The Influence of Pornography on Sexual Assault". (Eds. W.L. Marshal, D.R. Laws and H.E. Barbaree). Plenum Press, New York.

Nyborg, H. (1984). Performance and intelligence in hormonally different groups. *Progress in Brain Research*, **61**, 491-508.

Quinsey, V.L., Chaplin, T.C. and Varney, G.A. (1981). A comparison of rapists and non-sex offenders sexual preferences from mutually consenting sex, rape, and physical abuse of women. *Behavioural Assessment*, **3**, 127-135.

Rada, R.T. (1978). "Clinical Aspects of the Rapist". Grune & Stratton, New York.
Rattray, R.S. (1923). "Ashanti". Clarendon Press, Oxford.
Reiss, B.F. (1980). Psychological tests in homosexuality. *In* "Homosexual Behavior". (Ed. J. Marmor). Basic Books, New York.
Rekers, G.A., Mead, S.L., Rosen, A.C. and Bentler, P.M. (1979). Genetic and physical studies of male children with psychological gender disturbances. *Psychological Medicine*, **9**, 373-375.
Rekers, G.A., Mead, S.L., Rosen, A.C. and Brigham, S.L. (1983). Family correlates of male childhood gender disturbance. *Journal of Genetic Psychology*, **142**, 31-42.
Reynolds, V. and Kellett, M. (1991). "Mating and Marriage". Oxford University Press.
Rosen, A.C., Rekers, G.A. and Rogers Friar, L. (1977). Theoretical and diagnostic issues in child gender disturbances. *Journal of Sex Research*, **13**, 89-103.
Ross, M.W., Walinder, J., Lundstrom, B. and Thuwe, I. (1981). Cross-cultural approaches to transsexualism: A comparison between Sweden and Australia. *Acta Psychiatrica Scandinavica*, **63**, 75-82.
Saghir, M.T. and Robins, E. (1973). "Male and Female Homosexuality". Williams and Wilkins, Baltimore.
Sanday, P.R. (1981). The socio-cultural context of rape: A cross cultural study. *Journal of Social Issues*, **37**, 5-27.
Slijper, F.M.E. (1984). Androgens and gender role behaviour in girls with congenital adrenal hyperplasia (CAH). *Progress in Brain Research*, **61**, 417-422.
Stoller, R.J. (1985). "Presentations of Gender". Yale University Press.
Storr, C.A. (1990). Sadomasochism. *In* "Principles and Practice of Forensic Psychiatry". (Eds R. Bluglass and P. Bowden). Churchill Livingstone, London.
Van Wyk, P.H. and Geist, C.S. (1984). Psychosocial development of heterosexual, bisexual, and homosexual behavior. *Archives of Sexual Behavior*, **13**, 505-545.
Wells, E. (1986). The view from within. *In* "Transsexualism and Sex Reassignment". (Eds W.A.W. Walters and M.W. Ross), Oxford University Press.
Wilson, G.D. (1987). An ethological approach to sexual deviation. *In* "Variant Sexuality: Research and Theory". (Ed. G.D. Wilson). Croom Helm, London.
Zuger, B. (1976). Monozygotic twins discordant for homosexuality: Report of a pair and significance of the phenomenon. *Comprehensive Psychiatry.*

# 21. Awareness of body image, parietal lobe disturbances, neglect and agnosias

W.J.K. Cumming

The concept of a body schema as a permanent, albeit vague, perception one has of one's own body has been constructed by neurologists from observations made on impairments of recognition of parts of the body which can occur in those afflicted by lesions of the central nervous system (Cumming, 1988; Damasio and Tranel, 1992). The originators of the concept – Bonnier (1905), Head and Holmes (1911) – were interested in the central cortical representation of sensation, and the first notion of a body image was in essence a physiological explanation of how tactile or postural sensation was represented in the brain (Cutting, 1989).

Greater refinement of this concept has been realized as an important component of the gradual unification of neurobiology with areas of psychology, beginning in the early 1920s and 1930s with the merger of psychophysics and sensory physiology and continuing through the 1970s and 1980s with the neurobiological analysis of simple behavioural systems and elementary forms of learning. The concept of a body schema thus comes to lie along side, and as part of, the highest cognitive functions: the processes of perception, attention, language, memory and the organization of actions (Kandel and Squire, 1992).

The substrate for these advances has been made possible by techniques of brain imaging – in particular computerized tomography (CT), magnetic resonance imaging (MRI), and proton emission tomography (PET) – and from an understanding of the basic cytoarchitecture and anatomical pathways within the cortex (Knierim and Van Essen, 1992). In the monkey, and probably in the human, there are at least 30 visual areas in the neocortex belonging to a distinct hierarchy, consisting of two major parallel streams of processing. These streams originate in the retina, project to the laterogeniculate and then to the striate and extra-striate cortices. Eventually one stream projects from the striate area to the infra-temporal cortex and appears to be primarily concerned with visual pattern recognition (the analysis of visually presented objects) and the other projects dorsally to the parietal cortex and appears to be primarily concerned with location of objects in space and in the movements necessary to reach these locations.

Signals leading to visual perception can be enhanced by attention (Posner and Driver, 1992). Other distinct systems are presumably involved in spatial orienting, or attention to visual locations, in vigilance and in directing a specific visual feature or dimension among multiple targets.

The terms body schema, body concept, somatopsychic bodily image, "ego", and body awareness are often used indiscriminately and interchangeably; and may be used in either a neurological or psychological sense. In general terms: body schema refers to an awareness of spatial characteristics formed from current and stored sensory information; and body experience includes psychological and situational traits as well as emotional and intentional factors – thus body schema is a fact of perception whereas body experience is a fact of psychological experience.

In neurological practice the most striking impairment of a patient's body schema is the condition of unilateral neglect or misconception (Lhermitte, 1939). For example, the patient may be unaware of the left half of his body, dressing only the right sided limbs. He may claim that it is not his arm, but someone else's in the bed beside him. He may give it a name, e.g. Tom. If the hemisomatoagnosia is accompanied by a defect of vision to that side, he may even be terrified when the forgotten hand suddenly appears in front of his face (M. Critchley, 1953). The disorder may occur in full consciousness as a transient phenomenon in association with other paroxysmal cerebral events such as migraine or epilepsy. In the presence of a stroke or tumour the patient may behave as though one half of his body was non-existent (see Table I).

TABLE I. *Types of altered consciousness of one side of the body*

| | |
|---|---|
| Conscious neglect | Unconscious neglect |
| Sensory displacement | Illusory displacement |
| Delusional alienation | Denial of paralysis |
| Denial of disability | Personification of the limb |
| Morbid fear or dislike of affected limb | |

Gerstmann (1930) describes how the patient shows no apparent concern for one half of his body and, if asked to elevate the affected limb, his facial expression may suggest that he has accomplished the task successfully although no limb movement is seen to occur. A very prominent feature is the fact that, even under normal visual control, movement still remains absent. The lesion in most of these patients lies within the parietal lobe. Anton (1893-99) and Babinski (1918, 1923) stressed that, if the examiner was not familiar with the phenomenon, he would simply attribute the patient's ignorance of his hemiplegia to some non-specific mental impairment.

There have been various theories of the pathogenesis of anosognosia. Early writers (Goldstein, 1928; Weinstein and Khan, 1955; Ullmann, 1962) suggested that it was an expression of a general mental disorder resembling a diffuse cortical syndrome and that the patient's premorbid personality was the basis for the subsequent reaction to illness. Gerstmann (1930) believed that, like most agnosias, anosognosia for hemiplegia was an artificial creation due to a failure of communication – the result of a specific disconnection from the speech area of the brain. Weinstein and Khan (1955) extended this, suggesting that the fact that anosognosia occurred only in left sided hemiplegia, was explained by patients with right sided hemiplegia being confused, silent or using jargon. Lastly, Fredericks (1985) commented that denial of hemiplegia is brought on only when the pertinent question is asked by the examiner. When left to his own devices, the patient does not deny spontaneously the existence of hemiplegia. Even when the patient's limb is moved passively there is still no appreciation of hemiparesis, suggesting thereby a defect in the appreciation of sensory information from the hemiplegic limb, which, because of a stroke on the right side of the brain, is not being filtered and processed. The fact that in most patients the syndrome tends to disappear in 1-2 weeks could be explained by the improved information handling by the paretic limb.

A lesser form of impaired identification, usually from a lesion in the same part of the brain, can take the form of inability to name which finger is touched (finger agnosia) or right-left disorientation. Other forms of spatial disorientation which tend to be permanent are hemi-inattention and hemi-spatial neglect. In these patients the peripheral motor and sensory mechanisms are intact. The patient fails to report or respond to a stimulus presented to the side opposite to the brain lesion (Heilman, 1979; Heilman and Valstein, 1979). With visual neglect the patient may respond to a stimulus in the right visual field and to a stimulus in the left visual field, but presented with both simultaneously will ignore one of the stimuli. Similarly with sensory neglect, if touched on one side then the other, both stimuli will be recognized but if both arms (for example) are touched simultaneously he will recognize the touch on only one side. Although patients with unilateral neglect syndromes are most inattentive to stimuli contralateral to the lesion, they may also be inattentive to ipsilateral stimuli, although ipsilateral neglect is not as severe.

With hemi-spatial neglect patients asked to perform behaviour tasks in space they neglect the hemi-space contralateral to their lesion. For example, when asked to draw a picture of a flower, they draw only half a flower and if asked to draw a clock face, they draw one half of the clock face crowding the numbers into that half. Similarly a patient may eat food from only one half of his plate and a nurse recognizing this problem will turn the plate through 180° to enable him to complete the meal.

Benson and Geschwind (1969) described patients with paralexia as those who, if asked to read the word "cowboy" would read only "boy". A similar abnormality can be seen when they are using a typewriter in that they fail to type letters on the keyboard contra-lateral to their lesions. This was described as paragraphia (Valenstein and Heilman, 1979).

In hemi-spatial neglect, as in hemi-inattention, lesions can be produced by abnormalities in deeper structures.

Frontal lobe lesions, particularly those involving the supplementary motor area, frequently cause hemi-spatial neglect in both visual, auditory and somatosensory areas (Damasio et al., 1980,1985). If the frontal eye field is involved, then there is impairment of the gaze towards the contra-lateral side in the presence of neglect.

Lesions of the basal ganglia and internal capsule have again been implicated. Watson and Heilman (1979) and Vilkki (1984) reported contra-lateral hemineglect in patients who had undergone thalamotomy for the treatment of Parkinsonian tremor. Severe hemi-spatial neglect was reported by Ferro and Kertesz (1984) in a patient with a posterior internal capsule infarction.

Rubens (1985) thought that it was possible to improve inattention and neglect by optokinetic or vestibular stimulation directed towards the neglected side. Grüsser and colleagues (Grüsser, 1982; Grüsser et al., 1990a,b) believed that a network of the parietal-insular-vestibular cortex, which normally monitors head in space position, was activated, shifting the subjective co-ordinates towards the direction of the slow phase of optokinetic nystagmus. Although this is of theoretical interest, it is difficult to see a practical application in terms of management of patients.

The agnosias cover the different disorders of higher level perception that follow brain damage. The definition of agnosia is by exclusion. That is, there is impairment of object recognition not caused by sensory deficits or generalized intellectual loss.

Assessment of a patient with a presumed agnosia requires both clinical examination and specialized testing.

Bed-side examination includes discrimination between straight and curved lines, the ability to judge the shapes of forms made up to dotted lines, and using tests of line bisection or copying of a complex figure (Grüsser and Landis, 1991). The patient can be confronted by real objects and asked to name them or describe their use (clearly having excluded any impairment of language comprehension). The details of specialized testing are outside the scope of this chapter, but are discussed in detail by Grüsser and Landis (1991).

Within disorders of visual agnosia there are selected agnosias for face, object and printed word recognition. There are pair wise dissociations among face recognition, object recognition and printed word recognition suggesting that there is a division of labour for different types of stimuli within the visual recognition system (Farah, 1992). Analysis of a large group of patients has shown the existence of two types of visual pattern recognition processes: one that is essential for face recognition, not needed for reading and used for object recognition; another that is essential for reading, used for object recognition and not needed for face recognition (Farah, 1990, 1991). The former appears to depend on ventral temporo-occipital regions bilaterally but may occasionally be seen after a unilateral right hemisphere lesion; the latter appears to depend upon the left temporo-parieto-occipital cortex.

Non visual agnosias also exist, particularly tactile agnosia (Caselli, 1991). This work greatly expands the understanding of the syndrome and shows it to be consistent with object recognition in the visual and tactile modalities, relying on separate components of the functional architecture. Of particular interest within the agnosias has been the recent expansion of understanding of prosopagnosia, being an agnosia for facial recognition (Gross and Seergent, 1992), which brings together the developments in the field of single neuron studies in animals, imaging techniques and human neuropsychological studies.

Visual agnosia for form (apperceptive visual agnosia) is defined as the inability to distinguish two structures similar in all respects except for shape. This is a small group of patients seen usually after diffuse brain damage as, for example, that produced by carbon monoxide (Milner et al., 1991). These patients appear to overcome their difficulty to some extent by the use of tracing strategies in that, by tracing around the object, they are able to recognize its form.

Visual object agnosia (visual associative agnosia) is very much more common and patients have been described (Benson, 1989) with associated visual agnosia who cannot name on visual stimulation but can easily copy figures or written material. Tactile and auditory stimuli are named normally. Routine language testing shows no significant abnormality and the IQ is normal, except for those test modalities demanding visual identification.

Grüsser and Landis (1991) have laid down three major requirements in order to make the diagnosis; first, that elementary visual perception should be intact, or at least intact enough for the patient to be able to copy objects or drawings he cannot recognize or to match pairs as being the same or different; second, the presented visual stimulus should be normally recognized through modalities other than vision (i.e. by touch or hearing characteristic sounds); and third, the difficulty in recognizing meaningful visual stimuli should not be restricted to naming but should extend to classification into semantic and behavioural categories and also to recognition of meaning by function.

It is generally believed that bilateral occipitotemporal damage is required to produce this syndrome (Alexander and Albert, 1983), however, there are some cases where only posterior unilateral left sided damage has been described (McCarthy and Warrington, 1986) or unilateral right sided damage (Levin, 1978). Hecaen and Ajuriaguerra (1956) stressed that object agnosia, subsequent to lesions of the left hemisphere's visual system, was strongly associated with pure reading difficulty (alexia), while agnosia associated with lesions in the right hemisphere system was strongly associated with prosopagnosia.

## References

Alexander, M.P. and Albert, M.L. (Eds) (1983). The anatomical basis of visual agnosia. *In* "Localization in Neuropsychology". pp. 393-415. Academic Press, New York.
Anton, G. (1893). Beitrage zur klinischen Beurteilung und zur Localisation der Muskelsinnestorungen im Grosshirne. *Zeitschrift für Heilkunde*, **14**, 133-348.
Anton, G. (1898). Ueber Herderkrankungen des Gehirnes, welche vom Patienten selbst nicht wahrgenommen werden. *Wiener Klinische Wochenschrift,* **11**, 227-229.
Anton, G. (1899). Ueber die Selbstwahrnemung der Herderkrungen des Gehirns durch den

Kranken bei Rindenblindheit und Rindentaubheit. *Archiv für Psychiatrie und Nervenkrankheit*, **32**, 86-127.

Assal, G., Favre, C. and Anderes, J.P. (1984). Non-reconaissances d'animaux familiers chez un paysan. (Nonrecognition of familiar animals by a farmer: zooagnosia or prosopagnosia for animals). *Revue Neurologique*, **140**, 580-584.

Babinski, J. (1918) Anosognosie. *Revue Neurologique*, **31**, 365-367.

Babinski, J. (1923). Sur l'anosognosie. *Revue Neurologique*, **39**, 731-732.

Bauer, R.M. (1984). Autonomic recognition of names and faces in prosopagnosia: A neuropsychological application of the Guilty Knowledge Test. *Neuropsychologia*, **22**, 457-469.

Benson, D.F. (1989). Disorders of visual gnosis. *In* "Neuropsychology of Visual Perception" pp. 59-78. Erlbaum, New York.

Benson, D.F. and Geschwind, N. (1969). The alexias. *In* "Handbook of Clinical Neurology", pp.112-140. Elsevier, Amsterdam.

Benton, A. (1990). Face recognition. *Cortex*, **26**, 491-499.

Bonnier, P. (1905). l'Aschématie. *Revue Neurologique*, **13**, 605-609 .

Bornstein, B., Sroka, H. and Munitz, H. (1969). Prosopagnosia with animal face agnosia. *Cortex*, **5**, 164-169.

Caselli, R.J. (1991). Rediscovering tactile agnosia. *Mayo Clinic Proceedings*, **66**, 129-142.

Critchley, M. (1953). "The Parietal Lobes". Arnold, London.

Cumming, W.J.K. (1988). The neurobiology of the body schema. *British Journal of Psychiatry*, **153**, 7-11.

Cumming, W.J.K., Hurwitz, L.J. and Pearl, N.T. (1970). A study of a patient who had alexia without agraphia. *Journal of Neurology, Neurosurgery and Psychiatry*, **33**, 34-39.

Cutting, D.J. (1989). Body Image distribution in neuropsychiatry. *In* "The Bridge between Neurology and Psychiatry" (Eds E.H. Reynolds and M.R. Trimble), pp.106-134. Churchill Livingstone, London.

Damasio, A.R. and Damasio, H. (1983). The anatomic basis of pure alexia and color "agnosia". *Neurology*, **33**, 1578-1583.

Damasio, A.R. and Tranel, D. (1992). Knowledge systems. *Current Opinion in Neurobiology*, **2**, 186-190.

Damasio, A.R., Damasio, H. and Chang, H.C. (1980). Neglect following damage to the frontal lobe or basal ganglia. *Neuropsychologia*, **18**, 123-132.

Farah, M.J. (1990). "Visual Agnosia: Disorders of object recognition and what they tell us about normal vision". MIT Press, Cambridge, Mass.

Farah, M.J. (1991). Pattern a of co-occurence among the associative agnosias: Implications for visual object representations. *Cognitive Neuropsychology*, **8**, 1-19.

Farah, M.J. (1992). Agnosia. *Current Opinion in Neurobiology*, **2**, 162-164.

Ferro, J.M. and Kertesz, A. (1984). Posterior internal capsule infarction associated with neglect. *Archives of Neurology*, **41**, 422-424.

Fredericks, J.A.M. (1985). Disorders of body schema. *In* "Handbook of Clinical Neurology". pp. 373-393, Elsevier, Amsterdam.

Gerstmann, J. (1930). The symptoms produced by lesions of the transitional area between the inferior parietal and middle occipital gyri. *In* "Neurological Classics in Modern Translation". pp. 35-40. Hafner Press, New York.

Goldstein, K. (1928). Beobachtungen bei die Veranderungen des Gesamtverhaltens bei Gehirnschadigung. *Monatsschrift für Psychiatrie und Neurologie*, **68**, 217-242.

Head, H. and Holmes, G. (1911). Sensory disturbances from cerebral lesions. *Brain*, **34**,

102-254.

Hecaen, H. and Ajuriaguerra, J. de, (1956). Agnosie visuelle pour les objets inaimes par lesion unilaterale gauche. *Revue Neurologique,* **94**, 222-233.

Heilman, K.M. (1979). Neglect and related disorders. *In* "Clinical Neuropsychology". pp. 268-307. Oxford University Press, Oxford.

Heilman, K.M. and Valenstein, E. (1979). Mechanisms underlying hemispatial neglect. *Annals of Neurology,* **5**, 166-170.

Heilman, K.M., Valenstein, E. and Watson, R.T. (1985). The neglect syndrome. *In* "Handbook of Clinical Neurology". pp 153-183. Elsevier, Amsterdam.

Kandel, E. and Squire, L. (1992). Cognitive neuroscience: editorial overview. *Current Opinion in Neurobiology,* **2**, 143-145.

Knierim, J.J. and Van Essen, D.C. (1992). Visual cortex: cartography, connectivity, and concurrent processing. *Current Opinion in Neurobiology,* **2**, 150-155.

Lhermitte, (1939). L'image de notre corps... *Nouvelle Revue Critique.* Paris.

McCarthy, R.A. and Warrington, E.K. (1986). Visual associative agnosia: A clinico-anatomical study of a single case. *Journal of Neurology, Neurosurgery and Psychiatry.* **49**, 1233-1240.

Milner, A.D., Perrett, D.I. Johnston, R.S., Benson, P.J., Jordan, T.R., Heel Y.D.W., Bettuci, D., Mortara, F., Mutani, R. and Terazzi, E. (1991). Perception and action in visual form agnosia. *Brain,* **114**, 405-428.

Posner, M.I. and Driver, J. (1992). The neurobiology of selective attention. *Current Opinion in Neurobiology,* **2**, 165-169.

Rubens, A.B. (1985). Caloric stimulation and unilateral visual neglect. *Neurology,* **35**, 1019-1024.

Snowden, R.J. (1992). The perception of visual motion. *Current Opinion in Neurobiology,* **2**, 175-179.

Ullmann, M. (1962). "Behavioural Changes in Patients Following Strokes". Charles C. Thomas, Springfield, Illinois.

Valenstein, E. amd Heilman, K.M. (1979). Apraxic agraphia with neglect-induced paragraphia. *Archives of Neurology,* **36**, 406-408.

Vilkki, J. (1984). Visual hemi-inattention after ventrolateral thalamotomy. *Neuropsychologia,* **22**, 399-408.

Weinstein, E.A. and Khan, R.L. (1955). "Denial of Illness". Charles C. Thomas, Springfield, Illinois.

# 22. Childhood development of awareness of self

E. Rivlin

The development of self-awareness presents one of the most empirically challenging, complex and multi-faceted journeys of childhood. Neurological, developmental and psychoanalytic models, as well as more recent empirically based studies have shown development to be a dynamic interplay between the inner self, neurological modality and outside influences.

This chapter will examine:
1  models of development and childhood awareness, neuropsychological and development aspects;
2  play and imaginary friends;
3  the development of body image in children's drawings;
4  body image development in mentally retarded children;
5  body schema and the interior of the body image;
6  the effects of congenital and acquired disfigurement, illness and abusive life situations and the resultant personal distortion of body image.

## Models of Development and Childhood Awareness

The development of body schema, somatognosis and its disorders, have been succinctly summarized by De Ajuriaguerra and Stucki (1975). They emphasize two aspects of body schema: the body concept the child has or the body the child knows (le corps connu), based upon the body the child experiences preverbally (le corps vecu). "Le corps vecu" is analagous to the term "body awareness". The origins of such awareness lie in the consequences of the child's earliest experiences with his/her mother. Body awareness constitutes the child's own body and the extracorporeal space. The earliest affective experiences of preverbal body awareness arise from vestibular, visual, kinaesthetic and tactile information received in earliest infancy. This results in the body schema (le corps connu) as perceived between the ages 4 and 8 years.

Table I presents a development framework of life-span age-related tasks (Cicchetti et al., 1988). It also presents developing awareness of self and tasks expected.

TABLE I. *Life-span age-related tasks.*

| Approximate ages | Development |
| --- | --- |
| 1  0-3 months | Homeostatic regulation and the development of a reliable signalling system |
| 2  4-6 months | Management of "tension" (cognitively produced arousal) and the differentiation of affect. |
| 3  6-12 months | Development of a secure attachment |
| 4  18-24 months | Development of an autonomous self. Symbolic representation of further self – other differentiations |
| 5  24-36 months | Symbolic representation of further self – other differentiations |
| 6  Early childhood | Establishing peer relationships |
| 7  Middle childhood | Adapting to school |

Psychoanalytical theories encompass not only the works of Freud, but also the developmental views of Anna Freud, Melanie Klein, E.H. Erikson, M.S. Mahler, D.W. Winnicott and L. Sander. They follow Freud in conceptualizing the infantile psychological state as dominated by affects, of which anxiety and pleasure (Freud, 1926) are the most relevant. Anna Freud is concerned with the integrated use of an aggressive drive. Klein stresses the role of unconscious fantasies. These evolve as a series of developmental crises in Erikson's epigenetic theory. Mahler and Sander sequence the process of adaptation and separation from the mother; and Winnicott concentrates on the child's capacity to be alone and to play. Stern (1977) in reviewing psychoanalytic views as to the nature of infantile responses to stimulation and the quality of affects in babies, says, "What remains (of Freud's model) is a kernel concept: affect is related to the build-up and fall-off of stimulation and tension".

Winnicott (1957, 1958a,b, 1965), Balint (1968) and Kernberg (1975, 1980) embrace the "object-relations schools" of psychoanalysis, and view the infant from birth as both responsive and interactive in an adaptation to its own state and the nature of the actual maternal response. This is a very different picture from the tabula rasa view of the child as being a passive recipient of maternal responses and his/her environment. This more interactive viewpoint is in keeping with the motility, self-control and increasing autonomy that are evolving features of child development.

Contemporary investigators such as Minuchin (1977), Thomas and Chess (1977), Kohlberg (1967) and Shapiro and Perry (1976) suggest that significant discontinuities in development occur at 7 years (plus or minus 1 year) and are consistent with the presence of a distinctive phase between early, preschool phases and adolescence.

## From Early Experience of Body Image to Cohesion of Body Self

In Piaget's developmental stage theory of cognition (1950, 1970), body image plays a crucial role in the development of the person's affective and cognitive processes. Piaget divides the course of development into: a sensory motor period (0-2 years), pre-operational thinking (2-7 years), which culminates in a period of concrete operations (7-11 years), and a period of formal operations in early adolescence. He characterizes these periods within a stable cognitive structure that is restructured into the next.

Lerner (1986; Lerner and Kauffman, 1985) emphasizes that personal and social context interactions are central in the process of change. He uses the term "developmental contextualism" to explain how the body evokes differential reactions from interaction with others and as the object of feedback from other people. From this viewpoint, the person's appraisal of his/her own body (cognitions and feelings about his/her body) are really reactions which firstly derive in part from socializing external reactions to the person (Cooley, 1902; Meade, 1934). Cooley and Meade propose the concept of "the looking-glass self" to describe the self (a) as perceived through the reflections in the eyes of others; and (b) from the person's cognitive and emotional developments involving the body (Piaget, 1950). Thus the body image is a dual product of social interactions, feedback from others and psychological developments; and performs as an initiator of such interactions and developments.

Spitz (1957), and later Krueger (1990), conceptualize the development of a body self from infancy to a more complete integrated body schema. Such development is seen as a tri-partite process:

### 1 Early psychic experience of the body

The body the child experiences without words (le corps vecu) is essentially connected to the young child's affective experiences through the reflection of his/her self object, i.e. his/her mother. Initially, these experiences merge and are not separated from the mother figure.

### 2 Early awareness of a body image with an integration of inner and outer experience

This stage, beginning at a few months and extending until 2 years, is characterized by a sense of reality based on an integrated body self, emerging from initiated body boundaries and the infant's perception of differentiated bodily feelings. As the infant becomes more aware of the internal and external aspects of his/her own body, he/she develops a more coherent and defined level of understanding his/her own body experiences. Image formation commences at this time (Horowitz, 1983). This is also true for blind children. But interestingly, in children suffering from spina bifida, vision can replace kinaesthesia and somaesthesia in the development of body awareness (Robinson et al., 1986).

In each of six phases of sensory motor development, Piaget describes circular reactions which are elaborated in an increasingly cognitive complex way. Through knowledge of actions on his/her own body the infant can act on one external object to influence another, moving from primitive imaging capacities to identification of symbols of transitional objects, for example, a thumb to suck rather than a breast. The child thus moves from initially recognizing that the mirror in front of him imparts information about his/her body and actions in a definite and objectifiable manner, and the movement of that image is created directly by his/her own actions (Modaressi and Kinney, 1977) to full imaging capacity at about 18 months, corresponding with Piaget's description of "object permanence". After this age, the child can extend his/her conceptual capacity beyond himself/herself to include the body of others, as is shown in imaginative play, for example, drinking from his/her cup and offering the cup to a parent or doll (Nicholich, 1977).

## 3 Definition and cohesion of the body self as a basis of self-awareness

This third stage commences at about 15 months, as shown by the observational studies of the infant discovering himself/herself in the mirror at 15 to 18 months (Emde, 1983) and the acquisition of the semantic "no". Spitz (1957) cites the child's ability to say and understand the word "no" as evidence of the emerging distinctiveness of the "I" and "non I". At this stage, the child begins to become aware of his/her own autonomy and that his/her own body is his/her own. The essential developmental tasks to be achieved during this stage involve the synthesis of a stable, integrated unified mental representation of one's body. The child needs to understand what is outside with distinct boundaries and what is inside. From this vantage point, the child may progress to individual mastery. Both Spitz (1965) and Blatt (1974) indicate the importance of developing boundaries between inner and outer experience as well as between self and others. The establishment of the boundary distinctions are crucial for the later more complex differentiation and integration in the developmental process.

**Neuropsychological and Developmental Aspects**

One limitation of Piagetian theory (Wolff, 1960) is that the individual's own action in the organization of intelligence and the role of others in the environment subsumes a subsidiary role, ignoring the fact that the thinking of children is "social". Trevarthen (1979) emphasizes the shared "intersubjective" understandings that develop in the interchanges between mother and infant from the earliest period. He argues that such acts of communication "appear powerful enough to take charge of the process by which the cognitive processes of the mind develop". Further research by Hewson (1978) and Bruner (1978) show that patterns of human intercourse may shape the infant and child's patterns of thinking.

Visual perception is essential for the establishment of a schema of the surrounding space. As the infant develops, the differences between front and back, up and down, and left and right outside the body, are essentially significant, as is being able to visualize manipulations in the contralateral half field. A child needs to integrate his/her purposeful movement within the structure of a normal body schema development, with the visually perceived outside world. The infant learns to localize what he /she perceives; first close and far (as a baby in a cot), then up and down (at about 1 year), and thirdly, left and right and opposite diagonals (5-10 years). By 8 years, a body schema develops that has an extracorporeal and a corporeal modality. The child learns to estimate distances, time spans and speeds. However, blind children are unable to follow this normal development of body schema (Poeck and Orgass, 1964).

What is the neurological basis for left/right orientation? Between 5 and 8 years, children begin to understand the use of "left" and "right" as it pertains to the child's own body. Many children have problems crossing the mid-line "touch your left ear with your right hand" or completing tasks with their eyes closed (Benton 1985; Berges and Lezine 1972). The cerebral location of the left/right orientation may be closely associated with language, since such disorders usually accompany aphasia. Left/right orientation regarding another person and the outside world does not usually occur until 9 to 12 years (see Njiokiktjien, 1988).

Children have different capacities to rotate. For example, not all children sitting on mobile toys can steer them backwards and forwards. Both visualization and body awareness play a major role in the growth of motor concepts (Njiokiktjien, 1988).

Before 8 years, the right hemisphere is dominant for the recognition of familiar faces (Cohen, 1985). The capacity to recognize facial emotions is also initially asymmetrical but improves with age. Stoit (1986) examined emotional recognition of 6.5-, 9-, 11-, and 20-years-olds in the central, lateral and bilateral fields. He found that asymmetry did not change after 6.5, and attributed the improvement to an interhemisphere connection that appeared to be more efficient with age.

**Problems of Constructional Dyspraxia**

Constructional dyspraxia is evident when a child constructs or draws. Children with right sided brain damage produce drawings often containing several details without any recognizable whole, whereas children with left-sided lesions can draw a complete whole, but omit the details. After the age of 5, there is no lateralization effect, but visuo-spatial and perceptual construction of space progressively develop with age and depend on the child's active manipulation in the space around him. Kirk (1985) demonstrated in children aged 6 to 16 that the ability to produce a complex figure (the Rey-Osterreith Test) increases with maturation of specific areas in the left and right hemispheres, and developing integration by way of the corpus callosum. She found that the right hemisphere plays a central role in the spatial comprehension (posterior) and performance (anterior) of drawing tasks.

Children with a right hemisphere deficit show limitation of body schema, lack facial expression and show poor recognition of others and of their facial expressions.

## Play and Imaginary Friends

Play is the principal activity of childhood and has a much more personal significance than merely relief. Play has a special meaning for the child. Erikson believes that much of the unique meaning of play is concerned with the child's efforts to master himself, his body and body sensation, and the anxiety stimulated by the world and events around him. Thus play has a particular significance for the child's understanding of the boundaries between himself and others. Through play the child learns to master reality by experiment and planning. As Erikson elucidates it is a definite human trait at any age to deal with experience by creating modal situations.

Tizard and Harvey (1977) comment on the biological meaning of playing. Imaginary or fantasy play progresses through developmental processes (Cole and La Voie, 1985). There are some children however who have no capacity for imaginative play or who are unable to pretend (ideomotor dyspraxia) (Bauman and Kemper, 1985). Children start to play through fantasy at 2 years, but tragically there are some who fail to manage fantasy play. Autistic children, while playing in a perseverative manner, may be distinguished from the type of perseveration found in frontal lobe dysfunction (Beaumanoir, 1985; Bakkar, 1970).

Imaginary friends can be a source of help and comfort to a child. They can also assume many identities. As quoted by Christina Hardyment from "Arthur Ransome and Capt Flint's Trunk" (page 100, 1984):

"Nancy is still a bit of a muddle," said Daisy, "is she Taqui or is she Barbara Collingwood or is she Georgina Rawdon-Smith? There seem to be too many people being her."

"Peggy was just as much of a muddle, but they thought she was such a shadowy character anyway that she didn't matter so much." "I think he put her in so that Nancy would have someone to boss about, so she wouldn't just be alone", said Tilly.

Gallino (1991) studied the intelligence, creativity and social skills among children with and without imaginary friends. Of the 357 male and female Italian pre-school and school age children (4 – 10 years old) 147 had an imaginary friend which was determined during individual game-playing sessions. Somers and Yawkey (1984) contend that the uses and functions of imaginary play companions or friends in the lives of young children are linked with creative and intellectual growth. The development of sensitivity, elaboration and originality have been linked with such imaginary companions. They found that the key elements connected to intellectual growth appear to include symbolic functioning, decontextualization, object relations and symbolization. They suggest that the same elements can be used as guidance strategies by adults working with these children who have imaginary friends and their use has the potential for increasing creative and intellectual thought in both school and home settings.

Are imaginary playmates visual hallucinations or do they have a role to play in childhood? Weller and Wiedemann (1989) analysed the pathomechanisms involved in the development of visual hallucinatory experiences and argue that no single model served to explain all phenomena encountered in the field of visual hallucinations. They also question the validity of the current distinction between hallucination and illusion and eliminate conditions which are only appreciable psychologically, for example the imaginary playmates of childhood and visual hallucinations in the face of a severe grief reaction.

## Development of Body Image in Children's Drawings

Eye and hand coordination skills on pencil and paper tasks such as drawing a person follow a normal developmental course. At 4 years old a child can draw a primitive man and can draw a circle for a head or a body and add at least two other body features such as eyes, legs, arms, nose, mouth, feet or hands. By 6 years this has developed to a real representation with complete facial features and most limbs. At this stage the child can indicate clearly what is represented in addition to the circle or head. At least six other features should be present. By 7 years the child can produce a representation of people who are clothed. Trousers are drawn with double lines showing thickness rather than single line drawings for legs. There are also other features present such as hats, ribbons, clothing details. Figure 1 shows the developmental course of drawings from 4 to 8 years. Figure 2 is the family group of a 6-year-old child; notice the animated three-legged cat.

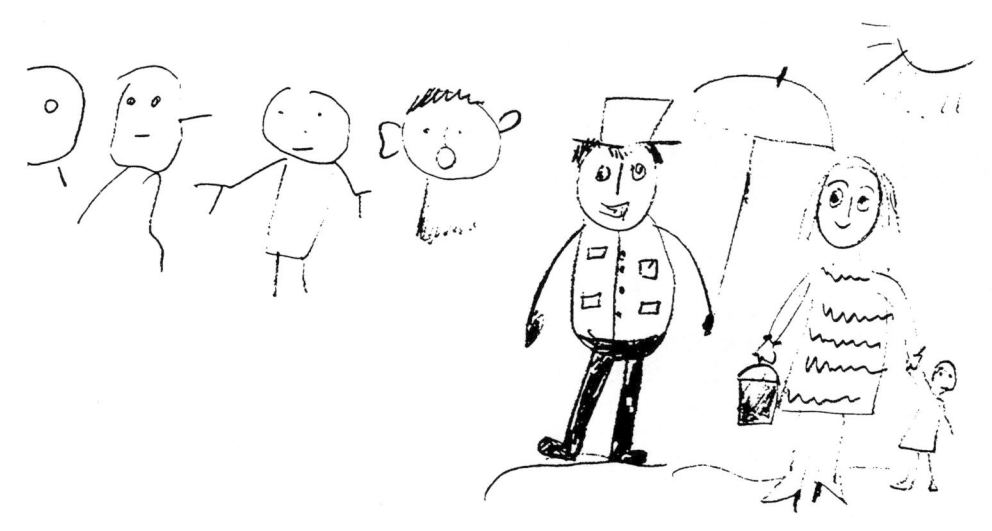

FIG. 1.

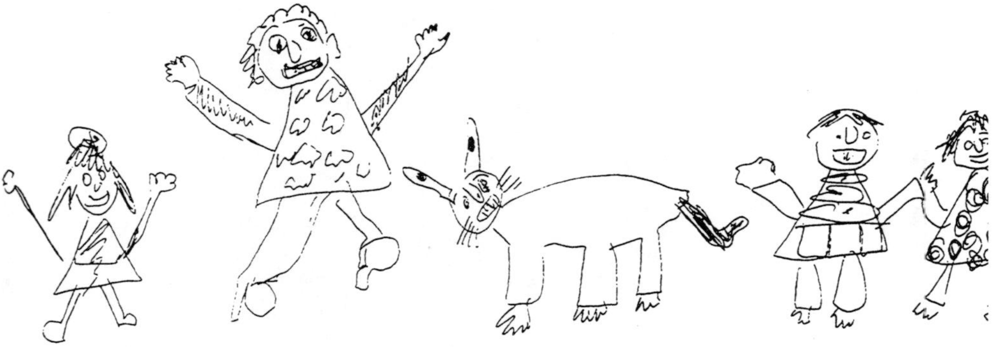

FIG. 2.

Fujimoto (1979) examined the hypothesis that body images are a more dominant factor in drawing performance than visual coordination or perceptual discrimination. He examined the drawings of 384 6- to 12-year-old kindergarten to 6th grade pupils and analysed at various points (e.g. face, shoulders, 3-dimensional expression of legs). He found that stereotype expressions change to realistic styles as follows:
1   from full face to side face (7-8 years),
2   2- to 3-dimensional shoulders (8-9 years),
3   and, 2- to 3-dimensional legs (11-12 years).

The developmental sequence of body part identification in young children follows a normal developmental course with a positive correlation between the number of parts correctly identified and increasing age (Witt et al., 1990). Such findings may be of diagnostic help for children with suspected delays in cognitive, language or body schema development. No significant differences exist between the ability to point to body parts on a doll and the ability to point to body parts on the self. More children named the body when it was pointed to than could point to the body when the examiner named it (Brittain and Chien, 1983).

Three developmental levels were identified in the acquisition of anatomical constancy in children between 2 – 6 years old (Feiner, 1987):
1   the integration of part images of the body into a whole body image,
2   the establishment of a cohesive and inviable body image, and
3   the capacity to retain a sense of the body's continuity over time.

Thus as children develop they acquire specific cognitive capacities, their body images become increasingly stable, cohesive and continuous.

Duncan (1985) observed the effects of the onset of puberty on body image, school behaviour and deviance. Taking a large sample of 12- to 17-year-old children, he found that early maturing males were most satisfied with height and weight, whereas early maturing females were most dissatisfied with weight, with 69% wishing to be thinner. The normal developmental process was viewed negatively by females and positively by males.

## Body Image Development in Mentally Retarded Children

Clapp (1972) investigated the body schema in organically mentally handicapped children compared to other impaired children and to normal children. The organic retardates had greatest difficulty in recognizing their body schema.

For young pre-verbal retarded children shown TV images of themselves, the emergence of self-recognition was closely related to the maturity of the children's general responsiveness to their reflections (Hill and Tomlin, 1981). Down's Syndrome children made a broad range of responses, including the curiosity and self-conscious behaviours characteristic of normal children during the second year of life, and almost all recognized their images. The range of behaviours displayed by multi-handicapped children was greatly restricted and similar to children in the first year of life. Less than half of this latter group showed an emergence of self-recognition.

## Body Schema and the Interior of the Body Image

Glaun and Rosenthal (1987) suggest that children's understanding of the interior of the body and its functioning develops in a regular sequence paralleling cognitive development. Two hundred and ten children aged 5 - 11 years were asked to draw the interior of the body inside a body outline provided. They were also questioned about the contents of the body, and the number and nature of the parts drawn was noted. There was a significant increase in conceptual sophistication with age, supporting a clear delineation of stages in the development of the child's thinking about the body's interior.

Amann-Gainotti *et al.* (1989) examined genital inner space and their identity formation in girls. Two hundred and seventy-five adolescent Italian girls (aged 11 to 18) were asked to make a drawing of the inside of their bodies and their sexual organs. The process of structuring and integrating genital inner space into the body image appeared to develop slowly with integration by 17 to 18 years.

Deaf and hearing children's concepts of the body's interior were found to differ at three age levels between 5 to 15 (Badger and Jones, 1990). Deaf children in each group knew significantly fewer body parts than the hearing children.

## Body Image and Abuse

The relationship between affect and cognition in maltreated infants, the quality of attachment and the development of visual self-recognition indicates that children as young as 19 months who evidenced visual self-recognition were significantly more likely to be more securely attached to their mothers (Schneider-Rosen and Cicchetti, 1984).

Hibbard and Hartman (1990) studied emotional indicators in human figure drawings of sexually victimized and non-abused children. The total number of emotional indicators did not differ significantly but the sexual abuse victims tended to draw some indicators more often, e.g. legs pressed together, big hands, and genitals. Drawings made by sexually abused children attending a child psychology clinic (Rivlin 1993b) often showed enlarged penile and genital areas of both the victim and the abuser. The genitals and hands are given specific significance as in Figs 3 and 4 drawn by 6- and 9-year-olds, respectively. Such drawings indicate precocious sexual knowledge and distortion of body image. The extreme distress may be clearly viewed for both victims.

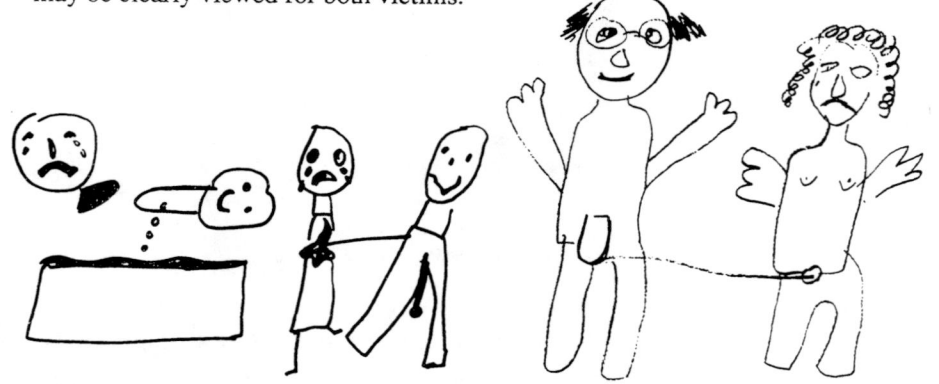

FIGS. 3 and 4.

Rape can also produce distorted drawings of body image. Figure 5 shows a 12-year-old girl raped by her mother's lover and how she feels towards him. Notice the distortion in the size of body. The girl while much smaller in real life than her rapist, draws herself in a powerful, dominating position with a phallic-shaped gun firing at her rapist who is drawn smaller than herself with very large hands.

What are the indicators of emotional abuse in children regarding body image? Children have been seen to draw their bodies isolated away from other members of the family, or often with the care-giver's back turned away from the child. The example below (Fig. 6) indicates drawings based on those of a grossly emotionally abused boy of borderline intelligence who was deserted by both his parents at 5 years old and seen in the clinic when aged 12. When requested to draw his parents from memory he indicated his father's teeth veering between menace and happiness. The child was unattached emotionally with some psychopathic personality features focused on cruelty to animals.

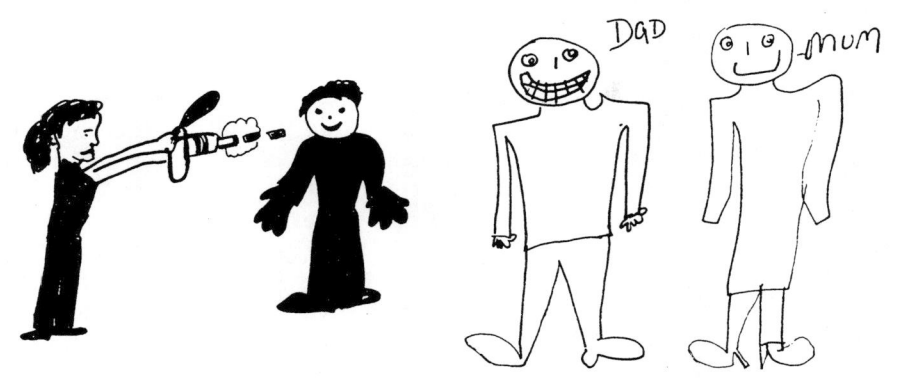

FIGS 5 and 6.

**Body Image and Illness**

Children and adolescents afflicted with chronic and life-threatening illness have frequently to grapple with issues involving treatment which may be disfiguring (chemotherapy with ensuing hair loss). Increased levels of control over themselves and their environment have been shown to have beneficial effects on body image development (Tull and Goldberg, 1984).

Human figure drawings by children with malignancies examined by the Goodenough-Harris Drawing test were significantly smaller in height, width and area than were the drawings of school children and general surgical patients. The test scores were also significantly lower than those of both the other groups. Paine et al. (1985) hypothesize that anxiety, lowered self-esteem and the effects of chemotherapy contributed to such findings.

Gordon et al. (1980) employed the Draw-A-Person test for investigating depressive symptoms in 166 boys and 182 girls. Depression was assessed by three independent methods: peer nominations, self-rating and teacher assessments. A significant negative relationship was obtained between size of figure drawn and teacher-rated depression. In another study, Robins et al. (1991) examined change in human figure drawing during the course of intensive treatment of seriously disturbed young adults finding that the drawings improved significantly with the course of treatment.

**Disfigurement**

For infants afflicted with visible disfigurement the child may not only react himself with anxiety but also evoke sadness and rejection in his carers. Droater et al. (1975) and Fajardo (1987) describe a muting of the child's environment evoked by his disfigurement. It was observed that the child's concept of self is influenced by the values the child evolves and connects in his/her mental world (Kagan, 1984) and that the mothers of disfigured infants cuddled and stimulated their children less than mothers of normal children (Rogers-Salyer et al., 1985).

Children at 5 years of age are at a critical stage in the development of attractiveness, discriminations and stereotyping. The unattractive child experiences negative and rejecting peer relations, which in turn lead to the perception of maladjustment by teachers and other peers and the belief of a lessened learning capacity. The child's development in such an interactional climate may foster the emergence of the very behaviours and characteristics expected by the unattractive child's "socializing other" (Lerner and Lerner, 1977; Rivlin, 1986).

The role of facial appearance in popularity, dating and marriage, persuasion politics and employment prospects has further been delineated by Bull and Rumsey (1988); as Harrison (1985) observed, "a body defect can affect self esteem directly, by causing negative feedback about appearance, and indirectly, by interfering with the developmental process... Children will focus on a physical attribute as the organizing factor for feelings of defectiveness."

The social consequences of deformity such as cleft lip and cranio-facial malformations, e.g. Cruzon's syndrome, are different at various ages also for gender. Deformity and disfigurement that are corrected surgically in early childhood may have a different social/psychological impact on the individual whose deformity or disfigurement cannot be improved until mid-adolescence or older. Many people suffering from cranio-facial deformity are stigmatized by others who label them as mentally retarded or odd. They are further isolated by the fact that their condition is rare, and potential support from those with the same condition is thus absent.

Social deficits with cranio-facial malformations (Pertschuk and Whitaker, 1988), with cleft palate patients (Peter et al., 1975a,b) and with burned patients (Rivlin, 1992) may persist or even increase as adolescence approaches and there are long term difficulties for all such patients with regard to friendship and marriage. The burned child who is injured by trauma or disfigured by operative procedures suffers the excruciating sadness of acquired disability. Not surprisingly, the child's estimates of scarring are significantly higher than both their mother's and the surgeon's estimate of scarring (Rivlin, 1993).

Figure 7 indicates a child presently aged 11 who suffered delay in treatment which led to deformation of the femoral head and dislocation of the hip. She drew one leg longer than the other and then told the examiner that she had made a mistake there. (Note the rejection of both legs coloured in black and her pronounced operation scar).

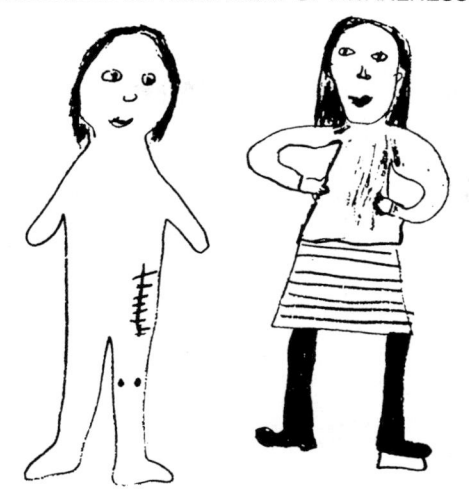

FIG. 7.

Figures 8 and 9 show the drawings of burned victims and their own self-image. Their distress is clear and one adolescent is screaming. Figures 10 and 11 indicate the traumatic disfigurement of two adolescent road traffic accident victims.

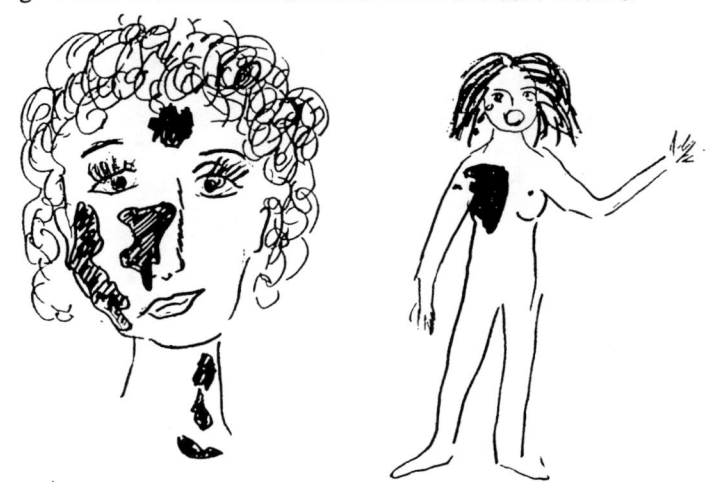

FIGS 8 and 9.

The self-image is a complex phenomenon; Douvan and Adelson (1966) wrote "the normal adolescent holds, we think, two conceptions of himself. What he is and what he will be or the way in which he integrates the future image into his current life will indicate a good deal about his current adolescent integration". The self concept is not only what an individual designs himself or herself from the view of others, but is also reflective in that it is learned from the reactions of others through role taking (Miller, 1963).

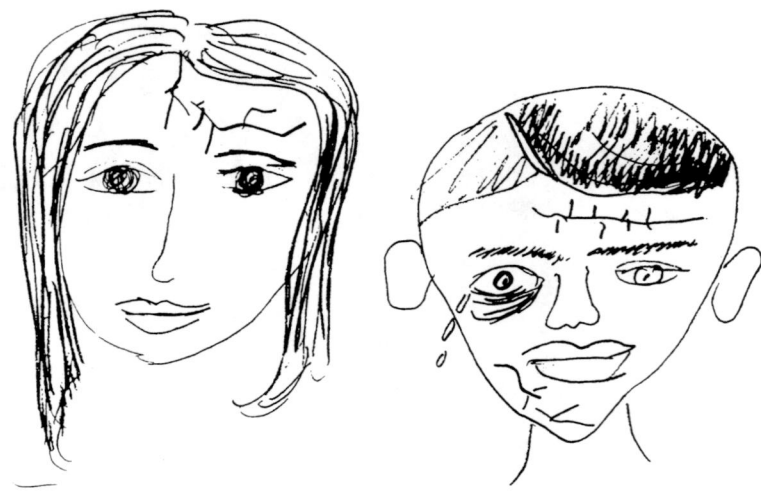

FIGS 10 and 11.

In formalizing the notions of a reflective self, Kinch (1963) specified the three components of self concept: an individual's self concept, his perception of the response of others towards him, and the actual responses of others towards him; or as stated by Miller (1963) "self-esteem", "subject public esteem", and "objective public esteem". Gordon (1966) observed that, as the child grows, different parts of him will become more important to him and different parts of his world will assume changing significance. Even a minor physical defect can be as damaging to a person's self-esteem as a major one (Macgregor *et al.*, 1953).

## Conclusions

Childhood development of awareness of self is a questing field for future research. We are still on the boundaries of discovering how a child views his persona, body image and the outside world. Developmentally, psychologically and neurologically progress has been made in describing possible mechanisms of how a child's cortex interprets reality. Yet this is only a beginning to understanding the uniqueness of childhood individual interpretation of reality.

Many uncomfortable and challenging questions remain. How do we cope with differences in others? Is our cortex programmed in such a way as to reject uniqueness, disfigurement, individual differences? To what extent are children influenced adversely by the stereotyping of the so-called cultural ideal? Are we so fettered by our own anxiety and conformity for "normality" that we do not strive creatively to engage with and discover the unusual, the unique self present in others?

Children afflicted with either congenital or acquired disfigurement and/or handicap are vulnerable and forced by society to carve for themselves an inner boundary of safety. Daily, such children and adolescents are deprived of their own privacy by revealing to the world the inner pain reflected from their scars or deformity. Other young people are shamed by their appalling abusive life experiences.

It is only by further developing thorough assessment procedures to predict areas of probable difficulty, by developing effective intervention strategies not only with the individual child, but also with his family, and by educating the public that children and young people, afflicted by the invisible wounds of psychological trauma and external mutilation from congenital and acquired disfigurement/deformity, may actualize themselves.

**References**

Amann-Gainotti, M. and Antenore, C. (1990). Development of internal body image from childhood to early adolescence. *Journal of Perceptual and Motor Skills*, 7, (2) 387-393.

Amann-Gainotti, M., Di-Prospero, B. and Nenci, A.M. (1989). Adolescent girls' representations of their genital inner space. *Adolescence*, 24, (94) 473-480.

Badger, T.A. and Jones, E. (1990). Deaf and hearing children's conceptions of the body interior. *Paediatric Nursing*, 16, (2) 201-205.

Bakkar, D.J. (1970). Temporal order perception and reading retardation. *In* "Specific Reading Disability. Advances in Theory and Method". (Eds D.J. Bakkar and P. Satz). pp. 81-98. Rotterdam University Press, Rotterdam.

Balint, M. (1968). "The Basic Fault". Tavistock Publications, London.

Bauman, M. and Kemper, T.L. (1985). Histoanatomic observation of the brain in early infantile autism. *Neurology*, 35, 866-874.

Beaumanoir, A. (1985). The Landau-Klefner syndrome *In* "Epileptic Syndromes in Infancy, Childhood and Adolescence". (Eds J. Roger, C. Dravet, M. Bureau, F.E. Dreifuss and P. Wolff). pp. 181-192. John Libbey Eurotext, Paris.

Benton, A. (1985). Body schema disturbances: Finger agnosia and right-left disorientation. *In* "Clinical Neuropsychology". (Eds K.M. Heilman and E. Valenstein). pp. 115-129.

Berges, J. and Lezine, I. (1972). Test d'imitation de gestes. Techniques d'exploration du schema corporel et des praxies chez l'enfants de 3 à 6 ans. Masson, Paris.

Blatt, S. (1974). Levels of object representation in analytic and intrajective depression. *Psychiatric Study of the Child*, 29, 107-157.

Brittain, W.L. and Chien, Y.I. (1983). Relationship between preschool children's ability to name body parts and their ability to construct a man. *Perceptual and Motor Skills*, 57, (1) 19-24.

Bruner, J.S. (1978). Learning how to do things with words. *In* "Human Growth and Development". (Eds J. Bruner and A. Garton). Clarendon Press, Oxford.

Bull, R. and Rumsey, N. (1988). "The Social Psychology of Facial Appearance". Springer, New York.

Cash, T.F., Winstead, B.A. and Janda, J.H. (1986). The great American shape-up. *Psychology Today*, 20, 30-37.

Cates, J.A. (1991). "Comparison of Human Figure Drawings by Hearing and Hearing-Impaired Children". *Indiana U-Purdue U, Doctoral Rehabilitation Psychology Programme, Indianapolis, USA.* 93, (1) 31-39.

Cavior, N. and Dokecki, P.R. (1973). Physical attractiveness, perceived attitude similarity, and academic achievement as contributors to interpersonal attraction among adolescents. *Developmental Psychology*, **9**, 44-54.

Clapp, R.K. (1972). The body schema of normal and mentally retarded children. *Journal of Psychology*, **80**, (1) 37-44.

Cohen, L.S. (1985). Developmental changes in right-hemisphere involvement in face recognition. *In* "Hemispheric Function and Collaboration in the Child". (Ed. C.T. Best), pp. 157-192. Academic Press, Orlando.

Cole, D. and LaVoie, J.C. (1985). Fantasy play and related cognitive development in 2-6 years olds. *Developmental Psychology*, **21**, 233-240.

Cooley, C.H. (1902). "Human Nature and the Social Order". Charles Scribner & Sons, New York.

De Ajuriaguerra, J. and Stucki, J.D. (1975). Developmental disorders of the body schema. *In* "Handbook of Clinical Neurology". Vol. 4, (Eds P.J. Vinken and G.W. Bruyn). pp. 392-406. North Holland, Amsterdam.

Douvan, E. and Adelson, J. (1966). "The Adolescent Experience". John Wiley, New York.

Drotar, D., Baskiewicz, A., Irvin, N., Kennell, J. and Klaus, M. (1975). The adaptation of parents to the birth of an infant with a congenital malformation: a hypothetical model. *Paediatrics*, **56**, 710-717.

Duncan, P.D. et al. (1985). The effects of pubertal timing on body image, school behaviour and deviance. Special Issue: Time of maturation and psychosocial functioning in adolescence: I. *Journal of Youth and Adolescence*, **14**, (3) 227-235.

Emde, R.N. (1983). The pre-representational self. *Psychoanalytic Study of the Child*, **38**, 165-192.

Erikson, E.H. (1950). "Childhood and Society". Norton, New York.

Erikson, E.H. (1959). "Identity and the Life Cycle". International Universities Press, New York.

Fajardo, B. (1987). Parenting the damaged child: Mourning, regression and disappointment. *The Psychoanalytic Review*, **74**, 19-43.

Feiner, K. (1987). Development of the concept of anatomical constency: 1. *Psychoanalytic-Psychology*, **4**, (4) 343-354.

Fisher, S. (1986). "Development and Structure of the Body Image". Vol. 2. Erlbaum, New Jersey.

Frazier, A. and Lisonbee, L.K. (1950). Adolescent concerns with physique. *School Review*, **58**, 397-405.

Freud, S. (1920). "Beyond the Pleasure Principle". Standard Edition 18. Hogarth Press, London.

Freud, S. (1923). "The Ego and the Id". Standard Edition 19. Hogarth Press, London.

Freud, S. (1926). "Inhibitions, Symptoms and Anxiety". Standard Edition 20. Hogarth Press, London.

Fujimoto, K. (1979). Developmental study on the drawings of the human figure in motion. *Japanese Journal of Educational Psychology*, **27**, (4) 245-252.

Gallino, T.G. (1991). Bambini "Con o Senza" Compagno Immaginario. Una Indagine. Imaginary Friend: Their creative and social abilities. *Eta-Evolutiva*, **39**, 33-44.

Giljohann, A. (1979). Adolescents burned as children. *Burns*, **7**, (2) 95-99.

Glaun, D. and Rosenthal, D. (1987). Development of children's concepts about the interior of the body. *Psychother-psychosom*, **48**, (1-4) 63-67.

Goffman, E. (1963). "Stigma, Notes on the Management of Spoiled Identity". Prentice-Hall,

Englewood Cliffs, New Jeresy.
Gordan, N., Lefkowitz, M.M. and Tesiny, E.P. (1980). Childhood depression and the Draw-A-Person Test. *Psychological Reports,* **47**, (1) 251-257.
Gordon, I.J. (1966). "Studying the Child in School". John Wiley, New York.
Hardyment, C. (1984). "Arthur Ransome and Captain Flint's Trunk". p.100. Jonathan Cape, London.
Harrison, A. (Eds). (1985). Body image and self-esteem. *In* "The Development and Sustenance of Self-esteem". (Eds J. Mack and M. Abalon). pp. 90-183. International University Press, New York.
Hibbard, R.A. and Hartman, G.L. (1990). Emotional indicators in human figure drawings of sexually victimized and non-abused children. *Journal of Clinical Psychology.*
Hill, S.D. and Tomlin, C. (1981). Self recognition in retarded children. *Child Development,* **52**, (1) 145-50.
Horowitz, M. (1983). "Image Formation and Psychotherapy". Aronson, New York.
Kagan, J. (1984). "The Nature of the Child". Basic Books, New York.
Kagan, J. and Moss, H. (1962). "Birth to Maturity". Wiley, New York.
Kernberg, O. (1975). "Borderline Conditions and Pathological Narcissism". Aronson, New York.
Kinch, J.W. (1963). A formalized theory of the self concept. *American Journal of Sociology,* **68**, 481-586.
Kirk, U. (1985). Hemispheric contributions to the development of graphic skill. *In* "Hemispheric Function and Collaboration in the Child". (Ed. C.T. Best). pp. 193-228. Academic Press, New York.
Krueger, D.W. (1990). Developmental and psychodynamic perspectives on body image change. Chapter 12. *In* "Body Images Development, Deviance and Change". (Eds T.S. Cash and T. Pruzinsky). pp. 256. The Guilford Press, New York.
Lerner, R.M. (1986). "Concepts and Theories of Human Development". 2nd Edn. Random House, New York.
Lerner, R.M. and Kauffmann, M.B. (1985). The concept of development in contextualism. *Development Review,* **5**, 309-333.
Lerner, R.M. and Lerner, J.V. (1977). The effects of age, sex and physical attractiveness on child-peer relations, academic performance and elementary school adjustment. *Developmental Psychology,* **13**, 585-590.
Lerner, R.M. and Lerner, J.V. (1987). Children in their contexts: A goodness of fit model. *In* "Parenting the Life Span: Biosocial Dimensions". (Eds J.B. Lancaster, J. Altmann, A.S. Rossi and L.R. Sherrod). pp. 377-404. Aldine, Chicago.
Luria, A.R. (1966). "Higher Cortical Functions in Man". Tavistock Publications, London.
MacGregor, F.C., Abel, T.M., Bryt, A. and Lauer, E. (1953). Facial deformities and plastic surgery. *In* "A Psychosocial Study". Springfield, Illinois.
Machtiger, H.G. (1985). Perilous beginnings: loss, abandonment and transformation. *Chiron,* 101-129.
Mahler, M.S. (1968). "On Human Symbiosis and the Vicissitudes of Individualism". International Universities Press, New York.
Mahler, M.S., Pine, S. and Bergman, A. (1975). "The Psychological Birth of the Infant". Hutchinson, London.
Maurin, C., Mennesson, J.F., Aussillouz, Ch. and Visier, J.P. (1980). Etude du schema corporel sur une population d'enfants psychologiquement perturbés. (A body image test in a population of children suffering from psychological disturbances). *Revue de*

*Psychologie Appliquée,* **30,** (4) 273-292.
Mead, G.H. (1934). "Mind, Self, and Society". University of Chicago Press, Chicago.
Miller, D.R. (1963). The study of social relationships: situation identity and social interaction. *In* "Psychology: A Study of a Science". Vol. 5. (Ed. S. Cotch). pp. 639-737. McGraw-Hill, New York.
Minuchin, P. (1977). "The Middle Years of Childhood". Brooks/Cole, Palo Alto.
Modaressi, T. and Kinney, T. (1977). Children's response to their true and distorted mirror images. *Child Psychiatry and Human Development,* **8,** 94-101.
Newson, J. (1978). Dialogue and development. *In* "Action, Symbol and Gesture". (Ed. A. Lock). pp 31-42. Academic Press, London and New York.
Nicholich, L. (1977). Beyond sensory motor intelligence: Assessment of symbolic maturity through analysis of pretend play. *Merrill-Palmer Quarterly,* **28,** 89-99.
Njiokiktjien, C. (1988). "Paediatric Behavioural Neurology". Suyi Publicaties. Amsterdam.
Paine, P., Alves, E. and Tubino, P. (1985). Size of human figure drawing and Goodenough-Harris scores of paediatric oncology patients: a pilot study. *Perceptual and Motor Skills,* **60,** (3) 911-914.
Pertschuk, M.J., Trisdorfer, A. and Whitaker, L.A. (1989). Longterm Follow-up of Cranio-Facial Surgery in Early Childhood. Paper presented at the American Cleft Palate Association Meetings, San Francisco.
Peter, J.P., Chinsky, R.R. and Fisher, M.J. (1975a). Sociological aspects of cleft palate adults: III. Vocational and economic aspects. *Cleft Palate Journal,* **12,** 193-199.
Peter, J.P. Chinsky, R.R. and Fisher, M.J. (1975b). Sociological aspects of cleft palate adults IV. Social integration. *Cleft Palate Journal,* **12,** 304-310.
Piaget, J. (1950). "The Psychology of Intelligence". Harcourt Brace, New York.
Piaget, J. (1951). "Play, Dreams and Imitation in Childhood". (Transl. C. Gattegno and F.M. Hodgson). Norton, New York.
Piaget, J. (1970). Piaget's theory. *In* "Carmichael's Manual of Child Psychology". Vol. 1. (Ed. P.H. Mussen). pp. 703-732. Wiley, New York.
Poeck, K. and Orgass, B. (1964). Ueber die Entwicklung des Korperschemas. Untersuchung an gesunden blinden und ampurierten Kindem. *Fortschritte der Neurologie und Psychiatrie,* **32,** 538-555.
Poeck, K. and Orgass, B. (1969). An experimental investigation of finger agnosia. *Neurology,* **19,** 801-807.
Rivlin, E. (1985). The Psychological Sequelae and Management of Severe Burns in Children and Families. Paper given to the Association of Child Psychology and Psychiatry, London, November 1985.
Rivlin, E. (1986). The psychological sequelae and management of severely burned children and their families. *Proceedings of the Annual Conference of the British Psychological Society.*
Rivlin, E. (1988). The psychological trauma and management of severe burns in children and adolescents. *British Journal of Hospital Medicine,* **40,** September 1988.
Rivlin, E. (1992). The psychological trauma, sequelae, and management of severe burns in children, adolescents and their families. *International Review of the Armed Forces Medical Services Quarterly,* **15,** September, pp 221.227.
Rivlin, E. (1993a). In process of submission for publication: "Self Esteem and Body Image in Severely Burned Adolescents".
Rivlin, E. (1993b). Unpublished paper: "Traumatized Children and their Drawings".
Robins, C.E., Blatt, S.J. and Ford, R.Q. (1991). Changes in human figure drawings during

intensive treatment. *Journal of Personality Assessment,* **57**, (3) 477-497.

Robinson, R.O., Lippold, T. and Land, R. (1986). Body schema: does it depend on bodily-deprived sensations? *Developmental Medicine in Child Neurology,* **28**, 49-52.

Rogers-Salyer, M.A. Jensen, A.G. and Borden, C. (1985). Effects of facial deformities and physical attractiveness on mother-infant bonding. *In* "Craniofacial Surgery, Proceedings of the First International Congress of the International Society of Cranio-Maxillo-Facial Surgery". (Ed. D. Marchac). Springer-Verlag, New York.

Sander, L. (1980). Panel Report. New knowledge about the infant from current research: implications for psychoanalysis. *American Journal of Psychoanalysis,* **28**, 181-198.

Schneider, R.K. and Cicchetti, D. (1984). The relationship between affect and cognition in maltreated infants: quality of attachment and the development of visual self-recognition. *Child Development,* **55**, 648-658.

Shapiro, T. and Perry, R. (1976). Latency revisited: the age 7+ or -1. *Psychoanalatical Study of Children,* **3**, 79-105.

Somers, J.U. and Yawkey, T.D. (1984). Imaginary play companions: Contributions of creative and intellectual abilities of young children. *Journal of Creative Behaviour,* **18**, (2) 77-89.

Spitz, R. (1957). "No and Yes". International Universities Press, New York.

Spitz, R. (1965). "The First Year of Life". International Universities Press, New York.

Stern, D. (1977). "The First Relationship: Infant and Mother". Fontana, London.

Stoit, A.M.B. (1986). Do onwikkeling van de herkenning van emoties in Het Gelaat, de lateralisatie en de interhemisfere uitwisseling ervan. "Scriptie Vakgrope Psychonomie". University of Amsterdam.

Thomas, A. and Chess, S. (1977). "Temperament and Development". Brunner/Mazel, New York.

Tizard, B. and Harvey, D. (1977). Biology of play. "Clinics in Developmental Medicine". no 62. Heineman, London and Lippincott, Philadelphia.

Trevarthen, C. (1979). Communication and co-operation in early infancy: A description of primary intersubjectivity. *In* "Before Speech". (Ed. M. Bullowa). pp. 321-347. Cambridge University Press, Cambridge.

Tull, R.M. and Goldberg, R.J. (1984). Life-threatening illness in youth. *Family Therapy Collections,* **8**, 73-81.

Weller, M. and Wiedemann, P. (1989). Visual hallucinations. An outline of etiological and pathogenetic concepts. *Journal of International Ophthalmology.*

Winnicott, D.W. (1957). "The Child and the Family". Tavistock Publications, London.

Winnicott, D.W. (1958). "Collected Papers: Through Paediatrics to Psychoanalysis". Tavistock Publications, London.

Winnicott, D.W. (1965). "The Maturational Process and the Facilitating Environment". Hogarth Press, London.

Witt, A., Cermak, S. and Coster, W. (1990). Body part identification in 1 to 2 year-old children. *American Journal of Occupational Therapy.* **44**, (2) 147-153.

Wolff, P.H. (1960). The developmental psychologies of Jean Piaget and psychoanalysis. "Psychological Issues". Vol II, 1. Monograph 5. IUP, New York.

# 23. Psychological correlates of disordered body image

T.M. Reilly

---

> Physical beauty is the sign of an interior beauty,
> a spiritual and moral beauty which is the basis,
> the principle and the unity of the beautiful.
> *Schiller. (Essays Esthetical and Philosphical: Introduction.)*

> A man's body and his mind, with the utmost
> reverence to both I speak it, are
> exactly like a jerkin and a jerkin's lining; –
> rumple the one, – you rumple the other.
> *Sterne. (Tristram Shandy, Book 111, Chapter 4).*

The experiential awareness of self would seen to be a fairly straightforward human function to explain and understand. After all, *cogito ergo sum* was sufficient for Descartes; "I am who am" provoked no demand for further elucidation when uttered by Clint Eastwood's menacing *alter ego* "The Man With No Name". Alas – or perhaps it should be "hoorah" – the reality is considerably more complex, with the influence of many disparate, self-directed factors, perceptual, cognitive and affective, coalescing into what is for many of us a rather fragile amalgam, of which physical self-awareness is but one component part.

It would be misleading to fail to acknowledge that a separate dimension of human existence – all that which is encompassed by the psychological, spiritual, noetic domains – makes a unique, yet complementary, contribution to sensory awareness in all its facets. The Atomist proposition that brain and mind are wholly separate entities is surely unconvincing in its simplest form, and a Gestaltist view, which regards each of these entities as possessing its own separate reality while being confluent for perceptual (and other) purposes into an interdependent functional dyad in which the instrumental whole is greater than the sum of its two constituent parts, is surely more appealing to a balanced exegesis and closer to the philosophical standpoint of this volume's editor.

Physical self-awareness loosely approximates to the term "body image", despite the desirability of distinguishing conceptually between "body image" and related notions such as "body schema", "body experience", "body concept", and so on (Cumming, 1988), not to mention the even trickier "external perception", "inner perception" and "self perception" (Scheler, 1966). Although "psychological correlates of disordered body image" may more or less embrace, albeit overinclusively, the content of this chapter, each section will touch upon a different psychological aspect of physical self-awareness in the context of three quite different psychiatric disorders. The first section will address disorders of part body image as opposed to total body image: that aspect of body image which has been referred to by some writers, particularly those assuming a psychoanalytical perspective, as "organ image" (Fenichel, 1946). This will be undertaken in the context of exploring the psychiatric syndrome "body dysmorphic disorder". The second section will examine disturbances of physical self-awareness which may occur in association with the eating disorders anorexia nervosa and bulimia nervosa. The third section will visit the strange world of transsexualism.

## Body Dysmorphic Disorder ("Dysmorphophobia")

*The absence of flaw in beauty is itself a flaw.*
*Havelock Ellis. (Impressions and Comments. Series 1, p.217.)*

*There is no excellent beauty that hath not some strangeness in the proportion.*
*Francis Bacon. (Essays: Of Beauty.)*

Despite these wise words the syndrome of the "ugliness worrier" (Jahrreiss, 1930) has been familiar to psychiatrists for many years. The term dysmorphophobia was elaborated in 1886 by the Italian neuropsychiatrist Morselli to describe a particular pattern of presentation of psychiatric disorder in which the patient insisted erroneously that some aspect of his facial appearance was disfigured or misshapen, with associated emotional distress. The original Italian spelling of the word – *dismorfofobia* – reflected its Greek origin in the tales of Herodotus, wherein the term "dismorfia", or facial ugliness, was used to describe "the ugliest girl in Sparta". Unfortunately, "dysmorphophobia" is a phenomenological misnomer, since the psychopathogical basis of the disorder is not a true phobia, or irrational *fear*, of ugliness, but a false *belief* that one's physical attractiveness is already marred by deformity or disproportion. The essence of the disorder as now defined is an exaggerated cognitive awareness of some aspect of bodily appearance, commonly though not necessarily facial, which is adjudged to be abnormal in some fashion, to a degree which evokes significant emotional distress. Usually there is no discernible abnormality to the objective eye, but in a few individuals some minor flaw or blemish may be detected. Any such disproportion which may exist, however, lies not so much in the "offending" bodily feature but rather in the excessive psychological reaction to the "imperfection".

Birtchnell (1988) has suggested that the quality of complaint, too, may suggest the presence of this disorder, with many of her patients being vague and imprecise in their description of subjective abnormality. She quotes the comment: "the skin under my eyes joins my nose in a funny way", juxtaposing for the sake of contrast a supposedly more "normal" presentation of awareness of facial abnormality: "the tip of my nose is rather bulbous". This feature is inconstant. The actual complaints made, and the organs or part-organs identified as the seat of abnormality, vary considerably from person to person. Dermatologists see many more such patients than do psychiatrists (Cotterill, 1981). This is partly because sufferers infrequently regard themselves as mistaken in their belief and they choose to consult a physician whose expertise would seem logically relevant to their perceived need for remedy. It is also partly because the skin – the largest single "organ" of the body – is the site of the majority of these false beliefs. This is hardly surprising given that the skin serves, both in a concrete and symbolic sense, as a boundary separating the inner person from the outer world, what is self from what is non-self. It is richly supplied with afferent sensory nerves and functions, therefore, as an important contributor to the perceptual databank which we continually access in order to construe, maintain or revise our cognitive elaboration of peripheral body image. Specific complaints commonly presented (Cotterill, 1981; Sneddon, 1971) include wrinkles; spots; moles; areas of pale, reddened or swollen skin; excessive hair, thinning hair or abnormal hair distribution; rashes; burning or itching patches; or some completely idiosyncratic focus of concern, perhaps akin to Birtchnell's previously quoted example. After the face, the most common sites of complaint are the breasts (too large, too small, misshapen or unequal in size); the scalp (redness, burning or excessive hair loss); and the perineum, in both sexes (burning, lumpiness, pain, misformed or undersized genitalia).

Plastic or cosmetic surgeons often encounter patients presenting with subjective physical (often facial) abnormality (Reich, 1969). The nose is the commonest site of complaint. Cosmetic surgeons have learned to be wary of operating on objectively absent or trivial defects associated with disproportionate subjective distress. Connolly and Gipson (1978) reported on two groups of patients 15 years following surgical nasal reconstruction. Of 101 who were operated upon because of disease or injury, nine had developed severe neurotic difficulties and one schizophrenia. Of 86 operated upon for cosmetic reasons, at their own request, 32 had become severely neurotic and six schizophrenic. This would appear to suggest (a) that "nose-type" dysmorphophobia – and by implication other forms of body dysmorphic disorder – carry an ominous long-term prognosis; and (b) that surgical intervention does not constitute a panacea for psychologically determined difficulties. Nevertheless, Hay and Heather (1973) followed up a smaller group of 17 patients two years after self-requested cosmetic rhinoplasty and found that 13 individuals were "satisfied in every way" with the outcome. Psychological test results were less straightforward to interpret, but seemed principally to reveal significant changes in measurements of "hostility".

Those who suffer from body dysmorphic disorder, whatever its specific content, are usually distressed by their abnormally perceived physical aspect. They assume that others, too, will share their considerable distaste for their flawed appearance, and are excessively self-conscious. Repeated mirror checking is a common feature and may almost have a compulsive quality. Reclusiveness and social avoidance often ensue. Frank depression frequently develops. "Doctor shopping" becomes the most prominent activity for many, while others spend hours each day in microscopic self-scrutiny. Hollander and colleagues (1989) described a lady who spent up to eight hours each day trimming her hair in an attempt to achieve symmetry.

Despite the bizarre nature of the disorder, its psychological meaning must be addressed in the context of wider social values. In many cultures physical attractiveness is an especially prized human attribute, and Dion and colleagues (1972) have described the "halo effect" whereby the external perception of beauty in an individual may positively influence overall evaluation of the person. The phrase "what is beautiful is good" has been attributed to many classical sources including Sappho and Plato. The facial beauty of Helen of Troy was sufficiently potent "to launch a thousand ships". Comedians have paraphrased this statement to refer to unattractive people as having "the face that launched a thousand quips"! The many schoolchildren who have been the butt of cruel teasing because of some unusual facial feature – for example, prominent teeth, strabismus, "Prince Charles ears" – painfully recognize this reality. Yet many "normal" individuals with no unusual physical attributes are also dissatisfied with some aspect of their appearance – 70% in one study of college students (Fitts *et al.*, 1989). After all, which one of us can honestly say that we would not prefer to be six inches taller, to have a "stronger" chin, a fuller bust, or some other conventionally attractive physical quality?

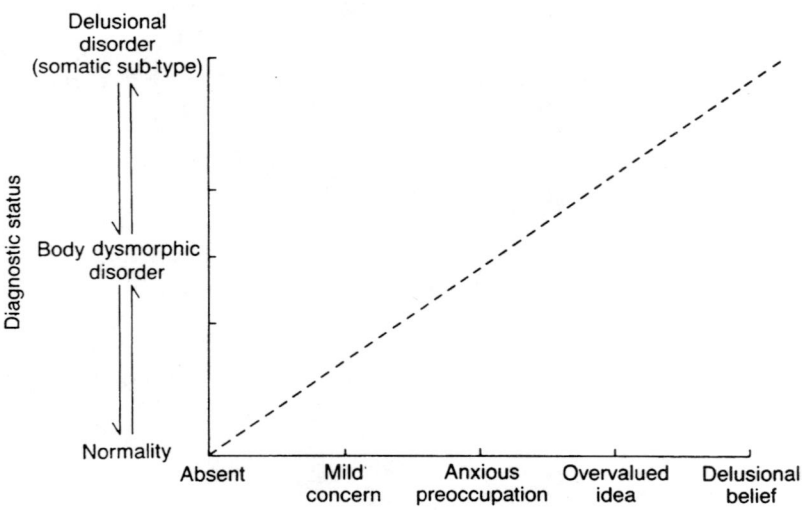

FIG. 1. Degree of conviction.

Patients suffering from body dysmorphic disorder do not present a static pattern of complaint. The intensity of conviction can vary at times. Emotional factors, particularly affective factors, and situational factors (for example, "quality of life" parameters) are probably only the most obvious influences. Given this fluctuating degree of conviction, many patients will at different times in their illness history manifest a fading of intensity to an anxious preoccupation, or an intensification of conviction bordering on the delusional. A separate category exists in DSM-III-R for those dysmorphic syndromes which are fully delusional. Figure 1 comprises a representational scheme of the resulting spectrum.

Psychodynamic explanations of dysmorphic symptomatology are, predictably, varied. Many theories focus upon the presumed symbolic significance of the incriminated organ or part-organ. For example when the nose is "targeted" by a male, this is often viewed as being symbolic of dissatisfaction with his phallus, and, by inference, represents a lack of confidence in his overall masculine adequacy. Similarly, a woman's request for breast enlargement is taken to indicate deeper feelings of maternal and/or sexual inadequacy; a request for reduction mammaplasty to represent a wish to retreat from the demands and responsibilities of adult sexuality. It may be more helpful to recognize in these individuals an incompletely developed sense of self-worth and consequent diffidence in interpersonal relationships which undermines their secure sense of adult adequacy. Many problematical personality traits have been identified in these individuals with sensitive, narcissistic and schizoid (introverted and withdrawn) features varying in significance from person to person. Obsessional traits are seldom absent. This characteristic may explain the persistence of the disorder over time; the repetitive almost compulsive quality of many of the associated behaviours; and the stubborn resistance to change often encountered in therapeutic transactions. With other abnormal traits it may partly explain, too, why the normal, though usually transitory, psychological phenomenon "attentional augmentation" (Reilly, 1984) may become enduring in sufferers from body dysmorphic disorder. The phenomenon of attentional augmentation is most simply explained by asking the reader to recall stubbing his toe in the bedroom, or hitting his thumb with a hammer. The assaulted "part organ" sends to the brain, through its afferent nerve supply, powerful messages of pain, heat and pressure which demand the conscious attention of the organism as a whole. For a limited time awareness of the injured part dominates the sensorium and it actually feels much larger than it really is, even allowing for traumatic swelling. In body dysmorphic disorder an analogous mechanism may be operative, perhaps because some minor flaw permits selection of the part as the "affective scapegoat", becoming the seat of powerful negative emotions which then demand disproportionate conscious attention. Since the ego-defence mechanism of displacement is a continuing process, the augmented demand for attention from the "offending" part is not self-limiting and its persistence over time is further guaranteed by the existence of obsessional, and other, personality traits. Fluctuating intensity over time may be explained largely by the occurrence of spontaneous mood changes or external life happenings. When the sufferer is feeling happier in himself, the power of negative emotions will temporarily subside rendering the "target organ" less demanding of central awareness. When a self-esteem reinforcing event occurs – for example, a promotion at work, a compliment, a successful date or meeting – a similar internal process temporarily ensues.

Treatment approaches to this spectral disorder include antipsychotic medication for the overtly delusional; antidepressant medication for frank depression; and psychotherapy, which will concentrate upon building self-esteem and may, depending upon ego strength, extend to an anamnestic exploration of childhood experiences. These latter may reveal evidence of inconsistent or inadequate parenting, often of a subtle nature, which contributed to an incompletely developed sense of value as a person for the child later to become a "dysmorphophobic" adult.

> What a strange illusion it is to suppose that beauty is goodness.
> Tolstoy. (The Kreutzer Sonata. Chapter 5)

### Anorexia Nervosa/Bulimia Nervosa

> A man must take the fat with the lean; that's what he must make up his mind to in this life.
> Dickens. (David Copperfield. Chapter 51)

These related eating disorders are now considered to be separate diagnostic entities in DSM-III-R, although there is a degree of overlap between the two. Anorexia nervosa – literally, nervous loss of appetite – is another terminological misnomer since appetite in this disorder is not reduced, and may often be intense. The principal psychopathological criterion of this disorder is a refusal on the part of the patient to maintain body weight over a minimally acceptable norm for her [the majority of patients is female] height and age; associated with an intense fear of gaining weight or becoming fat, even though underweight. Cessation of menstruation is also a diagnostic feature, due to the secondary effects of persistently low body weight on the hormonal function of the hypothalamo-pituitary axis. Many patients with anorexia nervosa will experience episodes of bulimia, or binge eating, often followed by vomiting.

When episodes of bingeing dominate the clinical picture, the diagnosis of bulimia nervosa is more appropriate, particularly if any weight loss which might occur does not surpass that which would be required to take them below the minimally acceptable norm. Furthermore, the periodic occurrence of weight reducing activities such as self-induced vomiting, use of laxatives or diuretics, strict dieting or fasting, or vigorous exercise also characterizes this disorder. Both anorexia nervosa and bulimia nervosa are approximately twenty times more common in females than males, and both disorders customarily begin in adolescence. Incidence figures are difficult to verify but perhaps 1% of the female population of Western countries may be affected at some point in their life. The occurrence of lesser forms of these disorders, or self-limiting one-off episodes, is probably very much commoner than even that figure. One other diagnostic criterion for both disorders has been loosely termed "disturbance of body image". Bruch (1962) suggested that patients with anorexia nervosa misperceived their body size leading to denial of excessive thinness. This early notion was interpreted in what might be seen to be a somewhat overliteral manner as a perceptual abnormality specific to patients with anorexia nervosa which leads them to overestimate their body size. Apparent confirmation came in 1973 when Slade and Russell asked a group of women to estimate the widths of various body parts using an apparatus consisting of two movable lights mounted on an horizontal bar. The anorexic women were much more likely to overestimate their body width (though not height) than the normal controls. Subsequent replication studies were unconvincing, however. Image distortion techniques employ adjustable photographs, mirrors or television pictures to measure total body size rather than part size. These whole body techniques have been even less consistent in demonstrating body size overestimation in anorexic women, with considerable individual variation in most studies (Hsu, 1982). It is, however, possible to determine a trend: anorexic patients are be more likely to overestimate their body size, with a small minority being highly abnormal in this respect (Whitehouse et al., 1988).

Slade (1988) now suggests that image distortion techniques may be measuring "a relatively fixed cognitive attitude to body size". In a minority of patients, this technique may reveal a clearly false belief of the type described by Bruch as delusional. These patients may constitute a sub-group (Reilly, 1977); they stand in the same relation to the larger, heterogeneous group of patients with anorexia nervosa as do patients manifesting delusional disorder, somatic sub-type to those suffering from body dysmorphic disorder. More subtle disturbances of body image in anorexia nervosa may be studied using size estimation techniques (for example, the movable caliper) which Slade (1985) suggests may measure "a fluid state of body size sensitivity, strongly influenced by affective/emotional factors and which is responsive to changes in both external and internal environment". Buvat and Buvat-Herbaut (1978) suggest that such abnormalities in anorexic populations constitute a form of "dysmorphophobia". Weight reduction in anorexia nervosa can be viewed as a way of rendering less conspicuous one, or more than one, body part which is thought to be disproportionately unattractive.

Extraneous aspects of the test environment, are now recognized to have a significant influence upon the results of experimental body image measurement (Cooper and Taylor, 1988). For example, the amount of lighting, the size of the adjustable image, the distance between subject and image, and the degree of distortion allowed by the particular equipment are only some of the variables to which subjective judgements are unexpectedly sensitive. Similarly, the "demand characteristics" of the test situation have been shown to influence the results of body size estimation (Proctor and Morley, 1986). Giving test instructions in four quite different ways significantly altered the resulting estimations in each case, both for anorexics and controls. Apart from demonstrating the intrinsic untrustworthiness of the measuring techniques employed, this study does tend to suggest that "ambiguous" instructions (open; non-directive) resulted in anorexics (though not controls) overestimating to a much greater extent than "confrontational" instructions ("you were wrong last time; try and be more accurate"). These findings suggest that anorexics in general find it more necessary than non-anorexics to "please" an external authority figure. Such a characteristic would be consonant with the hypothesis that eating and weight are felt by many anorexic adolescents to be the only areas of their life in which they can exert full self-control in the face of what they perceive to be a dominant critical maternal influence with oppressively high expectations of achievement and behaviour.

Such disturbances of body image as may exist in association with anorexia nervosa, however difficult consistently to demonstrate and define, are also often encountered in other populations. Normal controls (Hsu, 1982) and non-anorexic, psychiatrically disordered controls (Struber et al., 1979) also overestimate their body size, and similar findings have been reported for groups of obese (Glucksman and Hursch, 1969) and pregnant (Slade, 1987) women. Nylander (1971) reported that 53% of 20-year-old women feel themselves to be fat. Dolan and colleagues (1982) found that a group of 100 "normal" men and women using a visual size estimation apparatus consistently overestimated the width of chest, hips and waist by a factor varying from 15% to 24%. Body size overestimation is not, therefore, a particular defining characteristic of anorexia nervosa.

Findings for bulimia nervosa are similar, although rather more consistent. The trend towards overestimation is more marked. Cooper and Taylor (1988) reviewed eight previously published studies, using differing measurement technology, and reported that seven revealed a significant difference between bulimics and controls.

There remains some debate about the legitimacy of diagnostically separating anorexia nervosa and bulimia nervosa, since there is considerable overlap between the two disorders. It has been suggested that the level of psychopathological disturbance is greater in the latter, linked to the possibility that "successful" anorexics are more in control of both body weight and eating behaviour than normal weight bulimics, and feel less threatened by the possibility of loss of control and fantasized chaotic consequences. The opposing view is that the personality structure of the bulimic patient is disturbed in a more diffuse fashion. Lacey (1990), for example, has suggested that the type and degree of disturbance in bulimic patients identifies them with "multi-impulse" disordered individuals who may also abuse drugs or alcohol, gamble pathologically or steal compulsively.

It may be helpful to conceptualize a continuum of body image disturbance (Fig. 2) varying in degree from the relatively common concerns of normal populations through obese and anorexic populations to the severe perceptual distortions of patients suffering from bulimia nervosa and delusional dysmorphia (Schachter, 1971). Several studies now suggest that body size/shape dissatisfaction is a more consistent finding than body size overestimation in eating-disordered populations, and more relevant to an understanding of the psychopathological core of these disorders. Touyz and colleagues (1984) noted that the ideal body shape desired by the anorexic subjects was much thinner than that chosen by controls. Coker and Cooper (1991) generated an index of body size dissatisfaction (IBSD) based on the discrepancy between personal size estimation and desired size in a group of bulimic patients. The mean IBSD for controls was 14%; for patients, 42%. Several studies have revealed significantly higher scores for anorexics and bulimics than controls on the Body Dissatisfaction subscale of The Eating Disorder Inventory (Garner *et al.*, 1985) – a rating scale which assesses feelings concerning various body parts. In similar studies, utilizing the Body Shape Questionnaire, 84% of patients with bulimia nervosa expressed moderate or extreme dissatisfaction in contrast to 17% of the comparison group.

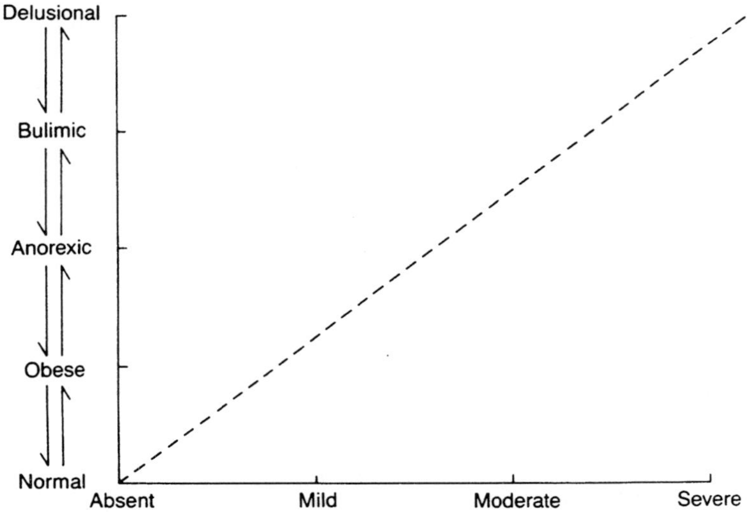

FIG. 2. Degree of body image disturbance.

We may have some clues as to the real nature of the disturbance of body image in eating-disordered populations. It is not primarily perceptual, but related much more to cognitive and affective factors. It has less to do with body size *per se* and more to do with body shape as a correlate of evaluative self-image. The association between indicators of depressed mood and body shape dissatisfaction (Cooper and Taylor, 1988) suggests that while concern over the possession of a socially desirable body shape is widespread throughout normal populations, some individuals, perhaps because of pre-existing personal or family overweight, or family conflicts centred on weight/eating issues related to loss of control, attribute an exaggerated importance to the maintenance of slimness and low body weight. When weight rises, even to the population norm, self-esteem declines, depression may follow, leading to generalized self-depreciation including body shape disparagement and a tendency, albeit less consistent, to overestimate body size.

## Transsexualism

> Come you spirits
> that tend on mortal thoughts! Unsex me here,
> And fill me from the crown to the toe top full
> of direst cruelty.
> Shakespeare. (Macbeth. Act I, Scene V)

One very specialized and specific aspect of self-awareness is gender identity: the belief/feeling (both cognitive and emotional components contribute) that one is a man or a woman. Subjective gender identity, of course, derives largely from the product of a variety of psychological influences operative within the self, but its consideration in relation to disorders of external body image is justified by the recognition that sexual and genital organs, and secondary sexual characteristics of the body, are also an essential determinant of assigned gender identity. It is conflict between these two different groups of determinants which underlies the presentation of gender dysphoria. It has been estimated that approximately 60 000 citizens of the USA are significantly gender dysphoric in this manner (Walker et al., 1985). Approximately 10% of this heterogeneous group are sufficiently seriously disturbed to meet the specific DSM-III-R criteria for the psychiatric disorder transsexualism.

Male transsexuals outnumber females by approximately 3:1, with the incidence of the former estimated to be 1:37000 of the general male population (Roberts, 1988).

Transsexuals encountered in clinical settings are commonly motivated principally, or indeed entirely, by the overriding desire for sex reassignment surgery (in males castration; in females hysterectomy and bilateral mastectomy) and/or opposite sex hormone treatment as a second best option. They are usually experienced in the "playing of the game" and may have consulted many previous medical practitioners. They reluctantly accept that seeing a psychiatrist is a necessary (though tiresome) prerequisite to surgical referral and often overemphasize, or indeed fabricate, aspects of their own feeling, behaviour and life experience in order to maximize the legitimacy of their goal. They are usually young or middle-aged and typically provide a history of cross-dressing of many years' duration. They may openly wear clothes appropriate to the other sex;

cultivate gender-inappropriate mannerisms; and admit to behaviour designed to minimize secondary sexual characteristics (for example, electrolysis, use of cosmetics or taking of illicitly obtained hormone preparations). Associated psychiatric pathology, current or previous, is a relatively common finding, reflecting, perhaps, frustration arising from society's "callous" insistence that "I, a woman (man) be forced to continue living in a man's (woman's) body"; perhaps more general psychological disturbance.

A distinction must be drawn between gender identity and sexual orientation. By no means all transsexuals manifest homosexual or bisexual preferences in their choice of sexual partner. In one recent study (Burns *et al.*, 1990) 45% of transsexual males and 13% of females were heterosexual. Nor must transsexualism be confused with transvestism, a purely fetishistic sexual disorder. Many authorities (Burns *et al.*, 1990) now believe that in "core" transsexualism, the most homogeneous and "pure culture" sub-group of the larger whole, an absence of sexual arousal during cross-dressing, and a low level of sexual activity generally, are virtually pathognomonic of "true" or "primary" transsexualism, highlighting the function of cross-dressing as but one behavioural practice of many designed to achieve congruence with the central theme of this disorder: the conviction of false gender assignment.

Inevitably, physical theories of causation have proved attractive but investigations of genetic, chromosomal, hormonal, enzymatic, antigenic, neurotransmitter and cerebral dysfunction factors have resulted in no convincing, replicable abnormal findings. The majority of theorists conceptualizes this disorder as arising in the first few years of life – the pre-Oedipal phase – as a result of seriously dysfunctional family dynamics. At a phase of his (generic usage) development during which the child is becoming aware of his gender identity he becomes the object of chaotic, aggressive and destructive parental (mainly maternal) input, often including overt physical and sexual abuse as well as more subtle forms of hostility, which has both a general quality but also a specific focus in "consistently expressing displeasure and disgust at the child's body image, genitals and emerging masculinity or femininity" (Lothstein, 1987). This might be based on envy in the case of a male child, or intragenerational transmission of learned anti-feminine attitudes in the case of a female child. The outcome is a generally insecure adult with an impaired sense of personal worth which he localizes in his gender identity. He seeks to overcome his self-loathing by the primitive ego defence mechanism of splitting off his bad feelings about himself into gender disparagement and then attempting to lose the physical encapsulation of these feelings by obtaining surgical castration. The desire to gain possession of the alternative gender identity represents an omnipotent and idealized fantasy, also psychologically primitive, in which being the opposite sex becomes equated with being lovable, worthwhile and all things good.

Lothstein (1987) has made a compelling plea for the use of psychotherapeutic techniques rather than surgical techniques. In fact, it is recognized that for the majority of transsexuals, surgical intervention is not appropriate. Yet many of these individuals cannot work effectively in a psychotherapeutic medium and there is increasing awareness that sex reassignment surgery is a viable option for a sizeable minority. The likelihood of a successful outcome is greater if (a) the candidate is required to live as completely as possible as a member of the opposite sex for a minimum of two years prior to surgery being recommended; (b) psychological and social support is provided consistently both before surgery and thereafter; (c) hormone therapy is provided to minimize secondary sexual characteristics appropriate to the anatomical gender. All of these criteria are mandatory in most specialized units. A successful outcome is alleged by Burns and co-workers (1990) to be more likely the closer the presentation and history approximate to the clinical profile of "core" transsexualism, thus excluding as far as possible "secondary" cases. Twenty-three per cent of their group of 106 patients were referred for surgery. Mate-Kole and co-workers (1990) have compared two groups of transsexuals two years after initial assessment, the first group having undergone surgery soon after initial assessment, the second group still being on the waiting list. During the intervening two years, the operated group as a whole had significantly improved on measures of social and sexual activity, and on measures of "neurotic disability" whereas the non-operated group showed no improvement in social or sexual activity and significant deterioration in measures of "neurotic disability". Careful patient selection for surgery is vital and even then, notwithstanding the provision of all appropriate support measures before and after surgery, the long term outcome may not be as satisfactory as early findings suggest. Lothstein (1987) has warned that in the short term all we may be doing (though appreciated by the patient) is relieving dysphoria, and that since the basic personality difficulties underlying the disorder remain essentially untouched it may only be a matter of time before serious problems re-emerge.

This chapter may have introduced readers to three areas of psychiatric dysfunction of which they may not previously have had knowledge in depth. Some feeling of the suffering associated with these disorders may have been conveyed. Greater empathy may be possible if the psychological substrates of these three very different disorders are more clearly glimpsed. They all share some degree of disturbance of body image, at least in so far as psychological factors contribute to animate that conceptual chimera. What they own in common is of greater importance than those superficial behavioural characteristics which separate them diagnostically and phenomenologically. That shared psychological nexus may be presumptuously equated with low self-esteem; feeling bad about the inner person is converted into feeling bad about the external person we expose to the scrutiny of others.

> We are not ourselves
> When nature, being oppress'd, commands the mind
> To suffer with the body.
> *Shakespeare. (King Lear. Act II, Scene IV)*

## References

Birtchnell, S.A. (1988). Dysmorphophobia – a centenary discussion. *British Journal of Psychiatry,* **153**, suppl. 2, 41-43.
Brown, G.R. (1990). A review of clinical approaches to Gender Dysphoria. *Journal of Clinical Psychiatry,* **51**, 57-64.
Bruch, H. (1962). Perceptual and conceptual disturbances in anorexia nervosa. *Psychosomatic Medicine,* **24**, 187-194.
Burns, A., Farrell, M. and Christie Brown, J. (1990). Clinical features of patients attending a gender identity clinic. *British Journal of Psychiatry,* **157**, 265-268.
Buvat, J. and Buvat-Herbaut, M. (1978). Misperception of body concept and dysmorphophobias. *Annales Medico-Psychologiques,* **136**, 563-580.
Coker, S. and Cooper, P.J. (1991). "The Specific Psychopathology of Bulimia Nervosa". Proceedings of a National Symposium on Bulimia Nervosa, pp. 7-9. Haymarket Publishing Services, London.
Connolly, F. and Gipson, M. (1978). Dysmorphophobia. A long term study. *British Journal of Psychiatry,* **132**, 458-470.
Cooper, P.J. and Taylor, M.J. (1988). Body image disturbance in bulimia nervosa. *British Journal of Psychiatry,* suppl. 2, 32-36.
Cotterill, J.A. (1981). Dermatological non-disease: a common and potentially fatal disturbance of cutaneous body image. *British Journal of Dermatology,* **104**, 611-619.
Cumming, W.J.K. (1988). The neurobiology of the body schema. *British Journal of Psychiatry,* **153**, suppl. 2, 7-22.
Dion, K., Berscheid, E. and Walster, E. (1972). What is beautiful is good. *Journal of Personal and Social Psychology,* **24**, 285.
Dolan, B.M., Birtchnell, S.A. and Lacey, J.H. (1987). Body image distortion in non-eating disordered women and men. *Journal of Psychosomatic Research,* **31**, 513-520.
Fenichel, O. (1946). "The Psychoanalytic Theory of Neurosis". Routledge and Kegan Paul, London.
Fitts, S.N., Gibson, P., Redding, C.A. and Deiter, P.J. (1989). Body dysmorphic disorder: implications for its validity as a DSM-III-R clinical syndrome. *Psychological Reports,* **64**, 655-658.
Garner, D.M., Garfinkel, P.E. and O'Shaughnessy, M. (1985). The validity of the distinction between bulimia with and without anorexia nervosa. *American Journal of Psychiatry,* **142**, 581-587.
Glucksman, M.L. and Hursch, J. (1969). The response of obese patients to weight reduction: III. The perception of body size. *Psychosomatic Medicine,* **31**, 1-17.
Hay, G.G. and Heather, B.B. (1973). Changes in psychometric test results following cosmetic nasal operations. *British Journal of Psychiatry,* **122**, 89-90.
Hollander, E., Liebowitz, M.R., Winchell, R., Klumker, A. and Klein, D.F. (1989). Treatment of body-dysmorphic disorder with serotonin reuptake blockers. *American Journal of Psychiatry,* **146**, 768-770.
Hsu, L.K.G. (1982). Is there a disturbance in body image in anorexia nervosa? *Journal of Nervous and Mental Disease,* **170**, 305-307.
Jahrreiss, W. (1930). Hypochondriacal thinking. *Archives of Psychiatric and Nervous Illness,* **92**, 686-823.
Lacey, J.H. (1991). "Multi-impulsive Bulimia". Proceedings of a National Symposium on

Bulimia Nervosa, pp. 12-13. Haymarket Publishing Services, London.
Lothstein, L. (1987). Theories of transsexualism. *In* "Sexuality and Medicine". Vol. 1. (Eds E.E. Shelp and D. Dordrecht). pp. 55-72. Reidel Publishing Co.
Mate-Kole, C., Freschi, M. and Robin, A. (1990). A controlled study of psychological and social change after surgical gender reassignment in selected male transsexuals. *British Journal of Psychiatry*, **157**, 261-264.
Morselli, E. (1886). Sulla dismorfofobia e sulla tafefobia. *Bolletino delle Scienze Mediche di Genova*, **vi**, 100-119.
Nylander, I. (1971). The feeling of being fat and dieting in a school population. *Acta Socio-Medica Scandinavica*, **1**, 17-26.
Proctor, L. and Morley, S. (1986). "Demand characteristics" in body-size estimation in anorexia nervosa. *British Journal of Psychiatry*, **149**, 113-118.
Reich, J. (1969). The surgery of appearance: psychological and related aspects. *Medical Journal of Australia*, **2**, 5-13.
Reilly, T.M. (1977). Monosymptomatic hypochondriacal psychosis: presentation and treatment. *Proceedings of the Royal Society of Medicine*, **70**, suppl. 10, 39-43.
Reilly, T.M. (1984). Monosymptomatic hypochondriacal psychosis: an introduction to the concept. Paper presented at Symposium: Monosymptomatic hypochondriacal psychosis: a diagnostic entity? Held at First European Conference on Recent Advances in Psychiatric Treatment, Vienna, March.
Roberto, L. (1983). Issues in diagnosis and treatment of transsexualism. *Archives of Sexual Behaviour*, **12**, 445-473.
Schachter, M. (1971). Dysmorphic neurosis (ugliness complexes) and delusions or delusional conviction of ugliness. *Annals of Medical Psychology*, **129**, 723-745.
Scheler, M. (1955). Die Idole der Selbsterkenntnis. *In* "Gesammelte Werke". Vol. III. pp. 215-292. Bern. Translated (1973) as The Idols of Self-Knowledge by D.R. Lachterman. *In* "Selected Philosophical Essays". Northwestern University Press, Evanston.
Slade, P.D. (1977). Awareness of body dimensions during pregnancy: an analogue study. *Psychological Medicine*, **7**, 245-252.
Slade, P.D. (1985). A review of body-image studies in anorexia nervosa and bulimia nervosa. *Journal of Psychiatric Research*, **19**, 255-266.
Slade, P.D. (1988). Body image in anorexia nervosa. *British Journal of Psychiatry*, **153**, suppl. 2, 20-22.
Slade, P.D. and Russell, G.D. (1973). Experimental investigations of bodily perception in anorexia nervosa and obesity. *Psychotherapy and Psychosomatics*, **22**, 359-363.
Sneddon, I.B. (1979). The presentation of psychiatric illness to the dermatologist. *Acta dermatovenereologica (Stockholm)*, **59**, suppl. 85, 177-179.
Strober, M., Goldenberg, I., Green, J. and Saxon, J. (1979). Body image disturbance in anorexia nervosa during the acute and recuperative phase. *Journal of Psychiatric Research*, **19**, (2-3), 239-246.
Touyz, S.W., Beumont, P.J.V., Collins, J.K., McCabe, M. and Jupp, J. (1984). Body shape perception and its disturbance in anorexia nervosa. *British Journal of Psychiatry*, **144**, 167-171.
Walker, P., Berger, J. and Green, R. (1985). Standards of care: The hormonal and surgical sex reassignment of GD persons. *Archives of Sexual Behaviour*, **14**, 79-90.
Whitehouse, A.M., Freeman, C.P.L. and Annandale, A. (1988). Body size estimation in anorexia nervosa. *British Journal of Psychiatry*, **153**, suppl. 2, 23-26.

# 24. Disorders of consciousness

David Bates and Niall Cartlidge

---

Examples of abnormalites of consciousness may be found in a wide variety of sources extending back to man's earliest written recordings, often described in vivid detail (Courville, 1955).

> Swift at his word his ponderous javelin fled;
> Nor miss'd its aim, but where the plumage danced
> Razed the smooth cone, and thence obliquely glanced,
> Safe in his helm (the gift of Phoebus' hands)
> Without a wound the Trojan hero stands;
> But yet so stunn'd that, staggering on the plain,
> His arm and knee his sinking bulk sustain;
> O'er his dim sight the misty vapours rise,
> And a short darkness shades his swimming eyes.

With these words Homer depicted the plight of Hector the Trojan hero. Concussion is a brief but widespread paralysis of the function of the brain which comes on as an immediate consequence of a blow to the head. Other dramatic portrayals of concussion may be found in legends such as the stories of King Arthur and his knights of the Round Table:

> Then the brains of Sir Gawaine swam like shallow water, and he reeled this way and that in his saddle, and would have fallen had it not been for Sir Galahad, who catched him ere he fell beneath the feet of his horse and so helped him up in the saddle.

Impairment of consciousness after blows to the head have occurred to a variety of important historical figures, such as Romulus, Alexander The Great, Montezuma and Captain Cook. Not all such characters with head injury recover spontaneously without perceptible brain damage. Charles VIII died on 7 April 1498 of what was probably an intracerebral haemorrhage. He was walking through a gallery, the opening of which was rather low, he struck his forehead and was rendered dizzy. A few hours later he collapsed unconscious and nine hours later he died.

Sussman (1967) refers to descriptions of cerebral haemorrhage and epilepsy resulting in impairment of consciousness in the Bible and the Talmud yet suggests that in both of these ancient texts there is no single case of a disease in man specifically related to the brain, spinal cord or nerves. In the Bible there are several descriptions of epileptic seizures, the most famous being that which occurred to Paul of Tarsus.

Probably the first known medical text book was those writings which we now know as the Edwin Smith Papyrus (Breasted, 1930). The papyrus itself is an incomplete copy of a work probably written during the period 2500-3000 BC. Case 22 describes an individual who suffered a head injury and was unable to speak. In the Hippocratic writings there are numerous accounts of impairment of consciousness. For example, in the so-called "Hippocratic Aphorisms" there is a reference "in cases of concussion of the brain produced by any cause the patients of necessity lose their speech" (Walker, 1951). In the Roman era, Galen and Celsus were aware of disorders of consciousness resulting from head injury (Major, 1961). Few medical writings of value are available until the 10th century and the time of the eminent physicians Rhazes and Avicenna from Arabia (Sigerist, 1967) both of whom described in detail the clinical effects of loss of consciousness.

During the next few centuries many examples of the effects of concussion are recorded (Courville, 1955) and in the 16th century Jean Fernel drew attention to the close relationship between concussion and sleep. Throughout this period there was clear recognition of the importance of the brain in maintaining consciousness.

In 1853, Carpenter recognized the importance of links between subcortical structures and the cortex but it was the development of the electroencephalogram (EEG) which led to the concept of a sub-cortical pace-maker (Berger, 1929). The site of this pace-maker was uncertain but Bremer in 1937 reported that coma resulted from transection of the mid-brain in cats whereas transection of the cervico-medullary region did not result in coma. He suggested that wakefulness required constant stimulation of the cerebral hemispheres by incoming sensory impulses and coma would result when such stimulation was silenced or interrupted.

The identification of the pace-maker was made in 1949 with the description of the ascending reticular activating system, "the reticular formation" (Moruzzi and Magoun, 1963). This structure was recognized to extend through the brain-stem and to have diffuse projections to the cerebral cortex.

**Normal Consciousness**

The term "consciousness" has been endowed with so many different meanings that it is almost impossible to define precisely. Fredericks (1969) gives an excellent account of the various concepts of normal consciousness. Indeed, it is not strictly a medical term but literary, philosophical and psychological as well. To the psychologist consciousness denotes a state of awareness of oneself and one's environment. Knowledge of the former includes all feelings, attitudes, emotions, impulses, volitions and activity or the striving actions of conduct – in short, an awareness of all one's mental functioning, particularly of the cognitive processes. This, in simple terms can be regarded as the state of the patient's awareness of self and environment. In practice this can be judged only by the individuals' accounts of their feelings and, indirectly, by their actions. To the physician, consciousness is defined by the observation of the patient's behaviour and reaction to stimuli.

Normal consciousness is the condition of a normal individual when awake. In this state the individual is fully responsive to stimuli and indicates awareness by behaviour and speech. This normal state may vary during the course of the day from keen alertness or deep concentration to mild general inattentiveness and drowsiness. There are two separate aspects of consciousness: the first is the arousal component of wakefulness which keeps the patient awake and relates to the physical manifestations of awakening from sleep, the eyes being open and purposive motor activity occurring; the second is the content of consciousness or the awareness of self and environment – the sum of the psychological functions of sensations, emotions and thoughts. It should be noted that the individual's awareness of self can be recognized only by an observer on the basis of responses made to external stimuli, especially verbal or motor responses.

## The reticular formation and consciousness

Our current ideas concerning consciousness and its abnormalities owe much to a better understanding of the reticular formation. A major step forward followed the work of Moruzzi and Magoun (1963) with the introduction of the term "ascending reticular activating system". Electrical stimulation of the brain-stem in anaesthetized cats produced changes in the EEG similar to those observed in man on transition from a drowsy state to a state of alertness. From these, and other observations, it was concluded that the brain-stem reticular system can best be regarded as a non-specific arousal system projecting to the cerebral cortex. Thus, the brain-stem reticular formation appears to be responsible for the arousal, alert and wakeful component of consciousness.

Our knowledge concerning the brain-stem reticular activating system has advanced considerably in recent years. Its functions and ramifications are widespread and extend beyond its role as a cortical arouser (Brodal, 1981). It can be regarded as a continuous isodentritic core traversing from the medulla through the pons to the midbrain, continuous caudally with the reticular intermediate grey lamina of the spinal cord and rostrally with the subthalamus, hypothalamus and thalamus. A variety of named cell groups can be identified, and there is a general arrangement such that the medial two-thirds have large cells as a prominent feature whereas the lateral one-third contains only smaller cells. It was thought that arousal depended on projections from the reticular formation to the midline thalamic nuclei and thence to the thalamic reticular nucleus and the cortex. More recent studies suggest that the thalamic reticular nucleus cannot be considered a final relay to the cortex and it is not possible to reach a definite conclusion as to the particular role in arousal played by the various links from reticular formation to thalamus (Brodal, 1981).

The neuro-pharmacological mechanisms involved in consciousness are ill understood, although it has been suggested that cholinergic mechanisms are important in arousal (Defeudis, 1974). Jouvet (1972) suggested that monoaminergic systems play a role in sleep arousal and neural pathways involving the neuro-transmitter gamma aminobutyric acid (GABA) may be important in controlling consciousness (Tinuper *et al.*, 1992).

## Cerebral hemispheres and consciousness

The latter half of the 20th century has seen a greater understanding of the function of the cerebral hemisphere and particularly the cerebral cortex. We now recognize that man's pre-eminence in evolutionary terms depends not only on the neuronal context of the cerebral cortex but also on the complexity of the neuronal connections (Hubal, 1979). Although many discrete cortical functions, such as language, are localized to specific areas of the cerebral cortex, the content of consciousness can best be regarded as the sum total of cognitive functions; thus the cortex as a whole mediates this aspect of consciousness.

Many areas of the neo-cortex, such as the frontal lobes which are hardly visible in lower animals (3.1% of cortex in cats), are considerably larger (13% in primates) and occupy up to 25% of the total hemispheres in man, were formally regarded as silent areas of the brain. Myelination of fibres within the frontal lobes is delayed until the child is between four and seven years old allowing prolongation of maturation to enable continued learning. Nowadays many physiologists consider the frontal regions of the brain to be the seat of conscious motivated and intellectualized behaviour. Recognition of the functions of the frontal lobe continues to be difficult in that they do not appear to be essential to life, only crude deficits can be recognized clinically and sophisticated tests such as those requiring delayed response solutions (Jacobson, 1936) are required to elicit essential functions. They are responsible for higher meta-functions: intentionality, initiation, complex sequencing, creation of plans, manipulation of representational systems – in short, they denote an awareness of the activity of the mind: the consciousness of being conscious. Consciousness becomes behaviour: the display of affect and spontaneity, the integration of expression, gesture and emotion with speech, the anticipatory preparation for action with the organization of goal-directed tasks and inhibitional control of potential interference, self-awareness associated with self-regulation, and memory pattern and sequence events (Perecman, 1987). These meta-functions relate to the reality of the person as an individual: as yet we cannot presume how they relate to man's understanding of "reality without" except in so far as feedback mechanisms – recognition of an empathic exchange of gestures or expressions, the tone of a speaker's voice, the feel for an audience – are fed back from the special sensors to the brain. With such a large structure as the frontal lobes, divided into the precentral (pre-motor areas), fronto-limbic and dorso-lateral or integrative cortex a wide variety of impairments may occur. The patient may become impulsive, disinhibitive, flat or facetious in affect, distractable, unreliable, "forgetting to remember", confabulating and clumsy. Fluctuations may occur in the level of activity, either over-active or apathetic, perseverating or shifting with impaired ability to initiate movements. If associated with criminality, crimes tend to show discontrol, impulsiveness and crudeness in planning an execution. Orbitofrontal leucotomies, dividing fibres subserving pain and emotional reactions, may overcome obsessional reactions or recognition of otherwise intractable pain; but do so at the price of a flattening of the personality and lessening of abilities. The mental capacity may be sufficient for executing routine work, but the attention span may be impaired, learning intricate material faulty, and they can lack initiative, foresight, fail to grasp the totality of a situation, or display inability to deal simultaneously with more than one source of information.

## The relationship of sleep to abnormalities of consciousness

Of the abnormalities of consciousness perhaps the most easy to define is that of coma (*vide infra*) and sleep and coma share many similarities. Conscious behaviour is suspended in both and behaviourally they resemble one another. The EEG can be slow in both and until a few years ago there was a widespread tendency amongst physiologists to regard sleep and coma as due to a damping down of the activity of the reticular activating system upon the cerebral hemispheres. We now recognize that sleep and coma are physiologically quite different. Sleep is an active physiological process associated with biological rhythms (circadian cycles) whereas coma can be regarded as a negative phenomenon. A patient in light coma, for example, might show sleep-wake cycles; indeed, this is a typical finding in patients with diffuse cortical damage showing features of the vegetative state (*vide infra*). This observation supports the view that in man the control of sleep and awakening resides in the brain-stem in proximity to the cyclically arranged centres that control respiration and cardiovascular homeostasis – blood pressure, vascular tone and heart rate. Other circadian rhythms such as those concerned with endocrine activities probably reside in the hypothalamus and are likewise linked to the reticular activating system.

## Abnormalities of Consciousness

### Definitions

The terminology in current usage derives from a Medical Research Council Brain Injuries Committee which reported in 1941.

*Confusion (clouding of consciousness)*
"Disturbance of consciousness characterized by impaired capacity to think clearly and with customary repetition and to perceive, respond to and remember current stimuli; there is also disorientation".

This definition implies that confusion and clouding of consciousness are one and the same. However, Plum and Posner (1980) have defined a confusional state as an advanced state of clouding of consciousness. In practice, confusion may be divided into quiet confusion or agitated confusion which is the term for delirium (*vide infra*). The term semi-coma is imprecise and should not be used. Confusion implies a generalized disturbance of cerebral function, particularly of the cerebral cortex, and it is usually associated with widespread EEG abnormalities.

*Delirium*
"A state of much disturbed consciousness (confusion) with motor restlessness, transient hallucinations, disorientation and perhaps delusions"; delirium can be regarded as agitated confusion.

*Obtundation*
"A disorder of alertness associated with psychomotor retardation". At times, this may be a feature of a confusional state and the term simply describes the clinical picture.

*Stupor*
"A state in which the patient, though not unconscious, exhibits little or no spontaneous activity". In this state, the individual appears to be asleep and yet, when vigorously stimulated, may become alert as manifest by eye opening and ocular movement. Other motor activities are limited and there is usually no speech.

*Coma*
"A state of absolute unconsciousness, as judged by the absence of any psychologically understandable response (including, for example, change of expression) to external stimuli or inner need".

A simple and more understandable definition of coma is that of unrousable unresponsiveness. This implies a defect not only in arousal but also in awareness of self and environment and therefore, inability to respond.

*Locked-in syndrome* (Feldman, 1971)
The ventral pontine or locked-in syndrome describes a condition of total paralysis below the level of the third nuclei. Such patients can open, elevate and depress their eyes. However, horizontal eye movements are lost and no other voluntary movement is possible. The diagnosis of this locked-in state depends on the recognition that the patient can open his eyes voluntarily rather than spontaneously as in the vegetative state. Patients with this condition usually die or remain tetraplegic, although there are reports of recovery. The neuropathological basis for such cases is usually infarction of the ventral pons and efferent motor tracts. A similar clinical picture may sometimes be seen in patients with pontine tumours, pontine haemorrhage, central pontine myelinolysis, head injury or brain-stem encephalitis.

*Vegetative state*
When the cortex of the cerebral hemispheres of the brain recovers more slowly than

the brain-stem or when it is irreversibly damaged there may arise a situation in which the patient enters a vegetative state as described in 1972 by Jennett and Plum. Patients will recover the arousal component of consciousness but not, as far as can be determined, awareness. They will show a return of wakefulness, respiration and the maintenance of blood pressure and temperature but a total lack of cognitive function. It may be a transient phase through which patients in coma pass as they recover or deteriorate but, and commonly after a hypoxic ischaemic injury to the brain following cardiac arrest or head injury, there develops a state in which the brain-stem recovers function but the cerebral hemispheres are incapable of recovery. This is then defined as a persistent vegetative state (Jennett and Plum, 1972). Such patients may survive for long periods, on occasion for decades, but never recover outward manifestations of higher mental activity. The viability of the brain-stem, despite the continued inactivity of the cerebral cortex, allows the continuation of breathing, eye movements and digestion as well as those functions of blood pressure, temperature and pulse rates. The criteria which are regarded as identifying brain-stem death (*vide infra*) are manifestly not fulfilled and to the lay person the patient remains ostensibly alive with eye-opening, sleep-wake cycles and evidence of respiration. Such patients are not dependent upon artificial respiration though many are ventilated at some period during their initial coma or following resuscitation. The vegetative state has appeared predominantly due to those advances in medical technology which have protected the brain-stem through a period of potential injury but have not been able to protect the cortex to the same extent. It is therefore a side-effect of the "success" of modern medical techniques.

In general patients in coma begin either to awaken or deteriorate within the first few days or weeks depending upon the severity of the injury. If they improve and sleep-wake cycles develop they are not strictly in coma though they may never again show evidence of conscious intelligence. Terms such as neo-cortical death, the apallic state, coma vigil, cerebral death and total dementia have been used for this syndrome. The term akinetic mutism is applied to a behaviourally-similar condition of unresponsiveness yet apparent alertness with reactive alpha and theta EEG rhythms consistent with consciousness. The striking difference from the vegetative state is the lack of motor signs of rigidity or spasticity despite a paucity of movement even in response to pain. This condition may be produced by bilateral frontal lobe lesions, diffuse cortical lesions or lesions of the deep grey matter.

When patients who are vegetative neither improve or deteriorate the adjective "persistent" may be added and should be taken as being descriptive of the current state of affairs and not necessarily predicting long-term outcome. Retrospectively, after post-mortem examination it may be possible to identify massive neo-cortical damage which will indicate that the patient was permanently in the vegetative state but there are no clinical or laboratory means of confirming this prior to post-mortem, and specialists in rehabilitation are concerned that physicians may take the attitude that there is no point in treating patients who develop the vegetative state, thereby creating a self-fulfilling prophecy of poor prognosis, no treatment and poor outcome (Andrews, 1992). There is continuing debate as to the potential for recovery for patients who are vegetative. In patients who have suffered non-traumatic injuries such as anoxia and ischaemia, the prognosis for recovery from the vegetative state is poor after the first few weeks. There are some examples of patients who suffered coma as a result of head trauma in whom an improvement from the vegetative state has been recognized after months, but those anecdotal cases of recovery from vegetative state after years are difficult to validate and it seems possible that such patients were not truly vegetative but rather in a state of profound disability but with cognition. One of the major factors in assessing outcome for patients in the vegetative state arises because those who are above the level of vegetation are recorded by inaccurate observers as being vegetative, and when they later show some elements of cognition, are regarded by their carers as having recovered from a vegetative state which was never truly established. The electroencephalogram does not help in identifying the vegetative state or the prognosis. Many varying types of EEG pattern have been recorded in the vegetative state from near normality to an essentially flat record.

**Brain Death**

The advent of cardiopulmonary resuscitation during the 1950s presaged the inevitable debate upon the definition of human death. If the criteria such as a beating heart and respiration can no longer be taken as the standard by which life and death are determined, it is necessary to establish other criteria upon which the ebb of life can be decided. In practice it is recognized that the death of the brain is the necessary and sufficient condition to establish the death of the individual and if one amends the word death to "irreversible loss of function" then one can accept that the "irreversible loss of function of the brain" is the criterion which shall identify the death of the individual.

Anatomically it is apparent that the area of the brain which determines viability is the brain-stem since it contains centres responsible for respiration, heart rate and blood pressure, and the ascending reticular activating system, which allows the capacity of consciousness, and is the route whereby both afferent and efferent pathways link the brain to the rest of the body. It follows that if the brain stem is not able to function there can be no capacity for consciousness and therefore content of consciousness which function lies within the cerebral hemispheres.

The first recognition of an irretrievable state of being dead before the heart and lungs brought physiological life to an end once artificial ventilation had been established, was by the French neurologists Mollaret and Goulon in 1959. They identified "coma dépassé": "a state beyond coma". They described patients who had irremediable damage to the brain stem, were incapable of breathing and had lost their ability to react not only to the external world, but also to their own internal environment. They therefore became unable to breathe, unable to monitor body temperature and unable to control their blood pressure or heart rate. At that time ventilation was continued until the heart beat ceased, usually within a few days.

In 1968 a committee of the Harvard Medical School published the first criteria for recognition of the "brain death syndrome". They identified the persistence of apnoeic coma without brain stem or spinal reflexes and a flat electroencephalogram for 24 hours as indicative of brain death, provided that the cause of the coma was known and that reversible causes of brain dysfunction had been excluded. The authors identified "death" as meaning "brain death" though they did not define the word death and endorsed the withdrawal of respiratory support. They did not provide evidence to prove that if artificial ventilation was continued no such patient had ever recovered consciousness and that in all the heart invariably ceased, but the contentions of this committee have been validated since that time and there is no recognized exception.

The diagnosis of brain stem death is now accepted in the UK and USA as being synonymous with brain death. It is made on clinical grounds and it is recognized that the clinician is not identifying that every neurone within the head shall be dead but simply establishing that there is irreversible loss of brain stem function. Studies of electroencephalography and cerebral blood flow do not contribute information towards the prognosis and tests of evoked potentials of somatosensory and auditory origin have nothing to add to the diagnosis.

Brain stem death is established by three important criteria:

1   The cause of coma must be ascertained and it must be known that the patient is suffering from irremediable structural brain damage.

2   All complicating factors such as drug intoxication, metabolic upset and, particularly, hypothermia shall have been corrected or excluded.

3   The absence of all brain stem reflexes must be demonstrated and the fact that the patient cannot breathe, however strong the stimulus, must be established.

It is important, given the need for organs for donation, that decisions about brain death are made by physicians distinctly separate from those involved in any transplant. In general neurologists, anaesthesiologists or intensive therapists are responsible for making the diagnosis of brain stem death and there is no urgency in making the diagnosis. It may take 24 or 48 hours to establish that there is brain stem death during which time the totality of apnoea is established by allowing the carbon dioxide level in the blood to rise above that which is sufficient to drive any respiratory centre cells which may still be viable.

It is interesting that the concept of brain stem death arose from the effectiveness of cardiopulmonary resuscitation. Until it was possible to re-establish circulation in patients who had suffered cardiac arrest, and undertake ventilation in those who were not spontaneously capable of breathing, the problem of defining death did not exist. Once these functions could be performed artificially it became important to identify those patients who were not capable of supporting a sentient life independently and from this developed the concept of brain stem death. The way in which the medical colleges of the United Kingdom and the United States have developed criteria which are now widely accepted as defining brain stem death is a model for future planning with respect to other ethical considerations in medicine and should be taken as an example of the way in which medical opinion can identify and manage those problems arising when a patient is in a state beyond coma without the necessity of litigation and political debate.

**Measurement or Assessment of Consciousness**

As stated above, the assessment of consciousness can be made only by the responses that a patient might give, and the actions that he or she makes or undertakes either spontaneously or as a response.

The alertness component of consciousness can be readily judged by observing that the patient's eyes are open, that he is attentive and that he is able to move and respond appropriately. The content of consciousness is most easily assessed by some form of formal psychological assessment such as the mini mental test score.

For patients with significant impairment of consciousness, and particularly, impairment of alertness, the Glasgow Coma Scale is perhaps the simplest and best validated method of assessment (Table 1). This is really a consciousness scale as patients at the top of the scale are probably normal. The scale has been widely used in a variety of studies of coma (Levy et al., 1981; Jennett et al., 1979) and patients can be easily scored by both paramedical and medical personnel. As can be seen below more detailed assessments need to be made of other neurological functions in patients with profound impairment of consciousness such as coma but the Glasgow Coma Scale remains the best method of assessing level of consciousness.

TABLE 1. *The Glasgow Coma Scale.*

| A. Eye opening | B. Motor Response | C. Verbal |
|---|---|---|
| 1. Nil | 1. Nil | 1. Nil |
| 2. Pain | 2. Abnormal Extension | 2. Incomprehensible |
| 3. Verbal | 3. Abnormal Flexion | 3. Inappropriate |
| 4. Spontaneous | 4. Weak Flexion | 4. Confused |
|  | 5. Localization | 5. Orientated fully |
|  | 6. Obeys command |  |

**Pathophysiology of the Major Categories of Disorders of Consciousness**

Confusion

Many demented patients are confused but the term acute confusional state is restricted to episodes of acute or subacute confusion characterized by abnormal attention with perceptual, cognitive and other behavioural disturbances. Acute confusion is one of the most common neurobehavioural disorders seen in general hospitals (Wells, 1985). Such states occur in about 5-15% of those on medical or surgical wards, 18-30% of those in Intensive Care Units and as many as 80% of those on geriatric wards (Lipowski, 1985).

Two separate types of confusional state may be seen: the lethargic type in which the patient may be somnolent and slow to respond and the delirious type where hyperkinesia agitation and overactivity of the autonomic nervous system is prominent (delirium). Patients with acute confusion do not necessarily remain in either the lethargic or delirious state and may alternate at times being somnolent and at other times being agitated.

## Clinical features (Table 2)

A disturbance of attention is the cardinal symptom of acute confusional states and the patients are often distractible switching their attention from one stimulus to another. Fluctuation in the degree of confusion is another important component, and worsening of confusion often occurs at night. Loss of the sleep wake cycle in confused patients often leads to particular problems when such patients start to wander and cause disruption at night.

TABLE 2. *Features of acute confusional states.*

Depressed or fluctuating level of consciousness
Impaired attention span
Inability to maintain coherent line of thought
Distractibility
Difficulty learning new material
Disorientation
Incoherent speech
Anomia or non aphasic misnaming
Agraphia
Perseveration and/or impersistence
Hallucination (visual and tactile most common)
Delusions
Mood alterations
Sleep disturbances
Autonomic disturbances
Psychomotor retardation and/or hyperactivity
Action tremor
Myoclonus
Asterixis
Dysarthria
Paratonic rigidity

Perceptual disturbances are also common in that patients often miss what is going on around them and may misinterpret their environment leading to illusions and frank hallucinations. Visual hallucinations are the most common and auditory hallucinations are unusual. Reduplicative paramnesia, the replacement of persons or places, results from decreased integration of recent observations with past memories. The stream of thought is disturbed and patients are unable to carry out sequenced activity and organize goal directed behaviour. In the lethargic type the stream of thought is slowed whilst in delirium it may be accelerated. Speech reflects the jumbled thoughts, shifting from subject with hesitations, repetitions and perseverations.

Disturbances occur in orientation, recent memory, higher visual processing and writing. Patients are disorientated first to time and then to place, whilst disorientation to person rarely, if ever, occurs. Behavioural and emotional abnormalities may occur with lability agitation and occasionally apathy.

TABLE 3. *Causes of confusional states.*

| |
|---|
| Infections |
| Intracranial tumours |
| Stroke |
| Ischaemia/anoxic brain damage |
| Metabolic encephalopathies |
| Non-convulsive status epilepticus |
| Toxins |
| Drugs |

Acute confusional states must be distinguished from dementia, Wernicke's aphasia and a variety of psychiatric conditions such as schizophrenia or mania.

The main differentiating features of dementia are the longer time course and the absence of prominent fluctuating attentional and perceptual deficits. Chronic confusion is a form of dementia. Acute confusional states in dementia may overlap because demented patients have an increased susceptibility for developing a superimposed confusional state, particularly at night.

The assessment of language should distinguish a Wernicke's aphasia from an acute confusional state. A patient with aphasia will usually have prominent paraphasias of all types including neologisms yet have relatively preserved axial or whole body commands.

In general patients with psychiatric conditions mimicking confusion lack the fluctuating attentional and related deficits. Schizophrenics may have a very disturbed verbal output but their speech often has an underlying bizarre theme. Schizophrenic hallucinations are more often auditory than visual.

## Coma

### Definition

The patient who appears to be asleep and is at the same time incapable of sensing or responding to external stimuli or inner needs is in a state of coma. A simple and understandable definition of coma (as above) is that of unarousable unresponsiveness. This implies not only a defect in arousal but also one of awareness of self and environment. A more practical definition may be obtained using the Glasgow Coma Scale (Table 1). Coma is defined as certain pattern of behavioural responses at the lower end of the scale. In precise terms, coma may be defined as the lower two responses of eye-opening, the lower two verbal responses and the lower three motor responses. At best, such patients do not open their eyes to voice or spontaneously, do not localize a painful stimulus and utter no recognizable words. The depth of coma may vary from a patient showing total absence of responses to the best responses as noted above.

## Pathophysiology

In general, disorders of consciousness almost invariably result from diffuse or multi-focal lesions of the cerebral hemispheres and cortex. The one exception to this rule is coma itself which may result from lesions in the brain-stem (Fig. 1). Unilateral lesions of the cerebral hemispheres produce impairment of consciousness only in proportion to their size. However, there is some evidence to suggest that the left hemisphere influences consciousness more than the right and occasionally a sudden unilateral, large, dominant hemisphere lesion may produce impairment of consciousness out of proportion to the size of the lesion. In such instances this is usually short-lived (Albert et al., 1976).

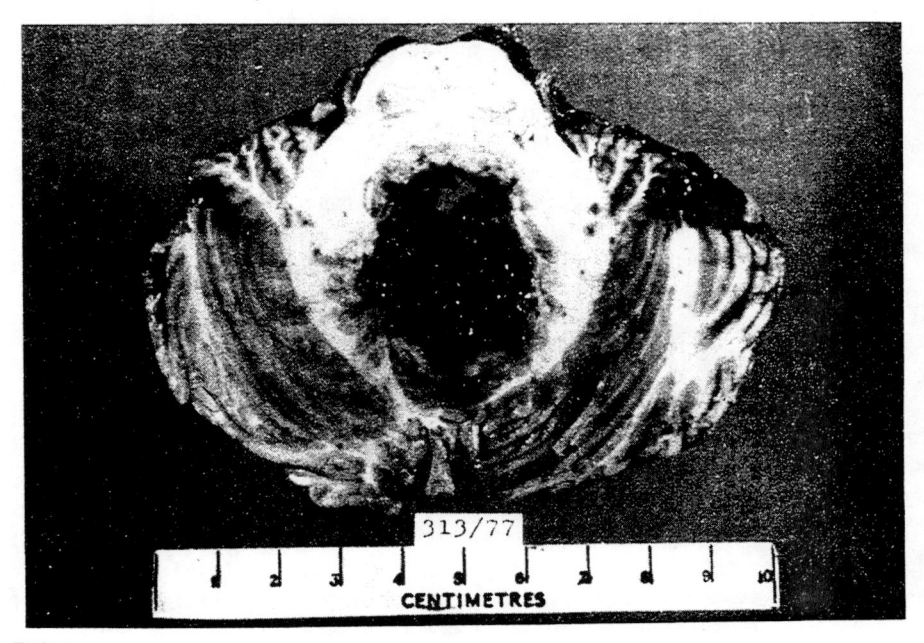

FIG. 1.

## Coma due to cerebral hemisphere lesions

To produce coma cerebral hemisphere disturbances must be diffuse and extensive. These may be structural such as diffuse anoxic damage, or metabolic such as hepatic dysfunction or hypoglycaemia.

## Coma due to lesions of the reticular formation

Discrete brain-stem lesions can readily damage the reticular formation. Lesions caudal to the lower pons do not produce coma but rostral to this level bilateral lesions, even if quite small, may cause coma. Brain-stem infarction or haemorrhage (Fig. 1) often causes coma though this is rare with brain-stem gliomas or brain-stem plaques of demyelination. Massive demyelination as seen in central pontine myelinolysis may impair consciousness.

Drug coma results largely from depression of the reticular formation though many drugs have additional effects on the cerebral cortex. Profound metabolic or anxic insults to the brain may also affect brain-stem structures as well as the cortex. Large diencephalic lesions interrupting ascending projections from the reticular formation to cortex may occasionally cause coma but, more often, such lesions are associated with akinetic mutism. Bilateral thalamic damage, though rare, may produce coma. It is usually due to occlusion of perforating arteries from the apex of the basilar artery.

## Coma from unilateral hemisphere or super-tentorial lesions

It is axiomatic that a localized unilateral supra-tentorial lesion will not in itself produce coma though it is common clinical experience that, for example, a patient with a unilateral cerebral haemorrhage is almost invariably unconscious. Whilst a unilateral hemisphere lesion may compromise consciousness by direct infiltration of ascending projections from the reticular formation, a more common mechanism is downward shift of the cerebral hemisphere with brain-stem distortion: the syndrome of rostro-caudal herniation (Figs 2 and 3).

## Differential diagnosis

The differential diagnosis of coma includes the locked-in syndrome in which the patient is alert and aware though tetraplegic with cranial nerve palsies below the level of eye movements, and the persistent vegetative state where patients are unaware though arousable and show spontaneous eye movements and eye-opening. A variety of psychiatric disorders, most particularly those associated with catatonia may be confused with coma though such patients usually have spontaneous eye-opening and are obviously aware, a factor which can be demonstrated by the preservation of a menace response to visual stimuli. Feigning of coma as in pseudo-coma is quite rare and readily diagnosed from true coma by the preservation of a normal oculovestibular response.

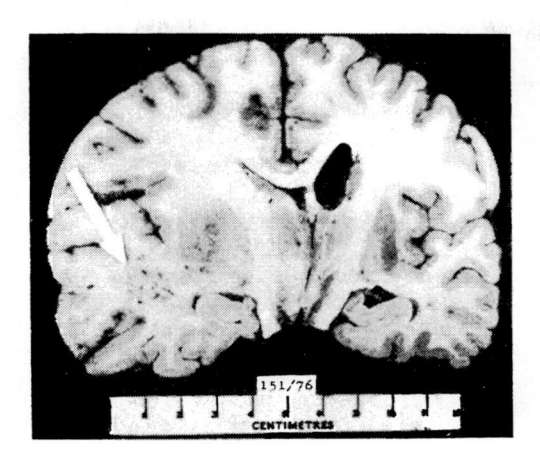

FIG.2.

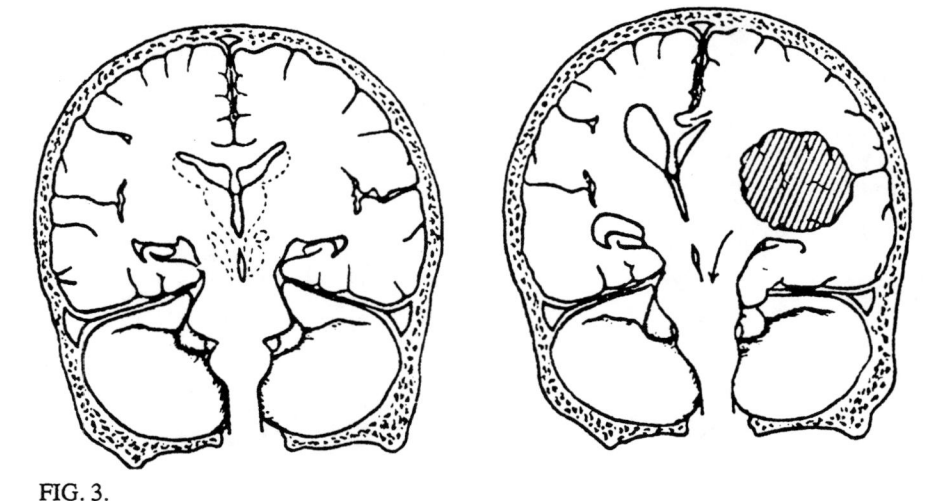

FIG. 3.

## References

Ad hoc committee of the Harvard Medical School to examine the definition of brain death. A definition of irreversible coma. *(1968). Journal of the American Medical Association,* **205**, 337-340.

Agardh, C.D., Folbergerova, J. and Siesjo, B.K. (1978). Cerebral metabolic changes in profound insulin induced hypoglycaemia and in the recovery period following glucose administration. *Journal of Neurological Chemistry,* **31**, 1135-1142.

Andrews, K. (1992). Managing persistent vegetative state. *British Medical Journal*, **305**, 486-7.
Berger, H. (1929). Uber das Elektrenkephalogramm des Menschen. *Archiv für Psychiatrishe Nervenkranktheit.*, **87**, 527-570.
Breasted, J.H. (1930). "The Edwin Smith Surgical Papyrus". The University of Chicago Press, Chicago, Illinois.
Bremer, F. (1937). l'Activite cérébrale au cours du sommeil et de la narcose. *Bulletin de l'Academie Royale Médicale Belgique*, **2**, 68-86.
Brodal, A. (1981). "Neurological Anatomy in Relation to Clinical Medicine". 3rd Edn. Oxford University Press, Oxford.
Carpenter, W.B. (1853). "Principles of Human Physiology". Blanchard and Lea, Philadelphia.
Cartlidge, N.E.F. (1981). Drug-induced coma. *Adverse Drug Reaction Bulletin*, **88**, 320-323.
Courville, C.B. (1955). "Commotio-Cerebri", San Lucas Press, Los Angeles.
Defeudis, F.V. (1974). Cholinergic roles in consciousness. *In* "Cholinergic Systems and Behaviour". (Ed. F.V. Defeudis). pp. 7-32. Academic Press, London.
Feldman, M.H. (1971). Physiological observations in a chronic case of locked-in syndrome. *Neurology*, **21**, 459-478.
Fischer, J.E. and Baldessarini, R.J. (1976). Pathogenesis and therapy of hepatic coma. *In* "Progress in Liver Disease." (Eds F. Schaeffner and H. Popper). Bruyn and Smith, New York.
Fredericks, J.A.M. (1969). Consciousness. *In* "Handbook of Clinical Neurology, Vol. 3. Disorders of Higher Nervous Activity". (Eds P.J. and G.W. Bruyn). North Holland Publishing Company, Amsterdam.
Grinker, I.M. (1945). Transtentorial herniation of the brain-stem: a characteristic clinico-pathologic syndrome: pathogenesis of haemorrhages in the brain-stem. *Archives of Neurology and Psychiatry*, **53**, 289-298.
Hubel, D.H. (1979). The brain. *Scientific American*, **241**, 38-48.
The International Consortium on Cerebral and Psychopathological Dysfunctions following Cardiac Surgery. Milwaukee County Mental Health Complex, Milwaukee, Wisconsin.
Jennett, B. and Teasdale, G. (1981). "Management of Head Injuries". F.A. Davis, Philadelphia.
Jennett, B., Teasdale, G., Braakman, R. *et al.* (1979). Prognosis of patients with severe head injury. *Neurosurgery*, **4**, 283-289.
Jennett, W.B. and Plum, F. (1972). The persistent vegetative state: A syndrome in search of a name. *Lancet*, **i**, 734-737.
Jorgensen, E.O. Malchow-Moller, A. (1981). Natural history of global and critical brain ischaemia. *Resuscitation*, **9**, 155-174.
Jouvet, M. (1972). The role of monoamines and acetyl choline containing neurones in the regulation of the sleep wake cycle. *Reviews of Physiology*, **64**, 166-307.
Larrabee, M.G. and Posternak, J.M. (1952). Selective action of anaesthetics on synapses and axons in mammalian sympathic ganglia. *Journal of Neurology and Physiology*, **15**, 91-114.
Lipowski, Z.J. (1985). Delirium (acute confusional state). *In* "Handbook of Clinical Neurology". Vol. 46. (Ed. J.A.M. Frederiks). pp. 523-559. Elsevier, Amsterdam.
Major, R.H. (1961). Galen as a neurologist. *World Neurology*, **2**, 372-376.
Medical Research Council Brain Injuries Committee. (1941). A glossary of psychological terms commonly used in cases of head injury. Medical Research Council War

Memorandum 4. London, HMSO.

Mollaret, P. and Goulon, M. (1959). Le coma dé passé. *Review of Neurology,* **101**, 3-15.

Moruzzi, G. and Magoun, H.W. (1963). Brain stem reticular formation and activation of the EEG. *Electroencephalography and Clinical Neurophysiology,* **1**, 455-473.

Perecman, E. (1987). "The Frontal Lobes Revisited". Lawrence Erlbaum, Hillsdale, New Jersey.

Przybyla, A.C. and Wang, S.C. (1968). Mechanisms of action of the benso-diazapines. *Journal of Pharmacology and Experimental Therapy,* **163**, 439-447.

Ripperger, E.A. (1975). The mechanics of brain injuries. *In* "Injuries of the Brain and Skull Part I. Handbook of Clinical Neurology". Vol. 23. (Eds P.J. Vinken and G.W. Bruyn). North Holland, Amsterdam.

Diagnosis of brain death (1976). A paper endorsed by the conference of the Royal Colleges and Faculties of the UK. *Lancet,* **ii**, 1069-1070.

Sigerist, H.E. (1967). "A History of Medicine" 1. Oxford University Press, New York.

Sussman, M. (1967). Diseases in the Bible and the Talmud, *In* "Diseases in Antiquity" Chapter 16. Brothwell and Sandison, Charles C. Thomas, Springfield, Illinois.

Tinuper P. *et al.* (1992). Idiopathic recurring Stupor: a case with possible involvement of the gamma-aminobutyric acid (GABA) ergic system. *Annals of Neurology,* **31**, 503-506.

Walker, A.E. (1951). "A History of Neurological Surgery". Haffner Publishing, New York.

Wells, C.E. (1985). Organic syndromes: delirium. *In* "Comprehensive Textbook of Psychiatry" Vol. 4. 4th Edn. (Eds H.I. Kaplan and B.J. Sadock). pp. 838-51. Williams and Wilkins, Baltimore.

# 25. Memory, disturbances of memory and human knowledge of reality and ourselves

Andrew R. Mayes

### Introduction

Our awareness of the outside world and of ourselves is clearly influenced by disturbances in our sensory and perceptual processes. It is not quite so obvious that disturbances of memory can affect awareness of ourselves and the outside world in a similarly dramatic way. Nevertheless, it is true. Our ability to make sense of what we perceive and of the outside world in general depends critically on our ability to acquire memories about the properties, functions and inter-relationships of things in the world such as hammers, cats and yachts, as well as our ability to acquire memories about the meanings of the words that are used to describe these things. These kinds of memory are known collectively as semantic memory. Semantic memory is progressively lost in patients with Alzheimer's disease, who suffer from an increasing difficulty in interpreting what they perceive and in understanding what other people are saying to them. For a patient with advanced Alzheimer's disease the world becomes a meaningless confusion. Some aphasic patients and patients who have suffered Herpes simplex encephalitis that has caused destruction of parts of the temporal association cortex also experience a more selective disturbance of their ability to make semantic sense of the world. For example, such patients may look at a picture of a frog and although they may know that it is an animal, they may still have no idea where it lives, how it reproduces, what it sounds like and how large it is. Clearly their experience of the world is seriously impoverished.

Other patients suffer from what is known as organic amnesia and forget much of what they experienced only minutes or even seconds earlier. This disturbance is known as anterograde amnesia. One famous patient with this condition, known by the initials H.M., had his medial temporal lobes removed in 1953 to treat an intractable epilepsy and consequently became severely amnesic. H.M. is aware that he is amnesic and in 1970 described his state in the following words "Every day is alone in itself, whatever enjoyment I've had, and whatever sorrow I've had... Right now, I'm wondering. Have I done or said anything amiss? You see at this moment everything looks clear to me, but what happened just before? That's what worries me. It's like waking from a dream; I just don't remember." H.M. and amnesic patients like him can make sense of the world they experience reasonably well at the time, but they rapidly forget what they have experienced so they frequently get confused about what situation they are in and how they got there. It has never been proved, but it seems likely that if a very young child had the same kind of brain damage as H.M., then it would acquire very few semantic memories and so would have great difficulty in making sense of the world as well as feeling that it was constantly waking from a dream. Amnesics also typically suffer from some degree of retrograde amnesia in which their ability to recall and recognize what happened before their brain damage is compromised. Although the condition can be mild, there are patients on record who still believe they are now as they were 20 or 30 years before and still doing the same thing. For example, one such patient (Hodges, personal communication) suffered a bilateral thalamic infarction in 1989 and became globally amnesic as a result. Although he left the navy in 1946, the most persistent feature of his autobiographical memory was that he was still in the navy, but currently on shore leave. Clearly, this patient was able only to access normally the earlier portions of his autobiography so that many of the intervening years of his personal history were typically impossible for him to recall. It seemed that all his memory searches used the guiding theme "I am in the navy and it is around 1945", and this inappropriate guide (which operated with almost delusional intensity) prevented him from accessing relevant and more recent episodes that were still held in storage.

Even when patients are not suffering from a severe organic amnesia, they may be showing one of a number of paramnesic disorders in which recall or recognition is in some way aberrant. The best known of these disorders is confabulation in which patients recall incorrect, sometimes bizarre, information in response to standard questions. For example, a patient of Barbizet (1970) suffered cranial damage in a car accident, but when asked about his accident two years later, he claimed that he had been piloting a plane which had crashed into a car that had strayed on to the runway. The patient persisted with this story even when shown a picture of his car, stating that he could not have crashed his car because he was in his plane at the time. He stuck with this story for many months eventually incorporating the truth about the car accident by saying "Would you believe my luck? On leaving the police station I had a second accident, in which my car was completely wrecked!" But he believed that this happened after his plane accident! More often, the patient's recall seems to be for genuine information for which the context has been confused. For example, a patient of Damasio *et al.* (1985) reported that she just graduated from a technical institute whereas it was, in fact, her daughter who had just graduated. Confabulators appear to believe that they are genuinely remembering. The condition shares certain features with reduplicative paramnesia and Capgras syndrome in which sufferers respectively believe that the place they are in is similar to, but distinct from the place that it actually is, and that the familiar-looking person they are with is, in fact an ingenious copy or an impostor of some kind. In these conditions, however, there appears to have been an inappropriate interpretation of a feeling of familiarity whereas with confabulation there appears to be an inappropriate feeling of familiarity associated with information that should not have been recalled. Inappropriate feelings of familiarity may arise in certain cases of temporal lobe epilepsy where déjà vu or jamais vu may be experienced as part of the aura. The notion of familiarity is not, however, a clear one. One might, for example, decide that one is genuinely remembering because one makes an automatic attribution that something has been experienced before because the "memory" has certain intrinsic features such as vividness or is processed with apparent ease. Or one might decide that the memory is genuine because it fits in so well with one's other memories and general knowledge. There may be no need to postulate the existence of a primitive feeling of familiarity that depends on activity in specific medial temporal lobe structures.

Although confabulation has been strongly associated with damage to the frontal lobes of the brain, it may constitute an exaggeration of processes that operate in normal human memory. Normal memory also seems to be subject to reconstructive distortions which occur after the time of initial learning. This process is illustrated in an experiment by Spiro (1980). He read to his subjects a short story about a couple, and, a few minutes after finishing the reading, he injected an apparently incidental afterthought either that the couple had or that they had not subsequently married. This detail either confirmed or conflicted with the story's theme. Recall of the story was tested two days, two weeks or six weeks later. At the longer intervals, subjects made "reconciling errors" in which the story was made consistent with the later conflicting detail. They were confident that they were accurately remembering these distortions just like confabulators. These distortions took time to develop because they were not present two days after the story was read. They were also abolished if subjects were told before the story was read to them that they would later be asked to remember the story. Although this immunization of reconstructive distortion is interesting, it is important to note that we do not deliberately set out to remember most things that we try to recall. Spiro's experiment, therefore, suggests that, when what happens does not make easy sense to us, what we later recall may contain several untrue components, but that we will be unable to distinguish these from genuine memories. Nevertheless, normal adults can accurately recall and recognize much of what has happened to them in their personal lives as well as about the world around them. But a screen comes down on all personal events experienced before the age of three or four in the average person. There appears to be no direct recall of anything experienced earlier than this, a phenomenon known as infantile amnesia.

The psychological literature contains studies of individuals who have exceptional memories. One such supermnemonist was the Russian journalist Shereshevskii, who was investigated by Luria (1968). This man could repeat back a list of 70 items without apparently reaching his limit. He was able to retain detailed memories of complex material for decades. Several features of Shereshevskii's memory are of interest. First, he had rich, multisensory imagery which he used to encode materials and later developed into a mnemonic system when he became a professional mnemonist. In fact, he had synaesthesia, an ability in which stimulation within one sensory modality evokes imagery in another. This undoubtedly increased the distinctiveness of the memories he created. Second, he could reorganize and elaborate on meaningless materials with great rapidity. These two features of Shereshevskii's memory are compatible with the view, held by many people, that supermnemonists do not differ in retentive power from the mass of humanity, merely in their ability to encode new information in a rich and distinctive fashion. For example, a man who started with the ability to repeat only seven digits was trained to encode in larger chunks so that he was eventually, after 18 months of practice, able to repeat back around 80 digits (Ericson et al., 1980). Gordon et al. (1984) have also described a man whose memory was as exceptional as other supermnemonists. After giving him detailed memory tests, however, they concluded that neither he nor some other supermnemonists, described in the literature, have unusual memory abilities. Rather, they argued that his and other supermnemonists' exceptional performance on tests depended on the use mnemonic techniques. However, Shereshevskii was able to retain memories perfectly for decades whereas most people find that even well rehearsed memories fade over such long time periods, so it seems more likely that he had exceptional retentive ability as well as unusual innate and acquired encoding abilities. People with rich encoding and powerful retentive abilities should have a much fuller access to their personal pasts and to useful information about the world than do most of us.

It is possible, however, that exceptional memory is a mixed blessing Shereshevskii's powerful imagery made it difficult for him to abstract the essential in a conversation, a problem that he described thus: "All this makes it impossible for me to stick to the subject we're discussing. It's not that I'm talkative. Say you ask me about a horse. There's also its colour and taste I have to consider. And this produces such a mass of impressions that if 'I' don't get the situation in hand, we won't get anywhere with the discussion. I have to deal not only with the word horse but with its taste, the yard it's penned in – which I can't seem to get away from myself.... It was only recently that I learnt to follow a conversation and stick to the subject." Although Shereshevskii's difficulty arose from his imagery, it is hard to identify to what extent this reflects a problem with a too copious memory. Nevertheless, it is interesting to note that in a short story, called "Funes, The Memorious" about a man who becomes a supermnemonist after a closed head injury (a good example of artistic licence – in real life, a head injury would be likely to have the opposite effect!), the Argentinian, Borges, suggests that an overly rich memory inhibits the ability to abstract: "Without effort, he had learned English, French, Portuguese, Latin. I suspect, nevertheless, that he was not very capable of thought. To think is to forget a difference, to generalize, to abstract. In the overly replete world of Funes there were nothing but details, almost contiguous details."

Memory can deteriorate because of stable or progressive damage to the brain or it can be exceptionally good, probably because an individual has a brain capable of rapid and distinctive encoding and great powers of retentiveness. But some individuals with relatively normal brains may suffer what is known as a psychogenic loss of memory. It is widely believed that this kind of forgetting is motivated although individuals do not realize that it is they who are blocking out particular memories. Certainly momentary lapses of memory occur at emotionally significant points during psychotherapy although this may result from arousal rather than repression. But more active repression may explain psychogenic amnesias or fugues in which the victim abruptly and totally forgets the events of a discrete period of time, linked to an emotional trauma. For example, a woman who was mischievously told that her husband had been killed was in extreme emotional turmoil for two days, and emerged from this state oblivious of the traumatic events. Even so, although the events were not consciously accessible, they were revealed in nightmares and through hypnosis (see Kihlstrom and Evans, 1979).

Fugue states have been related to several predisposing factors (Kopelman, 1987a). These include: (a) an emotional precipitating crisis that may involve marital, financial or battle stress, (b) the presence of a depressed mood, which may be associated with suicidal thoughts, and (c) a history of problems, such as head injury and alcoholic blackout, that could lead to some degree of organic amnesia. In convincing cases of fugue, however, an organic cause for the amnesia can be eliminated with some confidence although it is possible that the medical history may have provided the essential precondition for the occurrence of motivated forgetting. In severe fugue states of the kind typically represented in films, people may forget their past lives and even forget their personal identities, and go on to assume new identities with apparent lack of concern. This may be associated with a period of wandering away from the haunts frequented before the onset of the fugue state. Typically these amnesias are not permanent although they may persist for months or even years. It remains unclear to what degree the repression of so many personal memories is an unconscious process and to what degree consciousness of the repression enters the equation. It is certainly the case that lightly hypnotized subjects are aware that they are trying to repress target memories and many cases of apparent unconscious repression may involve frank malingering. One thing is clear: if and when fugue states are genuine they represent a massive distortion of a person's awareness of their personal history.

## A Simple Taxonomy of Organic Memory Disorders

The human brain does not only process sensory information, it also stores it. It is now generally believed that most regions of the brain (and possibly even the spinal cord) are plastic to some degree and are concerned with storing the kind of information that is represented by the neurons that they contain. If this heuristic is taken seriously (as it should be), one should not expect to find that memories are stored in brain structures which have nothing to do with processing the corresponding kind of information. Brain damage in different brain regions should also be expected to disturb different kinds of memory, and this is exactly what is found. There appear to be several groups of memory disorders that are caused by brain damage, which have more in common with each other then they do with memory disorders from the other groups (see Mayes, 1988).

The first group of disorders involves impairments of immediate memory for specific kinds of information that occur despite the fact that ability to encode the relevant information seems to be basically alright. For example, patients have been reported with selective immediate memory deficits for auditorily presented verbal material, visually presented verbal material, visuospatial material, and for colour information (see Mayes, 1987). These disorders are believed to be caused by lesions to the posterior association neocortex, the precise location of which will depend on the nature of the information for which immediate memory is disrupted. For example, with the best studied of these disorders, that which involves deficits in immediate memory for auditorily presented verbal information (or, more precisely, phonological information), lesions seem to concentrate particularly around the left inferior parietal lobe where it abuts the left temporal lobe (see McCarthy and Warrington, 1990) whereas impairments in immediate memory for visuospatial material are slightly more associated with right posterior association neocortex lesions (De Renzi and Nichelli, 1975). These disorders have been taken by some to provide evidence for the view that information passes in parallel into short-term and long-term memory systems rather than serially from a short-term into a long-term system. However, although patients with impaired phonological immediate memory show a normal ability to learn lists of spoken words and retain the gist of a spoken passage, Baddeley and Vallar have shown that an Italian woman with this deficit was completely unable to learn spoken associations between Italian numbers and Russian words (see Mayes, 1988). It seems very probable that her short- and long-term memory for phonological material was severely compromised, but that she was able to translate phonological representations into semantic ones rapidly and that her long-term memory for semantic information was preserved. The probability is that other immediate memory disorders are also accompanied by long-term memory deficits for the affected information. These disorders may not greatly affect patients' awareness of the outside world, largely because they involve only very specific kinds of information. For example, it is hard to show that patients with impaired immediate phonological memory are poor at understanding any kinds of spoken sentences although McCarthy and Warrington (1987) have argued that deficits are apparent when it is vital to backtrack over the information that has just been spoken.

Impairments of previously well-established memories concerned with semantic information about language and the world constitute the second group of memory disorders. Disorders of this group are caused by lesions in the posterior association neocortex, particularly in the temporal cortex (see Mayes, 1988). There is considerable controversy about (1) the degree of specificity shown by these disorders, and (2) whether they arise as a result of a storage or an access failure. Although patients with Alzheimer's disease typically have a global breakdown of their semantic memories, some surprisingly specific deficits have been reported. For example, Hart *et al.* (1985) described a patient with a selective inability to name fruits and vegetables. This patient could name in a normal fashion all other categories of objects, including food objects other than fruits and vegetables. He could also correctly categorize the written names of fruits and vegetables and correctly identify pictures corresponding to the spoken names of fruits and vegetables. It seems probable that this patient's semantic representations of fruits and vegetables were intact and that his deficit arose because of his difficulty in using these intact representations so as to access their corresponding names. Claims have been made about other specific deficits including selective impairments for previously familiar faces, colours, body parts, letters, numbers, abstract words, concrete words, grammatical words, inanimate objects, and animate objects. The bases for these claims are polemical and hard to assess as is illustrated by the claim that some patients show relatively selective impairments in their semantic memory for animate things. Although this is true at a descriptive level, in order to show that there is something special about living things it is necessary to compare knowledge of living and man-made objects that are matched not only in terms of the frequency with which they are encountered and their familiarity, but also of how complex they are and how similar they are to each other.

It is also very difficult to determine whether patients' deficits result from storage rather than access failures because there are no generally agreed criteria for deciding which is affected (see Mayes, 1988). The two most widely used criteria are (a) whether patients consistently succeed at, or fail to, retrieve specific items across occasions with consistency being taken as evidence that there has been a storage failure, and (b) whether patients can show normal memory for items that they cannot recall or recognize when memory is tested indirectly. Indirect memory tests make no reference to memory so that the presence of memory is inferred from a change in the way that subjects behave towards and process previously presented material. Most researchers believe that performance on such tests is mediated by item-specific implicit memory, an unconscious form of memory that depends on automatic retrieval processes. For example, if subjects are briefly shown words and non-words and have to decide when a word has been shown, this decision is facilitated if the target word is preceded by a semantically related word. If patients show such facilitation, then it seems likely that some of the semantic information is still stored even though their explicit memory, as indicated by recall and recognition, is grossly impaired. Whether or not one accepts that these criteria really do indicate whether storage or access has been degraded, it is certainly the case that patients with semantic memory disorders perform differently with respect to the criteria (see Mayes, 1988). It seems likely, therefore, that their memory deficits have somewhat distinct bases.

The third group of memory disorders is that associated with damage to the frontal lobes. The prefrontal association neocortex constitutes a substantial proportion of total neocortical volume and is subdivided into cytoarchitectonically distinct regions. It, therefore, seems likely that these regions will not have identical functions. Nevertheless, it has been suggested that the frontal lobes play a central role in planning behaviour (Luria, 1973) and, as planning must involve the operation of many subprocesses, this kind of view is compatible with different functions being located in different frontal lobe regions. One major view about the effects of frontal lobe lesions on memory functions states that all memory disturbances found are a result of disrupting planning operations. If frontal lobe lesions impair the ability to set up and maintain appropriate hypotheses, and use these to guide behaviour, as well as impairing the ability to shift hypotheses when the old ones no longer apply and inhibit now inappropriate tendencies, then they should cause difficulties in executing elaborative encoding and retrieval strategies. An alternative view, derived from work with monkeys, is associated with Goldman-Rakic (1992), who has postulated that the frontal lobes act as a working memory system. She believes that in different parts of the frontal lobes different kinds of representational memory (for example, spatial location memory) are kept activated or on line for long enough to modulate behaviour or allow further informational processing. This suggests that the frontal lobes must play a role in immediate memory. Nevertheless, if working memory is impaired, one would expect to see disturbances of the ability to plan so the predictions of the Goldman-Rakic model may not differ radically from the straightforward planning deficit model although some differences in the predictions of the two models have been suggested with the results favouring the working memory model (Daigneault *et al.*, 1992).

If planning abilities are disturbed either directly or because working memory is disrupted, then patients will be impaired on free recall, but not necessarily on recognition, of previously experienced information because recognition is much less influenced than recall by elaborative encoding and retrieval strategies. The hypothesis has received some support from studies showing that patients with frontal lobe lesions are impaired on free recall, but not on recognition of recently presented material (for example, see Janowsky *et al.*, 1989). There is also evidence that patients' recall can be improved so as to approach normal levels when they are given detailed directions about how to encode material (Signoret and Lhermitte, 1976). In this situation, the examiner substitutes for the patient's damaged frontal lobes. Although these findings support the planning deficit account of frontal lobe memory disorders, it has also been reported that a patient, RW, with a history of rupture and repair of an anterior communicating artery aneurysm, who was believed to have frontal damage, showed intact free recall and *impaired recognition* (Delbecq-Derouesne *et al.*, 1990). It is, however, possible to explain both selective free recall and selective recognition deficits in terms of planning deficits caused by frontal lobe lesions. In the words of Shallice (1988), "formulating the description of any memories that might be required and verifying that any candidate memories that are retrieved are relevant" are both clearly planning or supervisory operations. Selectively impaired recall would result if patients are poor at setting up suitable retrieval (or encoding) strategies whereas selectively impaired recognition would result if patients are poor at verifying or rejecting candidate memories. If correct, one implication would be that differently located frontal lobe lesions disrupt distinct planning operations (as has already been suggested) and these disruptions affect distinct aspects of memory.

Patient RW also confabulated and Shallice (1988) has argued that this disturbance, like the deficit in recognition, may be caused by a problem with the verification and rejection of candidate memories. Several points are worth noting about this interpretation. First, it may well be that frontal lobe lesions cause the form of confabulation, found in RW, because they disturb the feeling of familiarity that is essential to recognition. Specifically, the wrong memories feel to the patient to be as familiar as the correct ones. But this still needs to be proved. Second, other confabulators may also be impaired at setting up suitable retrieval strategies so that they generate inappropriate cues and consequently trigger the wrong memories. Once wrong memories are triggered, they may have great difficulty in rejecting them because, for unknown reasons, the false memories seem as familiar as correct ones. Third, although patients with large frontal lobe lesions have occasionally been reported to show very impaired recognition performance, similar impairments have been reported after large posterior cortex lesions (Warrington, 1984). These deficits could be amnesic in which case it is likely that the lesions must extend into the limbic-diencephalic regions traditionally associated with amnesia. Alternatively, they could be associated with cortical lesions with the frontal recognition deficit arising from an as yet unspecified deficit in familiarity and the posterior recognition deficit arising from a different, unknown cause.

Organic amnesia constitutes the fourth group of memory disorders. In its pure form it is a syndrome characterized by four symptoms: first, anterograde amnesia, which is a deficit in the ability to recall or recognize recently experienced facts and events; second, retrograde amnesia, which is a deficit in the ability to recall or recognize facts and events that were encountered up to decades before the brain damage that caused the amnesia; third, the preservation of intelligence; and fourth, the preservation of immediate memory. The detailed features of this syndrome will be discussed more fully in the next section, but it is worth noting here that it can be caused by lesions in several distinct brain regions. It is known to be caused by lesions to the medial temporal lobes, which may occur subsequent to an anoxic episode, Herpes Simplex encephalitis, or an infarction of the posterior cerebral artery. It can also be caused by lesions to the midline diencephalon, which may occur after paramedian artery infarctions or as a result of chronic alcoholism that is associated with poor diet. There is also more controversial evidence that it is caused by lesions to basal forebrain structures consequent upon rupture and repair of anterior communicating artery aneurysms (Gade, 1982). One interpretation of the fact that amnesia can be independently caused by lesions in several brain regions is that the disorder is functionally heterogeneous. This interpretation is not necessarily correct, however, because the medial temporal lobes have reciprocal connections to the midline diencephalon and both these regions have bilateral links with the basal forebrain which probably modulates their activity. There is some evidence that lesions to fibre tracts, such as the fornix, which connect medial temporal lobe structures to the midline diencephalon, can cause a mild amnesia (Hodges and Carpenter, 1991). So it remains possible that amnesia is the result of a single processing disorder although such a view is somewhat against the Zeitgeist of contemporary cognitive neuropsychology. Whether or not classical amnesia is caused by a single processing deficit, there may be closely related disorders which affect only some of the kinds of memory disrupted in the classical syndrome. For example, lesions to particular parts of the anterior temporal lobes cause a relatively selective retrograde amnesia. One young woman, who suffered damage to this region, but not to the regions usually associated with amnesia, showed a retrograde amnesia for both public events and autobiographical information, but only a mild and patchy anterograde amnesia (Kapur et al., 1992).

There are several other groups of memory disorders, but these involve disturbances of simpler kinds of memory and are unlikely to influence greatly the conscious experience of reality. These include disorders of classical conditioning, disorders of various kinds of skill memory, and disorders of what may be referred to as non-associative memory. All these kinds of memory are sometimes described as implicit because people are not aware directly of what is being remembered. This clearly applies to memory for skills where subjects learn to do something with great efficiency, but are unable to describe what it is that they are doing. This automatic form of memory seems to be mediated by the basal ganglia although other subcortical structures are also likely to be involved (see Mayes, 1988).

## Amnesia and Item-specific Implicit Memory

Although amnesics are very impaired at recalling and recognizing information about facts and events that they have recently experienced, it has long been known that other kinds of memory appear to be preserved in these patients. Thus, there is good evidence that amnesics show no impairment in acquiring classically conditioned responses, or in the acquistion and retention of motor, perceptual, and cognitive skills, or various kinds of perceptual after effects that must depend on memory (see Shimamura, 1989). For example, it has been shown that amnesics showed the same biasing effects in their judgements about the weights of objects as a result of having previously lifted a set of either heavy or light objects (Shimamura, 1989).

The most theoretically interesting kind of memory that it has been claimed may be preserved in amnesics is item-specific implicit memory. In indirect memory tasks, where no reference is made to the relevance of memory for performance, subjects frequently behave differently towards a repeated stimulus or an item that is related to a previously shown stimulus. The behavioural change indicates that the repeated item is being processed differently or more efficiently than equivalent non-repeated items. For example, if words are shown to subjects and then later those words together with other similar, but previously unshown words, are flashed very briefly on a screen, then the subjects will be better at identifying the repeated words. This increase in processing efficiency is hypothesized to be mediated by implicit memory, which depends on automatic retrieval processes and does not give rise to a direct awareness that the relevant item was experienced in the recent past.

There is no generally agreed theory of how implicit memory works or how it relates to explicit memory (recall and recognition, which to some degree involve effortful retrieval processes and which are, of course, associated with the awareness that the remembered items have been encountered before). At one extreme, it is held that implicit memory depends on automatic retrieval from newly created memories for episodes and at the other, it is believed that it depends on the continued activation (or biasing) of memory representations that either preceded the "priming" experience or were newly created (see Mayes, 1992 for a discussion). What is of perhaps most interest is that memory for the same information seems to be possible to tap either implicitly or explicitly. Although some workers have suggested that item-specific implicit and explicit memory depend on different memory systems, and, therefore, must presumably be mediated by separate memory representations, this view seems implausible and it is more parsimonious to assume, until it is proved otherwise, that both kinds of memory are mediated by a single kind of memory representation (see Mayes, 1992). If amnesics show preservation of item-specific implicit memory for all kinds of novel information, therefore, this would be strong support for the view that not only is their encoding of information normal, but so is their storage, and that their deficit must be one of retrieval.

There is now good support for the view that amnesics do show normal implicit memory for both verbal and nonverbal items, memory for which existed prior to any "priming" experience (see Mayes, 1992). The issue is more undecided with novel information. It could be claimed that studies have shown consistently that amnesics perform normally on indirect memory tasks that tap memory for novel nonverbal items (like unknown faces or complex and meaningless drawings), but that amnesics did not always show normal performance in indirect memory tasks that tapped memory for novel verbal information (for example, see Mayes and Gooding, 1989). It is, however, most unlikely that amnesics will show this kind of material-specificity with their implicit memory. What is more likely is that performance on indirect memory tasks is not usually mediated solely by implicit memory, but that, with normal people at least, performance is also influenced by explicit memory processes. If this is correct, then amnesics may perform subnormally on some indirect memory tasks even though they show complete preservation of implicit memory.

There is a need to develop indirect memory tasks that are likely to depend entirely or almost entirely on implicit memory. Two kinds of task fulfil this desideratum reasonably well. The first involves the use of reaction time reductions as an indication of the presence of implicit memory. For example, if subjects are shown pairs of novel faces and asked to decide as rapidly as possible whether the picture pairs represent one person or two different people, it has been shown that when the picture pairs are repeated, subjects make same/different judgements more rapidly (Paller et al., 1992). As the responses are made in this kind of task in around one second or just over, it is less probable that there will have been sufficient time for relevant information to have been retrieved explicitly so as to speed up the response. The second kind of task involves the use of changes in autonomic responses to indicate the presence of implicit memory. The assumption is that autonomic responses are automatically mediated and much less likely to be influenced by the kinds of effortful, aware processes that underlie explicit memory. There is a small amount of published evidence which suggests that amnesics, like normal people, show different skin conductance responses to repeated words and faces whether or not these words or faces are recognized (see Mayes, 1992). In unpublished work, a research student of mine, Bruce Diamond, has shown in two separate memory tasks, that amnesics can show completely normal discriminative autonomic responses to repeated words as indicated by changes in skin conductance, heart rate and pupillary dilation. This work now needs to be extended so that implicit memory for different kinds of novel information can be tested.

A third approach to the problem of obtaining purer measures of implicit memory can be derived from work of Jacoby (see Jacoby and Kelly, 1992). Using a modification of Jacoby's procedure, it is possible to develop a method of directly assessing the strength of implicit and explicit memory in particular tasks. The modification allows for the fact that subjects may use different decision criteria and gives independent estimates of memory strength and bias. Like Jacoby's original procedure, the modified procedure assumes that implicit and explicit memory are independent of each other rather than positively or negatively related. Using the modified procedure another of my research students, Claire Isaac, has found preliminary evidence that amnesics may show preserved implicit memory for recently perceived names even though they are very impaired at recollecting these names. If the three approaches give similar results, then one can be relatively confident about asserting whether or not amnesics show preservation of implicit memory for all kinds of novel information. At present, we do not know the answer, but the balance of evidence seems to be tipping in favour of the possibility of preservation.

Whether or not they show complete preservation of all kinds of implicit memory, amnesics certainly do seem to show considerable signs of unconsciously remembering many things that they are unable to recall or recognize. Their current behaviour is, therefore, being influenced by many past experiences that they are unable consciously to remember. This phenomenon may be far more common in amnesics than in normal people. Nevertheless, it seems probable that the behaviour, feelings, and attitudes of everyone are influenced to some extent by past experiences that can no longer be consciously remembered.

## Confabulation and Distortion in Normal Memory

One problem that some, but apparently not all, amnesic patients show is a disproportionate deficit in remembering the source from which information was derived. This has been shown in experiments where lists of trivial (and previously unknown) facts, such as "Bob Hope's father was a fireman", are taught to subjects. In these experiments, some amnesics are much poorer than normal people at remembering the source of the facts (for example, whether they heard them in the experimental situation or elsewhere) even when the normal people are tested at much longer delays so as to equate their explicit memory for the facts with that of the patients (for example, see Shimamura and Squire, 1991). One explanation of why problems of this kind are found in only some amnesics is that source amnesia is caused by frontal lobe lesions (see Shimamura et al., 1990). Source amnesia may occur in frontal lobe patients who show normal memory for the facts themselves (Janowsky et al., 1990). It also seems to be a feature of ageing (Rabinowitz, 1989), and there is a strong association between ageing and atrophy of the frontal lobes of the brain. As confabulation that may be very persistent is a feature of some patients with frontal lobe lesions (see Stuss et al., 1978), it is possible that source amnesia is causally related to confabulation, or at least, to some forms of confabulation.

Confabulation usually arises in situations where we are recollecting the past (or previously learnt factual information) either spontaneously or in response to question probes. Memories about our past or about factual information comprise a large number of associations between the components that were encoded together during the relevant learning experience. If storage has not been degraded so that most of these links have been lost, then the re-encoding of some of these components during recollection should automatically activate many of the other components of the relevant memory. If the components of the memory have fragmented to some extent as a result of decay (see Jones, 1979), then it may be necessary to re-encode several components of the original memory if most of the critical components of the original memory are to be re-activated. Effective recollection, therefore, involves operating a plan to maximize the chances of re-encoding key features of the target memory so as to re-activate the rest of it. Another way of characterizing it is as a process of generating memory cues that are initially extrinsic to a target memory in order to generate cues that are intrinsic to the memory (part of it) so as to re-activate the whole memory. This process is not necessarily just a simple unidirectional one because the encoding of an intrinsic cue may lead to the encoding of other extrinsic cues that are effective generators of further intrinsic cues. For example, in order to remember what you were doing on your 21st birthday you may have to determine where you were living at that stage of your life (extrinsic cue) so as to remember that you were with X (intrinsic cue). This may be insufficiently linked to the rest of your memory to re-activate it, but leads you to re-encode the information that you usually saw X and Y (extrinsic cue). You do not remember being with Y on this occasion, but you usually went to a particular pub with Y (intrinsic cue) and that is where you were on your birthday, having a party. However, it should be apparent from the experiment of Spiro (1980), described in the introduction to this chapter, that memories may not only be automatically reactivated via the re-encoding of intrinsic cues, but may also be reconstructed from extrinsic cues, and that people have great difficulty in knowing which one of these they are doing. Patients with frontal lobe lesions are likely to be impaired at operating an effective plan for recollection and so may engage in wild reconstructions from extrinsic cues much more often than normal people.

Once information comes to mind in the process of recollection it is necessary to decide whether it represents an appropriate and genuine memory. It is very often difficult to decide whether the recollected information is part of a target memory or comes from a similar, but distinct memory. In the extreme, it may even be hard to decide whether something that comes to mind in a recollective situation is related to any genuine memory, let alone the correct one. It has been suggested by Johnson (1991) that monitoring of the reality of a memory depends on two kinds of judgement processes. The first is a nondeliberative kind of evaluation of the characteristics of information that comes to mind, particularly with respect to its perceptual detail. For example, when what comes to mind seems vivid and detailed, we are more inclined to believe that what it represents is a genuine memory. We normally check this inclination against a second and more deliberative evaluation process that assesses the meaningful content of what comes to mind in the context of our other memories and knowledge. Johnson suggests that patients who have experienced a cingulectomy may sometimes slip into confabulation because they have unusually vivid mental experiences that pass an initial reality monitoring check. One such patient (Whitty and Lewin, 1957) believed at first that his wife had visited him earlier in the day because the scene of the visit presented itself so clearly to him. Only when he checked by using the second, more deliberative judgemental process did he realize that he had remembered falsely. Patients with frontal lobe lesions seem to confabulate more often because they are impaired at the second kind of judgemental process which enables one to determine that an apparent memory just does not fit in with one's other memories and knowledge. One kind of information that may be critical for this second kind of judgement process is that concerning the contextual markers of the target information or information about the source of that target material. It is possible to be recalling genuine episodes, but they may be from the wrong context or even drawn from a concatenation of several wrong contexts. The process of deciding whether information is drawn from a correct context involves complex reasoning of a kind at which patients with frontal lobe lesions may be particularly bad.

Normal people do not usually confabulate in the dramatic way that is apparent in some amnesics and patients with frontal lobe damage. But they do make reconstructive errors in recollection and these probably can be explained in the same way as confabulation in patients. In other words, normal people also sometimes fail to set up and execute adequate search plans during recollection so that false memories are produced, and these may sometimes not be eliminated because an adequate checking procedure is not performed. These failures are, however, far more common in patients, particularly those with frontal lobe lesions.

**Psychogenic Amnesia**

As discussed in the Introduction, there are situations where subjects, whose general ability to recollect seems unimpaired, forget specific episodes from their past life. Two examples, not considered before, further illustrate the phenomenon. The first is multiple personality as popularized by the story of Dr Jekyll and Mr Hyde. As with the Stevenson story, there are typically two personalities (although there may be more), one of whom represents the frustrated desires of the other. The characteristic of relevance here is that one personality may not know of the existence of the other. In other words, there may be an asymmetric amnesia, which is presumably motivated by a desire to avoid an intolerable reality. The amnesia is interesting because the person is only amnesic about the activities of personality B when in the role of personality A. The deficit is, therefore, a highly selective one. This disorder is rare and may be somewhat subject to fashion as reported cases became rarer at least up until the 1960s. As with all psychogenic amnesias, it is very hard to determine when the sufferer is malingering and when they are unaware that they are in some way repressing their recall. If genuine, the owner of personality A in the above example, just like Dr Jekyll, must live an existence with no proper continuity and some very disturbing gaps in it.

Amnesia is not uncommonly associated with crimes, and is seen most often with homicide cases. Between 25% and 45% of the perpetrators of homicide claim amnesia for the crime and although the length of the amnesic gap varies it usually includes an anterograde component as well as a retrograde one (that is, the forgetting covers a period after as well as before the crime). Non-violent crimes are only occasionally associated with claims of amnesia and this is perhaps because the amnesia is related to high levels of emotional arousal, which tends to be most extreme in cases of homicide. But the amnesia is also often associated with alcoholic intoxication and florid psychosis. Particularly when alcohol is involved, the amnesia may be caused largely by impaired initial encoding of the event itself, although the use of alcohol may also be associated with the kind of retrieval failure found in state-dependent forgetting. In this form of forgetting, recall is very poor because of the change in internal state (drug induced) between learning and test, which reduces the availability of relevant cues. State-dependent forgetting effects may also be associated with emotional changes between the crime and attempts at later recall. For example, it is reported that Sirhan Sirhan, who was in a state of extreme arousal when he killed Robert Kennedy, and who was subsequently amnesic for the crime, later apparently recovered his memory of it when hypnosis was used to induce a similar highly aroused state. Whether amnesia for crime is ever caused by an unconscious process of repression similar to that believed to underlie fugue states still needs to be convincingly demonstrated (see Kopelman, 1987*b*). Nevertheless, provided confounding factors like epilepsy (which would diminish responsibility) are absent, the presence of amnesia carries no legal implications so deceiving the authorities is not a reason for feigning the condition.

If psychogenic forms of amnesia can be caused by an unconscious process of repression that blocks retrieval of explicit memories, it is hard to prove when it is present and harder still to determine how it operates. Unlike the active processes that are involved in recollection, those involved in repression are not intended to lead to appropriate extrinsic and intrinsic cues so that target memories can be reactivated. Rather, they are intended to draw attention away from the identification of these appropriate cues. How this process operates may best be investigated through the examination of hypnotic amnesia, which may also help determine how such active processes can operate without the amnesic subject being aware of them.

## Conclusion

Memory processes are fallible even in people with healthy brains. This is partly because we cannot store all relevant information about the past and about the world and because even that which we store initially may fade from storage as time passes. But it is also because the process of reactivating memories about complex facts and events is an active process, which is subject to various kinds of distortion. These distortions are greatly exaggerated after certain kinds of brain damage such as that to the frontal lobes of the brain. The storage processes and storage sites themselves may be damaged by other kinds of brain damage, such as that to the posterior association cortices. But it remains controversial whether amnesia is caused by a storage deficit or a different kind of retrieval deficit from that caused by frontal lobe lesions. Even when all the normal memory processes are capable of operating, it seems to be the case that certain people may block the active processes of recollection without being fully aware that they are doing so. Everyone, therefore, has some problem in accessing the past and those items of factual information about the world that enable us to make sense of the present. This problem even applies to the supermnemonists. Even though these people may be able to access more information than most of us, some of them at least have more difficulty than most of us in abstracting those items that are most salient for the current situation.

## Acknowledgements

I would like to thank Dr John Downes for providing me with the Borges short story "Funes, The Memorious", for several helpful discussions and for his comments on the manuscript.

## References

Barbizet, J. (1963). Etude clinique sur la mémoire. *Semaine des Hôpitaux de Paris*, 39, (20), 931-950 and no. 21, 983-995.

Daigneault, S., Braun, C.M.J. and Whitaker, H.A. (1992). An empirical test of two opposing theoretical models of prefrontal function. *Brain and Cognition*, 19, 48-71.

Damasio, A.R., Graff-Radford, N.R., Eslinger, P.J., Damasio, H. and Kassell, N. (1985). Amnesia following basal forebrain lesion. *Archives of Neurology*, 42, 252-259.

De Renzi, E. and Nichelli, P. (1975). Verbal and nonverbal short term memory impairments following hemispheric damage. *Cortex*, 11, 341-353.

Delbecq-Derouesne, J., Beauvois, M.F. and Shallice, T. (1990). Preserved recall versus impaired recognition, *Brain*, 113, 1045-1074.

Ericson, K.A., Chase, W.G. and Faloon, S. (1980). Acquisition of a memory skill. *Science*, 208, 1181-1182.

Gade, A. (1982). Amnesia after operations on aneurysms of the anterior communicating artery. *Surgical Neurology*, 18, 46-49.

Goldman-Rakic, P.S. (1992). Working memory and the mind. *Scientific American*, 267, 72-79.

Gordon, P., Valentine, E. and Wilding, J. (1984). One man's memory: a study of a mnemonist. *British Journal of Psychology*, 75, 1-14.

Hart, J., Berndt, R.S. and Caramazza, A. (1985). Category-specific naming deficit following cerebral infarction. *Nature*, 316, 439-440.

Hodges, J.R. and Carpenter, K. (1991). Anterograde amnesia with fornix damage following removal of third ventricle colloid cyst. *Journal of Neurology, Neurosurgery and Psychiatry*, 54, 633-638.

Janowsky, J.S., Shimamura, A.P. and Squire, L.R. (1989a). Source memory impairment in patients with frontal lobe lesions. *Neuropsychologia*, 27, 1043-1056.

Janowsky, J.S., Shimamura, A.P., Kritchevsky, M. and Squire, L.R. (1989b). Cognitive impairment following frontal lobe damage and its relevance to human amnesia. *Behavioural Neuroscience*, 103, 548-560.

Johnson, M.K. (1991). Reality monitoring: evidence from confabulation in organic brain disease patients. *In* "Awareness of Deficit after Brain Injury: Clinical and Theoretical Issues". (Eds G.P. Prigatano and D.L. Schacter). Oxford University Press, New York.

Jones, G.V. (1979). Analysing memory by cuing: intrinsic and extrinsic knowledge. *In* "Tutorial Essays in Psychology: a guide to recent advances". Vol. 2. (Ed. N.S. Sutherland). Erlbaum, Hillsdale, New Jersey.

Kapur, N., Ellison, D., Smith, M.P., McLellan, D.L. and Burrows, E.H. (1992). Focal retrograde amnesia following bilateral temporal lobe pathology: a neuropsychological and magnetic resonance study. *Brain*, 115, 73-85.

Kihlstrom, J.F. and Evans, F.J. (1979). "Functional Disorders of Memory". Erlbaum, Hillsdale, New Jersey.

Kopelman, M.D. (1987a). Amnesia: organic and psychogenic. *British Journal of Psychiatry,* **148**, 517-525.

Kopelman, M.D. (1987b). Crime and amnesia: A review. *Behavioural Sciences and the Law,* **5**, 323-342.

Luria, A.R. (1968). "The Mind of a Mnemonist". Published by Penguin Education in 1975.

Luria, A.R. (1973). "The Working Brain". Penguin, Harmondsworth.

McCarthy, R.A. and Warrington, E.K. (1987). Understanding: a function of short-term memory? *Brain,* **110**, 1565-1578.

Mayes, A.R. (1987). Human organic memory disorders. *In* "Psychology Survey 6". (Eds H. Beloff and A.M. Colman). The British Psychological Society, Letchworth.

Mayes, A.R. (1988). "Human Organic Memory Disorders". Cambridge University Press. Cambridge.

Mayes, A.R. (1992). Automatic memory processes in amnesia: how are they mediated? *In* "The Neuropsychology of Consciousness". (Eds Milner A.D. and Rugg, M.D.). Academic Press, London.

Mayes, A.R. and Gooding, P. (1989). Enhancement of word completion priming in amnesics by cueing previously novel associates. *Neuropsychologia,* **27**, 1057-1072.

Paller, K.A., Mayes, A.R. Thompson, K.M., Roberts, J. and Meudell, P.R. (1992). Priming of face matching in amnesia. *Brain and Cognition,* **18**, 46-59.

Rabinowitz, J.C. (1989). Judgements of origin and generation effects: Comparison between young and elderly adults. *Psychology and Aging,* **4**, 259-268.

Shallice, T. (1988). "From Neuropsychology to Mental Structure". Cambridge University Press, Cambridge.

Shimamura, A.P. (1989). Disorders of memory: the cognitive science perspective. *In* "Handbook of Neuropsychology". Vol. 3. (Eds L. Squire and Gainotti). Elsevier, Amsterdam.

Shimamura, A.P. and Squire, L.R. (1991a). What is the role of frontal lobe damage in memory disorder? *In* "Frontal Lobe Function and Injury" (Eds H.S. Levin, H.M. Eisenberg and A.L. Benton). Oxford University Press, New York.

Shimamura, A.P. and Squire, L.R. (1991b). The relationship between fact and source memory: findings from amnesic patients and normal subjects. *Psychobiology,* **19**, 1-10.

Signoret, J.L. and Lhermitte, F. (1976). The amnesic syndromes and the encoding process. *In* "Neural Mechanisms of Learning and Memory". (Eds M.R. Rosenzweig and E.L. Bennett). MIT Press, Cambridge, Mass.

Spiro, R.J. (1980). Accommodative reconstruction in prose recall. *Journal of Verbal Learning and Verbal Behaviour,* **19**, 84-95.

Stuss, D.T., Alexander, M.P., Lieberman, A. and Levine, H. (1978). An extraordinary form of confabulation. *Neurology,* **28**, 1166-1172.

Warrington, E.K. (1984). "Recognition Memory Test". NFER Publishing Company, Windsor.

Whitty, C.W.M. and Lewin, W. (1957). Vivid day-dreaming: an unusual form of confusion following anterior cingulectomy. *Brain,* **80**, 72-76.

# 26. The constraints of language

E.M.R. Critchley

If we regard communication as the exteriorization of the innate capacities of the human brain, the hypothetical possibilities for future development are boundless, exceeding the predictions of our wildest imagination. Man has in his possession a delicate and intricate instrument whose potential he has yet to realize, with which he tinkers without understanding. In a series of unanticipated evolutionary strides the human brain has been transformed, surpassing that of other animals. The phenomenon of prolonged fetalization represents one of the most far-reaching life-thrusts within the evolution of the animal kingdom. The increase in the capacity of the skull, the result of delayed closure of the sutures in the neonatal period, enables a threefold increase in brain size to be effected in infancy. By avoiding a rapid maturation and elaboration of structure, previously dictated by the necessities of survival of the fittest, the pluripotency of the cell provides a greater compass of development than hitherto. The child, up to and well beyond puberty, is nurtured through years of perpetuated immaturity wherein myelination is delayed, the receptivity of boutons terminaux is repeatedly modified, synaptic connexions increase in complexity, and the modulation of neurotransmitter substances is finely tuned. Thus the foundations are laid for prolonged receptivity of the learning process: receiving, storing and learning to utilize information and instruction from other members of the species.

A comparable fecund serendipity applies to the spectacular creation of hierarchies of language as a component of the evolutionary process. "The natural law governing the formulation of guttural laryngeal sounds and mouth clicks do not account for the combinations of sounds into words controlled by a vocabulary. Similarly the rules regulating the development of vocabulary do not presuppose the formation of sentences controlled by syntax and grammar. At each stage the principles governing the isolated particulars of a lower level leave indeterminate conditions to be controlled by a higher principle. Consequently, the operation of a higher level cannot be accounted for by the laws governing its particulars on the next lower level" (Polyani, 1968). Vocabulary is not derived automatically from phonetics, nor grammar from vocabulary: a correct use of grammar does not anticipate style or content as in the prose or poetry of Shakespeare or Milton. Speech did not lead inevitably to writing or the written word to the advanced audio-visual devices of today.

We may continue on this tide of evolutionary optimism. Language thrives on change becoming a more flexible and powerful instrument for the expression of new propositions and ideas. The whole vocabulary of language has moved from the designation of what is coarse, gross, more material, to the designation of what is finer, more abstract and conceptual, more formal (Dwight Whitney). The proportion of verbs used in everyday speech has lessened with a corresponding increase in the number of nouns and adjectives. Compared to our ancestors, both our formal and vernacular speech have become simpler, freer, and more generic. Neologisms, acronyms and other vogue words are constantly created to add to or enlarge our experience. Foreign languages are open to us from travel, cassettes and the media. Dead languages such as Latin and Greek provide the stems from which we can synthesize novel terminologies to provide the framework for discoveries in the sciences. Algebra and computer languages are merely the starting point for a galaxy of new symbolism.

There is a price for almost every advance in the technology of communication. Even speech lacks the warmth of tactile communication. Writing does not reflect the beauty of the voice nor the wealth of gesture and expression which may enhance the spoken word. But, with greater elaboration and refinement, nuances of speech can reciprocate emotional feelings previously confined to touch, and a more extensive written vocabulary replicate in print inflexions previously expressible only through speech. Thus the mutations of language mimic the mutations of the natural world confering initially a form of balanced polymorphism before a more distinctive advantage is apparent.

Whilst emphasizing the potential of language, it needs to be stated that man does not possess an unrestrained ability to make full use of that potential; indeed the constraints are enormous. Psychic processes are involved at each stage in the initiation and interpretation of communication. Anatomical structures are activated in the act of speaking, and even hearing is not entirely a passive function. The brain is the site not only of conceptual thought but also of automatic behaviours. What is exteriorized through speech is rarely a distillate of the intellect but more commonly a mishmash of propositional and non-propositional utterances, articulated and vocalized. In certain circumstances – as in the dark or speaking on the telephone – articulation alone must suffice: at other times it may be enhanced by facial expression and gesture. Similarly comprehension is dependent upon hearing, aided by the expressions and mannerisms of the speaker. Sounds cannot be excluded from hearing, but through vigilance certain sounds may appear more meaningful than others; thus a mother may recognize the cry of her baby or a party-goer realize that someone is mentioning his own name on the other side of a crowded room. Ease of understanding can be helped by observation of the facial expression of the speaker and by lip-reading; but even the most skilful lip-reader needs to guess 9 out of 10 words (Sutcliffe, 1964).

## The Motor Mechanism for Speech

The motor apparatus required for speech has evolved in a more readily understandable way than that discussed hitherto but necessarily imposes limitations as well as freedom on speech production.

The ululations, cries and calls of the higher vertebrates depend on a bellows and reed system involving the lungs and laryngeal sphincter. Sound is produced by phonation – the release of controlled bursts of air by the larynx. The release of phonated air provides the requisite volume for the sound. The rate at which the vocal cords open and close determines the fundamental frequency of phonation. In order to convert the phonated breath into speech it is modified by movement of the muscles of articulation and given resonance by passage through the pharynx, nasal and buccal cavities.

We owe our present knowledge of the comparative anatomy of the respiratory passages to the outstanding contributions of Sir Victor Negus. The stages of evolution he adumbrated, and his principal suppositions, are still accepted with a minimum of criticism. He found that the laryngeal sphincter of the lung fish was relatively crude. It was not until a much later stage of evolution was reached, when animals first took to an arboreal habitat, that a more delicate control over this sphincter appears. A monkey swinging from branch to branch relies upon his arms to grip firmly and support the whole weight of his body. The unyielding grip must be matched by the secure connection of the shoulder girdle to the rest of the body. The arms must be fastened securely to the animal's trunk to obtain full purchase from the muscles. The muscles fixing the shoulder girdle take origin from the rib cage and, if the ribs are to form a stable base from which to contract the muscles, the ribs must also be held firm relative to the rest of the body. Theoretically, this might have been achieved by more powerful abdominal muscles fixing the ribs to the pelvic girdle but to do so would require an enormous expenditure of muscular energy. A strong laryngeal sphincter closing to contain a fixed amount of air within the lungs achieves exactly the same effect with great economy of effort.

Among arboreal monkeys the inlet valve (the inferior thyroartenoid folds or false vocal cords) is particularly effective as a valve able to exclude all but a definite volume of air. By comparison, although the control is still highly developed, the inlet valve of terrestrial anthropoids which have abandoned life in the trees is structurally less efficient. In man this valve is more rounded and lacks the sharp edge of the valve of lemurs or chimpanzees.

In most animals the vocal cords function essentially as a sphincter situated high in the pharynx and protecting the lungs and trachea. However, the sound quality of a larynx in close proximity to the tongue is very limited. Human speech is helped by the descent of the vocal cords and larynx enabling the frequencies of phonation to be modified within the hypopharynx. The larynx is high at birth when its sphincter functions are most needed but descends during childhood. Thus the child gradually acquires facility for speech in the first years of life. In monkeys, and in humans in the presence of certain cranio-facial anomalies, e.g. Down's syndrome, Cri du chat, Trisomy 18 and the Cornelia de Lange syndrome, the larynx remains in an elevated position and normal human speech is not possible. Neither Australopithecus nor Neanderthal man possessed a supralaryngeal vocal tract, but intermediate forms are found among other fossils such as Cro-Magnon man.

The main source of phonetic differentiation in human languages, arises from the dynamic properties of the supralaryngeal vocal tract acting as an acoustic filter. Its length and shape determine the frequencies at which maximum energy will be transmitted to the air adjacent to the speaker's lips (Lieberman, 1973). These frequencies, at which maximum acoustic energy will be transmitted, are known as format frequencies. A speaker can vary the format frequencies by changing the length and shape of his hypopharynx. He can manipulate his tongue within the buccal cavity. He can raise or lower his larynx and retract or extend his lips. He can open or close the passage of air through the nasal cavity to add resonance to his voice from the nasal antra and sinuses by altering the position of the velum. It is even possible for patients whose larynx has been removed to make use of oesophageal speech. With training they are able to hold a bolus of air in their gullet and release it at will.

Deformities of the soft palate, the tongue, the teeth or the lips can affect the clear enunciation of speech. Dyslalic disabilities, particularly involving certain consonants such as the, z, r, l, and s, may occur physiologically in the learning period but may persist particularly among certain speakers commensurate with a genetic defect in pronunciation. The control of the rate of speech may also be defective leading to cluttering, stammering or stuttering resulting in confused, hurried, slurred or halting diction. However, most aspects of speech fluency and prosody are centrally determined and do not primarily involve the articulatory apparatus.

**The Reception of Speech**

At first glance it would appear that the hearing apparatus of man represents a regression rather than an evolutionary advance. Most mammals, hunters and hunted, possess a fine sense of hearing over a wide frequency range. Binaural hearing with two mobile pinnae permits sound to be precisely localized and funnelled down a wide external auditory meatus. The three-ossicled mammalian middle ear enables sound energy impinging upon the tympanic membrane to be transmitted to the oval window of the inner ear with relatively little loss of efficiency. The tympanic membrane lies between two air-filled spaces and vibrates at low impedance to the incoming sound; but if the sound is loud its effect may be dampened by a strong reflex contraction of the tensor tympani muscle. By contrast the oval window, with an air-filled cavity exteriorly and the fluid-filled inner ear within, has a surface area one-twentieth that of the drum and presents a high impedance to incoming sound. In isolation the oval window would reflect most of the sound energy reaching it; thus, in pathological conditions, where there is destruction of the ossicles, appreciable deafness results. The malleus, attached to the inner surface of the tympanic membrane, the incus, and the stapes, the footplate of which is attached to the oval window by means of a cartilaginous surround or annular ligament, interarticulate and form an impedance-matching device maintained in a remarkable state of equilibrium by a number of ligaments.

Man's ear is immobile and atavistic in appearance; the meatus is tortuous, of variable diameter and readily blocked by wax; the Eustachian tubes may be readily blocked and are liable to infection which may then spread, affecting the tympanic membrane and middle ear; man's appreciation of the higher frequencies of sound is reduced compared to that of most other mammals.

Despite its odd appearance and almost total immobility, the anatomical configuration of the external ear remains relevant to the collection and localization of sounds. In order to collect and deflect sound into the ear, physical acoustics require that the dimensions of the pinna should be at least comparable to or larger than the wave length of the sound reaching it. Wave length varies inversely with frequency and in man this condition prevails only at the highest audible frequencies. The ridges and valleys of the pinna contribute to the directional localizations of sounds. The convolutions introduce time delays in arrival between direct sound and sound reflected from its folds which can be meaningfully interpreted by the central nervous system in directional terms, providing a stereophonic appreciation of individual sounds in a melange of noise.

Small mammals, such as mice, with their ears in close proximity, are best able to localize high frequency sounds. The development of low frequency hearing below 1 kHz in primates and large mammals is a secondary adaptation at the expense of detecting higher frequencies. The relative bias towards high and low frequency hearing generally correlates with head size and consequently dictates the cue (interaural intensity versus tone differences) most useful in sound localization. Since low frequency sounds are less attenuated over distance, low frequency hearing facilitates long distance communication. Human hearing extends from about 160 Hz to at most 20 kHz and within this range that of speech is centred upon 1 kHz and, on a logarithmic scale, extends an equal distance to either side.

The human ear has undergone some specific adaptions for speech. The modulation of impedance is performed by the tension of the tensor tympani on the tympanic membrane and the stapedius muscle exerts a similar reflex control upon the equilibrium of the footplate. The reflex regulation of the state of the tympanic membrane and ossicles is imperfect in the presence of loud noises, being too slow to afford protection against a sudden bang and fatiguing where noises are sustained for a period. However, a more physiological function of the regulatory mechanism occurs prior to vocalization and reinforces the feedback control of the voice in the presence of other sounds when speaking. We hear the sound of our own voice by two routes: air conduction and bone conduction. Bone conduction implies that the skull itself is set into vibration and the subsequent vibrations are transmitted directly to the inner ear, by-passing the middle ear mechanisms. Contraction of the middle ear muscles, while reducing the efficiency of transmission by the air conduction route, will tend to increase bone conduction thereby preferentially enhancing the hearing of the speaker's own voice. Thus we hear our own voices at a higher level than would be perceived by a listener nearby (Hood, 1977).

One can but marvel at the tremendous versatility of the cochlea. High pitched sounds vibrate a small portion of the basilar membrane but, when low pitched sounds set the whole membrane into vibration, the complex innervation of the external hair cells enables the various characteristics of the sound – intensity, frequency, quality and direction and the enormous variation within each category – to be conveyed to the brainstem and cortex. From the complexity of arborizations within the brainstem and the elaboration of the relay centres, it is at once apparent that the cochlear nerve mediates many functions connected with hearing besides that of speech. These include vigilance, alerting responses and directional responses to speech sounds. Likewise auditory evoked responses alert many areas of cortex besides the temporal lobe acoustic area. The second order neurones within the brainstem appear to be arranged tonotopically so that the frequency organization of the cochlear is maintained at all levels from the auditory nerve to the cortex. Most auditory neurones are spontaneously active and in response to cochlear stimulation their activity may be either excited, suppressed or even unchanged. Interactions occur in such a way that two or more frequencies can often produce exquisite resolution by a neurone that would otherwise be indifferently responsive to only a single tone.

## The Brain and Speech

There are limitations of speed imposed on speaking, writing, typing and other means of communication such that most of us think faster than we express our thoughts. Hearing and sight enable a much faster intake of information, added to which is an ability to guess at much of what is said or to speed read, gaining the sense from only a portion of what is written. But having dealt with the expressive and receptive aspects of language, we must now turn to the analysis of man's use of language to appreciate the boundaries or constraints which the "gift of tongues" imposes.

To what extent is language innate? The belief in a lingua adamaica – that in the beginning man possessed the word – takes many forms. King James believed that a child brought up in isolation would speak pure Hebrew – a notion not substantiated in the experiences of feral children. A modern equivalent is Chomsky's more scientific hypothesis that there is an innate syntax to all languages upon which the acquisition of one's native language is based. The early cries are often reflex noises such as gulps, sneezes, coughs, burps and pain signals. Pleasurable sucking and cooing sounds develop, and as the reflex sounds diminish so the noise-making process loses its infantile quality and contains a quotient of more mature sounds that possess a speech-like inflection. This is the beginning of babbling, but without social stimulation and hearing, babbling will dry up (Critchley, 1967; Lenneberg, 1967). Babbling, lallation and echolalia represent a tremendous advance because these playful repetitions lay the foundations of a repertoire of sound complexes that will eventually be reproducible at will. At this time the relatively small infantile cochlea is more receptive to higher pitched than lower pitched sounds, thus the mother's stimulation is more valuable than that of the father. Hearing and understanding heard speech is always in advance of the ability to speak. Nonetheless, it is remarkable that a child born clumsy and muscle-bound in its use of a few simple muscles in its arms and legs, is usually able to master the complex articulation of speech at a rate commensurate with that of its more healthy contemporaries.

In the animal kingdom many cries and calls have a hormonal basis, so much so that the ability to reproduce them may be confined to the mating or rutting period. Hormones can certainly influence voice production (Luchsinger and Arnold, 1965), and the greatest contrast is seen between the monosyllabic teenage male and his loquacious female counterpart: Hamstrung – He; Incessant – She: Swift, high and flowing. He with a groan replies.

Hughlings-Jackson (1884) drew attention to the ability of patients rendered aphasic with loss of intellectual speech to produce emotional, involuntary utterances; and there is evidence to suppose that Pithecanthropus and even Australopithicines were capable of the production of some meaningful sounds and noises despite their small brain size (Stein, 1942). In the same way microcephalic and nanocephalic dwarfs may acquire a few words. Sounds can be obtained in a number of species of animals by stimulating parts of the brain away from the site of the human dominant hemisphere language zone; and stereotactic stimulation in the region of the basal ganglia of man can arrest or accelerate speech (Guiot et al., 1961) or evoke compulsory utterances (Schlaternbrand, 1975). Thus Myers (1968) has suggested that in man two mechanisms may function in parallel producing a dual control of social communication: a phylogenetic older system more emotional in expression, emptier in content and less open to modification by feedback mechanisms, and a neocortical system for more intellectual speech. Such a proposition would fit the early theories of the development of speech.

Muller (1861) was the principal advocate of a series of hypotheses concerning the origin of speech from natural sounds: from the intestine, from expressions of pain or delight, from muscular effort, from gesture and from mimicry of animal cries. For the hunter, especially in poor visibility, sounds evoke vigilance, aid mutual recognition, encourage concerted action, and cause the prey to panic. Some form of command or combined effort is possible using the simplest sounds – "slow", "hurry", "wait", "scatter". More sophisticated orders such as "go right" or "left" are likely to have arisen at a much later stage of development. To early man sounds probably had an awesome quality.

"Words have never seemed to be earthly. They belong to the spirit or soul, and rest uneasily on the earthly. They departed with the breath of life. They are man's link with the supernatural. In more regions than not, it has been supposed that language is the direct gift of the immortals to their chosen creation – to mankind at large.

"The earlier gods were gruesome. The words they spake were terrifying and mighty. Man was subjugated by language. He faltered when he came to reply. He strove for a greater share of the secret of language, and even today the mystique remains; for ability to harness the full power of language for the benefit of mankind eludes us still" (Critchley, 1967).

We could add that even among the ancient Greeks the Delphic oracle was noted for its omnipotent and deliberately obscure sayings leaving those who consulted it to crave for an understanding.

This theme can be extended through discussion of the conventionality of language today. Primitive man and native speakers today, who have had little contact with foreigners, cope very badly with people who do not speak their tongue exactly: i.e. those who do not introduce themselves correctly, mispronounce words or flounder over grammar. The correct portmanteau phrase is expected and required – a pride of lions, a covey of partridges, a sege of herons, a flight of doves, a claterynge of choughes, a muster of pacockys, a herde of cranys. If we turn to our own society, many deaf people taught to speak at school rapidly lose speech when they leave a protected environment because people will not listen to speech that is an effort, sounds awkward, and may be accompanied by extraneous noises which the deaf speaker has been unable to eliminate. People do not bother to look at the listener so that he can make use of his lip-reading ability.

Language has prospered, grammar and syntax have adapted to express thoughts more clearly in situations where several races speaking different languages have come together; thus the interchange of Saxon, Jute and Dane laid the foundations for modern day English; and languages evolve quicker in cities – New York, London, Liverpool – and particularly in sea-ports than in the countryside or in small, isolated island communities. The oldest English is to be found among the Ozarks and Appalachians, in Smith and Tangier islanders of Chesapeake Bay, on Tristan Da Cunha, Prince Edward Island, New Zealand and parts of Australia. Exiles speak an older language than their contemporaries who remain behind.

Let us divide modern speech into high speech and low speech. Low speech is often falsely regarded as degenerate, spoken among equals, an argot. But high speech with its correct nuances, polite expressions, has a social phraseology which humbles the speaker rendering him subservient and belittled. What purpose is served by writing "Dear Sir"? Is he "dear" to you? Do you even know him? What is achieved by calling someone his worship, his eminence, the venerable, your excellency? These add purposely to the awkwardness of communication and achieve little more than providing a pecking order. In the tittle-tattle of everyday speech empty phrases are responses – so that speech does not dry up through lack of response. In propositional terms they are verbal garbage or sympathetic circulatory sequences: "One does, doesn't one?", "Yes, you know", "Well, I never",

" You see; well it's like this, you see". This platitudinous garrulousness has been dubbed phatic communication. Among uncivilized peoples speech scarcely serves as a vehicle for profound thought; early man, like the modern savage, probably talked a lot but had little to say. However, it is not only primitive man who succumbs to speech as a means merely of establishing social intimacy. The lives of present-day men are largely controlled by jargon. Bertrand Russell in "The Analysis of Mind" (1921) wrote that "Behaviourists say that the talk they have to listen to can be explained without supposing that people think. Where you might expect a chapter on 'thought process' you come instead upon a chapter 'the language of habit'. It is humiliating to find how terribly adequate this hypothesis turns out to be."

Almost certainly, there is some propositional input into most speech – though it may be considerably diluted. According to Langer (1942), all forms of mystical incantation, most poetry, the use of repetitions, slogan calling to generate mass hysteria, and the babbling phase of infancy can be termed generically "voice-play". It is necessary to realize that there are other purposes to speech than the propositional: placing ourselves in society as through small talk; the feeling of togetherness at a football match, a sing-song or when performing a liturgy; and the aesthetic delight of poetry, a beautiful voice, music. Incantation, strict metre, rhymes, alliterations – help the flow of a monologue or dialogue as when the story-teller of old recites the sagas accurately and at length. Conventions – though they can be broken as necessary – mostly function as helpmates in everyday life.

Mastery of language is incomplete even for the most educated and civilized man. One has only to observe a person prepare to speak in difficult circumstances, or in a foreign tongue, or puzzle out an awkward proposition to note how readily he depends on the help of gesture. His lips move silently before he formulates his words, accessory facial muscles come into play, a physiological tremor might be evident. When thinking his dominant hand may be held above waist height, the fingers upright and slightly cupped. The hand will move from the wrist in time with lip movements, the thumb be in apposition to the fingers and touch each in turn. The non-dominant hand, held below the waist, will make cruder synergistic movements, mirror movements of the dominant hand. A child, puzzling over an equation or piece of translation will suck at a pencil, or more symbolically move the pencil tranversely across moistened lips as if to facilitate the task.

The average man has only a limited capacity for language. His heard vocabulary is greater than that which he speaks and his reading vocabulary greater than his written. But even highly intelligent speakers tend to build their sentences up from a relatively small number of set clauses. This fact can be recognized in listening to any public person – politician, judge, or communicator. If we take any famous writer, he or she will tend to have stock phrases and use grammar and syntax in a certain way. Shakespeare may have a wider vocabulary than the average man but a computer can be used to pick up his limitations and "finger-print" his works to authenticate his writings. Even the most advanced languages are riddled with apparent lacunae. In English there is no appropriate mode of address for a father- or mother-in-law, the bride or bridegroom must await the birth of their first child before designating their in-law as "grandma" or some equivalent word.

Language is an inexact means of communication. There is a falsity and fickleness to words, an ambiguity. Each word and its place in a sentence has to convey approximately the same meaning to speaker and listener. At times the sense of a word may transcend its meaning. A speaker can set out to make matters deliberately ambiguous. Words can be defined and their role in sentences learnt and understood, but this is not always so; and what we say is to a large extent wrapped in conventions of usage, expression and association. We tend to keep our use of language within artificial but explicable bounds.

The constraints of language are best understood when a fluent linguist switches from one language to another. His behaviour and personality may appear to alter as he adapts to the requirements of each language with a different stress, a different syntax, the acceptable use of gesture and the directness of address. His use of familiarity clauses, polite expressions, religious symbolism and swear words may vary considerably. Each language provides a different framework for thought: some must necessarily be rigid with placement of the verbs at the end of long sentences, others have a free and comparatively lax grammatical structure. The extremes of this are apparent if one is attempting to add, subtract or multiply using Roman rather than Arabic numerals, or if one considers the way numbers are spoken in different languages.

## Conclusion

This final chapter introduces a new, even futuristic, dimension to the neurological discussion of the boundaries of reality. It began with an assessment of the capacious expectations – the pluripotentiality – of the human brain with respect to language, showing the development of language and communication skills by a series of unexpected evolutionary strides. The constraints of language, also discussed, such as the limited range of the human voice and our mediocre capacity to hear, have meant that in many respects we have failed to take advantage of the full potential of our brains. However, in the realm of communication we have been able to circumvent some physical restrictions through the development of megaphones, telephones and telecommunications. Audio-aids increase our capacity to learn foreign languages and to familiarize ourselves before we travel into the unknown. At work, mechanical devices can translate data from one system to another.

In a similar fashion, the pooled "brain-power" of the human race, not only from our own era but from previous generations, has enabled us to go beyond the limitations of our sense organs to extend and explore our environment through the use of telescopes, microscopes, radar, sonar, radio-beams, etc. The practical application of each new invention extends our understanding of reality, creating new realities and new situations, which in turn test our concept of reality. Man is an unstable being who must forever experiment. Sometimes he does so for his own pleasure, creating new tastes, new smells, new art, new music. Sometimes he does so to improve his environment and bodily comfort, to improve his health, to improve his mobility, even to help others. At other times he inflicts harm on himself or upon others, he creates new weapons of terror or destruction, he places himself, or others, in unsupportable situations. In everyday situations we extend our body image as we drive a car or manipulate instruments. Drugs taken medically or experimentally can provoke hallucinatory states. In training pilots or astronauts, weightlessness can be simulated. Our world of reality is one of shifting contours demanding of us frequent adjustment. Conflicts of reality can, and do, arise. Are we stationary or falling when in a lift? The discussion of our grasp of reality will forever remain fluid.

## References

Critchley, E.M.R. (1967a). Hearing children of deaf parents. *Journal of Laryngology*, **81**, 51-61.
Critchley, E.M.R. (1967b). "Speech Origins and Development". C.C. Thomas, Springfield, Illinois.
Guiot, G., Hertoz, E., Rondet, P. and Molinar, P. (1961). Arrest or acceleration of speech evoked by thalamic stimulation in the course of stereotaxic procedures for Parkinsonism. *Brain,* **84**, 363-379.
Hood, J.D. (1977). Psychological and physiological aspects of hearing. *In* "Music and the Brain". Chapter 3. (Eds. M. Critchley and R.A. Henson), pp. 32-47. Heinemann, London.
Jackson, J.H. (1884). *See* "Selected Works of John Hughlings Jackson". (1958). Basic Books, New York.
Langer, S. (1942). "Philosophy of the New Key". Cambridge, Mass.
Lenneberg, E.H. (1967). "Biological Foundations of Language". Wiley, New York.
Lieberman, P. (1973). On the evolution of language: a unified view. *Cognition*, **2**, 59-94.
Luchsinger, R. and Arnold, G.E. (1965). "Voice-Speech-Language". Constable, London.
Muller, M. (1991). "Lectures on the Science of Language". Longman, Green, Longman and Roberts, London.
Myers, R.E. (1968). Neurology of social communication in Primates. *Proceedings of the 2nd International Congress of Primatology, Atlanta,* **3**, 1-91.
Negus, V.E. (1949). "Comparative Anatomy of the Larynx". Heinemann, London.
Polyani, M. (1968). Evolution of language. *Science*, **160**, 1308-1312.
Russell, B. (1921). "The Analysis of Mind". Allen and Unwin, London.
Schlaterbrand, G. (1975). The effects on speech and language of stereotactical stimulation in thalamus and corpus callosum. *Brain and Language*, **2**, 70-77.
Stein, L. (1942). "Speech and Voice, their Evolution, Pathology and Therapy". Methuen, London.
Sutcliffe, T.H. (1964). "Conversation with the Deaf". Royal National Deaf Institute.

# Index

Abnormal belief system, 261
Abused children, 358
Acceleration, 24
Acupuncture, 8, 12
Agnosia, 343
Agoraphobia, 38
Ajuriaguerra, J. de, 349
Akinetic mutism, 389
Alcohol, 37, 181, 195, 202
Alien hand syndrome, 171
Alzheimer's disease, 51, 240, 399, 405
Ambiguous stimuli, 102
Amnesia, 73, 399
Amygdala, 44
Anderson (Capgras variant), 95
Anglesea, Marquis of, 8
"Animal Farm", 17
Anomia, 87
Anorexia, 373
Anosoagnosia, 343
Apallic state, 389
Apperception, 216
Aquinas, T., 207, 328
Arctica, 68
Arieti, S., 274
Aristotle, 1, 3, 207, 208, 232, 274
Arp, J, 118
Art, 175-190
Arthur, King, 383
Assessment of consciousness, 392
Astral trial, 103
St Augustine, 207, 208, 214, 328
Aurier, A., 177
Australopithecus, 420
Autistic, 354
Autochthonous delusions, 273
Autoeroticism, 184
Automatism, 137
  poetry, 180
Avicenna, 384

Babbling, 423
Bach, J.S., 196-7
Bacon, F., ("Essays of Beauty"), 370
Bacon, F., (painter), 4
Baillarger, J., 208, 255
Balance, 6
Barbiguier, A., 229
Barbizon school, 187
Baron-Cohen, S., 106
Baudelaire, C., 116
Beardsley, A., 180
Beeckman, I., 208
Beethoven, L. Van, 192, 197-8
Bell, C., 242
Bell and Ritti, 255
Bell's theorem, 121
la Belle indifference, 294
Bel-Magendie Law, 12
Belousov-Zhabotinsky chaotic chemical
  reactions, 147
Benign positional vertigo, 37
Benson, F., 83, 262, 343
Berkeley, G., 108, 143, 144, 221
Berlioz, H., 195, 198
Berrios, G.E., 200
Bilocation, 235
Biopositive, 252
Bissiere, R., 185
Black hallucinations, 176
Blackmore, S., 103
Blake, W., 11, 113, 176, 180, 185
Bleuler, E., 113, 116, 261, 273, 275, 277, 282
Blind sight, 166, 216
  "to smell", 43
Bliss, A., 115
Blount, J., 252
Body schema, 7, 11, 148-150, 234, 341-9, 355, 357, 369-382
Body Shape Questionnaire, 377
Boenhoffer, K., 279

Bogen, J.E., 163
Bogen-Vogel patients, 166-168
Boismount, B., 233, 236
Bonnard, P., 184
Bonnet, Charles (visions), 185, 200, 202, 231, 240
Borderline personality disorder, 277
Borges, J.L., 181, 402
Bosch, H., 183-4
Bouchard, T.J., 316
Boyle, J., 224
Brahms, J., 199
Braille, 2
Brain dead, 389
 in a vat, 101, 151
 injuries (MRC), 387
 washing, 68
Braque, G., 184
Brauner, V., 176
Breast enlargement, 373
Bresdin, R., 179
Breton, A., 181
Briquet's hysteria, 230
British Empiricists, 221
Bucknill, J.C., 252
Bulimia, 373
Burned children, 360

*le Cadavre equis,* 180-1
Callot, J., 178
Capgras syndrome, 88-95, 257, 400
Caravaggio, M. 179
Carpenter W. 256, 389
Carter, A., 304
Castel, L.B., 115
Castor and Pollux, 303
Cataracts, 185, 199
St Catherine of Ricci, 125
Causalgia, 9
Celsius, 384
Cénesthopathie, 233
Cercle Chromatique, 112
Cezanne, P., 184
Chagall, M., 113, 177
Charcot, J.M., 294
Charles VIII, 383
Chaslin, P., 258
Chatwin, B., 304

Chavannes, P., 180
Chiaroscuro, 179
Childhood art/drawings, 187, 355, 358
 awareness, 349-360
 trauma, 325
de Chirico, G., 173, 181
Chomsky, N., 422
Chronic pain, 8
Circadian rhythms, 324
Clairaudience, 129
Clang associations, 111
Claustrophobia, 38
Cleft palate, 360
de Clerambault, G., 233, 332
Coenesthesiae, 234
Cognition, 351
Coleridge, S.T., 179
Colour constancy, 102
 perception, 70
Coma, 388
Comfort zone, 77
Commissurotomy, 161
Computerized Tomography (CT), 341
Concentration camp syndrome, 76-7, 319
Condillac, E., 230
Confabulation, 83, 161, 400, 407, 410
Confinement, 77
Confusion, 387, 392
Conscious awareness, 121-142, 383-400
 cosmic, 120
 experience, 161
 neglect, 342
Consciousness, 143-160
Constructional dyspraxia, 353
Contextualism, 351
Conversion disorder, 294
Cordotomy, 6, 12
Coriolis effect, 35
Cornelia de Lange, 422
Corollary discharge, 39
le corps connu/vecu, 349

Dada movement, 180
Dadd, R., 186
Dali, S., 176, 181, 184, 189
Darwin, C., 232, 233
*Dead Ringers* (film), 305
Deafness, 55-66, 202

concept of body, 357
Debriefing, 71, 78
Debussy, C., 192
Déjà vu, 401
Dejerine-Roussy syndrome, 109
Délire, 251, 255
Delirium, 181, 183, 389
Delius, F., 191
Delusional misidentification, 88, 238
  persecution, 93, 234
Denial of disability, 342
Dennett, H.C., 122, 155
Depersonalization, 70, 236
Deprivation, 75
Derain, A., 184
Derride, J., 228
Descartes, R., 121, 144, 148, 155, 157, 207-209, 22, 369
Diatonic scale, 198
Dickens, C., 136, 183, 185, 373
Direct realism, 150, 152
Discords, 193
Disfigurement, 359
Disney, W., 115
Dissociation, 71, 209, 291
Distortion, 70
Divine intervention, 303
Doppelganger, 235, 242
Dostoevsky, F., 9, 124
Doubles, 88, 235
Down's syndrome, 357, 420
Dreams, 105, 135, 147, 171, 180
  fugue, 72
  mood, 273
  objects, 181
Dr Jekyll, 413
Drug induced states, 70, 185, 240
DSM-III, 67
Dualism, 293
Dumas, A., 304
Dupré, M., 237, 257
Dürer, A., 183, 186
Dvorak, A., 105, 192
Dyadic interaction, 306
Dysmorphophobia, 234, 370

Eastwood, Clint, 369
Eating disorder inventory, 372

Eddington, T., 136
Education of the Deaf (congress), 58
Ego, 143
Eidetic, 113
Electrical phenomena, 13
Electro-cortical therapy (ECT), 12
El Greco, 115
Ellis, H., 148, 370,
Emotional numbing, 67
Encephalitis, 181
Ensor, J., 177
Entopic visions, 179
Epicureanism, 207, 217
Epileptic aura, 125
  experiences, 126, 200, 202, 414
  pseudoseizures, 295
  synaesthesia, 117
Ernst, M., 181-182
Erotomania, 332
Esquirol, J.E., 229, 232, 242, 254
Euclid, 153
Eusebius, 196
Eustachian tube, 36
Everyday errors, 87
Exhibitionism, 332
Existential dilemma, 75
Expressionism, 187
Extracampine hallucinations, 238
Extrasensory perception (*see* Telepathy), 318
Ey, H. 229, 252

Facial expression, 169, 353, 360
Familiarity, 95
Fantasmata, 189
Fatigue, 26, 45
Femininity, 291
Fernel, J., 384
Fetalization, 417
Fetishism, 331
Fevers, 189
Fibre size, 4
Flaret, J.P., 254, 263
Flashbacks, 67, 73, 200
Flatlines, 103
Florestan, 196
Flor-Henry, P., 334
Fodor, J.A., 155

## INDEX

Formication, 242
Fra Angelico, 175
Frankenstein, 182
Freeman, W.J., 45-6, 52, 145
Freud, Anna, 350
Freud, S. 70, 72, 143, 146, 156, 177, 180, 181, 230, 273, 276, 329, 333,
Frey, M. Von, 2
Friedreich, D., 177
Frontal lobes, 83, 145, 261, 344, 386, 406
Fry and Whetnall, 57
Fugues, 73, 403
Fulford, K., 276, 280
Fuseli, H., 180

Galen, 384
Galileo, G., 121-207
Galton, F., 113
Gassendi, P., 217
Gate control theory, 3-5, 12
Gauguin, P., 177
Gautier, T., 116
Gender identification, 323, 357, 374
Genital inner space, 357
Genuineness test, 107
Geomagnetic fields, 14
Geometry, 153, 222
Georget, E.J., 254, 264
Gerstmann, J., 342
Gestalt, 150, 369
Geulinx, A., 262
Gibbons, E., 314
Glasgow coma scale, 392
Goethe, J., 243
Gogh, V van, 113, 116, 176, 185, 186
Goldman-Rakic model, 406
Gombrich, E.H., 111, 176
Goodenough Harris Draw-a-man Test, 309
Goya, F., 179
Graves, R., 69
Gravity, 29
Gregory, R.L., 155
Griesinger, W., 255
Grosz, G., 184
Guillain-Barre syndrome, 11
Guilleminault, W., 182
Guilty knowledge test, 85
Gurney, E., 231, 242

Hallucinations, 52, 69, 70, 83, 178, 229-250
  auditory, 62, 294
  black, 61
  dissociated, 70
  haptic 61
  hypnagogic, 70
  in the elderly, 239
  intrinsic, 52
  reflex, 70
Handel, G.F., 197-199
Hardyment, C., 354
Harmony, 193
Harrison's story, 151
Hartley, A., 179
Hartley, D., 253
Hashish, 116
Haslam, J., 252
Hay, D., 120, 308
Haydn, J., 194
Head, H., 341
Head injury, 383
Hearing apparatus, 420
Hebbian synapses, 68, 69, 145
  hedonic odours, 45
  height vertigo, 31
Heilman, K., 343
Heidegger, M., 145
Heim, A., 113, 131
Helmholtz, V.H., 2
Hemifield tachiscopy, 170
Hemineglect, 165, 343
Hemispheric learning, 166
  specialization, 164
Henry, C., 112
Herpes simplex encephalitis, 399
Hierarchies, 417
Higher functions, 142
Hill, C.F., 187
Hindemith, P., 193
Hindu music, 113
  philosophy, 113
Hippocrates, 384
Histrionic, 230
Hobbes, T., 217, 251
Hoffert, M.J., 3
Holmes, S., 197
Holst, G., 193
Homer, 383

Homosexuals, 326, 328-30
Homunculus, 155
Horowitz, M.J., 178
Hostages, 71, 74, 78
Hudson River artists, 184
Hughlings-Jackson, J., 52, 143, 241, 252, 423
Hugo, V., 180
Hüg-Hellmuth, H., 117
Humour, 180
Hunger, 185
Huysmans, J.K., 48, 116, 184
Hyperarousal, 67
Hypersomnia, 51
Hypnagogia, 104, 135, 183
Hypnosis, 73
Hysteria, 185, 287-298

Iconic memory, 163
Icons, 175
Id, 143
Ideomotor apraxia, 168, 354
Idioglossia, 311
Illness and body image, 354
Illusions, 27, 70, 178
 dynamic, 35
 movement, 155
 self-motion, 31
Illusory displacement, 342
Image formation, 351

Klee, P., 113, 116, 182
Klein, M., 350
Klüver, H., 147-8
Koestler, A., 188
Korsakoff psychosis, 51
Köhler, W., 153
Kokoschka, O., 182
Kraepelin, E., 273
Krafft-Ebing, R., 184, 328
Kray twins, 312
Kretschmer, E., 273
Kubin, A., 116, 186

Language, 417-429
Lasègue, E.C., 255, 263
La Trobe Twin Study, 308
Laer, P.V., 178

Leans, 35
Lear, E., 186
Learning, 20
Left-right disorientation, 352
Leibnitz, G., 214, 216, 222
Leonardo, da Vinci, 178-9, 186, 211
Lesbians, 330
Leviathan, 251
Lewis, A., 287, 294
Life after Life, 131
Lilliputian dreams/hallucinations, 178, 238
Limbic system, 44
Linde, A., 157
Linear vection, 92
Lingua adamaica, 424
Lip read, 418
Liszt, F., 115
Locke, J., 113, 143, 232, 251
Locked-in syndrome, 388
Looking-glass self, 351
Lorry drivers, 68
LSD (lysergic acid), 148
Lucretian, 297
Ludwig (the brain in a vat) 101, 151
Luminism, 184
Luria, A.R., 113, 401

McQueen, C., 106
Madness, 189, 272, 323
Magic, 176
Magnan, V., 232, 257
Magnesco, A., 178
Magnetic phenomena, 13
Mahler, G., 197
Malebranche, W., 211, 224
Malignancies, 359
Manifesto (Surrealist), 188
"Man in the Iron Mask", 304
Marsden, C.D., 295
Martha's Vineyard, 58
Martin, J., 179
Masson, A., 176, 177
Masters and Johnson, 330
Matisse, H., 155, 181, 184
Melzack, R., 4, 8
Memory, 101, 162, 169
 iconic, 163
 lapses, 403

smells, 48
Mendelssohn, F., 197
Meniere's disease, 38
Mentally retarded children, 357
Mental state in deaf, 60
Mersenne, M., 205
Merskey, H., 295
Mescaline, 148
Messiaen, O., 114, 191
Messonier, E., 179
Metaphysical art, 178
Michelangelo, B., 179
Millet, J.F., 176
Milton, J., 417
Miró, J., 181, 185
Mitchell, Weir, 9-10, 148
Mneumonist, 113, 401
Modigliani, A., 185
Monad, 214
Mondrian, P., 116, 184
Monet , E., 185
Moore, G.E., 108
Moore, H., 186
More, H., 224
Moreau, G., 179-180
Moreau de Tours, 233, 255, 263
Morris, Jan, 326
Motion sickness, 36, 183
Moussorgsky, M.P., 196
Mozart, W.A., 148, 194, 197, 199
Muller, M., 423
Multiple personalities, 73, 290
Munch, E., 178-9
Music, 191-206
"Music and the Brain", 115
Musical hallucinations, 191-206, 238
  scales, 49
Musset, A. de, 195
Myopia, 185
Mystics, 68, 121, 124
Mythology, 176
Mythomania, 257

Nabakov, V., 106
Nagel, T., 122
Narcolepsy, 181-182
*National Geographic Magazine*, 50
Neanderthal man, 420

Near death experiences (NDEs), 103, 131
Negus, Sir V., 419
Neocortical death, 389
Neoimpressionism, 112
Nero, 328
Nervel, G. de, 181
Neuralgias, 9
Neuromatrix, 8
Neuronal cell assemblies (nerve circuits), 8,
  10, 145
Neuroses, 269, 287
Newton, I., 114, 222
Nicolai, C., 229
Night terrors, 136, 182, 183
Nose-type dysmorphism, 371

Obscene phone calls, 333
Obsessions, 146, 177, 253, 373
Occurrents, 144
Odours, perception, 45
Ogden, C.K., 112
Olfaction, 43-54
  demography, 50, 145, 239
  evoked potentials, 48
  reference syndrome, 52
Oneirism, 183
Opium, 49
Organ image, 370
O'Reilly, J.B., 175
Orff, C., 192
Orientation, 162, 167
Orwell, G., 17
Osmones, 49
Out of body experiences (OOBEs), 103, 235
"Oxford Companion to Music", 115

Paedophilia, 333
Pain, 3-11
Paleologic, 274
Papez circuits, 44, 46
Papyrus (Edwin Smith), 381
Parachuting, 73
Paralexia, 342
Paranoid states, 195
Paranormal, 127
Paraphilias, 320
Parasitosis, 234
Paré, A., 242

Pareidolia, 70, 178
Partially sighted, 184
St Paul, 126
Peduncular hallucinations, 238
Penfield, W., 200, 230
Penrose, R., 157
Perfumes, 48-9
Peripheral neuropathy, 5, 7
Peripheral vision, 184
Personality destruction, 74, 186, 277
Personification of a limb, 342
Phallus, 373
Phantasmal voices, 60
Phantom limb, 10, 11, 116, 239
"Phantasms of the Living", 232
Phantosmia, 51
Phenomenal space, 157
Pheromone receptors, 45
Philosophy, 207-228
Phobic behaviours, 75, 146
Phocomelia, 10
Phosphenes, 199
Photisms, 114
Phrensy, 254
Piaget, J., 351
Picasso, P., 179
Piesse's classification, 48
Pineal, P., 254
Piranesi, G.B., 1985
Pitch, 190
Plato, 143, 148, 207, 221
Play, 354
Poltergeist, 103
Pornographic art 181
Pornography, 335
Positional vertigo, 37
Positivism, 223
Positron emission tomography (PET), 108, 279, 341
Posthypnotic suggestion, 146
Post-traumatic stress disorder (PTSD), 67, 78
Precognition, 129
Predelusional state, 260
Pressure, 13
Primitive art, 187
Proprioception, 26
Prosopagnosia, 85, 91, 165

Proust, M., 49, 269, 283-4
Pryse-Phillips, W., 52
Psychedelic states, 143
Psychic gifts, 127
Psychogenic amnesia, 413
Psychoneural identity (IT), 144
*Psychopathia Sexualis,* 184, 328
Psychopathy, 379
Psychotherapy, 379
Public esteem, 362
Purkinjee effect, 184

Quadratura, 179
Quality of life, 172
Quincey, T. de, 72, 179, 181, 195
Quine, W., 228

Rage, 113
Ransome, A., 354
Rape, 75, 334, 358
Raphael, 186
Rationalists, 214
Ravel, M., 182
Read, H., 176
Reality dissociation, 83
Reception of speech, 420
Recognition 83-100, 171
  preference, 84, 353
Redon, O., 173, 180
Reduplicative paramnesia, 88, 94, 400
Referred pain, 6
Religious conversion, 125
  experience, 120, 189
Representative theory (RT), 153
*Res cogitans,* 149
Resuscitation, 103
Reticular formation, 385
Retinal mind, 143
Reynolds, Sir J., 185
Rey-Osterreith test, 353
Rhazes, 384
Rhythm, 193
Ribot, T., 253
Richter, J.P., 236
Riemann, G., 153
Right cerebral hemisphere, 85, 129, 162, 165, 169, 261, 304, 353, 354
Rimbaud, A., 106

# INDEX

Rimington, A.W., 115
Rimsky-Korsakof, N.A., 115
Ring, K., 103
Ritti, A., 228
Ruskin, J., 175-6
Russell, B., 108, 152, 155, 425
Russolo, L., 115
Rutter, M., 308
Ryder, A.P., 184
Ryle, G., 155

Sado-masochism, 333
Saint-Saens, C., 194, 198
Sambia, New Guinea, 327
Sargeant, J.S., 180
Sargent, W., 68
Scepticism, 207
Schilder, P., 150
Schiller, J.C.F., 198, 369
Schizophrenia, 61, 186, 196, 261, 269, 277
Schneider (first rank symptoms) 61, 273, 278
Scholes, P.A., 115
Schopenhauer, A., 180
Schrödinger, E., 121-2
Schubert, F., 192, 197
Schumann, R., 195, 199
Scipione, G.B., 185
Searle, J.R., 122
Secondary gain, 292
Secret language, 311
Self-awareness, 352
 esteem, 362
 perception, 370
 recognition, 75
Seligmann, K. 176
Semantic memory, 398
Senilis, S. de, 177
Sense
 fifth, 2, 32
 of existence, 234
 sentinel of, 43
Sensory
 categories, 2
 deprivation, 67-82
 displacement, 342
 motor development, 252
Seraut, G., 113

Serieux, P., 257
Sexuality, 323-340
 experiences, 117, 168, 358
 preference, 329
Sfumato, 179
Shakespeare, W., 304, 323, 378, 417, 425
Shallice, T., 407
Shemesherskii (*see* Mneumonist)
Sherrington, Sir C., 3, 121
Sibelius, J., 196
Sibling rivalry, 313
Sidgwick, H., 231
Sigmond, G., 233
Sign language, 59, 64
Signac, P., 113
Sirhan Sirhan, 414
Sitwell, E., 116
Skriabin, A., 115, 116
Slater, E., 293
Sleep, 135
 apnoea, 181
 walking, 73, 136, 183, 188
Small world phenomenon, 316
Smell
 blindness, 47
 stereochemical theory, 45
Smetena, B., 194
Smith, Sir M., 185
Sneezing, 44
Social learning theory, 335
Society for Psychical Research, 231
Solitary confinement, 76
Somaesthesia, 1
Somatoform disorder, 290
Sound, 59
 induced vertigo, 35
Soutine, C., 185
Spatial orientation, 342
Special powers, 302
Speed estimation, 32, 57
Spinoza, B., 213, 216
Spiro, R.S., 401
Split brain, 161-174
Spontaneous pain, 9
Sterne, L., 369
Stevenson, R.L., 413
Stidwandel, 186
Stockholm syndrome, 71, 77

# INDEX

Stoicism, 207
Stöller, R.J., 327
Strauss, J., 198, 199
Stravinsky, I.F., 196
Stuss, D.T., 83
Subjective experience, 122
Sudden infant death syndrome (SIDS) 317
Sully, J., 232, 242
Super-ego, 143
Supersaturated colours, 148
Surrealism, 180
Surrogate parentage, 312
Süskind, P., 49
Symbolism, 180
Synaesthesia, 105, 111-120, 191
Synaesthetes, 114
Syphilis, 9, 194, 196

Tactile hallucinations, 232
Talmud, 383
Tamburini, A., 230, 238, 258
Tartini, G., 196
Tchaikovsky, P.I., 193, 198
Telepathy, 127, 129, 302, 316
Temporal lobe, 47, 124, 200, 261, 401
Thalamic syndrome, 9
St Theresa of Lisieux, 62, 126
Tilt, 17-42
Timbre, 193
Titian, V., 185
Tolstoy, L., 373
Tomboys, 325
Tone painting, 196
Torture, 74, 75
Touch, 1-16
Trance states, 73
Transcendental idealism, 225
Transsexual, 325, 378
Transvestism, 331
Trickery, 189
*Trompe l'oeil*, 179
Tuberculosis, 185
Tullio phenomenon, 35
Tuke, D.H., 233, 252
Tumours, 201
Turner, W., 173
TV, 83
Twain, M., 304

Twins, 299-322
Typhoid vigil, 181

Ugliness worrier, 370
Uncinate seizures, 52
Unconsciousness, 143-160, 181
Unilateral hallucinations, 238
Universal love, 123
University of Pennsylvania Smell
   Identification test (UPSIT), 47
Unlawful sex, 380

Vaughan Williams, R., 197-9
Vector illusions, 31
Vegetative state, 388
Veith, I., 287
Velasquez, D.R., 176, 187
Venn diagram, 194
Verdi, G., 198
Vernet, C.L., 176
Vernon, M.D., 154
Vertigo, 20, 31
   sound indeed, 35
Vestibular neuronitis, 37
   system, 18
Vestibulo-ocular reflex (VOR), 24-26, 37
Vibration, 13
Vigilance, 7
Visual Reality, 101-110
   self-recognition, 358
   space, 152, 343
Visuo-limbic pathways, 86, 161
Vivaldi, A., 192, 197
Vlaminck, M., 184
Voice play, 425
Voices, hearing, 62

Wagner, R., 180, 192
Wain, L., 186
Walpole, H., 181
*Wanderleben*, 258
Warrington, E., 467
Watches, 14
Wave particle duality theory, 126
Weber, E.H., 232
Wells, E., 327
Wiertz, A., 115
Wilder, T., 304

Wilfred, T., 115
Wines, 48
Winnicott, D.W., 250
Wittgenstein, L., 228
Wolfenden report, 324
Wolffi, A. 183, 187
Woolhouse, T., 105, 113
World Congress of Psychiatry, 254

Yang and Yin, 13
Y-chromosome, 325

Zajonc, R.B., 84
Zazzo, R., 300
Z-lens, 171
Zola, E., 49
Zollner illusion, 28
Zutt, J., 243

# About the Author

Edmund Michael Rhys Critchley, DM Oxford, MA, BM, BCh, FRCP Ed., FRCP London, is a Consultant Neurologist, Royal Preston Hospital, Preston, Lancashire, United Kingdom.